Handbook of Applied Nutrition, Dietotherapy and Diet Management

Handbook of Applied Nutrition, Dietotherapy and Diet Management

Mangala Punekar
Jerry D'Souza

2010

SBS Publishers & Distributors Pvt. Ltd.
New Delhi

ISBN: 13-9789380090092

First Published in 2010

Published by:

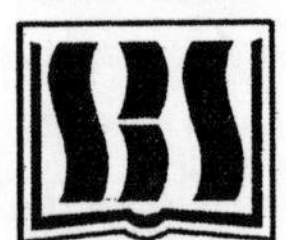

SBS PUBLISHERS & DISTRIBUTORS PVT. LTD.
2/9, Ground Floor, Ansari Road, Darya Ganj,
New Delhi - 110002,
INDIA
Tel: 0091.11.23289119 / 41563911 / 32945311
Email: mail@sbspublishers.com
www.sbspublishers.com

Printed in India by Chaman Enterprises, New Delhi.

Preface

Nutrition is the provision to cells and organisms of the materials necessary, in the form of food, to support life. Many common health problems can be prevented or alleviated with a healthy diet. The diet of an organism is what it eats, and is largely determined by the perceived palatability of foods. Dietitians are health professionals who specialize in human nutrition, meal planning, economics, and preparation. They are trained to provide safe, evidence-based dietary advice and management to individuals (in health and disease), as well as to institutions. A poor diet can have an injurious impact on health, causing deficiency diseases such as scurvy, beriberi, and kwashiorkor; health-threatening conditions like obesity and metabolic, and such common chronic systemic diseases as cardiovascular disease, diabetes, and osteoporosis. In nutrition, the diet is the sum of food consumed by a person or other organism. Dietary habits are the habitual decisions an individual or culture makes when choosing what foods to eat. Although humans are omnivores, each culture holds some food preferences and some food taboos. Individual dietary choices may be more or less healthful. Proper nutrition requires the proper ingestion and equally important, the absorption of vitamins, minerals, and food energy in the form of carbohydrates, proteins, and fats. Dietary habits and choices play a significant role in health and mortality, and can also define cultures and play a role in religion. A particular diet may be chosen to seek weight gain, weight loss, sports training, cardio-vascular health, and avoidance of cancers, food allergies and for other reasons. Changing a subject's dietary intake, or "going on a diet", can change the energy balance and increase or decrease the amount of fat stored by the body. Some foods are specifically recommended, or even altered, for conformity to the requirements of a particular diet. These diets are often recommended in conjunction with exercise.

Applied nutrition deals with the tools and techniques of developing science-based nutritional supplements at clinically researched levels. Major research areas in applied nutrition include diet, cleansing and sexual health product categories by providing customers high-quality, effective products at a reasonable price. Use of the latest delivery system technology has been in practice. A dietary supplement, also known as food supplement or nutritional supplement, is a preparation intended to provide nutrients, such as vitamins, minerals, fiber, fatty acids or amino acids, that are missing or are not consumed in sufficient quantity in a person's diet. Some countries define dietary supplements as foods, while in others they are defined as drugs. Supplements containing vitamins or dietary minerals are included in the Codex Alimentarius Commission, a guidebook on food safety sponsored by the United Nations. Diet therapy can be regarded as a change in the diet we normally consume in order to treat an illness or disease in our body. Basic nutrition for your specific needs is vital for dietary treatments aimed at getting you back to normal, healthy eating patterns.

The modification in your diet may mean change in several dietary factors. For instance, modification in consistency may mean a liquid diet, modification in texture often means a low fiber diet and likewise. Specific diet therapies can also be practiced in order to maintain good nutritional status while losing weight and often increasing fitness. Other reasons for diet therapy often include the following: It is often used in order to afford rest to the entire body or to certain organs. It can be practiced to maintain the correct vitamin levels that may have been compromised due to illness or poor diet.

Dietary therapy is often used to avoid or treat obesity, post-surgery treatment and fighting or controlling symptoms of disease. For beginning diet therapy, it is necessary to start with a normal or goal diet and mapping a plan to achieve it. In other words we can say that diet therapy is the modification of your normal diet in which this modified diet is taken in such a way that it is nutritional and acceptable at the same time to the patient. During times of illness, a person moves from one type of modified diet to the other diet gradually and thus ultimately leading to your normal or goal diet. For instance, if a person has under gone a surgery, a liquid diet is very essential and eventually it becomes a stepping stone that leads to your everyday, base diet.

The main intention of providing this kind of diet plan is to help the patient to return to the normal absorption and digestion patterns. A liquid diet may include many clear liquids, fruit drinks, fruit waters and possibly specialized sport drinks. For example, water, fruit juices, sugarcane juice, clear gatorade or vitamin water and other clear beverages. These liquids provide clear fluids to relieve thirst and prevent dehydration. They maintain the electrolyte balance in our body and provide minimum bowel residue. The liquid diets are recommended only for shorter periods of time, typically after a surgery. This is because of the fact that a liquid diet contains inadequacies in all types of nutrients and usually causes fast weight loss; however that fact may be a desired result of a liquid diet. The soft diet is often called a low fiber diet. It contains only materials and foods that are soft in consistency and easily chewable. They are free from most of the fibers of a normal diet and are easily digestible. These soft diets contain adequate nutrition and serves as an intermediate diet between liquid and normal diet. This diet is very helpful when you have gastrointestinal problems. These diets also contain nutrition that is adequate and sufficient for most people. The fluid diet contains liquefied foods as well as clear liquids, milk and milk products. A fluid diet may include food like milk, fruit and vegetable juices. The fluid diet is the recommended diet therapy for patients who cannot tolerate solid food or are unable to chew and swallow their food.

This "Handbook of Applied Nutrition, Dietotherapy and Diet Management" follows a new approach to deal with the said subject. It provides an introduction to nutrition, nutrients, dietitian and nutritional genomics with special focus on prebiotic nutrition, nutritional facts and labels, micronutrients, dietary minerals, non-nutritive foods, nutritional gatekeeper, gastroenterology and molecular gastronomy. In addition, this handbook also addresses issues related to nutritional disorders, malnutrition, food allergy, healthy diet, food fortification and dietotherapy. Select case studies are also made about few famous global food industry trade groups, institutes, guilds, associations, councils and research centres. This publication also outlines select aerobic and anaerobic organisms, saturated and unsaturated fats and food groups. The concepts, services and test's related to applied nutrition are discussed. The microbiological aspects of food safety are touched briefly. Select systems of medicine and related dietary laws are dealt in detail. Related issues concerned with global food scarcity, famine, foodgrains' management, food security and food policy are also touched upon. These are further substantiated with relevant case studies from around the world. This handbook also evaluates the role of food aid and food security vis-a-vis global hunger crisis. The role of agricultural production, demand and trade in providing global food/livelihood security and mitigating food shortage challenges has been discussed in an elaborate fashion.

This book also provides readers with a holistic approach towards healthy diet, nutrition and physical fitness. Extensive resource material is provided on applied nutrition, dietotherapy and diet management. Necessary case studies are also made on relevant issues. This book also provides necessary list of abbreviations, glossary of terms, bibliography, and a detailed index to make this book more user friendly. This handbook will be useful for all kinds of readers as it covers the whole subject area in an integrated fashion.

Contents

Abbreviations

ACP African, Caribbean and Pacific
AMS Aggregate Measurement of Support
AoA Agreement on Agriculture
ATC Agreement on Textiles and Clothing
BSE bovine spongiform encephalopathy
CAP Common Agricultural Policy (of EC)
CARICOM Caribbean Community
CET Common External Tariff
CIS Commonwealth of Independent States
EC European Community
EU European Union
FAO Food and Agriculture Organization of the United Nations
GATS General Agreement on Trade in Services
GATT General Agreement on Tariffs and Trade
GDP gross domestic product
GMOs genetically modified organisms
GSP Generalized System of Preferences
HFTA high temperature forced air
HS Harmonized System (Harmonized Commodity Description and Coding System)
IIASA International Institute for Applied Systems Analysis
IFPRI International Food Policy Research Institute
IMF International Monetary Fund
LDC least developed country
LIFDC low-income food-deficit country
MERCOSUR Southern Common Market (Mercado Común del Sur)
MFA Multifibre Arrangement

MFN	most favoured nation
NFIDC	net food-importing developing country
NGO	non-governmental organization
NTB	non-tariff barrier
NTC	non-trade concern
OECD	Organization for Economic Cooperation and Development
PSE	Producer Support Estimate (of OECD)
PVP	plant variety protection
SACN	Southern African Customs Union
SADC	Southern African Development Community
SAP	structural adjustment programme
SARD	sustainable agricultural and rural development
SDT	special and differential treatment
SPARTECA	South Pacific Regional Trade and Economic Cooperation Agreement
SPS	Sanitary and Phytosanitary
SSG	special safeguard (measures)
TBT	technical barriers to trade
TRIMS	trade-related investment measures
TRIPS	trade-related aspects of intellectual property rights
TRQ	tariff rate quota
UNCTAD	United Nations Conference on Trade and Development
UR	Uruguay Round
USDA	United States Department of Agriculture
WFS	World Food Sue Organization

1

Nutrition, Nutrients, Dietitian and Nutritional Genomics: An Introduction

NUTRITION

The "Nutrition Facts" table indicates the amounts of nutrients which experts recommend you limit or consume in adequate amounts.

Nutrition (also called nourishment or aliment) is the provision, to cells and organisms, of the materials necessary (in the form of food) to support life. Many common health problems can be prevented or alleviated with good nutrition.

The diet of an organism refers to what it eats. Dietitians are health professionals who specialize in human nutrition, meal planning, economics, preparation, and so on. They are trained to provide safe, evidence-based dietary advice and management to individuals (in health and disease), as well as to institutions.

Poor diet can have an injurious impact on health, causing deficiency diseases such as scurvy, beriberi, and kwashiorkor; health-threatening conditions like obesity and metabolic syndrome, and such common chronic systemic diseases as cardiovascular disease, diabetes, and osteoporosis.

Overview

Nutritional science investigates the metabolic and physiological responses of the body to diet. With advances in the fields of molecular biology, biochemistry, and genetics, the study of nutrition is increasingly concerned with metabolism and metabolic pathways, the sequences of biochemical steps through which the many substances of living things change from one form to another.

The human body contains chemical compounds, such as water, carbohydrates (sugar, starch, and fiber), amino acids (in proteins), fatty acids (in lipids), and nucleic acids (DNA/RNA). These compounds, in turn, consist of elements such as carbon, hydrogen, oxygen, nitrogen, phosphorus, calcium, iron, zinc, magnesium, manganese, and so on. All of these chemical compounds and elements occur in various forms and combinations (e.g. hormones/vitamins, phospholipids, hydroxyapatite), both in the human body and in organisms (e.g. plants, animals) that humans eat.

The human body consists of elements and compounds ingested, digested, absorbed, and circulated through the bloodstream. Except in the unborn fetus, it is the digestive system which carries out the first steps in feeding the cells of the body. In a typical adult, about seven liters of digestive juices enter the lumen of the digestive tract. They break chemical bonds in ingested molecules and modulate their conformations and energy states. Though some molecules are absorbed into the bloodstream unchanged, digestive processes release them from the matrix of foods in which they occur. Unabsorbed matter is secreted in the feces.

Studies of nutritional status must take into account the state of the body before and after experiments, as well as the chemical composition of the diet and the products of excretion. Comparing the food to the waste can help determine the specific compounds and elements absorbed in the body. Their effects may only be discernible after an extended period of time, during which all food and waste must be analyzed. The number of variables involved in such experiments is high, making nutritional studies time-consuming and expensive, which explains why the science of human nutrition is still slowly evolving.

In general, eating a wide variety of fresh, whole (unprocessed), foods has proven favourable compared to monotonous diets based on processed foods. In particular, the consumption of whole plant foods slows digestion and provides higher amounts, and a more favourable balance, of essential nutrients per Calorie, resulting in better management of cell growth, maintenance, and mitosis (cell division), as well as better regulation of appetite and blood sugar.

Regularly scheduled meals (every few hours) have also proven more wholesome than infrequent, haphazard ones.

Nutrients

There are seven major classes of nutrients: carbohydrates (saccharides), fats (triglycerides), fiber (cellulose), minerals, proteins, vitamins, and water.

These nutrient classes can be generally grouped into the categories of macronutrients (needed in relatively large amounts), and micronutrients (needed in smaller quantities). The macronutrients are carbohydrates, fats, fiber, proteins and water. The other nutrient classes are micronutrients.

The macronutrients (excluding fiber and water) provide energy, which is measured in kilocalories, often called "Calories" and written with a capital C to distinguish individual calories. Carbohydrates and proteins provide four (4) Calories of energy per gram, while fats provide nine (9) Calories per gram. Vitamins, minerals, fiber, and water do not provide energy, but are necessary for other reasons.

Molecules of carbohydrates and fats consist of carbon, hydrogen, and oxygen atoms. Carbohydrates may be simple monomers (glucose, fructose, galactose), or large polymers polysaccharides (starch). Fats are triglycerides, made of various fatty acid monomers bound to glycerol. Some fatty acids are essential, but not all. Protein molecules contain nitrogen atoms in addition to the elements of carbohydrates and fats. The nitrogen-containing monomers of protein, called amino acids, fulfill many roles other than energy metabolism, and when they are used as fuel, getting rid of the nitrogen places a burden on the kidneys. Similar to fatty acids, certain amino acids are essential.

Other micronutrients not categorized above include antioxidants and phytochemicals.

Most foods contain a mix of some or all of the nutrient classes. Some nutrients are required on a regular basis, while others are needed less frequently. Poor health can be caused by an imbalance of nutrients, whether an excess or a deficiency.

Carbohydrates

A pack of toasted bread is a cheap, high nutrient (usually unbalanced i.e. deficient in essential minerals and vitamins, because of removal of grain bran) food source (which also has a long shelf life).

Carbohydrates may be classified as monosaccharides, disaccharides, or polysaccharides by the number of monomer (sugar) units they contain. They are found in large proportion in foods such as rice, noodles, bread and other grain-based products. Monosaccharides contain 1 sugar unit, disaccharides contain 2, and polysaccharides contain 3 or more. Polysaccharides are often referred to as complex carbohydrates because they are long chains of sugar units, whereas monosaccharides and disaccharides are simpler. The difference is important because complex carbohydrates take longer to digest and absorb since their sugar units are processed one-by-one off the ends of the chains; the spike in blood sugar levels caused by substantial amounts of simple sugars is thought to be at least part of the cause of increased heart and vascular disease associated with high simple sugar consumption. Simple carbohydrates are absorbed quickly and thus raise blood sugar levels more quickly.

Fat

Calories/Gram: 9

Fats are composed of fatty acids (long carbon/hydrogen chains) bonded to a glycerol; they are typically found as triglycerides (three fatty acids attached to one glycerol backbone). Certain fatty acids are essential. Fats may be classified as saturated or unsaturated. Saturated fats have all of their carbon atoms bonded to hydrogen atoms, whereas unsaturated fats have some of their carbon atoms double-bonded in place of a hydrogen atom. In humans, multiple studies have shown that unsaturated fats are to be preferred for health reasons, particularly mono-unsaturated fats. Saturated fats, typically from animal sources, are next, while 'trans' fats are to be avoided; they have been banned in several locations (e.g., New York City). Saturated and trans fats are typically solid at room temperature (such as butter or lard), while unsaturated fats are typically liquids (such as olive oil or flaxseed oil). Unsaturated fats may be further classified as monounsaturated (one double-bond) or polyunsaturated (many double-bonds). Trans fats are saturated fats but are typically created from unsaturated fat by adding the extra hydrogen atoms in an industrial process called hydrogenation; they are also called hydrogenated fat. They are very rare in nature, but have properties useful in the food processing industry.

Essential Fatty Acids

Most fatty acids are non-essential, meaning the body can produce them as needed from other fats and some energy. However, in humans, at least two fatty acids are essential and must be consumed in the diet. An appropriate balance of essential fatty acids—omega-3 and omega-6 fatty acids—has been discovered to be important in reducing risk of some chronic diseases and conditions. Both of these "omega" long-chain polyunsaturated fatty acids are substrates for a class of eicosanoids known as prostaglandins which have uses throughout the human body; they are in some respects, hormones. The omega-3 eicosapentaenoic acid (EPA) (which can be made in the human body from the omega-3 essential fatty acid alpha-linolenic acid (LNA), or taken in through marine food sources), serves as a building block for series 3 prostaglandins (e.g. weakly-inflammation PGE3). The omega-6 dihomo-gamma-linolenic acid (DGLA) serves as a building block for series 1 prostaglandins (e.g. anti-inflammatory PGE1), whereas arachidonic acid (AA) serves as a building block for series 2 prostaglandins (e.g. pro-inflammatory PGE 2). Both DGLA and AA can be made from the omega-6 linoleic acid (LA) in the human body, or can be taken in directly through food. An appropriately balanced intake of omega-3 and omega-6 partly determines the relative production of different prostaglandins, which partly explains the importance of omega-3/omega-6 balance for cardiovascular health. In industrialised societies, people typically consume large amounts of processed vegetable oils that have reduced amounts of the essential fatty acids along with a too high ratio of omega-6 fatty acids relative to omega-3 fatty acids.

The conversion rate of omega-6 DGLA to AA largely determines the production of the respective prostaglandins PGE1 and PGE2. Omega-3 EPA prevents AA from being released from membranes, thereby skewing prostaglandin balance away from pro-inflammatory PGE2 made from AA toward anti-inflammatory PGE1 made from DGLA. Moreover, the conversion (desaturation) of DGLA to AA is controlled by the enzyme delta-5-desaturase, which in turn is controlled by hormones such as insulin (up-regulation) and glucagon (down-regulation). Because the amount and type of glucose and starch) plus some amino acid types) in food affect insulin, glucagon and other hormones, not only the amount of omega-3 versus omega-6 eaten but also the general composition of the diet, are implicated in general health regarding the essential fatty acids, inflammation (e.g. immune function) and mitosis (i.e. cell division).

Good sources of essential fatty acids include: fish, flax seed oils, hemp seeds and oils, soy beans, pumpkin seeds, sunflower seeds, and walnuts.

Fiber

Calories/Gram: 0

Dietary fiber consists mainly of cellulose, a large carbohydrate polymer, that is indigestible because humans do not have enzymes to digest it. There are two subcategories, soluble and insoluble fiber. The first means fiber which absorbs water, the second does not. Whole grains, fruits (especially plums, prunes, and figs), and vegetables are rich in dietary fiber. It provides bulk to the intestinal contents and stimulates peristalsis (rhythmic muscular contractions passing along the digestive tract). Consequently, a lack of dietary fiber in the diet tends toward constipation. There is also some evidence that dietary fiber is helpful in other ways, e.g., reducing the incidence of some cancers.

Protein

Most meats such as chicken contain all the essential amino acids needed for humans. Proteins are the basis of animal body structures (e.g., muscles, skin, hair etc.). They are composed of amino acids, sometimes many thousands, which are characterized by inclusion of nitrogen and sometimes sulphur. The body requires amino acids to produce new body protein (protein retention) and to replace damaged proteins (maintenance). Amino acids not needed are discarded, typically in the urine. In animals, amino acid requirements are classified in terms of essential (an animal cannot produce them internally) and non-essential (the animal can produce them from other nitrogen containing compounds) amino acids. Humans use about 20 amino acids, and about ten are essential in this sense. Consuming a diet that contains adequate amounts of essential (but also non-essential) amino acids is particularly important for growing, pregnant, nursing, or injured animals, all of whom have a particularly high requirement. Protein nutrition which contains the essential amino acids is a complete protein source, one missing one or more is called incomplete. It's possible to combine two incomplete protein sources (e.g., rice and beans) to make a complete protein source. Dietary sources of protein include meats, tofu and other soy-products, eggs, grains, legumes, and dairy products such as milk and cheese. A few amino acids from protein can be converted into glucose and used for fuel through a process called gluconeogenesis. The remaining amino acids are discarded.

Minerals

Calories/Gram: 0

Dietary minerals are the chemical elements required by living organisms, other than the four elements carbon, hydrogen, nitrogen, and oxygen which are present in common organic molecules. The term "mineral" is archaic, since the intent of the definition is to describe ions, not chemical compounds or actual minerals. Some dietitians recommend that these heavier elements should be supplied by ingesting specific foods (that are enriched in the element(s) of interest), compounds, and sometimes including even minerals, such as calcium carbonate. Sometimes these "minerals" come from natural sources such as ground oyster shells. Sometimes minerals are added to the diet separately from food, such as mineral supplements, the most famous being iodine in "iodized salt". .

Macrominerals

A variety of elements are required to support the biochemical processes, many play a role as electrolytes or in a structural role. In human nutrition, the dietary bulk "mineral elements" (RDA > 200 mg/day) are in alphabetical order (parenthetical comments on folk medicine perspective):

- Calcium (for muscle and digestive system health, builds bone, neutralizes acidity, clears toxins, helps blood stream)
- Chloride
- Magnesium required for processing ATP and related reactions (health, builds bone, causes strong peristalsis, increases flexibility, and increases alkalinity)
- Phosphorus required component of bones and energy processing and many other functions (bone mineralization)
- Potassium required electrolyte (heart and nerves health)
- Sodium electrolyte
- Sulfur for three essential amino acids and many proteins and cofactors (skin, hair, nails, liver, and pancreas health)

Trace Minerals

A variety of elements are required in trace amounts, unusually because they play a role in catalysis in enzymes. Some trace mineral elements (RDA < 200 mg/day) are (alphabetical order):

- Cobalt required for biosynthesis of vitamin B12 family of coenzymes
- Copper required component of many redox enzymes, including cytochrome c oxidase
- Chromium required for sugar metabolism
- Iodine required for the biosynthesis of thyroxin
- Iron required for many proteins and enzymes, notably hemoglobin
- Manganese (processing of oxygen)
- Molybdenum required for xanthine oxidase and related oxidases

- Nickel present in urease
- Selenium required for peroxidase (antioxidant proteins)
- Vanadium (There is no established RDA for vanadium. No specific biochemical function has been identified for it in humans, although vanadium is found in lower organisms.)
- Zinc required for several enzymes such as carboxypeptidase, liver alcohol dehydrogenase, and carbonic anhydrase. Zinc is pervasive.

Iodine is required in larger quantities than the other trace minerals in this list and is sometimes classified with the bulk minerals. Sodium is not generally found in dietary supplements, despite being needed in large quantities, because the ion is very common in food.

Vitamins

Calories/Gram: 0

Mineral and/or vitamin deficiency or excess may result in disease conditions such as goitre, scurvy, osteoporosis, impaired immune system, disorders of cell metabolism, certain forms of cancer, symptoms of premature aging, and poor psychological health (including eating disorders), among many others.

As of 2005, twelve vitamins and about the same number of minerals are recognized as "essential nutrients", meaning that they must be consumed and absorbed—or, in the case of vitamin D, alternatively synthesized in the skin via UVB radiation to prevent deficiency symptoms and possibly death. Certain vitamin-like substances found in foods, such as carnitine, have also been found essential to survival and health, but these are not strictly "essential" to eat because the human body can produce them from other compounds. Moreover, thousands of different phytochemicals have recently been discovered in food (particularly in fresh vegetables), which may have desirable properties including antioxidant activity. Other essential nutrients include essential amino acids, choline and the essential fatty acids.

Water

Calories/Gram: 0

About 70 per cent of the non-fat mass of the human body is made of water. To function properly, the body requires between one and seven liters of water per day to avoid dehydration; the precise amount depends on the level of activity, temperature, humidity, and other factors. With physical exertion and heat exposure, water loss will increase and daily fluid needs may increase as well.

It is not clear how much water intake is needed by healthy people, although some experts assert that 8-10 glasses of water (approximately 2 liters) daily is the minimum to maintain proper hydration. The notion that a person should consume eight glasses of water per day cannot be traced back to a scientific source. The effect of water intake on weight loss and on constipation is also still unclear. Original recommendation for water intake in 1945 by the Food and Nutrition Board of the National Research Council read: "An ordinary standard for diverse persons is 1 milliliter for each calorie of food. Most of this quantity is contained in prepared foods." The latest dietary reference intake report by the United States National Research Council in general recommended (including food sources): 2.7 liters of water total for women and 3.7 liters for men. Specifically, pregnant and breastfeeding women need additional fluids to stay hydrated. According to the Institute of Medicine—who recommend that, on average, women consume 2.2 litres and men 3.0 litres—this is recommended to be 2.4 litres (approx. 9 cups) for pregnant women and 3 litres (approx. 12.5 cups) for breastfeeding women since an especially large amount of fluid is lost during nursing.

For those who have healthy kidneys, it is rather difficult to drink too much water, but (especially in warm humid weather and while exercising) it is dangerous to drink too little. People can drink far more water than necessary while exercising, however, putting them at risk of water intoxication, which can be fatal. In particular large amounts of de-ionized water are dangerous.

Normally, about 20 per cent of water intake comes in food, while the rest comes from drinking water and assorted beverages (caffeinated included). Water is excreted from the body in multiple forms; including urine and feces, sweating, and by water vapor in the exhaled breath.

Other Nutrients

Calories/Gram: 0

Other micronutrients include antioxidants and phytochemicals. These substances are generally more recent discoveries which: have not yet been recognized as vitamins; are still under investigation; or contribute to health but are not necessary for life. Phytochemicals may act as antioxidants, but not all phytochemicals are antioxidants.

Antioxidants

Antioxidants are a recent discovery. As cellular metabolism/energy production requires oxygen, potentially damaging (e.g. mutation causing) compounds known as free radicals can form. Most of these are oxidizers 9ie, (acceptors of electrons) and some react very strongly. For normal cellular maintenance, growth, and division, these free radicals must be sufficiently neutralized by antioxidant compounds. Some are produced by the human body with adequate precursors (glutathione, Vitamin C) and those that the body cannot produce may only be obtained through the diet through direct sources (Vitamin C in humans, Vitamin A, Vitamin K) or produced by the body from other compounds (Beta-carotene converted to Vitamin A by the body, Vitamin D synthesized from cholesterol by sunlight). Phytochemicals and their subgroup polyphenols are the majority of antioxidants; about 4,000 are known. Different antioxidants are now known to function in a cooperative network, e.g. vitamin C can reactivate free radical-containing glutathione or vitamin E by accepting the free radical itself, and so on. Some antioxidants are more effective than others at neutralizing different free radicals. Some cannot neutralize certain free radicals. Some cannot be present in certain areas of free radical development (Vitamin A is fat-soluble and protects fat areas; Vitamin C is water soluble and protects those areas). When interacting with a free radical, some antioxidants produce a different free radical compound that is less dangerous or more dangerous than the previous compound. Having a variety of antioxidants allows any byproducts to be safely dealt with by more efficient antioxidants in neutralizing a free radical's butterfly effect.

Phytochemicals

A growing area of interest is the effect upon human health of trace chemicals, collectively called phytochemicals. These nutrients are typically found in edible plants, especially colourful fruits and vegetables, but also other organisms including seafood, algae, and fungi. The effects of phytochemicals increasingly survive rigorous testing by prominent health organizations. One of the principal classes of phytochemicals are polyphenol antioxidants, chemicals which are known to provide certain health benefits to the cardiovascular system and immune system. These chemicals are known to down-regulate the formation of reactive oxygen species, key chemicals in cardiovascular disease.

Perhaps the most rigorously tested phytochemical is zeaxanthin, a yellow-pigmented carotenoid present in many yellow and orange fruits and vegetables. Repeated studies have shown a strong correlation between ingestion of zeaxanthin and the prevention and treatment of age-related macular degeneration (AMD). Less rigorous studies have proposed a correlation between zeaxanthin intake and cataracts. A second carotenoid, lutein, has also been shown to lower the risk of contracting AMD. Both compounds have been observed to collect in the retina when ingested orally, and they serve to protect the rods and cones against the destructive effects of light.

Another carotenoid, beta-cryptoxanthin, appears to protect against chronic joint inflammatory diseases, such as arthritis. While the association between serum blood levels of beta-cryptoxanthin and substantially decreased joint disease has been established, neither a convincing mechanism for such protection nor a cause-and-effect has been rigorously studied. Similarly, a red phytochemical, lycopene, has substantial credible evidence of negative association with development of prostate cancer.

The correlations between the ingestion of some phytochemicals and the prevention of disease are, in some cases, enormous in magnitude.

Even when the evidence is obtained, translating it to practical dietary advice can be difficult and counter-intuitive. Lutein, for example, occurs in many yellow and orange fruits and vegetables and protects the eyes against various diseases. However, it does not protect the eye nearly as well as zeaxanthin, and the presence of lutein in the retina will prevent zeaxanthin uptake. Additionally, evidence has shown that the lutein present in egg yolk is more readily absorbed than the lutein from vegetable sources, possibly because of fat solubility. At the most basic level, the question "should you eat eggs?" is complex to the point of dismay, including misperceptions about the health effects of cholesterol in egg yolk, and its saturated fat content.

As another example, lycopene is prevalent in tomatoes (and actually is the chemical that gives tomatoes their red colour). It is more highly concentrated, however, in processed tomato products such as commercial pasta sauce, or tomato soup, than in fresh "healthy" tomatoes. Yet, such sauces tend to have high amounts of salt, sugar, and other substances a person may wish or even need to avoid.

The Table 1.1 presents phytochemical groups and common sources, arranged by family.

Intestinal Bacterial Flora

It is now also known that animal intestines contain a large population of gut flora. In humans, these include species such as Bacteroides, L. acidophilus and E. coli, among many others. They are essential to digestion, and are also affected by the food we eat. Bacteria in the gut perform many important functions for humans, including breaking down and aiding in the absorption of otherwise indigestible food; stimulating cell growth; repressing the growth of harmful bacteria, training the immune system to respond only to pathogens; producing vitamin B12, and defending against some diseases.

Balanced Diet

Balanced diet is a diet which consists of all the essential nutrients in a required proportion.

Table 1.1

Family	Sources	Possible Benefits
flavonoids	berries, herbs, vegetables, wine, grapes, tea	general antioxidant, oxidation of LDLs, prevention of arterio-sclerosis and heart disease
isoflavones (phytoestrogens)	soy, red clover, kudzu root	general antioxidant, prevention of arteriosclerosis and heart disease, easing symptoms of menopause, cancer prevention
isothiocyanates	cruciferous vegetables	cancer prevention
monoterpenes	citrus peels, essential oils, herbs, spices, green plants, atmosphere	cancer prevention, treating gallstones
organosulfur compounds	chives, garlic, onions	cancer prevention, lowered LDLs, assistance to the immune system
saponins	beans, cereals, herbs	Hypercholesterolemia, Hyper-glycemia, Antioxidant, cancer prevention, Anti-inflammatory
capsaicinoids	all capiscum (chile) peppers	topical pain relief, cancer pre-vention, cancer cell apoptosis

Junk Food

Junk food is a slang name for food items containing limited nutritional value. It includes food high in salts, fats, sugar, calories, and low nutrient content.

Sports Nutrition

Protein

The protein requirements of athletes, once the source of great controversy, have settled into a current consensus. Sedentary people and recreational athletes have similar protein requirements, about 1 gram of protein per kilogram of body mass. These needs are easily met by a balanced diet containing about 70 grams of protein for a 70 kg (150 pound) man or 60 grams of protein for a 60 kg (130 pound) woman.

People who exercise at greater intensity, and especially those whose activity grows muscle bulk, have significantly higher protein requirements. According to *Clinical Sports Nutrition,* active athletes playing power sports (such as football), those engaged in muscle-development training, and elite endurance athletes, all require approximately 2 grams of protein per day per kilogram of body weight, roughly double that of a sedentary persons. Older athletes seeking primarily to maintain developed muscle mass require 2 to 3 g per day per kg.

Protein intake in excess of that required to build muscle (and other) tissue is broken-down by gluconeogenesis to be used as energy.

Water and Salts

Water is one of the most important nutrients in your sports diet. It helps eliminate food waste products in your body, regulates body temperature during activity, helps digest, is involved in converting food into energy and helps lubricate joints. Athletes should drink as much water as they comfortably can. Maintaining hydration during periods of physical exertion is key to peak performance. While drinking too much water during activities can lead to physical discomfort, dehydration in excess of 2 per cent of body mass (by weight) markedly hinders athletic performance. Some studies have shown that an athlete that drinks before they feel thirsty stays cooler and performs better than one who drinks on thirst cues, although recent studies of such races as the Boston Marathon have indicated that this recommendation can lead to the problem of overhydration. Additional carbohydrates and protein before, during, and after exercise increase time to exhaustion as well as speed recovery. Dosage is based on work performed, lean body mass, and environmental factors, especially ambient temperature and humidity.

Carbohydrates

The main fuel used by the body during exercise is carbohydrates, which is stored in muscle as glycogen—a form of sugar. During exercise, muscle glycogen reserves can be used up, especially when activities last longer than 90 min. Because the amount of glycogen stored in the body is limited, it is important for athletes to replace glycogen by consuming a diet high in carbohydrates. Meeting energy needs can help improve performance during the sport, as well as improve overall strength and endurance. There are different kinds of carbohydrates—simple or refined, and unrefined. A typical American consumes about 50 per cent of their carbohydrates as simple sugars, which are added to foods as opposed to sugars that come naturally in fruits and vegetables. These simple sugars come in large amounts in sodas and fast food. Over the course of a year, the average American consumes 54 gallons of soft drinks, which contain the highest amount of added sugars. Even though carbohydrates are necessary for humans to function, they are not all equally healthful. When machinery has been used to remove bits of high fiber, the carbohydrates are refined. These are the carbohydrates found in white bread and fast food.

Longevity

Whole Plant Food Diet

Heart disease, cancer, obesity, and diabetes are commonly called "Western" diseases because these maladies were once rarely seen in developing countries. One study in China found some regions had essentially no cancer or heart disease, while in other areas they reflected "up to a 100-fold increase" coincident with diets that were found to be entirely plant-based to heavily animal-based, respectively. In contrast, diseases of affluence like cancer and heart disease are common throughout the United States. Adjusted for age and exercise, large regional clusters of people in China rarely suffered from these "Western" diseases possibly because their diets are rich in vegetables, fruits and whole grains.

The United Healthcare/Pacificare nutrition guideline recommends a whole plant food diet, and recommends using protein only as a condiment with meals. A National Geographic cover article from November, 2005, entitled The Secrets of Living Longer, also recommends a whole plant food diet. The article is a lifestyle survey of three populations, Sardinians, Okinawans, and Adventists, who generally display longevity and "suffer a fraction of the diseases that commonly kill people in other parts of the developed world, and enjoy more healthy years of life. In sum, they offer three sets of 'best practices' to emulate. The rest is up to you." In common with all three groups is to "Eat fruits, vegetables, and whole grains."

The National Geographic article noted that an NIH funded study of 34,000 Seventh-day Adventists between 1976 and 1988 "...found that the Adventists' habit of consuming beans, soy milk, tomatoes, and other fruits lowered their risk of developing certain cancers. It also suggested that eating whole grain bread, drinking five glasses of water a day, and, most surprisingly, consuming four servings of nuts a week reduced their risk of heart disease."

The French "Paradox"

It has been discovered that people living in France live longer. Even though they consume more saturated fats than Americans, the rate of heart disease is lower in France than in North America. A number of explanations have been suggested:

- Reduced consumption of processed carbohydrate and other junk foods;
- Ethnic genetic differences allowing the body to be harmed less by fats;
- Regular consumption of red wine; or
- Living in the South requires the body to produce less heat, allowing a slower, and therefore healthier, metabolic rate.
- More active lifestyles involving plenty of daily exercise, especially walking; the French are much less dependent on cars than Americans are.
- Higher consumption of artificially produced trans-fats by Americans, which has been shown to have greater lipoprotein impacts per gram than saturated fat.

However, a growing number of French health researchers doubt the theory that the French are healthier than other populations. Statistics collected by the WHO from 1990-2000 show that the incidence of heart disease in France may have been underestimated and in fact is similar to that of neighboring countries.

Malnutrition

Malnutrition refers to insufficient, excessive, or imbalanced consumption of nutrients. In developed countries, the diseases of malnutrition are most often associated with nutritional imbalances or excessive consumption. Although there are more people in the world who are malnourished due to excessive consumption, according to the United Nations World Health Organization, the real challenge in developing nations today, more than starvation, is combating insufficient nutrition — the lack of nutrients necessary for the growth and maintenance of vital functions.

Mental Agility

Research indicates that improving the awareness of nutritious meal choices and establishing long-term habits of healthy eating has a positive effect on a cognitive and spatial memory capacity, potentially increasing a student's potential to process and retain academic information.

Illnesses Caused by Improper Nutrient Consumption

Table 1.2

Nutrients	*Deficiency*	*Excess*
Calories	Starvation	Obesity, diabetes mellitus, Cardiovascular disease
Simple carbohydra-tes	Marasmus, starvation	diabetes mellitus
Complex carbohydrates	Marasmus, starvation	Obesity
Saturated fat/trans fat	none	Cardiovascular disease,

(Contd.)

Nutrients	Deficiency	Excess
Unsaturated fat	Rabbit starvation	Obesity
Cholesterol	none	Cardiovascular disease
Protein	Marasmus	Ketoacidosis, Rabbit starvation, kidney disease
Sodium	hyponatremia	Hypernatremia, hypertension
Iron	Anemia	Hepatitis C, cirrhosis, heart disease
Iodine	Goiter, hypothyroidism	Iodine Toxicity (goiter, hypothyroidism)
Vitamin A	Xerophthalmia and Night Blindness	Hypervitaminosis A (cirrhosis, hair loss, birth defects)
Vitamin B1	Beri-Beri	
Vitamin B2	Cracking of skin and Corneal Unclearation	
Niacin	Pellagra	dyspepsia, cardiac arrhythmias, birth defects
Vitamin B12	Pernicious Anemia	
Vitamin C	Scurvy	diarrhea causing dehydration
Vitamin D	Rickets	Hypervitaminosis D (dehydration, vomiting, constipation)
Vitamin E		Hypervitaminosis E (anticoagulant: excessive bleeding)
Vitamin K	Hemorrhage	

Some organizations have begun working with teachers, policymakers, and managed foodservice contractors to mandate improved nutritional content and increased nutritional resources in school cafeterias from primary to university level institutions. Health and nutrition have been proven to have close links with overall educational success (Behrman, 1996). Currently less than 10 per cent of American college students report that they eat the recommended five servings of fruit and vegetables daily. Better nutrition has been shown to have an impact on both cognitive and spatial memory performance; a study showed those with higher blood sugar levels performed better on certain memory tests. In another study, those who consumed yogurt performed better on thinking tasks when compared to those who consumed caffeine free diet soda or confections. Nutritional deficiencies have been shown to have a negative effect on learning behaviour in mice as far back as 1951.

> "Better learning performance is associated with diet induced effects on learning and memory ability".

The "nutrition-learning nexus" demonstrates the correlation between diet and learning and has application in a higher education setting.

> "We find that better nourished children perform significantly better in school, partly because they enter school earlier and thus have more time to learn but mostly because of greater learning productivity per year of schooling."

> 91 per cent of college students feel that they are in good health while only 7 per cent eat their recommended daily allowance of fruits and vegetables.

> Nutritional education is an effective and workable model in a higher education setting.

> More "engaged" learning models that encompass nutrition is an idea that is picking up steam at all levels of the learning cycle.

There is limited research available that directly links a student's Grade Point Average (G.P.A.) to their overall nutritional health. Additional substantive data is needed to prove beyond a shadow of a doubt that overall intellectual health is closely linked to a person's diet, rather than just another correlation fallacy.

Mental Disorders

Nutritional supplement treatment may be appropriate for major depression, bipolar disorder, schizophrenia, and obsessive compulsive disorder, the four most common mental disorders in developed countries.

Cancer

Cancer is now common in developing countries. According a study by the International Agency for Research on Cancer, "In the developing world, cancers of the liver, stomach and esophagus were more common, often linked to consumption of carcinogenic preserved foods, such as smoked or salted food, and parasitic infections that attack organs." Lung cancer rates are rising rapidly in poorer nations because of increased use of tobacco. Developed countries "tended to have cancers linked to affluence or a 'Western lifestyle' — cancers of the colon, rectum, breast and prostate — that can be caused by obesity, lack of exercise, diet and age."

Metabolic Syndrome

Several lines of evidence indicate lifestyle-induced hyperinsulinemia and reduced insulin function (i.e. insulin resistance) as a decisive factor in many disease states. For example, hyperinsulinemia and insulin resistance are strongly linked to chronic inflammation, which in turn is strongly linked to a variety of adverse developments such as arterial microinjuries and clot formation (i.e. heart disease) and exaggerated cell division (i.e. cancer). Hyperinsulinemia and insulin resistance (the so-called metabolic syndrome) are characterized by a combination of abdominal obesity, elevated blood sugar, elevated blood pressure, elevated blood triglycerides, and reduced HDL cholesterol. The negative impact of hyperinsulinemia on prostaglandin PGE1/PGE2 balance may be significant.

The state of obesity clearly contributes to insulin resistance, which in turn can cause type 2 diabetes. Virtually all obese and most type 2 diabetic individuals have marked insulin resistance. Although the association between overweight and insulin resistance is clear, the exact (likely multifarious) causes of insulin resistance remain less clear. Importantly, it has been demonstrated that appropriate exercise, more regular food intake and reducing glycemic load all can reverse insulin resistance in overweight individuals (and thereby lower blood sugar levels in those who have type 2 diabetes).

Obesity can unfavourably alter hormonal and metabolic status via resistance to the hormone leptin, and a vicious cycle may occur in which insulin/leptin resistance and obesity aggravate one another. The vicious cycle is putatively fuelled by continuously high insulin/leptin stimulation and fat storage, as a result of high intake of strongly insulin/leptin stimulating foods and energy. Both insulin and leptin normally function as satiety signals to the hypothalamus in the brain; however, insulin/leptin resistance may reduce this signal and therefore allow continued overfeeding despite large body fat stores. In addition, reduced leptin signalling to the brain may reduce leptin's normal effect to maintain an appropriately high metabolic rate.

There is a debate about how and to what extent different dietary factors— such as intake of processed carbohydrates, total protein, fat, and carbohydrate intake, intake of saturated and trans fatty acids, and low intake of vitamins/minerals—contribute to the development of insulin and leptin resistance. In any case, analogous to the way modern man-made pollution may potentially overwhelm the environment's ability to maintain homeostasis, the recent explosive introduction of high glycemic index and processed foods into the human diet may potentially overwhelm the body's ability to maintain homeostasis and health (as evidenced by the metabolic syndrome epidemic).

Hyponatremia

Excess water intake, without replenishment of sodium and potassium salts, leads to hyponatremia, which can further lead to water intoxication at more dangerous levels. A well-publicized case occurred in 2007, when Jennifer Strange died while participating in a water-drinking contest. More usually, the condition occurs in long-distance endurance events (such as marathon or triathlon competition and training) and causes gradual mental dulling, headache, drowsiness, weakness, and confusion; extreme cases may result in coma, convulsions, and death. The primary damage comes from swelling of the brain, caused by increased osmosis as blood salinity decreases. Effective fluid replacement techniques include Water aid stations during running/cycling races, trainers providing water during team games such as Soccer and devices such as Camel Baks which can provide water for a person without making it too hard to drink the water.

Processed Foods

Since the Industrial Revolution some two hundred years ago, the food processing industry has invented many technologies that both help keep foods fresh longer and alter the fresh state of food as they appear in nature. Cooling is the primary technology used to maintain freshness, whereas many more technologies have been invented to allow foods to last longer without becoming spoiled. These latter technologies include pasteurisation, autoclavation, drying, salting, and separation of various components, and all appear to alter the original nutritional contents of food. Pasteurisation and autoclavation (heating techniques) have no doubt improved the safety of many common foods, preventing epidemics of bacterial infection. But some of the (new) food processing technologies undoubtedly have downfalls as well.

Modern separation techniques such as milling, centrifugation, and pressing have enabled upconcentration of particular components of food, yielding flour, oils, juices and so on, and even separate fatty acids, amino acids, vitamins, and minerals. Inevitably, such large scale upconcentration changes the nutritional content of food, saving certain nutrients while removing others. Heating techniques may also reduce food's content of many heat-labile nutrients such as certain vitamins and phytochemicals, and possibly other yet to be discovered substances. Because of reduced nutritional value, processed foods are often 'enriched' or 'fortified' with some of the most critical nutrients (usually certain vitamins) that were lost during processing. Nonetheless, processed foods tend to have an inferior nutritional profile compared to whole, fresh foods, regarding content of sugar and high GI starches, potassium/sodium, vitamins, fibre, and of intact, unoxidized (essential) fatty acids. In addition, processed foods often contain potentially harmful substances such as oxidized fats and trans fatty acids.

A dramatic example of the effect of food processing on a population's health is the history of epidemics of beri-beri in people subsisting on polished rice. Removing the outer layer of rice by polishing it removes with it the essential vitamin thiamine, causing beri-beri. Another example is the development of scurvy among infants in the late 1800s in the United States. It turned out that the vast majority of sufferers were being fed milk that had been heat-treated (as suggested by Pasteur) to control bacterial disease. Pasteurisation was effective against bacteria, but it destroyed the vitamin C.

As mentioned, lifestyle-and obesity-related diseases are becoming increasingly prevalent all around the world. There is little doubt that the increasingly widespread application of some modern food processing technologies has contributed to this development. The food processing industry is a major part of modern economy, and as such it is influential in political decisions (e.g. nutritional recommendations, agricultural subsidising). In any known profit-driven economy, health considerations are hardly a priority; effective production of cheap foods with a long shelf-life is more the trend. In general, whole, fresh foods have a relatively short shelf-life and are less profitable to produce and sell than are more processed foods. Thus the consumer is left with the choice between more expensive but nutritionally superior whole, fresh foods, and cheap, usually nutritionally inferior processed foods. Because processed foods are often cheaper, more convenient (in purchasing, storage, and preparation), and more available, the consumption of nutritionally inferior foods has been increasing throughout the world along with many nutrition-related health complications.

Advice and Guidance

Governmental Policies

The updated USDA food pyramid, published in 2005, is a general nutrition guide for recommended food consumption for humans.

In US, "dietitians". are registered (RD) or licensed (LD) with the Commission for Dietetic Registration and the American Dietetic

Association, and are only able to use the title "dietitian," as described by the business and professions codes of each respective state, when they have met specific educational and experiential prerequisites and passed a national registration or licensure examination, respectively. In California, registered dietitions must abide by the "Business and Professions Code of Section 2585-2586.8". Anyone may call themselves a nutritionist, including unqualified personnel, as this term is unregulated. Some states, such as the State of Florida, have begun to include the title "nutritionist" in state licensure requirements. Most governments provide guidance on nutrition, and some also impose mandatory disclosure/labeling requirements for processed food manufacturers and restaurants to assist consumers in complying with such guidance.

In the US, nutritional standards and recommendations are established jointly by the US Department of Agriculture and US Department of Health and Human Services. Dietary and physical activity guidelines from the USDA are presented in the concept of a food pyramid, which superseded the Four Food Groups. The Senate committee currently responsible for oversight of the USDA is the *Agriculture, Nutrition and Forestry Committee.* Committee hearings are often televised on C-SPAN as seen here.

The U.S. Department of Health and Human Services provides a sample week-long menu which fulfills the nutritional recommendations of the government.

Canada's Food Guide is another governmental recommendation.

Teaching

Nutrition is taught in schools in many countries. In England and Wales the Personal and Social Education and Food Technology curricula include nutrition, stressing the importance of a balanced diet and teaching how to read nutrition labels on packaging. In many schools a Nutrition class will fall within the Family and Consumer Science or Health departments. In some American schools, students are required to take a certain number of FCS or Health related classes. Nutrition is offered at many schools, and if it is not a class of its own, nutrition is included in other FCS or Health classes such as: Life Skills, Independent Living, Single Survival, Freshmen

Connection, Health etc. In many Nutrition classes, students learn about the food groups, the food pyramid, Daily Recommended Allowances, calories, vitamins, minerals, malnutrition, physical activity, healthy food choices and how to live a healthy life.

A 1985 US National Research Council report entitled *Nutrition Education in US Medical Schools* concluded that nutrition education in medical schools was inadequate. Only 20 per cent of the schools surveyed taught nutrition as a separate, required course. A 2006 survey found that this number had risen to 30 per cent.

History

Humans have evolved as omnivorous hunter-gatherers over the past 250,000 years. The diet of early modern humans varied significantly depending on location and climate. The diet in the tropics tended to be based more heavily on plant foods, while the diet at higher latitudes tended more towards animal products. Analysis of postcranial and cranial remains of humans and animals from the Neolithic, along with detailed bone modification studies has shown that cannibalism was also prevalent among prehistoric humans.

Agriculture developed about 10,000 years ago in multiple locations throughout the world, providing grains such as wheat, rice, and maize, with staples such as bread and pasta. Farming also provided milk and dairy products, and sharply increased the availability of meats and the diversity of vegetables. The importance of food purity was recognized when bulk storage led to infestation and contamination risks. Cooking developed as an often ritualistic activity, due to efficiency and reliability concerns requiring adherence to strict recipes and procedures, and in response to demands for food purity and consistency.

Antiquity through 1900

The first recorded nutritional experiment is found in the Bible's Book of Daniel. Daniel and his friends were captured by the king of Babylon during an invasion of Israel. Selected as court servants, they were to share in the king's fine foods and wine. But they objected, preferring vegetables (pulses) and water in accordance with their Jewish dietary restrictions. The king's chief steward reluctantly agreed to a trial. Daniel and his friends received their diet for 10 days and were then compared to the king's men. Appearing healthier, they were allowed to continue with their diet.

In around 475 BC, Anaxagoras stated that food is absorbed by the human body and therefore contained "homeomerics" (generative components), thereby deducing the existence of nutrients. Around 400 BC, Hippocrates said, "Let food be your medicine and medicine be your food."

In the 1500s, scientist and artist Leonardo da Vinci compared metabolism to a burning candle. In 1747, Dr. James Lind, a physician in the British navy, performed the first scientific nutrition experiment, discovering that lime juice saved sailors who had been at sea for years from scurvy, a deadly and painful bleeding disorder. The discovery was ignored for forty years, after which British sailors became known as "limeys." The essential vitamin C within lime juice would not be identified by scientists until the 1930s.

Around 1770, Antoine Lavoisier, the "Father of Nutrition and Chemistry" discovered the details of metabolism, demonstrating that the oxidation of food is the source of body heat. In 1790, George Fordyce recognized calcium as necessary for fowl survival. In the early 1800s, the elements carbon, nitrogen, hydrogen and oxygen were recognized as the primary components of food, and methods to measure their proportions were developed.

In 1816, François Magendie discovered that dogs fed only carbohydrates and fat lost their body protein and died in a few weeks, but dogs also fed protein survived, identifying protein as an essential dietary component. In 1840, Justus Liebig discovered the chemical makeup of carbohydrates (sugars), fats (fatty acids) and proteins (amino acids.) In the 1860s, Claude Bernard discovered that body fat can be synthesized from carbohydrate and protein, showing that the energy in blood glucose can be stored as fat or as glycogen.

In the early 1880s, Kanehiro Takaki observed that Japanese sailors (whose diets consisted almost entirely of white rice) developed beriberi (or endemic neuritis, a disease causing heart problems and paralysis) but British sailors and Japanese naval officers did not. Adding various types of vegetables and meats to the diets of Japanese sailors prevented the disease.

In 1896, Baumann observed iodine in thyroid glands. In 1897, Christiaan Eijkman worked with natives of Java, who also suffered from beriberi. Eijkman observed that chickens fed the native diet of white rice developed the symptoms of beriberi, but remained healthy when fed unprocessed brown rice with the outer bran intact. Eijkman cured the natives by feeding them brown rice, discovering that food can cure disease. Over two decades later, nutritionists learned that the outer rice bran contains vitamin B1, also known as thiamine.

1900 through Present

In the early 1900s, Carl Von Voit and Max Rubner independently measured caloric energy expenditure in different species of animals, applying principles of physics in nutrition. In 1906, Wilcock and Hopkins showed that the amino acid tryptophan was necessary for the survival of rats. He fed them a special mixture of food containing all the nutrients he believed were essential for survival, but the rats died. A second group of rats to which he also fed an amount of milk containing vitamins. Gowland Hopkins recognized "accessory food factors" other than calories, protein and minerals, as organic materials essential to health but which the body cannot synthesize. In 1907, Stephen M. Babcock and Edwin B. Hart conducted the single-grain experiment. This experiment runs through 1911.

In 1912, Casimir Funk coined the term vitamin, a vital factor in the diet, from the words "vital" and "amine," because these unknown substances preventing scurvy, beriberi, and pellagra, were thought then to be derived from ammonia. The vitamins were studied in the first half of the twentieth century.

In 1913, Elmer McCollum discovered the first vitamins, fat soluble vitamin A, and water soluble vitamin B (in 1915; now known to be a complex of several water-soluble vitamins) and names vitamin C as the then-unknown substance preventing scurvy. Lafayette Mendel and Thomas Osborne also perform pioneering work on vitamin A and B. In 1919, Sir Edward Mellanby incorrectly identified rickets as a vitamin A deficiency, because he could cure it in dogs with cod liver oil. In 1922, McCollum destroyed the vitamin A in cod liver oil but finds it still cures rickets, naming vitamin D Also in 1922, H.M. Evans and L.S. Bishop discover vitamin E as essential for rat pregnancy, originally calling it "food factor X" until 1925.

In 1925, Hart discovered that trace amounts of copper are necessary for iron absorption. In 1927, Adolf Otto Reinhold Windaus synthesized vitamin D, for which he won the Nobel Prize in Chemistry in 1928. In 1928, Albert Szent-Györgyi isolated ascorbic acid, and in 1932 proves that it is vitamin C by preventing scurvy. In 1935 he synthesizes it, and in 1937 he wins a Nobel Prize for his efforts. Szent-Györgyi concurrently elucidates much of the citric acid cycle.

In the 1930s, William Cumming Rose identified essential amino acids, necessary protein components which the body cannot synthesize. In 1935, Underwood and Marston independently discover the necessity of cobalt. In 1936, Eugene Floyd Dubois showed that work and school performances are related to caloric intake. In 1938, Erhard Fernholz discovered the chemical structure of vitamin E. It was synthesised by Paul Karrer.

In 1940, rationing in the United Kingdom during and after World War II took place according to nutritional principles drawn up by Elsie Widdowson and others. In 1941, the first Recommended Dietary Allowances (RDAs) were established by the National Research Council.

In 1992, The U.S. Department of Agriculture introduced the Food Guide Pyramid. In 2002, a Natural Justice study showed a relation between nutrition and violent behaviour. In 2005, a study found that obesity may be caused by adenovirus in addition to bad nutrition.

NUTRITIONAL ANALYSIS

Nutrition analysis refers to the process of determining the nutritional content of foods and food products. The process can be performed through a variety of certified methods.

Methods

Laboratory Analysis

Traditionally, food companies would send food samples to laboratories for chemical testing. Chemical testing involves the incineration of the foods to test the ash for exact nutritional content.

Software

Software is available as an alternative to laboratory nutrition analysis. This software typically utilizes a database of ingredients that have previously been laboratory tested. The user can input ingredient data by matching their ingredients to ingredients found in the database; the analysis can then be calculated.

Online Nutrition Analysis

In recent years, web-based nutrition analysis software services have become more popular. Online nutrition analysis allows users to access online databases and draw from certified ingredients to product instant nutrition information.

Applications

In the United States, nutrition information is required on packaged retail foods in the form of nutrition facts panels as a result of food labeling regulations. In recent years, many restaurants have begun posting nutrition information as a result of both customer demand and menu-labeling laws.

Nutrition Facts Label

Menu-labeling

Recently many state and local menu-labeling laws have been passed requiring restaurants to post nutrition information on menus and menu boards, or have it readily available upon customer request. Restaurants have had to perform nutrition analysis in order to generate nutrition information and conform to these laws. More recently national legislation has been introduced that would set a national standard for menu labeling, the most popular of which is the LEAN act.

PREBIOTIC NUTRITION

Prebiotics are non-digestible food ingredients that stimulate the growth and/or activity of bacteria in the digestive system which are beneficial to the health of the body. They were first identified and named by Marcel Roberfroid in 1995. They are considered a functional food.

Typically, prebiotics are carbohydrates (such as oligosaccharides), but the definition does not preclude non-carbohydrates. The most prevalent forms of prebiotics are nutritionally classed as soluble fiber. To some extent, many forms of dietary fiber exhibit some level of prebiotic effect.

Roberfroid offered a refined definition in the 2007 Journal of Nutrition stating:

> "A prebiotic is a selectively fermented ingredient that allows specific changes, both in the composition and/or activity in the gastrointestinal microflora that confers benefits upon host well-being and health."

Additionally, in his 2007 revisit of Prebiotics, Roberfroid clarified that only two particular fructooligosaccharides fully meet this definition: oligofructose and inulin. Caution may be in order when referring to other substances as "Prebiotic," and it is increasingly common to refer to other similar substances as "possible" or "likely" Prebiotics in order to distinguish.

Researchers now also focus on the distinction between short-chain, long-chain, and full-spectrum prebiotics. "short-chain" prebiotics, e.g. oligofructose, contain 2-8 links per saccharide molecule, are typically fermented more quickly in the right-side of the colon providing nourishment to the bacteria in that area. Longer-chain prebiotics, e.g. Inulin, contain 9-64 links per saccharide molecule, and tend to be fermented more slowly, nourishing bacteria predominantly in the left-side colon. Full-spectrum prebiotics provide the full range of molecular link-lenghts from 2-64 links per molecule, and nourish bacteria throughout the colon, e.g. Oligofructose-Enriched Inulin (OEI). The majority of research done on prebiotics is based on full-spectrum prebiotics, typically using OEI as the research substance.

Function

The prebiotic definition does not emphasize a specific bacterial group. Generally, however, it is assumed that a prebiotic should increase the number and/or activity of bifidobacteria and lactic acid bacteria. The importance of the bifidobacteria and the lactic acid bacteria (AKA lactobacillus or LABs) is that these groups of bacteria have several beneficial effects on the host, especially in terms of improving digestion (including enhancing mineral absorption) and the effectiveness and intrinsic strength of the immune system. A product that stimulates bifidobacteria is considered a bifidogenic factor. Some prebiotics may thus also act as a bifidogenic factor and vice versa, but the two concepts are not identical.

Sources

Traditional dietary sources of prebiotics include soybeans, inulin sources (such as Jerusalem artichoke, jicama, and chicory root), raw oats, unrefined wheat, unrefined barley and yacon. Some of the oligosaccharides that naturally occur in breast milk are believed to play an important role in the development of a healthy immune system in infants.

It is becoming more common to properly distinguish between prebiotic substances and the food that contains them. References to Almonds, honey and other foods (most commonly in promotional materials from growers of those foods) as "a prebiotic" are not accurate. No plant or food is a prebiotic: Wheat, honey and many other foods contain prebiotics to a greater or lesser extent, ranging from fairly large portions (chicory root, jerusalem artichoke) to only trace quantities (thousands of other plant-based foods). Referring to a food as "a prebiotic" is no more accurate than calling a food "a vitamin."

Jerusalem Artichoke is a frequently referred to as a rich source of prebiotic fiber. This is true, but it should be pointed out that jerusalem artichoke is not the traditional spiky green artichoke found in most groceries stores, but another plant altogether (and a far-from-common offering at most food merchants).

Prebiotic oligosaccharides are increasingly added to foods for their health benefits. Some oligosaccharides that are used in this manner are fructooligosaccharides (FOS), xylooligosaccharides (XOS), polydextrose and galactooligosaccharides (GOS). Some monosaccharides such as tagatose are also used sometimes as prebiotics.

In petfood also mannooligosaccharides are being used for prebiotic purposes.

Again, one may wish to recall that Roberfroid, whom many consider the pre-eminent authority on Prebiotics, states that only two specific fructooligosaccharides—oligofructose and inulin—meet his seminal definition of "Prebiotic."

Genetically engineering plants for the production of inulins has also become more prevalent, despite the still limited insight into the immunological mechanisms activated by such food supplementation.

Effects

Studies have demonstrated positive effects on calcium and other mineral absorption, immune system effectiveness, bowel pH, reduction of colorectal cancer risk, inflammatory bowel disorders (Crohn's Disease and Ulcerative Colitis) and intestinal regularity. Recent human trials have reinforced the role of Prebiotics in preventing and possibly stopping early stage colon cancer. It has been argued that many of these health effects emanate not just from bifidogenic function of prebiotics, but also from increased production of short-chain fatty acids by the stimulated beneficial bacteria. Thus food supplements specifically enhancing the growth of intestinal bacteria are widely recognized to be beneficial.

While research does clearly demonstrate that prebiotics lead to increased production of these SCFA's, more research is required to establish a direct causal connection. It has been argued that prebiotics are beneficial to Crohn's Disease through production of SCFAs to nourish the colon walls, and beneficial to Ulcerative Colitis through reduction of Hydrogen Sulfide gas due to reduction of sulfate-reducing bacteria, which do not thrive in the slightly acidic environment SCFAs create.

The immediate addition of substantial quantities of prebiotics to the diet may result in a temporary increase in gas, bloating or bowel movement. It has been argued that chronically low consumption of prebiotic-containing foods in the typical Western diet may exaggerate this effect.

PREBIOTIC SCORES

A prebiotic score is a term sometimes used to estimate the health effects of prebiotics in humans or animals. There is no definition of prebiotic scores. The idea is that prebiotics may have many different effects in the human gut; some of these may be quantified and combined to an overall score. For example, an increase in bifidobacteria or a decrease in Clostridium perfringens can be quantified. Also increases and reductions of certain enzymes may be used as factors in a prebiotic score.

NUTRITIONAL SCALE

Nutrition scale is a weighing instrument that output precise nutritional information for foods or liquids. Most scales calculate calories, carbohydrates, and fats, with more sophisticated scales calculating additional nutrients such as Vitamin K, potassium, magnesium, and sodium.

Scales often use USDA information on food to ensure accuracy. The products are used primarily as a weight management tool, but have found a user base with diabetics and hypertensive people.

Nutritional Facts and Labels

The nutrition facts label (also known as the nutrition information panel, and various other slight variations) is a label required on most pre-packaged foods in many countries (Fig. 1.1).

Regional Manifestations

Australia and New Zealand

Australia and New Zealand use a nutritional information panel of the format shown in Fig. 1.1.

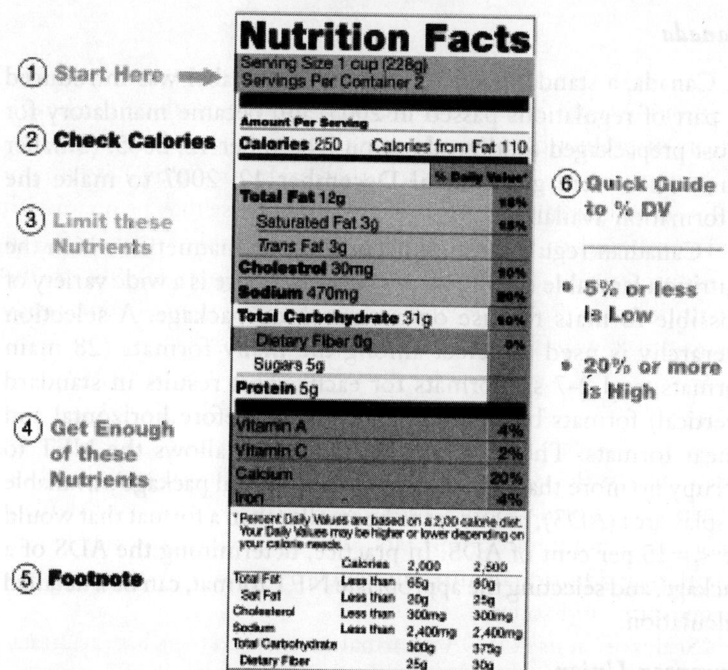

Fig. 1.1: A Sample Nutrition Facts Label with Instructions from the US FDA

Table 1.3: Nutrition Information

Servings per package: x		
Serving size: y g (or mL etc.)		
	Quantity per Serving	*Quantity per 100 g (or 100 mL etc.)*
Energy	n1 kJ (n'1 Cal)	m1 kJ (m'1 Cal)
Protein	n2 g	n2 g
Fat, total	n3 g	n3 g
—saturated	n4 g	n4 g
Carbohydrate	n5 g	n5 g
—sugars	n6 g	n6 g
Sodium	n7 mg	n7 mg

Other items are included as appropriate, and the units may be varied as appropriate.

Canada

In Canada, a standardized "Nutrition Facts" label was introduced as part of regulations passed in 2003, and became mandatory for most prepackaged food products on December 12, 2005. (Smaller businesses were given until December 12, 2007 to make the information available).

Canadian regulation tightly controls the manner in which the nutrition fact table (NFT) data is laid out. There is a wide variety of possible formats for use on a given food package. A selection hierarchy is used to select among the many formats (28 main formats, and 2-7 subformats for each). This results in standard (vertical) formats being considered for use before horizontal and linear formats. The selection hierarchy also allows the NFT to occupy no more than 15 per cent of the physical package's available display area (ADS), but never to be smaller than a format that would be <=15 per cent of ADS. In practice, determining the ADS of a package, and selecting the appropriate NFT format, can be a detailed calculation.

European Union

In the European Union the information (usually in panel format) is most often labeled "Nutrition Information" (or equivalent in other EU languages). The panel is optional, but if provided, the prescribed content and format must be followed. It will always give values for a set quantity — usually 100 g (3.5 oz) or 100 ml (3.5 imp fl oz; 3.4 US fl oz) of the product — and often also for a defined "serving". First will come the energy values, in both kilocalories and kilojoules, although the SI measurement is still little used by the general public.

Then will come a breakdown of constituent elements: usually most or all of protein, carbohydrate, starch, sugar, fat, fibre and sodium. The "fat" figure is likely to be further broken down into saturated and unsaturated fat, while the "carbohydrate" figure is likely to give a subtotal for sugars.

For most foods, there are no specific legal definitions of terms such as "low fat" or "high fibre", although spreadable fats (e.g. butter and margarine) do have statutory requirements for the quantity of fat they contain. However, terms such as "reduced calorie" may not be used unless they can be shown to be considerably lower in calories than the "usual" version of the product.

Provided the full nutrition information is shown on the packet, additional nutritional information and formats (e.g. a traffic light rating system) may be included and this falls outside the scope of regulation.

The United Kingdom regulations are given in Schedules 6 and 7 of the Food Labelling Regulations 1996.

Mexico

Food products sold in Mexico use the NOM-051-SCFI-1994 "Información nutrimental" product labelling standard (which is very similar to "Nutrition Facts" in the U.S.). The Official Mexican Standard, or NOM (Norma Oficial Mexicana), was developed by the Mexican Secretary of Commerce and Industrial Promotion (Secretaría de Comercio y Fomento Industrial, or SCFI), now a part of the Secretary of the Economy (SECOFI). It entered into effect on January 24, 1996, and defines "General specifications for labelling foods and pre-bottled non-alcoholic beverages".

United States

In the U.S., the nutritional facts label lists the percentage supplied required in one day of human nutrients based on the average 2000 calorie a day diet. With certain exceptions, such as foods meant for babies, the following Daily Values are used. These are called Reference Daily Intake values and were originally based on the highest 1968 Recommended Dietary Allowances for each nutrient in order to assure that the needs of all age and sex combinations were met.5 Notice that these are older than the current Recommended Dietary Allowances of the Dietary Reference Intake. For Vitamin C, Vitamin D, Vitamin E, Vitamin K, calcium, phosphorus, magnesium, and manganese, the current maximum RDA's (over age and sex) are up to 50 per cent higher than the Daily Values used in labeling, whereas for other nutrients the estimated maximal needs have gone down.

Nutrient	*Daily Value for Label*	*highest RDA of DRI*
Vitamin A	5000 IU	3000 IU
Vitamin C	60 mg	90 mg
Calcium	1000 mg	1300 mg
Iron	18 mg	18 mg
Vitamin D	400 IU	600 IU
Vitamin E	30 IU	15 mg (33 IU of synthetic)
Vitamin K	80 µg	120 µg
Thiamin	1.5 mg	1.2 mg
Riboflavin	1.7 mg	1.3 mg
Niacin	20 mg	16 mg
Vitamin B6	2 mg	1.7 mg
Folate	400 µg	400 µg
Vitamin B12	6 µg	2.4 µg
Biotin	300 µg	30 µg
Pantothenic acid	10 mg	5 mg
Phosphorus	1000 mg	1250 mg
Iodine	150 µg	150 µg
Magnesium	400 mg	420 mg
Zinc	15 mg	11 mg
Selenium	70 µg	55 µg
Copper	2 mg	900 µg
Manganese	2 mg	2.3 mg
Chromium	120 µg	35 µg
Molybdenum	75 µg	45 µg
Chloride	3400 mg	2300 mg

In certain cases this label is not yet required by law, so a list of ingredients should be present instead. Ingredients are listed in order from highest to lowest quantity.

The label was mandated for most food products under the provisions of the 1990 Nutrition Labeling and Education Act (NLEA), per the recommendations of the United States Department of Health and Human Services' Food and Drug Administration. It was one of several controversial actions taken during the tenure of FDA Commissioner Dr. David Kessler. The law required food companies to begin using the new food label on packaged foods beginning May 8, 1994. (Meat and poultry products were not covered by NLEA, though the U.S. Department of Agriculture proposed similar regulations for voluntary labeling of raw meat and poultry.) Foods labeled before that day could use the old label. This appeared on all products in 1995. The old label was titled "Nutrition Information per Serving" or simply, "Nutrition Information".

The label begins with a standard serving measurement, calories are listed second, and then following is a break down of the constituent elements. Always listed are total fat, sodium, carbohydrates and protein; the other nutrients usually shown may be suppressed if they are zero. Usually all 15 nutrients are shown: calories, calories from fat, fat, saturated fat, trans fat, cholesterol, sodium, carbohydrates, dietary fiber, sugars, protein, vitamin A, vitamin C, calcium, and iron.

Products containing less than 5 g of fat show amounts rounded to the nearest 0.5 g. Amounts less than 0.5 g are rounded to 0 g. For example, if a product contains 0.45 g of trans fat per serving, and the package contains 18 servings, the label would show 0 g of trans fat, even though the product actually contains a total of 8.1 g of trans fat.

Products that claim to be classified as low-fat and high-fiber must achieve uniform definitions between products of similar labels.

The nutrition facts label currently appears on more than 6.5 billion food packages. President Bill Clinton issued an award of design excellence for the nutrition facts label in 1997 to Burkey Belser in Washington, DC.

The FDA does not require any specific typeface be used in the Nutrition Facts label, mandating only that the label "utilize a single easy-to-read type style", though its example label uses Helvetica.

In 2009, a federal appellate court rejected the New York State Restaurant Association's challenge to the city's 2007 regulation requiring most major fast-food and chain restaurants to prominently display calorie information on their menus. The rule applies to restaurants that are part of chains with at least 15 establishments doing business nationally.

ESSENTIAL NUTRIENTS

An essential nutrient is a nutrient required for normal body functioning that either cannot be synthesized by the body at all, or cannot be synthesized in amounts adequate for good health (e.g. niacin, choline), and thus must be obtained from a dietary source. Some categories of essential nutrients include vitamins, dietary minerals, essential fatty acids, and essential amino acids. Water and oxygen are also essential for human health and life, as oxygen cannot be synthesized by the body, and water, while a biochemical reaction product of metabolism, is not created in sufficient amounts. Both are necessary as biochemical reactants in some processes, and water is used in various ways such as a solvent, carrier, coolant, and integral polar structural member, but both are often not included as nutrients.

Different species have very different essential nutrients. For example, most mammals synthesize their own ascorbic acid, and it is therefore not considered an essential nutrient for such species. It is, however, an essential nutrient for human beings, who require external sources of ascorbic acid (known as Vitamin C in the context of nutrition).

Many essential nutrients are toxic in large doses. Some can be taken in amounts larger than required in a typical diet, with no apparent ill effects. Linus Pauling said of vitamin B_3, (either niacin or niacinamide), "What astonished me was the very low toxicity of a substance that has such very great physiological power. A little pinch, 5 mg, every day, is enough to keep a person from dying of pellagra, but it is so lacking in toxicity that ten thousand times as much can [sometimes] be taken without harm."

Amino Acids

- Isoleucine
- Lysine
- Leucine
- Methionine
- Phenylalanine
- Threonine
- Tryptophan
- Valine
- Essential amino acids necessary for human children but not adults:
  - Histidine
  - Arginine

Vitamins

- Biotin (vitamin B7, vitamin H)
- Choline (vitamin Bp)

- Folate (folic acid, vitamin B9, vitamin M)
- Niacin (vitamin B3, vitamin P, vitamin PP)
- Pantothenic acid (vitamin B5)
- Riboflavin (vitamin B2, vitamin G)
- Thiamine (vitamin B1)
- Vitamin A (retinol)
- Vitamin B6 (pyridoxine, pyridoxamine, or pyridoxal)
- Vitamin B12 (cobalamin)
- Vitamin C (ascorbic acid)
- Vitamin D (ergocalciferol, or cholecalciferol)
- Vitamin E (tocopherol)
- Vitamin K (naphthoquinoids)

Dietary Minerals

- Calcium (Ca)
- Chloride (Cl^-)
- Cobalt (Co) (as part of Vitamin B-12)
- Copper (Cu)
- Iodine (I)
- Iron (Fe)
- Magnesium (Mg)
- Manganese (Mn)
- Molybdenum (Mo)
- Nickel (Ni)
- Phosphorus (P)
- Potassium (K)
- Selenium (Se)
- Sodium (Na)
- Sulfur (S) numerous roles
- Zinc (Zn)

The body's requirements vary widely. At one extreme, a 70 kg human contains 1.0 kg of calcium, but only 3 mg of cobalt.

Elements with Speculated Role in Human Health

Many elements have been implicated at various times to have a role in human health. For none of these elements has a specific protein or complex been identified:

- Boron (B)
- Chromium (Cr)
- Silicon (Si)
- Arsenic (As)

MICRONUTRIENTS

Micronutrients are nutrients needed throughout life in small quantities. They are dietary minerals needed by the human body in very small quantities (generally less than 100micrograms/day) as opposed to macrominerals which are required in larger quantities. The Microminerals or trace elements include at least iron, cobalt, chromium, copper, iodine, manganese, selenium, zinc and molybdenum. Note that the use of the term "mineral" here is distinct from the usage in the geological sciences.

Vitamins are organic chemicals that a given living organism requires in trace quantities for good health, but which the organism cannot synthesize, and therefore must obtain from its diet.

The Promise of Micro-Enriched Fertilization

The returns of applying micronutrient-enriched fertilizers could be huge for human health, social and economic development. Research has shown that enriching fertilizers with micronutrients had not only an impact on plant deficiencies but also on humans and animals, through the food chain. A report by the World Bank and the Asian Development Bank stated that eliminating micronutrient deficiencies could:

- improve GDP by more than 5 per cent;
- enhance the intellectual capacity of populations by more than 10 per cent;
- enhance worker productivity by 30 to 70 per cent;
- reduce maternal deaths by up to 50 per cent.
- Food biofortification using plant breeding (genetic

biofortification) and/or micronutrient fertilizers (agronomic biofortification) can contribute to this goal.

Addressing Zinc Deficiencies through Zinc Fertilization

Experiments show that soil and foliar application of zinc fertilizer can effectively reduce the phytate : zinc ratio in grain. People who eat bread prepared from zinc enriched wheat show a significant increase in serum zinc, suggesting that the zinc fertilizer strategy is a promising approach to address zinc deficiencies in humans.

Where zinc deficiency is a limiting factor, zinc fertilization can increase crop yields. Balanced crop nutrition supplying all essential nutrients, including zinc, is a cost effective management strategy. Even with zinc-efficient varieties, zinc fertilizers are needed when the available zinc in the topsoil becomes depleted.

Micronutrients for Plants

There are about eight nutrients essential to plant growth and health that are only needed in very small quantities. These are manganese, boron, copper, iron, chlorine, cobalt, molybdenum, and zinc. Some consider sulfur a micronutrient, but it is listed here as a macronutrient. Though these are present in only small quantities, they are all necessary.

- Boron is believed to be involved in carbohydrate transport in plants; it also assists in metabolic regulation. Boron deficiency will often result in bud dieback.
- Chlorine is necessary for osmosis and ionic balance; it also plays a role in photosynthesis.
- Cobalt is essential to plant health. Cobalt is thought to be an important catalyst in nitrogen fixation. It may need to be added to some soils before seeding legumes.
- Copper is a component of some enzymes and of vitamin A. Symptoms of copper deficiency include browning of leaf tips and chlorosis.
- Iron is essential for chlorophyll synthesis, which is why an iron deficiency results in chlorosis.

- Manganese activates some important enzymes involved in chlorophyll formation. Manganese deficient plants will develop chlorosis between the veins of its leaves. The availability of manganese is partially dependent on soil pH.
- Molybdenum is essential to plant health. Molybdenum is used by plants to reduce nitrates into usable forms. Some plants use it for nitrogen fixation, thus it may need to be added to some soils before seeding legumes.
- Zinc participates in chlorophyll formation, and also activates many enzymes. Symptoms of zinc deficiency include chlorosis and stunted growth.

Micronutrient Deficiencies in Crops

Micronutrient deficiencies are widespread. Fifty per cent of world cereal soils are deficient in zinc and 30 per cent of cultivated soils globally are deficient in iron. Steady growth of crop yields during recent decades (in particular through the Green Revolution) compounded the problem by progressively depleting soil micronutrient pools.

In general, farmers only apply micronutrients when crops show deficiency symptoms, while micronutrient deficiencies decrease yields before symptoms appear. Some common farming practices (such as liming acid soils) contribute to widespread occurrence of micronutrient deficiencies in crops by decreasing the availability of the micronutrients present in the soil. Also, extensive use of glyphosate is increasingly suspected to impair micronutrient uptake by crops, especially with regard to manganese, iron and zinc.

MICRONUTRIENT DEFICIENCY

A micronutrient deficiency (or trace mineral deficiency) is a physiological plant disorder which occurs when a micronutrient is deficient in the soil in which a plant grows. Micronutrients are distinguished from macronutrients (such as Nitrogen, Phosphorus, and Potassium) by the relatively low quantities needed by the plant. A number of elements are known to be needed in these small amounts for proper plant growth and development. Nutrient deficiencies in these areas can adversely affect plant growth and development. Some of the best known trace mineral deficiencies include: Boron deficiency, Calcium deficiency, Iron deficiency, Magnesium deficiency, and Manganese deficiency.

List of Essential Trace Minerals for Plants

- Boron is believed to be involved in carbohydrate transport in plants; it also assists in metabolic regulation. Boron deficiency will often result in bud dieback.
- Chlorine is necessary for osmosis and ionic balance; it also plays a role in photosynthesis.
- Cobalt is essential to plant health. Cobalt is thought to be an important catalyst in nitrogen fixation. It may need to be added to some soils before seeding legumes.
- Copper is a component of some enzymes and of vitamin A. Symptoms of copper deficiency include browning of leaf tips and chlorosis.
- Iron is essential for chlorophyll synthesis, which is why an iron deficiency results in chlorosis.
- Manganese activates some important enzymes involved in chlorophyll formation. Manganese deficient plants will develop chlorosis between the veins of its leaves. The availability of manganese is partially dependent on soil pH.
- Molybdenum is essential to plant health. Molybdenum is used by plants to reduce nitrates into usable forms. Some plants use it for nitrogen fixation, thus it may need to be added to some soils before seeding legumes.
- Zinc participates in chlorophyll formation, and also activates many enzymes. Symptoms of zinc deficiency include chlorosis and stunted growth.

NUTRITIONISTS

A nutritionist is a health specialist who devotes professional activity to food and nutritional science, preventive nutrition, diseases related to nutrient deficiencies, and the use of nutrient manipulation to enhance the clinical response to human diseases.

They can also advise people on dietary matters relating to health, well-being and optimal nutrition. Nutritionists have varying levels of education from someone with little or no education to an individual who has obtained a bachelor's, master's, or doctoral degree. This is because the term "nutritionist" is not a legally protected term in most parts of the world. As a result, the term "nutritionist" is subject to several interpretations. Many nutritionists appear on television, in newspapers and magazines, and write nutritional books, which may or may not have any real informational value regarding diet.

Training

There are a wide range of courses available which vary in duration from several days to several years. A person who represents him or herself as a nutritionist may have several different levels of education including a degree in nutrition or dietetics from a university (of which several may be accredited by nutritionist governing bodies such as the Nutrition Society accrediting degree courses in the UK) or certification in nutrition education and/or counseling from a private vocational/professional training school.

Regulation of the Title "Nutritionist"

Canada

The title "nutritionist" is protected in Quebec and Nova Scotia. It is not protected in British Columbia. There were discussions about this when the dietitian designation was protected in British Columbia, but as of March 2008 "nutritionist" is not currently protected there.

United Kingdom

Nutritionist, unlike dietician, is not currently a protected term. Anyone in the UK can refer to himself or herself as a nutritionist without any formal qualifications. Different organisations promoting holistic and alternative therapies may use their own criteria to define a nutritionist. According to one of these, the Nutrition Society of the UK , *the function of a nutritionist is to elicit, integrate, disseminate and apply scientific knowledge drawn from the relevant sciences, to promote an understanding of the effects of nutrition, and to enhance the impact of food on health and well-being of animals and/or people.* They accredit nutritionists, conferring the titles *Associate Nutritionist (ANutr), Associate Public Health Nutritionist (APHNutr), Registered Nutritionist, (R Nutr.),* and *Registered Public Health Nutritionist (RPHNutr).* For these they consider an undergraduate training sufficient to be entered on their Register of Nutritionists.

United States

The term "dietitian" is legally protected. Dietitians are registered with the American Dietetic Association and are only able to use the title "dietitian" when they have met strict, specific educational and experiential prerequisites and passed a national registration examination.

The title "nutritionist" is protected and designated by many but not all states in the United States. It is important that a person seeking the counsel of a nutritionist, check with their local state's licensing agency to find out if prospective practitioners are duly licensed.

Traditionally, dietitians work in institutional settings, such as hospitals, schools and prisons, rather than in private practice. Nutritionists sometimes work in such instititions but more often work in private practice, in education and research. Some overlap exists within the two professions.

Development of a Certified Registry

The Certification Board For Nutrition Specialists (CBNS) was founded in 1993 by the American College of Nutrition (ACN) to help meet the growing demand for knowledgeable, responsible professional nutritionists. The protected title of Certified Nutrition Specialist (CNS) is awarded by CBNS to those nutritionists meeting defined educational, experience and examination requirements. Similarly and as mentioned above, the Nutrition Society of the United Kingdom has established a Register of Nutritionists. This is to recognize and encourage high standards of professional training in nutrition as well as to protect the public.

Types of Nutritionist

Nutrition Scientists

Nutrition scientists are those individuals who use the scientific method to study nutrients, both as individual compounds and as they interact in food and nutrition. The role of the nutrition scientist is to develop new knowledge related to nutrients or nutrition or to develop new processes or techniques to apply existing knowledge. For example, nutrition scientists have been involved in developing food preservation processes, determining nutrient requirements for various animal species, describing how individual nutrients function within the cells of the human body, and identifying nutrition-related problems in various populations.

Nutritionist scientists may have their basic training in nutrition or in a related field such as biochemistry, microbiology, cell biology, epidemiology, toxicology, agriculture, or food science, chemistry.

Public Health Nutritionists

Public health nutritionists are professionals who view the community as their client. They specialize in diagnosing the nutritional problems of communities and in finding solutions to those problems. Some classic examples of public health nutrition interventions include the fortification of salt with iodine to prevent Goitre or the enrichment of grain products with B vitamins to prevent deficiency diseases.

DIETITIANS

A dietitian (also 'dietician' (UK spelling), though 'dietitian' is used consistently by professionals in the US) is an expert in food and nutrition.

Dietitians help promote good health through proper eating. They supervise the preparation and service of food, develop modified diets, participate in research, and educate individuals and groups on good nutritional habits. In a medical setting, a dietitian may provide specific artificial nutritional needs to patients unable to consume food normally. Dietary modification to address medical issues involving dietary intake is also a major part of dietetics. The goals of the dietary department are to provide medical nutritional intervention, obtain, prepare, and serve flavorsome, attractive, and nutritious food to patients, family members, and health care providers.

In many countries only people who have specified educational credentials can call themselves "dietitians" — the title is legally protected. The term "nutritionist" is also widely used; however, the term nutritionist is not regulated as dietitian is. People may call themselves nutritionists without the educational and professional requirements of registered dietitians.

Dietetic technicians are not the same as dietitians in terms of responsibilities and qualifications. Different professional terms are used in different countries. Dietitians are a valuable member of the medical multi-disciplinary team providing nutritional knowledge and acting as consultants to other health care professionals.

Types of Dietitians

The majority of dietitians are *clinical,* or *therapeutic,* dietitians. Clinical dietitians review medical charts and talk with patients' families. They work with other health care professionals and community groups to provide nourishment, nutritional programmes and instructional presentations to benefit people of all ages, and with a variety of health conditions. This is accomplished by developing individual plans to meet nutritional needs. These plans include nourishment, tube feedings (called enteral nutrition), intravenous feedings (called parenteral nutrition) such as total parenteral nutrition (TPN) or peripheral parenteral nutrition (PPN), diets, and education. Clinical dietitians provide individual and group educational programmes for patients and family members about their nutrition and health.

Dietitians in Practice

Clinical Dietitians

Clinical dietitians work in hospitals and other health care facilities to provide nutrition therapy to patients according to the disease processes, provide individual dietary consultations to patients and their family members and also conduct group educations for other health workers, patients and the public. They coordinate both medical records and nutritional needs to assess the patients and make a plan based on their findings. Some clinical dietitians have dual responsibilities with medical nutrition therapy and in foodservice, described below. In addition, clinical dietitians in smaller facilities will also provide or create outpatient education programmes. They work as a team with the physicians, physical therapists, occupational therapists, pharmacists, speech therapists, social workers and nurses to provide care to the patients.

Community Dietitians

Community dietitians work with wellness programmes and international health organizations. These dietitians apply and distribute knowledge about food and nutrition to specific life-styles and geographic areas. They coordinate nutritional programmes in public health agencies, daycare centers, health clubs, and recreational camps and resorts. Some community dietitians carry out clinical based patient care in the form of home visits for patients who are too physically ill to attend consultation in health facilities.

Foodservice Dietitians

Foodservice dietitians or managers are responsible for large-scale food planning and service. They coordinate, assess and plan foodservice processes in health care facilities, school food service programmes, prisons, cafeterias and restaurants. These dietitians will also perform audits of their departments, train other food service workers and use marketing skills to launch new menus and various programmes within their institution. They direct and manage the operational and nutrition services staffs such as kitchen staffs, delivery staffs and dietary assistants or diet aides.

Gerontological Dietitians

Gerontological dietitians are specialist in nutrition and aging. They are Board certified in Gerontological Nutrition with the American Dietetic Association. They work in government agencies in aging policy, and in a regulatory capacity in the oversight of nursing homes and community-based care facilities. They work as Consultants in Nursing Homes, and in higher education in the field of Gerontology (the study of Aging.)

Pediatric Dietitians

Pediatric dietitians provide health advice for persons under the age of 18.

Research Dietitians

Research dietitians are mostly involved with dietary related research in the clinical aspect of nutrition in disease states, public aspect on primary, secondary and sometimes tertiary health prevention and foodservice aspect in issues involving the food prepared for patients. Many registered dietitians also work with the biochemical aspects of nutrient interaction within the body. Research Dietitians normally work in a hospital or university research facilities. It should be noted that some Clinical dietitian's roles also involve research other than the normal clinical workload. Quality improvement in dietetics services is also one area of research.

Administrative Dietitians

Administrative, or manager or Director of Dietetics Department or Nutrition Services are sometimes also known as Manager instead of Director depending on the size, number of dietitians in the department and also the organizational structure adopted by the Health facilities or Hospital. Director or Manager acts as head of the dietitians. They also hire, train, direct and supervise employees and manage dietary departments. Administrative dietitians may also apply procedure and policy as part of their management job.

Business Dietitians

Business dietitians serve as resource people for the media. Dietitians' expertise in nutrition is often taped for TV, radio, and newspapers—either as an expert guest opinion, regular columnist or guest, or for resource, restaurant, or recipe development and critique. Dietitians have served as show hosts on major television stations and as drive-time radio news anchors. Dietitians write books, appear on television cooking channels, and author corporate newsletters on nutrition and wellness. They also work as sales representatives for food manufacturing companies that provide nutritional supplements and tube feeding supplies.

Consultant Dietitians

Consultant dietitians work under private practice. The title 'consultant' in this case should not be confused with the identical title given to certain medical doctors in countries such as the United Kingdom and Ireland. The term consultant in this instance is synonymous with the title attending as used in countries such as the United States. Consultant dietitians contract independently to provide nutrition services and educational programmes to individuals, nursing homes, and in health care facilities. As recent studies have shown the importance of diet in both preventing and managing disease, many US states have moved towards covering medical nutrition therapy under the Medicaid/Medicare making consulting a much more lucrative option for dietitians due to insurance reimbursement.

Other Nutrition Workers

These designations apply principally to the US although the generic classifications are likely to be applicable elsewhere.

Registered Dietetic Technicians

Dietetic Technicians, Registered (DTR), also commonly known as "Diet Techs", possess a specialized Associate Degree from Community College programmes which are accredited by the Commission on Accreditation of Dietetics Education (CADE) of the American Dietetic Association. In many settings they work alongside Registered Dietitians, and like Registered Dietitians, they have in-depth knowledge of nutrition. They must complete a dietetic internship with a minimum of 450 supervised practice hours in the areas of Food Service Theory and Management, Community Dietetics, and Clinical Dietetics. They must also complete a national registration examination administered by the Commission on Dietetics Registration (CDR) of the ADA. Although the DTR is an independently credentialed nutrition practitioner, when performing clinical dietetics, they must work under the supervision of a Registered Dietitian. In addition, some states have current legislation specifying the scope of practice for the DTR.

Dietetic Technicians (Unregistered)

Dietetic Technicians (DT), have obtained a Bachelors or Masters Degree in Human Nutrition from an accredited university. Dietetic Technicians are not required to be registered and have the same job duties as DTRs. Some working DTs are awaiting entry into dietetic internship programmes on their career path to become dietitians, benefiting from valuable work experience as Diet Techs.

Dietary Assistants or Dietary Aides

are responsible for assisting and carrying out the medical nutrition therapy prescribed by the Dietitians and to ensure that food for the patients as instructed by the Dietitians are carried out correctly by checking menus against recent diet orders before tray assembly begins and being physically present in the kitchen plating-lines at meal hours. Dietary aides in some countries might also carry out a simple initial health screening for newly admitted patients and only inform the Dietitians if any screened patients requires a dietitian's expertise for further assessments or interventions.

Dietary Clerks

Dietary clerks perform clerical tasks such as entry and maintenance of dietary requirements to a database. They also track financial information, such as the number of meals served each day.

Dietary Managers

Dietary managers are responsible for retail, catering and tray lines. If an operation is large, there may be one or more managers to help in directing the dietary workers.

Dietary Workers

Dietary workers prepare the food and meal trays in the kitchen. They check for accuracy and completeness. They also maintain the storage area for food supplies and ensure practice of sanitary procedures.

Dietary workers are trained on the job and can work in any commercial kitchen.

Dietary Hosts

Dietary hosts or *hostesses* deliver and bring back the meal trays to patients. They distribute and collect menus and help the patients to make complete selections.

Required Qualifications and Professional Associations

A dietitian's education in health science involves significant scientific based knowledge in anatomy, chemistry, biochemistry, biology, physiology, nutrition, medical science. It is these strong foundations in advanced scientific knowledge and an internship that equipped with counseling skills and aspects of psychology enable a Registered Dietitian to assess, analyze, intervene, and educate a patient in relation to the diet and disease.

There are a few different academic routes to becoming a fully qualified registrable dietitian:

- A professional bachelor degree in Dietetics which requires four years of studies; or
- A bachelor of science degree and a postgraduate diploma in Dietetics; or
- A bachelor of science degree and a master's degree in Dietetics
- Internship is also essential to become a fully qualified Dietitian. The internship process differs in different countries.

USA

In the US nutrition professionals include the registered dietitian (RD) and the "dietetic technician, registered" (DTR). These terms, as well as simply dietitian, are legally protected terms regulated by the American Dietetic Association (ADA).

Dietitians are registered with the Commission on Dietetic Registration (the certifying agency of the ADA) and are only able to use the label "Registered Dietitian" when they have met strict, specific educational and professional prerequisites and passed a national registration examination.

Besides academic education, registered dietitians must complete at least 1200 hours of practical, supervised experience through an accredited programme before they can sit for the registration examination. In a coordinated programme (CP) students acquire internship hours concurrently with their coursework. In a didactic programme (DP) these hours are obtained through a dietetic internship that is completed after obtaining a degree. In both programmes the student is required to complete several areas of competency including rotations in clinical, community, long-term care nutrition as well as food service, public health and a variety of other worksites.

Once the degree is earned, the internship completed, and registration examination passed, the individual can now use the nationally recognized legal term, Registered Dietitian and is able to work in a variety of professional settings. Most states require additional licensure to work in most settings. To maintain the RD credential, professionals must participate in and earn continuing education units 75 hours every 5 years.

Canada

In the United States and Canada the Dietitian, Registered Dietitian (RD), etc. are similarly protected titles. The professional association in Canada is the Dietitians of Canada. The US equivalent of it is American Dietetic Association.

In Canada, each province has an independent professional college (for example, The College of Dietitians of Ontario) which is responsible for protecting the public and regulating the profession. The colleges are entirely funded from licencing fees collected from dietitians. Each college must have both public and professional members, and is empowered to investigate and censure (when malpractice/negligence is found) members of the profession who breach either their scope of practice or harm/endanger the health of a patient/client, and receive a complaint against them from a member of the public or another health care professional. To practice as a registered dietitian within a province, a dietitian must register with the college and obtain a licence. The activities of the college are governed by legislation passed by the provincial government. It is the presence of this regulatory body which distinguishes registered dietitians from nutritionists in Canada.

In Canada, the colleges also set the minimum entry requirements for admission into practice as a registered dietitian. Requirements to entry into practice as a dietitian include a four year undergraduate degree from an accredited university (which includes courses in science, foods, nutrition, management, communication and psychology/sociology, among others), a 10-12 month supervised practice period (called an internship) and successfully passing a board exam in nutrition and dietetics.

Australia

Accredited Practising Dietitians (APDs) in Australia gain their qualifications through university courses accredited by the DAA (Dietitian's Association of Australia). In order for patients to receive a rebate from Medicare or Private Health insurance APD status is required. APDs are Dietitians engaged in the Continuing Professional Development programme offered by the DAA and commit to uphold the DAA Code of Professional Conduct and Code of Ethics.

Dietitians who do not wish to join the DAA may participate in DAA's Continuing Professional Development Programme without being a member of DAA and in this way can still hold APD status. However, under new rules (which commence 1 July 2009), health care providers must either have statutory registration or be members of their national, professional association to obtain a provider number. This means all private health funds will require private practitioners applying for provider numbers to be DAA members (not just 'eligible' for membership).

DIETARY MINERAL

Dietary minerals are the chemical elements required by living organisms, other than the four elements carbon, hydrogen, nitrogen, and oxygen present in common organic molecules. The term "mineral" is archaic, since the intent of the definition is to describe ions, not chemical compounds or actual minerals.

Dietitians may recommend that minerals are best supplied by

ingesting specific foods rich with the element(s) of interest. Sometimes minerals are ingested as mineral dietary supplements, the most common being iodine in iodized salt.

The dietary focus on minerals derives from an interest in supporting biochemical reactions with the required elemental components. Appropriate intake levels of certain chemical elements are thus required to maintain optimal health. According to nutritional experts, the requirements are met simply with a conventional balanced diet.

Essential Minerals

Some sources state that sixteen minerals are required to support human biochemical processes by serving structural and functional roles as well as electrolytes: Sometimes a distinction is drawn between this category and micronutrients. Most of the essential minerals are of relatively low atomic weight:

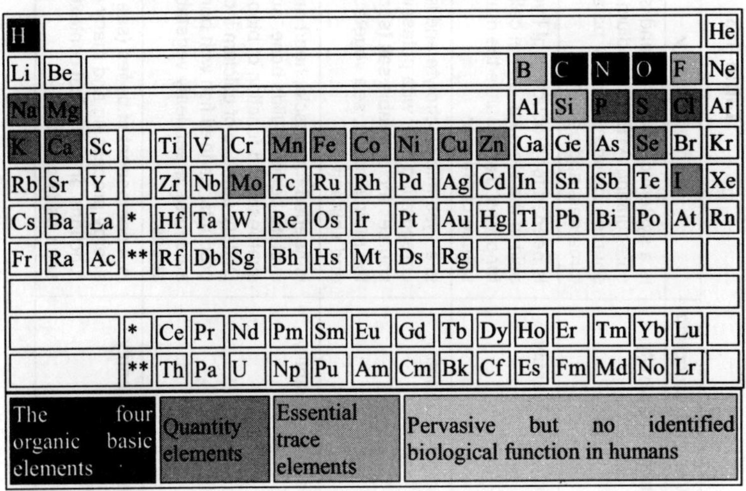

The Table 1.3 play important roles in biological processes:

Other Elements

Many elements have been suggested as essential, but such claims have usually not been confirmed. Definitive evidence for efficacy

Table 1.3

Mineral	*RDA/AI*	*Description*	*Category*	*Insufficiency*	*Excess*
Potassium	4700 mg	Quantity	is a systemic electrolyte and is essential in coregulating ATP with sodium. Dietary sources include legumes, potato skin, tomatoes, and bananas.	hypokalemia	hyperkalemia
Chloride	2300 mg	Quantity	is needed for production of hydrochloric acid in the stomach and in cellular pump functions. Table salt is the main dietary source of chloride.	hypochloremia	hyperchloremia
Sodium	1500 mg	Quantity	is a systemic electrolyte and is essential in coregulating ATP with potassium. Dietary sources include table salt (sodium chloride, the main source), sea vegetables, milk, and spinach.	hyponatremia	hypernatremia
Calcium	1000 mg	Quantity	is needed for muscle, heart and digestive system health, builds bone, supports synthesis and function of blood cells. Dietary sources of calcium include dairy products, canned fish with bones (salmon, sardines), green leafy vegetables, nuts and seeds.	hypocalcaemia	hypercalcaemia
Phosphorus	700 mg	Quantity	is a component of bones (see apatite) and energy processing and many other functions. In biological contexts, usually seen as phosphate.	hypophosphatemia	hyperphosphatemia

(*Contd.*)

Mineral	*RDA/AI*	*Description*	*Category*	*Insufficiency*	*Excess*
Magnesium	420 mg	Quantity	is required for processing ATP and for bones. Dietary sources include nuts, soy beans, and cocoa.	hypomagnesemia, magnesium deficiency	hypermagnesemia
Zinc	11 mg	Trace	is pervasive and required for several enzymes such as carboxypeptidase, liver alcohol dehydrogenase, and carbonic anhydrase.	zinc deficiency	zinc toxicity
Iron	8 mg	Trace	is required for many proteins and enzymes, notably hemoglobin. Dietary sources include red meat, leafy green vegetables, fish (tuna, salmon), eggs, dried fruits, beans, whole grains, and enriched grains.	anaemia	iron overload disorder
Manganese	2.3 mg	Trace	is a cofactor in enzyme functions.	manganese deficiency	manganism
Copper	900 µg	Trace	is required component of many redox enzymes, including cytochrome c oxidase.	copper deficiency	copper toxicity
Iodine	150 µg	Trace	is required for the biosynthesis of thyroxine.	iodine deficiency	
Selenium	55 µg	Trace	a cofactor essential to activity of antioxidant enzymes like glutathione peroxidase.	selenium deficiency	selenosis
Molybdenum	45 µg	Trace	the oxidases xanthine oxidase, aldehyde oxidase, and sulfite oxidase	molybdenum deficiency	

comes from the characterization of a biomolecule containing the element with an identifiable and testable function. One problem with identifying efficacy is that some elements are innocuous at low concentrations and are pervasive, so proof of efficacy is lacking because deficiencies are difficult to reproduce.

- Relatively large quantities of sulfur are required, but there is no RDA, as the sulfur is obtained from and used for amino acids, and therefore should be adequate in any diet containing enough protein.
- Cobalt is required in the synthesis of vitamin B12, but because bacteria are required to synthesize the vitamin, it is usually considered part of vitamin B12 deficiency rather than its own mineral deficiency.
- There have been occasional studies asserting the essentiality of nickel, but it currently has no known RDA.
- Chromium is sometimes described as essential. It is implicated in sugar metabolism in humans, leading to a market for the supplement, chromium picolinate, but definitive biochemical evidence for a physiological function is lacking.
- Fluoride has been described as conditionally essential, depending upon the importance placed upon the prevention of chronic disease.
- Arsenic, boron, bromine, cadmium, silicon, tungsten, and vanadium have established, albeit specialized, biochemical roles as structural or functional cofactors in other organisms. These elements appear not to be utilized by humans.

ESSENTIAL FATTY ACID

Essential fatty acids, or EFAs, are fatty acids that cannot be constructed within an organism (generally all references are to humans) from other components by any known chemical pathways, and therefore must be obtained from the diet. The term refers to fatty acids involved in biological processes, and not those which may just play a role as fuel. As many of the compounds created from essential fatty acids can be taken directly in the diet, it is possible that the amounts required in the diet (if any) are overestimated. It is also possible they can be underestimated as organisms can still survive in non-ideal, malnourished conditions.

There are two families of Fats from each of these families are essential, as the body can convert one omega-3 to another omega-3, for example, but cannot create an omega-3 from omega-6 or saturated fats. They were originally designated as Vitamin F when they were discovered as essential nutrients in 1923. In 1930, work by Burr, Burr and Miller showed that they are better classified with the fats than with the vitamins.

Functions

> The biological effects of the ω-3 and ω-6 fatty acids are mediated by their mutual interactions.

In the body, essential fatty acids serve multiple functions. In each of these, the balance between dietary ω-3 and ω-6 strongly affects function.

- They are modified to make
  - the classic eicosanoids (affecting inflammation and many other cellular functions)
  - the endocannabinoids (affecting mood, behaviour and inflammation)
  - the lipoxins from ω-6 EFAs and resolvins from ω-3 (in the presence of aspirin, downregulating inflammation.)
  - the isofurans, neurofurans, isoprostanes, hepoxilins, epoxyeicosatrienoic acids (EETs) and Neuroprotectin D
- They form lipid rafts (affecting cellular signaling)
- They act on DNA (activating or inhibiting transcription factors such as NFêB, which is linked to pro-inflammatory cytokine production)

Nomenclature and Terminology

Fatty acids are straight chain hydrocarbons possessing a carboxyl (COOH) group at one end. The carbon next to the carboxylate is known as α, the next carbon β, and so forth. Since biological fatty acids can be of different lengths, the last position is labelled as a "ω", the last letter in the Greek alphabet. Since the physiological properties of unsaturated fatty acids largely depend on the position of the first unsaturation relative to the end position and not the carboxylate, the position is signified by (ω minus n). For example, the term ω-3 signifies that the first double bond exists as the third carbon-carbon bond from the terminal CH_3 end (ω) of the carbon chain. The number of carbons and the number of double bonds is also listed. ω-3 18:4 (stearidonic acid) or 18:4 ω-3 or 18:4 n–3 indicates an 18-carbon chain with 4 double bonds, and with the first double bond in the third position from the CH_3 end. Double bonds are cis and separated by a single methylene (CH_2) group unless otherwise noted. So in free fatty acid form, the chemical structure of stearidonic acid is:

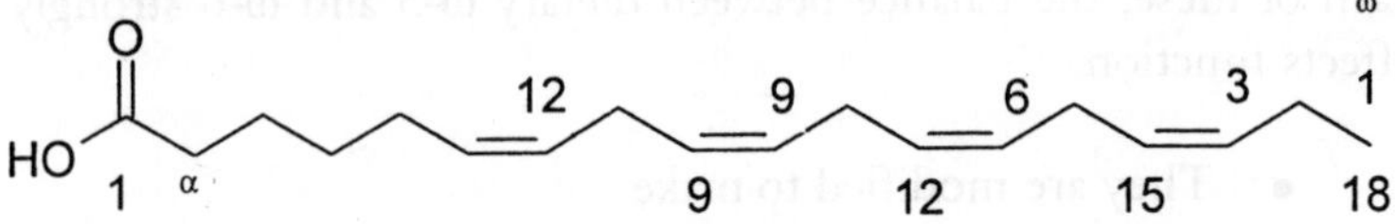

Fig.1.2: Chemical Structure of Stearidonic Acid Showing Physiological and Chemical Numbering Conventions

Examples

The essential fatty acids start with the short chain polyunsaturated fatty acids (SC-PUFA):

- -3 fatty acids:
  - Linoleic acid or LA (18:2)

These two fatty acids cannot be synthesised by humans, as humans lack the desaturase enzymes required for their production.

They form the starting point for the creation of longer and more desaturated fatty acids, which are also referred to as long-chain polyunsaturated fatty acids (LC-PUFA):

ω-3 fatty acids:

- eicosapentaenoic acid or EPA (20:5)
- docosahexaenoic acid or DHA (22:6)

ω-6 fatty acids:

- gamma-linolenic acid or GLA (18:3)
- dihomo-gamma-linolenic acid or DGLA (20:3)
- arachidonic acid or AA (20:4)

ω-9 fatty acids are not essential in humans, because humans generally possess all the enzymes required for their synthesis. Exceptions do occur in older people or people with a liver problem that do not completely produce a sufficient amount, and hence many supplement companies market Omega 3-6-9 blends.

Essentiality

Between 1930 and 1950, arachidonic acid and linolenic acid were termed 'essential' because each was more or less able to meet the growth requirements of rats given fat-free diets. Further research has shown that human metabolism requires both ω-3 and ω-6 fatty acids. To some extent, any ω-3 and any ω-6 can relieve the worst symptoms of fatty acid deficiency. Particular fatty acids are still needed at critical life stages (e.g. lactation) and in some disease states. In nonscientific writing, common usage is that the term essential fatty acid comprises all the ω-3 or -6 fatty acids. Authoritative sources include the whole families, without qualification. The human body can make some long-chain PUFA (arachidonic acid, EPA and DHA) from lineolate or lineolinate.

Traditionally speaking the LC-PUFA are not essential. Because the LC-PUFA are sometimes required, they may be considered "conditionally essential", or not essential to healthy adults.

A 2005 study has shown evidence that gamma-linolenic acid, GLA has been shown to inhibit the breast cancer promoting gene of Her2/neu.

Biologist Ray Peat has pointed out flaws in the studies purportedly showing the need for n-3 and n-6 fats. He notes that so-called EFA deficiencies have sometimes been reversed by adding

B vitamins or a fat-free liver extract to the diet. In his view, 'the optional dietary level of the "essential fatty acids" might be close to zero, if other dietary factors were also optimized.'

ESSENTIAL AMINO ACID'

An essential amino acid or indispensable amino acid is an amino acid that cannot be synthesized de novo by the organism (usually referring to humans), and therefore must be supplied in the diet.

Essentiality vs. Conditional Essentiality in Humans

Essential	Nonessential
Isoleucine	Alanine
Arginine*	
Lysine	Aspartate
Methionine	Cysteine*
Phenylalanine	Glutamate
Threonine	Glutamine*
Tryptophan	Glycine*
Valine	Proline*
Histidine*	Serine*
Tyrosine*	Asparagine*
Leucine	

(*) Essential only in certain cases.

Eight amino acids are generally regarded as essential for humans: phenylalanine, valine, threonine, tryptophan, isoleucine, methionine, leucine, and lysine. Additionally, cysteine (or sulphur-containing amino acids), tyrosine (or aromatic amino acids), histidine and arginine are required by infants and growing children. Essential amino acids are so called not because they are more important to life than the others, but because the body does not synthesize them, making it essential to include them in one's diet in order to obtain them. In addition, the amino acids arginine, cysteine, glycine, glutamine, histidine, proline, serine and tyrosine are considered conditionally essential, meaning they are not normally required in the diet, but must be supplied exogenously to specific populations that do not synthesize it in adequate amounts. An example would be with the disease phenylketonuria (PKU).

Individuals living with PKU must keep their intake of phenylalanine extremely low to prevent mental retardation and other metabolic complications. However, phenylalanine is the precursor for tyrosine synthesis. Without phenylalanine, tyrosine cannot be made and so tyrosine becomes essential in the diet of PKU patients.

The distinction between essential and non-essential amino acids is somewhat unclear, as some amino acids can be produced from others. The sulfur-containing amino acids, methionine and homocysteine, can be converted into each other but neither can be synthesized de novo in humans. Likewise, cysteine can be made from homocysteine but cannot be synthesized on its own. So, for convenience, sulfur-containing amino acids are sometimes considered a single pool of nutritionally-equivalent amino acids as are the aromatic amino acid pair, phenylalanine and tyrosine. Likewise arginine, ornithine, and citrulline, which are interconvertible by the urea cycle, are considered a single group.

The above list of 20 amino acids is the traditional one, but in fact there are now more than 20 amino acids that are routinely found in proteins. At this link from 2002 report on discovery of the 22nd amino acid, pyrrolysine is made.

On a related note, recently in Science it has also been reported that, in addition to the 22+ alpha-amino acids, scientists are finding far more beta-amino acids in bacteria with a variety natural functions, such as contributing to antibiotic resistance.

Recommended Daily Amounts

Estimating the daily requirement for the indispensable amino acids has proven to be difficult; these numbers have undergone considerable revision over the last 20 years. The following Table 1.4 lists the WHO recommended daily amounts currently in use for essential amino acids in adult humans, together with their standard one-letter abbreviations.

The recommended daily intakes for children aged three years and older is 10 per cent to 20 per cent higher than adult levels and those for infants can be as much as 150 per cent higher in the first year of life.

Table 1.4

Amino Acid	*mg per kg Body Weight*	*mg per 70 kg*	*mg per 100 kg*
I Isoleucine	20	1400	2000
L Leucine	39	2730	3900
K Lysine	30	2100	3000
M Methionine + C Cysteine	10.4 + 4.1 (15 total)	1050	1500
F Phenylalanine + Y Tyrosine	25 (total)	1750	2500
T Threonine	15	1050	1500
W Tryptophan	4	280	400
V Valine	26	1820	2600

Use of Essential Amino Acids

Foodstuffs that lack essential amino acids are poor sources of protein equivalents, as the body tends to deaminate the amino acids obtained, converting proteins into fats and. Therefore, a balance of essential amino acids is necessary for a high degree of net protein utilization, which is the mass ratio of amino acids converted to proteins to amino acids supplied.

Complete proteins contain a balanced set of essential amino acids for humans. Animal sources such as meat, poultry, eggs, fish, milk, and cheese provide all of the essential amino acids. Near-complete proteins are also found in some plant sources such as quinoa, buckwheat, hempseed, and amaranth, among others. Soya appears as lower in sulfur-containing amino acids (methionine and cysteine) , which instead are abundant in many other plant protein sources. It is not necessary to consume plant foods containing complete proteins as long as a reasonably varied diet is maintained. By consuming a wide variety of plant foods, a full set of essential amino acids will be supplied and the human body can convert the amino acids into proteins.

The net protein utilization of a human eating only one protein source (only wheat, for instance) is affected by the limiting amino acid content (the essential amino acid found in the smallest quantity in the foodstuff) of that source. Adequate protein utilization, however, will readily be obtained if a balanced variety of protein sources is eaten within a reasonable time (say, 4 hours), and/or the total (limited) protein consumed is greater than the requirement.

Protein Source	*Limiting Amino Acid**
Wheat	lysine
Rice	lysine
Legumes	tryptophan or methionine (or cysteine)
Maize	lysine and tryptophan
Egg, chicken	none; the reference for absorbable protein

Mnemonics

Using the one letter designation shown above, mnemonic devices have been developed for students wanting or needing to memorize the essential amino acids. Previous devices have utilized the first letter of the amino acids' names, and in general did not include arginine which is not always essential. One mnemonic device that has been used in the past is PVT TIM HALL.

Another method uses the first letter of each essential amino acid to begin each word in a phrase, such as: "Any Help In Learning These Little Molecules Proves Truly Valuable." This method begins with the two amino acids that need some qualifications as to their requirements.

NON-NUTRITIVE FOODS

Many Junk and Traditional Foods Require Statutory Warning "Non-Nutritive" Instead of Nutritional Information

Currently the notification G.S.R. 664(E) published in the Gazette of India, extra-ordinary, part II, section 3(i), and released by G. Balachandran, Additional Secretary, Ministry of Health and Family Welfare on 19th September 2008 is being discussed among food products manufacturers who want to know which type of nutritional information is to be printed on the labels of a food product and in which cases it is not necessary.

The new PFA 5th amendment rules likely to come into force from 19th March 2009 vide the notification, stipulate that all ingredients in packed food product must be listed in a descending order in terms of weight or volume. Significantly, the label of food products must also include the nutritional profile such as its energy value in kcal; the amount of protein, carbohydrates, including sugar and fat in grams; and any other nutrient for which nutrition claim or health claim is made like "rich in vitamins, fibers and potassium minerals" or "cholesterol, saturated fat and trans fat free" in metric units. However exemption from printing nutritional information on label has been granted to the food articles that belong to raw agricultural commodity or are non-nutritive in nature or are served for immediate consumption. The rules also lay down that a fruit juice, squash, beverage that does not contain a specified amount of a fruit juice or pulp cannot be described as a fruit product. Therefore, an item that contains only fruit flavours must make a mention of Added (Name of fruit) Flavour on the label.

The amendments made in "rule 32, clause (b) paragraph (2) list ingredients, sub-clause (vi) provided that (a)" are related to a provision of some exemption from printing nutritional information on the labels of certain food products. This particular sub-clause of rule 32 maintains that, "the nutritional information may not be necessary, in case of foods such as raw agricultural commodities, like, wheat, rice, cereals, spices, spice mixes, herbs, condiments, table salt, sugar, jaggery, or non-nutritive products, like, soluble tea, coffee, soluble coffee, coffee-chicory, mixture, packaged drinking water, packaged mineral water, alcoholic beverages or fruit and vegetables, processed and pre-packaged assorted vegetables, fruits, vegetables and products that comprise of single ingredient, pickles, papad or foods, served from immediate consumption such as served in hospitals, hotels or by food services vendors or halwais, or food shipped in bulk which is not for sale in that form to consumers"

The rationale behind exemption from printing nutritional information on labels of raw agricultural commodities, non-nutritive products or immediate consumption products is quite understandable. But the term "non-nutritive products" covering very low calorie products, unusual calorie source or alcoholic products, single ingredient products and imbalanced diet products (containing very high fat, salt, sugar etc.) has been introduced without any explanation.

In India a number of territorial traditional foods like Snacks (Bhujia, Namkeen, Khara, Farsan, Chanachur), Desi sweetmeats and syrups that claim for taste only and not for nutrition or health at all, exist in the market. Therefore if all the traditional foods that contain high amount of fat or salt or sugar be treated as non-nutritive and hence liable for grant of exemption from printing of nutritional information on labels as granted to pickles and papad, it would be more reasonable and lead to a uniformly applicable law.

Not only the junk foods but the traditional foods too particularly fried items including both snacks and sweets contain high enough fat and salt or sugar contents and so may be harmful for a number of people particularly hypertensive and diabetic patients or prone to be affected of such diseases in future. The doctors too advise patients to avoid such foods. Therefore any nutritional information regarding fat, carbohydrate, protein, salt and sugar contents on the labels of traditional foods would be misleading to consumers. To print "Non-Nutritive" instead of misleading nutritional information, as a statutory warning, would be more beneficial to consumers.

Thus exemption from printing of nutritional information on labels of traditional foods particularly sweets, snacks and syrups which don't make any nutritional claim, would cut unnecessary cost and reduce the burden on consumers' pockets too.

NUTRIOMICS

Nutriomics is an omics study for nutrition and energy metabolism related genes and proteins. Nutriomics is a new field where traditional nutrition researchers adopt genomics technology such as large scale microarray analysis with food intake.

NUTRITIONAL GENOMICS

Nutritional genomics is a science studying the relationship between human genome, nutrition and health. It can be divided into two disciplines:

- Nutrigenomics: studies the effect of nutrients on health through altering genome, proteome, metabolome and the resulting changes in physiology.

- Nutrigenetics: studies the effect of genetic variations on the interaction between diet and health with implications to susceptible subgroups. More specifically, nutrigenomics studies how individual differences in genes influence the body's response to diet and nutrition. For example, people with mutations in an enzyme deficiency in the enzyme phenylalanine hydroxylase cannot metabolize foods containing the amino acid phenylalanine and must modify their diets to minimize consumption. With modern genomic data, severe gene mutations with less severe effects are being explored to determine whether dietary practices can be more closely personalized to individual genetic profiles. However, there have been few validated studies for these kinds of classical gene mutation effects.

Gene-Diet-Disease Interaction

97 per cent of the genes known to be associated with human diseases result in monogenic diseases, i.e. a mutation in one gene is sufficient to cause the disease. Modifying the dietary intake can prevent some monogenic diseases. One example is phenylketonuria, a genetic disease characterized by a defective phenylalanine hydroxylase enzyme, which is normally responsible for the metabolism of phenylalanine to tyrosine. This results in the accumulation of phenylalanine and its breakdown products in the blood and the decrease in tyrosine, which increases the risk of neurological damage and mental retardation. Phenylalanine-restricted tyrosine-supplemented diets are a means to nutritionally treat this monogenic disease.

In contrast, many common diseases, such as obesity, cancer, diabetes, and cardiovascular diseases, are polygenic diseases, i.e. they arise from the dysfunction in a cascade of genes, and not from a single mutated gene. Dietary intervention to prevent the onset of such diseases is a complex and ambitious goal.

Recently, it was discovered that the health effects of food compounds are related mostly to specific interactions on molecular level, i.e. dietary constituents participate in the regulation of gene expression by modulating the activity of transcription factors, or through the secretion of hormones that in turn interfere with a transcription factor.

Nutrigenomics

Nutrigenomics refers to the prospective analysis of differences among nutrients in the regulation of gene expression i.e., it studies the effect of nutrients on the genome, proteome, and metabolome. It involves the application of high-throughput genomic tools such as DNA microarray technology in nutrition research. Nutrigenomics is a discovery science which aims at understanding how nutrition influences metabolic pathways and homeostatic control and how this regulation is disturbed in the early phase of a diet-related disease.

Biomics Technologies

The recent advances in nutrigenomics studies are owed to the completion of human genome project and the new biomics technologies that provide means for the simultaneous determination of the expression of many thousands of genes at the mRNA (transcriptomics), metabolites (metabolomics) and protein (proteomics) levels. Genomic and transcriptomic studies are mostly conducted by DNA microarray technologies. Proteomics and metabolomics have no standardized procedures yet, but usually, proteome analysis is done by two-dimensional gel electrophoresis and Liquid chromatography-mass spectrometry, while metabolome analysis is conducted through gas chromatography-mass spectrometry, liquid chromatography-mass spectrometry and liquid chromatography-nuclear magnetic resonance. Usually, these technologies are applied in a "differential display" mode, i.e. by comparing two situations (e.g. diseased versus healthy) in order to reduce the complexity in data by examining only differences.

Example of Applications

An example of the application of the nutrigenomic approach was a study that simultaneously identified a mechanism for the regulation of sterol uptake in the intestine and the basis for sitosterolemia (a genetic disorder characterized by hyperabsorption of dietary sterols leading to hypercholesterolemia with a high risk of developing atherosclerosis). In the study, a group of mice was treated with a lipid metabolism-altering drug and DNA microarray technology was used for mRNA expression profiling of various tissues. Differential display mode was used by comparing differences in expression levels with a control group of mice. This led to the discovery of an unknown gene. Through computer simulation techniques, it was found that two proteins produced by the newly discovered gene were responsible for the regulated reverse transport of animal and plant dietary sterols out of the apical surface of intestinal cells. By exploring human gene databases, a human homologue of the mouse gene was identified. This explained why dietary sterols, which are structurally similar to cholesterol, are not absorbed in normal individuals. By scanning sitosterolemic individuals for this gene, it was found that all of them had a mutation in this gene responsible for their uncontrolled hyperabsorption of dietary sterols.

Nutrigenetics

Nutrigenetics is the retrospective analysis of genetic variations among individuals with respect to the interaction between diet and disease. It is an applied science that studies how the genetic makeup of an individual affects the response to diet and the susceptibility to diet-related diseases. This necessitates the identification of gene variants associated with differential responses to nutrients and with higher susceptibility to diet-related diseases. The ultimate goal of nutrigenetics is to provide nutritional recommendations for individuals in what is known as *personalized or individualized nutrition.* A number of companies have begun offering nutrigenetic testing, but the recommendations are often highly generic, and could provide a false sense of security. As these companies are not offering specific clinical advice, they do not qualify for regulation beyond the accuracy of the genetic test applied. Objections to such testing kits in the UK have led to the voluntary suspension of commercial testing activity there, and in the US severe criticisms have been leveled against various testing companies by the Government Accountability Office.

Applications

A number of genetic variations have been shown to increase the susceptibility to diet-related diseases. These include variants that have been associated with Type 2 diabetes mellitus, obesity, cardiovascular diseases, some autoimmune diseases and cancers. Nutrigenetics aims to study these susceptible genes and provide dietary interventions for individuals at risk of such diseases. Some examples are shown below:

Nutrigenetics and Type 2 Diabetes Mellitus

A number of genes are involved in regulating lipid metabolism and insulin sensitivity, and thereby affecting the susceptibility to type 2 diabetes mellitus. Among them is the gene responsible for sterol response element binding protein-1c or SREBP-1c (a membrane-bound transcription factor which can directly activate the expression of several genes involved in the synthesis and uptake of cholesterol, fatty acids, triglycerides and phospholipids). In mice models, overexpression of SREBP-1c led to fatty livers, hypertriglyceridemia, severe insulin resistance and finally type 2 diabetes mellitus. Later, SREBP-1c was identified as a candidate gene in the regulation of human insulin resistance. Two missense mutations in exons coding the aminoterminal transcriptional activating domain of SREBP-1c were found in individuals displaying severe insulin resistance. Another association was found between an intronic single nucleotide polymorphism (C/T) between exons 18c and 19c and the onset of diabetes in men, but not in women. These studies suggest that mutations in SREBP-1c may increase the sensitivity to developing diabetes.

Furthermore, SREBP-1c appears to be susceptible to diet, and thus it can be a target for nutritional intervention. Studies in mice have shown that SREBP-1c mRNA expression was highly induced in mice having one polymorphism (-468 A/G) after the consumption of high fructose diets. This implies that a single nucleotide polymorphism can also modulate the sensitivity of a gene to dietary intervention.

Nutrigenetics and Cardiovascular Diseases

Hyperlipidemia is usually associated with atherosclerosis and coronary heart disease. Therapy includes lifestyle changes as alterations in the patient's diet, physical activity and treatment with pharmaceuticals such as statins. However, individuals respond differently to the treatment. This was attributed to genetic variations within the population. Genetic variations in genes encoding for apolipoproteins, some enzymes and hormones can alter individual sensitivity to developing cardiovascular diseases. Some of these variants are susceptible for dietary intervention, for example:

- Individuals with the E4 allele in the apolipoprotein E gene show higher low-density lipoprotein-cholesterol (bad cholesterol) levels with increased dietary fat intake compared with those with the other (E1, E2, E3) alleles receiving equivalent amounts of dietary fat.
- One single nucleotide polymorphism (-75 G/A) in the apolipoprotein A1 gene in women is associated with an increase in High density lipoprotein-cholesterol levels with the increase in the dietary intake of polyunsaturated fatty acids (PUFA). Individuals with the A variant showed an increase in the protective HDL (good cholesterol) levels following an increased consumption of PUFA compared with those with the G variant taking similar amounts of PUFA.
- One polymorphism (-514 CC) in the hepatic lipase gene is associated with an increase in protective HDL levels compared with the TT genotype (common in certain ethnic groups such as African-Americans) in response to high fat diet.

Nutrigenetics and Cancer

Nutrients can contribute to the development of cancers especially colon, gastric and breast cancer. Several gene variants have been identified as susceptibility genes. One example is the N-Acetyltransferase (NAT) gene. NAT is a phase II metabolism enzyme that exists in two forms: NAT1 and NAT2. Several polymorphisms exist in NAT1 and NAT2, some of which have been associated with NAT capabilities of slow, intermediate or fast acetylations. NAT is involved in acetylation of heterocyclic aromatic amines found in heated products especially well cooked red meat.

During cooking of muscle meat at high temperature, some amino acids may react with creatine to give heterocyclic aromatic amines (HAA). HAA can be activated through acetylation to reactive metabolites which bind DNA and cause cancers. Only NAT2 fast acetylators can perform this acetylation. Studies have shown that the NAT2 fast acetylator genotype had a higher risk of developing colon cancer in people who consumed relatively large quantities of red meat.

NUTRIGENOMICS

Nutrigenomics is the study of the effects of foods and food constituents on gene expression. It is about how our DNA is transcribed into mRNA and then to proteins and provides a basis for understanding the biological activity of food components. Nutrigenomics has also been described by the influence of genetic variation on nutrition by correlating gene expression or single-nucleotide polymorphisms with a nutrient's absorption, metabolism, elimination or biological effects. By doing so, Nutrigenomics aims to develop rational means to optimise nutrition, with respect to the subject's genotype. By determining the mechanism of the effects of nutrients or the effects of a nutritional regime, Nutrigenomics tries to define the causality| relationship between these specific nutrients and specific nutrient regimes (diets) on human health. Nutrigenomics has been associated with the idea of personalized nutrition based on genotype. While there is hope that nutrigenomics will ultimately enable such personalised dietary advice, it is a science still in its infancy and its contribution to public health over the next decade is thought to be minor.

Definitions

Nutrigenomics is applying the sciences of genomics, transcriptomics, proteomics and metabolomics to human nutrition in order to understand the relationship between nutrition and health. Nutrigenomics is a new science and has several different definitions. Nutrigenomics has been defined as the application of high-throughput genomic tools in nutrition research. The term high throughput tools in nutrigenomics refers to genetic tools that enable literally millions of genetic screening tests to be conducted at a single time. When such high throughput screening is applied in nutrition research, it allows the examination of how nutrients affect the thousands of genes present in the human genome. Nutrigenomics involves the characterization of gene products and the physiological function and interactions of these products. This includes how nutrients impact on the production and action of specific gene products and how these proteins in turn affect the response to nutrients.

Background and Preventive Health

Throughout the 20th century, nutritional science focused on finding vitamins and minerals, defining their use and preventing the deficiency diseases that they caused. As the nutrition related health problems of the developed world shifted to overnutrition, obesity and type two diabetes, the focus of modern medicine and of nutritional science changed accordingly.

In order to address the increasing incidence of these diet-related-diseases, the role of diet and nutrition has been and continues to be extensively studied. To prevent the development of disease, nutrition research is investigating how nutrition can optimize and maintain cellular, tissue, organ and whole body homeostasis. This requires understanding how nutrients act at the molecular level. This involves a multitude of nutrient-related interactions at the gene, protein and metabolic levels. As a result, nutrition research has shifted from epidemiology and physiology to molecular biology and nutrigenomics was born.

The emergence and development of nutrigenomics has been possible due to powerful developments in genetic research. Inter-individual differences in genetics, or genetic variability, which have an effect on metabolism and on phenotypes, were recognized early in nutrition research, and such phenotypes were described. With the progress in genetics, biochemical disorders with a high nutritional relevance were linked to a genetic origin. Genetic disorders which cause pathological effects were described. Such genetic disorders include the polymorphism in the gene for the hormone Leptin which results in gross obesity. Other gene polymorphisms were described with consequences for human nutrition. The folate metabolism is a good example, where a common polymorphism exists for the gene that encodes the methylene-tetrahydro-folate reductase (MTHFR).

It was realized however, that there are possibly thousands of other gene polymorphisms which may result in minor deviations in nutritional biochemistry, where only marginal or additive effects would result from these deviations. The tools to study the physiological impact were not available at the time and are only now becoming available enabling the development of nutrigenomics. Such tools include those that measure the transcriptome—DNA microarray, Exon array, Tiling arrays, single nucleotide polymorphism arrays and genotyping. Tools that measure the proteome are less developed. These include methods based on gel electrophoresis, chromatography and mass spectrometry. Finally the tools that measure the metabolome are also less developed and include methods based on nuclear magnetic resonance imaging and mass spectrometry often in combination with gas and liquid chromatography.

Rationale and Aims of Nutrigenomics

In nutrigenomics, nutrients are seen as signals that tell a specific cell in the body about the diet. The nutrients are detected by a sensor system in the cell. Such a sensory system works like sensory ecology whereby the cell obtains information through the signal, the nutrient, about its environment, which is the diet. The sensory system that interprets information from nutrients about the dietary environment includes transcription factors together with many additional proteins. Once the nutrient interacts with such a sensory system, it changes gene, protein expression and metabolite production in accordance with the level of nutrient it senses. As a result, different diets should elicit different patterns of gene and protein expression and metabolite production. Nutrigenomics seeks to describe the patterns of these effects which have been referred to as *dietary signatures.* Such dietary signatures are examined in specific cells, tissues and organisms and in this way the manner by which nutrition influences homeostasis is investigated. Genes which are affected by differing levels of nutrients need first to be identified and then their regulation is studied. Differences in this regulation as a result of differences in genes between individuals are also studied.

It is hoped that by building up knowledge in this area, nutrigenomics will promote an increased understanding of how nutrition influences metabolic pathways and homeostatic control, which will then be used to prevent the development of chronic diet related diseases such as obesity and type two diabetes. Part of the approach of nutrigenomics involves finding markers of the early phase of diet related diseases; this is the phase at which intervention with nutrition can return the patient to health. As nutrigenomics seeks to understand the effect of different genetic predispositions in the development of such diseases, once a marker has been found and measured in an individual, the extent to which they are susceptible to the development of that disease will be quantified and personalized dietary recommendation can be given for that person.

The aims of nutrigenomics also includes being able to demonstrate the effect of bioactive food compounds on health and the effect of health foods on health, which should lead to the development of functional foods that will keep people healthy according to their individual needs.

Nutrigenomics is a rapidly emerging science still in its beginning stages. It is uncertain whether the tools to study protein expression and metabolite production have been developed to the point as to enable efficient and reliable measurements. Also once such research has been achieved, it will need to be integrated together in order to produce results and dietary recommendations. All of these technologies are still in the process of development.

NUTRITIONAL GATEKEEPER

Nutritional gatekeeper has been used to refer to the person in a household who typically makes the purchasing and preparation decisions related to food. Nutritional gatekeepers can be a parent, grandparent, sibling, or caregiver. The term nutritional gatekeeper was first used by Kurt Lewin in 1943. Before that time, most past efforts to study nutrition education had focused on the individuals eating the food.

Based on Lewin's research, food reaches the household through "channels" such as grocery store, the garden, and the refrigerator. The selection of the channels and the food that passes through them is under control of the gatekeeper.

For sixty-five years since Lewin's work, many dietetics and nutrition textbooks have referred, in the discussions of children's and adolescents' dietary habits, to the gatekeeper role played by women.

Home Nutritional Gatekeeper

A home's nutritional gatekeeper usually has the biggest food influence in the nutrition life of most people. They are the biggest food influence in the lives of their children as well as in the life of their spouse or partner. Regardless of the gatekeeper's sex or age and regardless of whether they are a great cook or whether they are "culinarily challenged", the gatekeeper has a huge day-to-day influence on his or her family's nutrition.

An average of 72 per cent of what and how much children eat is estimated to be either directly or indirectly determined by these nutritional gatekeepers. In addition, the gatekeeper has a direct and an indirect impact on what the children eat outside the home. This happens every time they make their children's lunches and every time they give them enough money to afford whatever lunch or snack they want. They also influence the restaurant orders of their family by what they recommend or order themselves.

It has been proven that children without regular family dinners ate sweets and fast foods more often, and had more behavioural problems than those having regular family dinners.

Cooks as Nutritional Gatekeepers

Gatekeeper research starting in the 1940s suggests that the cooks are also responsible for nutrition. Cooking family dinners can expand the nutritional gatekeeper's influence. Eating family dinner has been associated with healthful dietary patterns, better fruit and vegetable intake, lower intake of fried food and soda. Cooks are not only gatekeepers, but opinion leaders as well.

Growing Role of Caregivers outside the Home as Nutritional Gatekeeper

Greater numbers of children are relying on caregivers to provide a significant portion of their nutritional needs or act as nutritional gatekeepers. Currently, child care in the United States is varied — child care homes (both regulated and unregulated) — and other placement such as care in the child's home by a relative or other caregiver.

Providing healthful meals and snacks to children during the day (and sometimes the early evening as well) in a pleasant eating environment is a major responsibility for the child care facility. In other words, the child care facility have joined the family as the nutritional gatekeepers'. As stated in Briley, Mcbride, & Roberts-Gray, 1997, Caregivers-are being asked to take the role of the nutritional gatekeeper for children.

Government Involvement

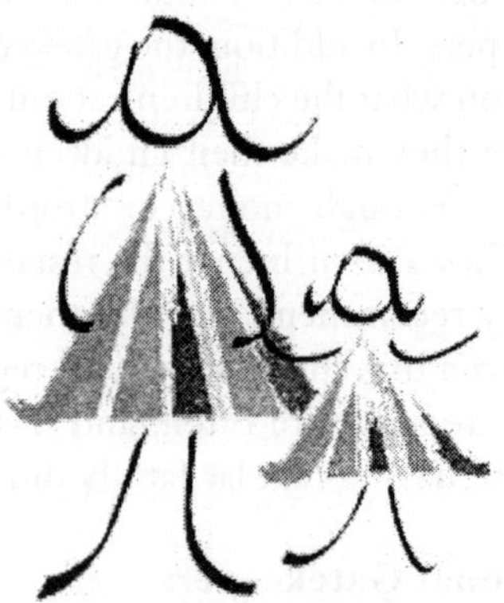

Fig.1.3: ProjectMOM

The USDA has taken note on the powerful influence of nutritional gatekeepers. They have launched an initiative called,

"Project M.O.M." (Mothers & Others & MyPyramid) to help improve eating habits by focusing on the nutritional gatekeepers. The idea behind the project is as follows: If we can collectively connect with a family's nutritional gatekeeper, in ways that help the family eat more nutritiously and be more physically active, we could make an immediate change, with lasting impact.

GASTROENTEROLOGY

Gastroenterology (MeSH heading) is the branch of medicine whereby the digestive system and its disorders are studied. Etymologically, the name is a combination of three Ancient Greek words *gastros* (stomach), *enteron* (intestine), and *logos* (reason).

Diseases affecting the gastrointestinal tract, which includes the organs from mouth to anus, along the alimentary canal, are the focus of this specialty. Physicians practicing in this field of medicine are called gastroenterologists. They have usually completed the eight years of pre-medical and medical education, the yearlong internship (if this is not a part of the residency), three years of an internal medicine residency, and two to three years in the gastroenterology fellowship. Specialists in GI radiology, hepatobiliary or gastric medicine, or in GI oncology will then complete a two-or three-year fellowship. Gastroenterology is not the same as gastroenterological surgery or of colon and rectal (proctology) surgery, which are specialty branches of general surgery. Important advances have been made in the last fifty years, contributing to rapid expansion of its scope.

Hepatology, or hepatobiliary medicine, encompasses the study of the liver, pancreas, and biliary tree and is traditionally considered a sub-specialty.

History

Citing from Egyptian papyri, Nunn identified significant knowledge of gastrointestinal diseases among practising physicians during the periods of the pharaohs. Irynakhty, of the tenth dynasty, c. 2125 B.C., was a court physician specialising in gastroenterology and proctology.

Among ancient Greeks, Hippocrates attributed digestion to

concoction. Galen's concept of the stomach having four *faculties* was widely accepted up to modernity in the seventeenth century.

Eighteenth Century

- Italian Lazzaro Spallanzani (1729-99) was among early physicians to disregard Galen's theories, and in 1780 he gave experimental proof on the action of gastric juice on foodstuffs.
- In 1767, German Johann von Zimmermann wrote an important work on dysentery.
- In 1777, Maximilian Stoll of Vienna described cancer of the gallbladder.

Nineteenth Century

- In 1805, Philip Bozzini made the first attempt to observe inside the living human body using a tube he named *Lichtleiter* (light guiding instrument) to examine the urinary tract, the rectum, and the pharynx. This is the earliest description of endoscopy.
- Charles Emile Troisier described enlargement of lymph nodes in abdominal cancer.
- In 1823, William Prout discovered that stomach juices contain hydrochloric acid.
- In 1868, Adolf Kussmaul, a well-known German physician, developed the gastroscope. He perfected the technique on a sword swallower.
- In 1871, at the society of physicians in Vienna, Carl Stoerk demonstrated an esophagoscope made of two telescopic metal tubes, initially devised by Waldenburg in 1870.
- In 1876, Karl Wilhelm von Kupffer described the properties of some liver cells now called Kupffer cell.
- In 1883, Hugo Kronecker and Samuel James Meltzer studied oesophageal manometry in humans.

Twentieth Century

- In 1915, Jesse McClendon tested acidity of human stomach *in situ*.
- In 1921-22, Walter Alvarez did the first electrogastrography research.

- Rudolph Schindler described many important diseases involving the human digestive system during World War I in his illustrated textbook and is portrayed by some as the "father of gastroscopy". He and Georg Wolf developed a semiflexible gastroscope in 1932.
- In 1932, Burrill Bernard Crohn described Crohn's disease.
- In 1957, Basil Hirschowitz introduced the first prototype of a fibreoptic gastroscope.

Twenty-first Century

- In 2005, Barry Marshall and Robin Warren of Australia were awarded the Nobel Prize in Physiology or Medicine for their discovery of *Helicobacter pylori* (1982/1983) and its role in peptic ulcer disease. James Leavitt assisted in their research, but the Nobel Prize is not awarded posthumously so he was not included in the award.

Disease Classification

1. International Classification of Disease (ICD 2007)/WHO classification:
    - Chapter XI, Diseases of the digestive system, (K00-K93)
2. MeSH subject Heading:
    - Gastroenterology (G02.403.776.409.405)
    - Gastroenterological diseases (C06.405)
3. National Library of Medicine Catalogue (NLM classification 2006):
    - Digestive system (W1)

Gastroenterological Societies

- World Gastroenterology Organisation
- American College of Gastroenterology
- American Gastroenterological Association
- American Society for Gastrointestinal Endoscopy
- British Society of Gastroenterology

MOLECULAR GASTRONOMY

A classic example of molecular gastronomy is the investigation of the effect of specific temperatures on the yolk and white when cooking an egg. Many cookbooks provide the instructions of boiling eggs 3-6 minutes for soft yolks, 6-8 minutes for a medium yolk and so on. Molecular gastronomy reveals that the amount of time is less important to cooking the eggs than specific temperatures—which always yields the desired result.

Molecular gastronomy is a scientific discipline involving the study of physical and chemical processes that occur in cooking. It pertains to the mechanisms behind the transformation of ingredients in cooking and the social, artistic and technical components of culinary and gastronomic phenomena in general (from a scientific point of view).

Term Origination

The term "Molecular and Physical Gastronomy" was coined in 1988 by Hungarian physicist Nicholas Kurti and by the French physical chemist Hervé This as the title for a set of workshops held in Erice, Italy that brought together primarily scientists and some professional cooks for discussions of the science behind traditional cooking preparations. Prof. Kurti had previously coined the term "Molecular Gastronomy" at a meeting at Oxford in May, 1980, of what was to become the Oxford Symposium on Food and Cookery; and he used the expression again at a meeting of the same group in June, 1985, when the subject of the meeting was "Science, Tradition and Superstition in the Kitchen," and the keynote speaker was Harold McGee. Hervé This, on his side, used this term since 1980, when he was exploring scientifically culinary old wive tales (now called "culinary precisions") and when he was lecturing, such at the Laboratory of Physics of the Ecole normale supérieure in 1984.

Kurti and This met in 1986, and soon they had the idea that they could create a scientific discipline.. In order to promote it, they decided to organize workshops. In March 1988, Kurti and This approached the director of the Ettore Majorana center, physicist Antonino Zichichi who liked the idea and imposed a condition that first class scientists would attend. As This was a friend of the Nobel Prize winner Pierre Gilles de Gennes, and as Kurti knew some scientists like Arnold Burgen, for example, they had no difficulty to get the approval. Together they invited the American food science writer Harold McGee to be a co-director of the first meeting, in 1992. Some years later, this was asked by the French Academy of sciences to present a PhD entitled: "Molecular and Physical Gastronomy", at the University of Paris. He also gave lectures in many places on this subject, including the Clarendon Laboratory, Oxford, invited by his friend Kurti.

After Kurti's death in 1998, the name of the conference was changed by Hervé this to "The International Workshop on Molecular Gastronomy 'N. Kurti'". This remained the sole director of the subsequent workshops from 1999 through 2004.

Terminology Confusion

The term molecular gastronomy has been adopted by a number of people and applied to both the scientific investigation of cooking and to cooking itself, both modern cooking that uses scientific principles in its creations as well as traditional cooking that re-examines its methods through experimentation in order to discard incorrect or irrelevant information. Though molecular gastronomy is by definition a science and science is generally practiced by scientists, the existence of the interdisciplinary occupations of "food scientist" and "Research Chef" have blurred the lines between the disciplines. This, coupled with the fact that the original objectives of molecular gastronomy included the "inventing of new dishes" and the fact that some chefs have created experimental research facilities, such as El Bulli Taller , for their restaurants has served to further blur these lines and propagate confusion between what is and isn't "molecular gastronomy".

In the late 1990s and early 2000s, the term started to be used to describe a new style of cooking in which some chefs began to explore new possibilities in the kitchen by embracing science, research, technological advances in equipment and various natural gums and hydrocolloids produced by the commercial food processing industry. It has since been used to describe the food and cooking of a number of famous chefs.

Some chefs do engage in the scientific investigation of cooking It is also true that the work of some scientists (particularly food scientists) involves cooking. "Chef scientists" also exist, and have for many years, particularly in the research and development departments of commercial food companies.

Despite the best efforts of many to separate and distinguish the scientific investigation of cooking (molecular gastronomy) from the creative use of recently available information, technology and ingredients by cooks to produce non-traditional dishes in non-traditional forms, textures and flavor combinations (e.g. "New Cuisine", "Progressive Cuisine", "Nueva Cocina", "Culinary Constructivism", "Modern Cuisine", "Avant-Garde Cuisine", "Experimental Cuisine" etc...), molecular gastronomy continues to be used, in many cases, as a blanket term to refer to any and all of these things—particularly in the media. As well, the terms "Molecular Cuisine" and "Molecular cooking" have been derived from the term and used by some to describe food and cooking produced with information, tools and ingredients associated with science or food science in general.

Chefs often associated with molecular gastronomy because of their embrace of science include: Pierre Gagnaire, Ferran Adrià, Heston Blumenthal, Homaro Cantu, Wylie Dufresne, Grant Achatz, Sat Bains, Sean Wilkinson, Richard Blais, Kevin Sousa/Pittsburgh, Sean Brock, Marc Lepine/Ottawa, Will Goldfarb/NYC, and Alton Brown.

Adoption and Repudiation of the Term

Some of the chefs and scientists often associated with molecular gastronomy at one time adopted the term or acknowledged the movement. Some of these people had connections to or directly collaborated with Hervé This, which may have contributed-in part-to the mis-application of the term "molecular gastronomy" to their food and cooking. For instance, Hervé This and Pierre Gagnaire are collaborators and publish the products of their collaboration on Gagnaire's website. As well, El Bulli and The Fat Duck are listed as partners in the EU funded European Research Project INICON, a project for the sustainable collaboration between chefs, science and the food industry for the modernization of cooking. The INICON project publishes a manual on molecular gastronomy co-authored by Hervé This, and generally uses molecular gastronomy as the term to refer to the work of the organization throughout its website.

Heston Blumenthal was once a Hervé This collaborator, publishing This's recipe for "Chocolate Chantilly" in his first installment of recipe writing for the UK newspaper The Guardian in 2001, followed by an account of his visit to This's laboratory in France in 2002 during which they developed a recipe for chocolate fondant containing egg whites instead of yolks and no sugar. Blumenthal, at one time, adopted the term molecular gastronomy to describe some of the research going on at his restaurant, The Fat Duck. He was also a participant in 2001 and 2004 International Workshop on Molecular Gastronomy in Erice. The 2001 meeting being where he met many of the scientists he works with today.

Harold McGee, noted kitchen science writer, was a co-director (along with Kurti and This, who were the organizers) of the first of the International School of Molecular and Physical Gastronomy meetings in Erice and has "known Hervé This for over a decade". Though he stepped down as organizer after the first meeting, he attended all the meetings from 1992 through 2004. He at one time defined molecular gastronomy as "the scientific study of deliciousness" in a contribution to the 2004 KVL Workshop on Molecular Gastronomy, in which he also proposed areas of focus for a university programme in molecular gastronomy. Harold's book, On Food and Cooking, mentions molecular gastronomy on pages 2 and 3 of the introduction.

Ferran Adria notes in a document published in the 2003 history section of the El Bulli website entitled "About Molecular Cuisine" that up until 2003 his contact with the scientific world had been "sporadic". He goes on to explain that this is why he had "never ascribed to any scientific origin of their (El Bulli's) creations" until his scientific collaborations in 2003. He notes that he had known Harold McGee and Hervé This through conferences since 2000. In a 2004 online Q&A, he made a distinction between his work and molecular gastronomy and went on to comment on the potential longevity of what he saw as a molecular gastronomy "movement":

> "I don't understand the characterization of molecular gastronomy as a type of cuisine. It's happening the same that happened years ago with fusion, it's becoming a common place. There isn't a molecular cuisine. There's a molecular movement, the molecular gastronomy, where some scientists cooperate with the world of cooking. Clearly, the move acts upon cooking, but I don't think it's a cuisine per se. In twenty years, we could look back and see how many new techniques, more than concepts, were introduced thanks to this movement. Having said this, whoever says that this movement doesn't have a future, only has to pick up a phone, turn on the TV or log-in the internet. Science has changed the world."

Perhaps frustrated with the common mis-classification of their food and cooking as "molecular gastronomy", several chefs often associated with the movement have since repudiated the term, releasing a joint statement in 2006 clarifying their approach to cooking. Still, other modern chefs have embraced molecular gastronomy. An organization known as "The Experimental Cuisine Collective" in New York which holds monthly workshops at which Hervé This has been a featured speaker and whose website lists works by This on the resources page has members including some of the most well known chefs in the city. In July 2008, New York University biochemist Kent Kirshenbaum, one of the founders of the Experimental Cuisine Collective, gave a lecture at the New York Academy of Sciences explaining the philosophy of the group. The lecture was detailed in this podcast.

Other interpretations of the Term

- "The application of scientific principles to the understanding and improvement of domestic and gastronomic food preparation."—Peter Barham
- "The art and science of choosing, preparing and eating good food."—Thorvald Pedersen
- "The scientific study of deliciousness"—Harold McGee

Nicholas Kurti and Hervé This

The Hungarian born physicist Nicholas Kurti (1908-1998) became Professor of Physics at Oxford in 1967, a post he held until his retirement in 1975. He was also visiting Professor at City College in New York, the University of California, Berkeley, and Amherst College in Massachusetts. His hobby was cooking, and he was an enthusiastic advocate of applying scientific knowledge to culinary problems. He was one of the first television cooks in the UK, hosting a black and white television show in 1969 entitled "The Physicist in the Kitchen" where he demonstrated techniques such as using a syringe to inject hot mince pies with brandy in order to avoid disturbing the crust. That same year, he held a presentation for the Royal Society of London (also entitled "The Physicist in the Kitchen") in which he is often quoted to have stated:

> "I think it is a sad reflection on our civilization that while we can and do measure the temperature in the atmosphere of Venus we do not know what goes on inside our soufflés."

During the presentation Kurti demonstrated making meringue in a vacuum chamber, the cooking of sausages by connecting them across a car battery, the digestion of protein by fresh pineapple juice, and a reverse baked alaska—hot inside, cold outside—cooked in a microwave oven. Kurti was also an advocate of low temperature cooking, repeating 18th century experiments by the English scientist Benjamin Thompson by leaving a 2 kg lamb joint in an oven at 80°C. After 8.5 hours, both the inside and outside temperature of the lamb joint were around 7°C, and the meat was tender and juicy. Together with his wife, Giana Kurti, Nicholas Kurti edited an anthology on food and science by fellows and foreign members of the Royal Society, "But the crackling is superb".

Hervé This started collecting "culinary precisions" (old kitchen wives' tales and cooking tricks) in the early 1980s and started testing these precisions to see which ones held up; his collection now numbers some 25,000. He also has received a PhD in Physical Chemistry of Materials for which he wrote his thesis on molecular and physical gastronomy, served as an adviser to the French minister of education, lectured internationally, and was invited to join the lab of Nobel Prize winning molecular chemist Jean-Marie Lehn. This has published several books in French, three of which have been translated into English, including "Molecular Gastronomy: Exploring the Science of Flavor", "Kitchen Mysteries: Revealing the Science of Cooking" and "Coóking, an quintessential art". He currently publishes a series of essays (in French) on Amabilia.com and hosts free monthly seminars on molecular gastronomy at the INRA in France. He is giving free and public Seminars on Molecular gastronomy any month, and once a year, he is giving a public and free Course on Molecular Gastronomy.

The idea of using techniques developed in chemistry to study food is not a new one, it dates back to 18th century, and the discipline of food science has existed for many years. Kurti and This were colleagues and decided that a new, specific, discipline should be created within food science that investigated the processes in regular cooking (as food science was primarily concerned with the nutritional properties of food and developing methods to process food on an industrial scale).

Fundamental Objectives According to Herve This

The objectives of molecular gastronomy, as defined by Herve This are:

Current Objectives

Looking for the mechanisms of culinary transformations and processes (from a chemical and physical point of view) in three areas:

1. the social phenomena linked to culinary activity
2. the artistic component of culinary activity
3. the technical component of culinary activity

Original Objectives

The original fundamental objectives of molecular gastronomy were defined by This in his doctoral dissertation as:

1. Investigating culinary and gastronomical proverbs, sayings, and old wives' tales
2. Exploring existing recipes
3. Introducing new tools, ingredients and methods into the kitchen
4. Inventing new dishes
5. Using molecular gastronomy to help the general public understand the contribution of science to society

However, This later recognized points 3, 4 and 5 as being not entirely scientific endeavours (more application of technology and educational), and has since revised the primary objectives of molecular gastronomy.

- How ingredients are changed by different cooking methods
- How all the senses play their own roles in our appreciation of food
- The mechanisms of aroma release and the perception of taste and flavor
- How and why we evolved our particular taste and flavor sense organs and our general food likes and dislikes
- How cooking methods affect the eventual flavor and texture of food ingredients
- How new cooking methods might produce improved results of texture and flavor
- How our brains interpret the signals from all our senses to tell us the "flavor" of food
- How our enjoyment of food is affected by other influences, our environment, our mood, how it is presented, who prepares it, etc.

Example Myths Debunked

- You need to add salt to water when cooking green vegetables
- Searing meat seals in the juices
- The cooking time for roast meat depends on the weight
- When cooking meat stock you must start with cold water

International Meetings in Erice, Italy

Up until 2001, The International Workshop on Molecular Gastronomy "N. Kurti" (IWMG) was named the "International Workshops of Molecular and Physical Gastronomy" (IWMPG0). The first meeting was held in 1992 and the meetings have continued every few years there after until the most recent in 2004. Each meeting encompassed an overall theme broken down into multiple sessions over the course of a few days, including more than 12 sessions during the meeting in 2004.

The focus of the workshops each year was as follows:

- 1992—First Meeting
- 1995—Sauces, or dishes made from them
- 1997—Heat in cooking
- 1999—Food flavors—how to get them, how to distribute them, how to keep them
- 2001—Textures of Food: How to create them?
- 2004—Interactions of food and liquids

Examples of sessions within these meetings have included:

- Chemical Reactions in Cooking
- Heat Conduction, Convection and Transfer
- Physical aspects of food/liquid interaction
- When liquid meets food at low temperature
- Solubility problems, dispersion, texture/flavour relationship.
- Stability of flavour

Precursors to Molecular Gastronomy

In the second century BC, the anonymous author of a papyrus kept in London used a balance to determine whether fermented meat was lighter than fresh meat. Since then, many scientists have been interested in food and cooking. In particular, the preparation of meat stock—the aqueous solution obtained by thermal processing of animal tissues in water—has been of great interest. It was first mentioned in the fourth century BC by Apicius (André (ed), 1987), and recipes for stock preparation appear in classic texts (La Varenne,

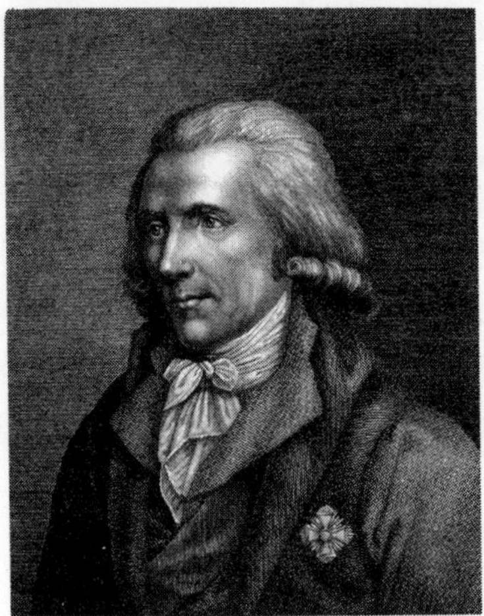

Fig.1.4: Sir Benjamin Thompson, Count Rumford (1753-1814) was One of the Early Pioneers in the Science of Food and Cooking.

1651; Menon, 1756; Carême & Plumerey, 1981) and most French culinary books. Chemists have been interested in meat stock preparation and, more generally, food preparation since the eighteenth century (Lémery, 1705; Geoffrey le Cadet, 1733; Cadet de Vaux, 1818; Darcet, 1830). Antoine-Laurent de Lavoisier is perhaps the most famous among them—in 1783, he studied the processes of stock preparation by measuring density to evaluate quality (Lavoisier, 1783). In reporting the results of his experiments, Lavoisier wrote, "Whenever one considers the most familiar objects, the simplest things, it's impossible not to be surprised to see how our ideas are vague and uncertain, and how, as a consequence, it is important to fix them by experiments and facts" (author's translation). Of course, Justus von Liebig should not be forgotten in the history of culinary science (von Liebig, 1852) and stock was not his only concern. Another important figure was Benjamin Thompson, later knighted Count Rumford, who studied culinary transformations and made many proposals and inventions to improve them, for example by inventing a special coffee pot for better brewing. There are too many scientists who have contributed to the science of food preparation to list here.—Hervé This, 2006

The concept of molecular gastronomy was perhaps presaged by Marie-Antoine Carême, one of the most famous French chefs, who said in the early 19th century that when making a food stock "the broth must come to a boil very slowly, otherwise the albumin coagulates, hardens; the water, not having time to penetrate the meat, prevents the gelatinous part of the osmazome from detaching itself."

2

Nutritional Disorders, Malnutrition, Food Allergy, Healthy Diet, Food Fortification and Dietotherapy

NUTRITION DISORDERS

Deficiency diseases are diseases in humans that are directly or indirectly caused by a lack of essential nutrients in the diet. Deficiency diseases are commonly associated with chronic malnutrition. Additionally, conditions such as obesity from overeating can also cause, or contribute to, serious health problems. Excessive intake of some nutrients can cause acute poisoning.

Overnutrition

Metabolic

Obesity is caused by consuming too many calories compared to the amount exercise the body is performing, causing a distorted energy balance. It can lead to diseases such as cardiovascular disease and diabetes. Obesity is a condition in which the natural energy reserve, stored in the fatty tissue of humans and other mammals, is increased to a point where it is associated with certain health conditions or increased mortality.

The low-cost food that is generally affordable to the poor in affluent nations is low in nutritional value and high in fats, sugars and additives. In rich countries, therefore, obesity is oftentimes a sign of poverty and malnutrition while in poorer countries obesity is more associated with wealth and good nutrition. Other non-nutritional causes for unhealthy obesity included: sleep deprivation, stress, lack of exercise, and heredity.

Acute overeating can also be a symptom of an eating disorder.

Goitrogenic foods can cause goitres by interfering with iodine uptake.

Vitamins and Micronutrients

Vitamin poisoning is the condition of overly high storage levels of vitamins, which can lead to toxic symptoms. The medical names of the different conditions are derived from the vitamin involved: an excess of vitamin A, for example, is called "hypervitaminosis A".

Iron overload disorders are diseases caused by the overaccumulation of iron in the body. Organs commonly affected are the liver, heart and endocrine glands.

Deficiencies (Eating Too Little)

Proteins/Fats/Carbohydrates

- Protein-energy malnutrition
  - Kwashiorkor
  - Marasmus
  - Mental retardation

Dietary Vitamins and Minerals

- Calcium
  - Osteoporosis
  - Rickets
  - Tetany
- Iodine deficiency
- Selenium deficiency
- Iron deficiency
  - Iron deficiency anemia
- Zinc
  - Growth retardation
- Thiamine (Vitamin B1)
  - Beriberi
- Niacin (Vitamin B3)
  - Pellagra

- Vitamin C
    - Scurvy
- Vitamin D
    - Osteoporosis
    - Rickets

Complex Disorders

In some cases, eating too much of one thing can induce an apparent deficiency of something else. A common example occurs when livestock eat locoweed: locoweed contains a toxin that inhibits an enzyme, simulating a deficiency of the enzyme.

OBESITY

Obesity is a medical condition in which excess body fat has accumulated to the extent that it may have an adverse effect on health, leading to reduced life expectancy and/or increased health problems. Body mass index (BMI), a measurement which compares weight and height, defines a person as overweight (pre-obese) when their BMI is between 25 kg/m^2 and 30 kg/m^2, and obese when it is greater than 30 kg/m^2.

Obesity increases the likelihood of various diseases, particularly heart disease, type 2 diabetes, breathing difficulties during sleep, certain types of cancer, and osteoarthritis. Obesity is most commonly caused by a combination of excessive dietary calories, lack of physical activity, and genetic susceptibility, although a few cases are caused solely by genes, endocrine disorders, medications or psychiatric illness. Evidence to support the view that some obese people eat little yet gain weight due to a slow metabolism limited; on average obese people have a greater energy expenditure than their thin counterparts due to the energy required to maintain an increased body mass.

The primary treatment for obesity is dieting and physical exercise. To supplement this, or in case of failure, anti-obesity drugs may be taken to reduce appetite or inhibit fat absorption. In severe cases, surgery is performed or an intragastric balloon is placed to reduce stomach volume and or bowel length, leading to earlier satiation and reduced ability to absorb nutrients from food.

Obesity is a leading preventable cause of death worldwide, with increasing prevalence in adults and children, and authorities view it as one of the most serious public health problems of the 21st century. Obesity is stigmatized in the modern Western world, though it has been perceived as a symbol of wealth and fertility at other times in history, and still is in many parts of Africa.

Classification

Obesity is a medical condition in which excess body fat has accumulated to the extent that it may have an adverse effect on health. It is defined by body mass index (BMI) and further evaluated in terms of fat distribution via the waist-hip ratio and total cardiovascular risk factors. BMI is closely related to both percentage body fat and total body fat.

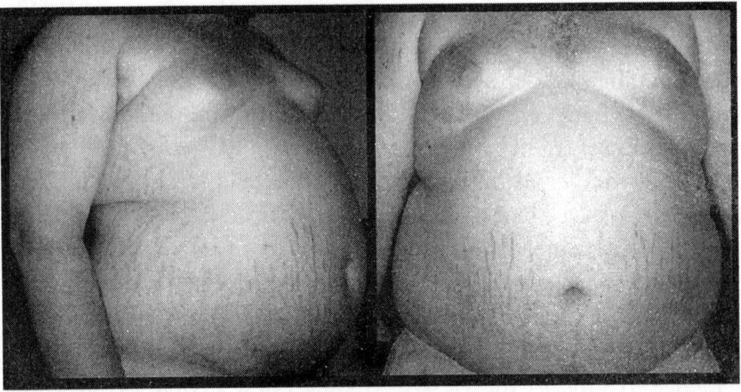

Fig. 2.1: An Obese Male with a Body Mass Index of 46 kg/m^2: Weight 146 Kg (322 lb), Height 177 cm (5 ft 10 in)

In children a healthy weight varies with age and sex. Obesity in children and adolescents is defined not as an absolute number but in relation to a historical normal group, such that obesity is a BMI greater than the 95th percentile. The reference data that these percentiles are based on is from 1963 to 1994 and thus has not been affected by the recent increases in weight.

BMI	*Classification*
< 18.5	underweight
18.5-24.9	normal weight
25.0-29.9	overweight
30.0-34.9	class I obesity
35.0-39.9	class II obesity
> 40.0	class III obesity

BMI is calculated by dividing the subject's mass by the square of his or her height, typically expressed either in metric or US "Customary" units:

Metric:

$$\text{BMI} = \text{kilograms/meters}^2$$

US/Customary and imperial:

$$\text{BMI} = \text{lb} \times 703/\text{in}^2$$

where '*lb*' is the subject's weight in pounds and '*in*' is the subject's height in inches.

The most commonly used definitions, established by the World Health Organization (WHO) in 1997 and published in 2000, provide the values listed in the table at right.

Some modifications to the WHO definitions have been made by particular bodies. The surgical literature breaks down "class III" obesity into further categories whose exact values are still disputed.

- Any BMI = 35 or 40 is *severe obesity*
- A BMI of = 35 or 40-44.9 or 49.9 is *morbid obesity*
- A BMI of = 45 or 50 is *super obese*

As Asian populations develop negative health consequences at a lower BMI than Caucasians, some nations have redefined obesity; the Japanese have defined obesity as any BMI greater than 25 while China uses a BMI of greater than 28.

Effects on Health

Excessive body weight is associated with various diseases, particularly cardiovascular diseases, diabetes mellitus type 2, obstructive sleep apnea, certain types of cancer, and osteoarthritis. As a result, obesity has been found to reduce life expectancy.

Mortality

Obesity is one of the leading preventable causes of death worldwide. Large-scale American and European studies have found that mortality risk is lowest at a BMI of 22.5-25 kg/m^2 in nonsmokers and at 24-27 kg/m^2 in current smokers, with risk increasing along with changes in either direction. A BMI above 32 has been associated with a doubled mortality rate among women over a 16-year period. In the United States obesity is estimated to cause an excess 111,909 to 365,000 death per year, while 1 million (7.7%) of deaths in the European Union are attributed to excess weight. On average, obesity reduces life expectancy by six to seven years: a BMI of 30-35 reduces life expectancy by two to four years, while severe obesity (BMI>40) reduces life expectancy by 10 years.

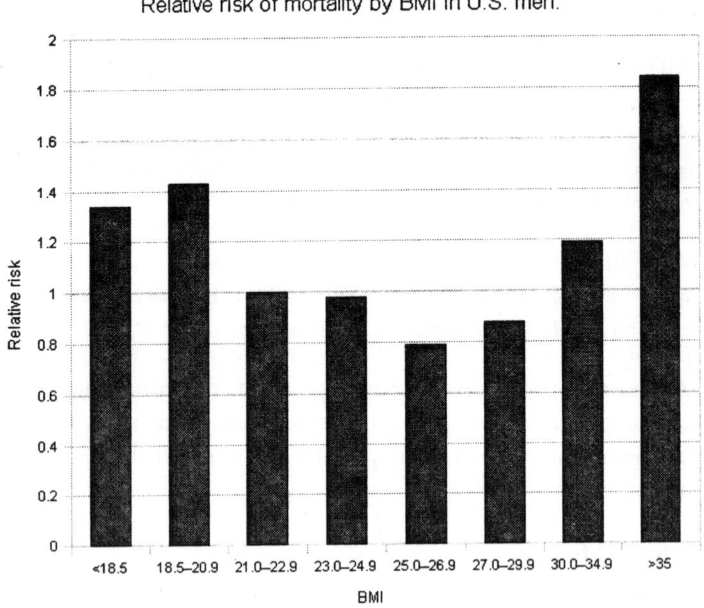

Fig.2.2: Relative Risk of Death for Men in United States by BMI

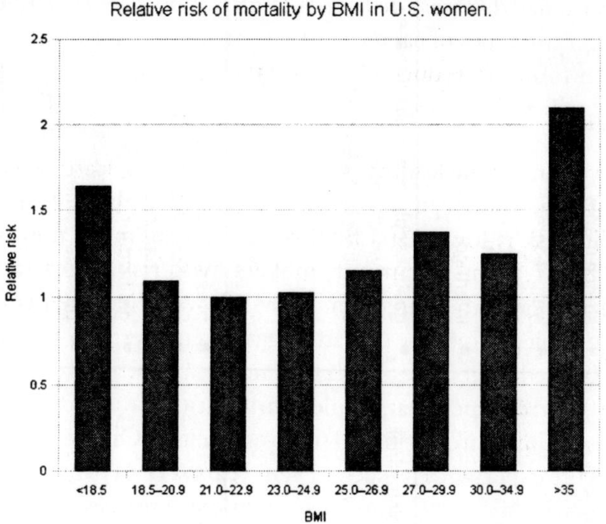

Fig. 2.3: Relative Risk of Death for Women in United States by BMI

Morbidity

Obesity increases the risk of many physical and mental conditions. These comorbidities are most commonly shown in metabolic syndrome, a combination of medical disorders which includes: diabetes mellitus type 2, high blood pressure, high blood cholesterol, and high triglyceride levels.

Complications are either directly caused by obesity or indirectly related through mechanisms sharing a common cause such as a poor diet or a sedentary lifestyle. The strength of the link between obesity and specific conditions varies. One of the strongest is the link with type 2 diabetes. Excess body fat underlies 64 per cent of cases of diabetes in men and 77 per cent of cases in women.

Health consequences can be categorized by the effects of increased fat mass (osteoarthritis, obstructive sleep apnea, social stigmatization) or by the increased number of fat cells (diabetes, cancer, cardiovascular disease, non-alcoholic fatty liver disease). Increases in body fat alter the body's response to insulin, potentially leading to insulin resistance. Increased fat also creates a proinflammatory state, increasing the risk of thrombosis.

Medical Field	*Condition*	*Medical Field*	*Condition*
Cardiology	• ischemic heart disease: angi-na and myocardial infarction • congestive heart failure • high blood pressure • abnormal cholesterol levels • deep vein thrombosis and pulmonary embolism	Dermatology	• stretch marks • acanthosis nigricans • lymphedema • cellulitis • hirsutism • intertrigo
Endocrinology and Reproductive medicine	• diabetes mellitus • polycystic ovarian syndrome • menstrual disorders • infertility • complications during pregnancy • birth defects • intrauterine fetal death	Gastrointestinal	• gastroesophageal reflux disease • fatty liver disease • cholelithiasis (gallstones)
Neurology	• stroke • meralgia paresthetica • migraines • carpal tunnel syndrome • dementia • idiopathic intracranial hypertension	Oncology	• breast, ovarian • esophageal, colorectal • liver, pancreatic • gallbladder, stomach • endometrial, cervical • prostate, kidney • non-Hodgkin's lymphoma, multiple myeloma

(*Contd.*)

Medical Field	*Condition*	*Medical Field*	*Condition*
Psychiatry	• depression in women • social stigmatization	Respirology	• obstructive sleep apnea • obesity hypoventilation syndrome • asthma • increased complications during general anaesthesia
Rheumatology and Orthope-dics	• gout • poor mobility • osteoarthritis • low back pain	Urology and Nephrology	• erectile dysfunction • urinary incontinence • chronic renal failure • hypogonadism

Obesity Survival Paradox

Although the negative health consequences of obesity in the general population are well supported by the available evidence, health outcomes in certain subgroups seem to be improved at an increased BMI, a phenomenon known as the obesity survival paradox. The paradox was first described in 1999 in overweight and obese people undergoing hemodialysis, and has subsequently been found in those with heart failure, and peripheral artery disease (PAD).

In people with heart failure, those with a BMI between 30.0-34.9 had lower mortality than those with a normal weight. This has been attributed to the fact that people often lose weight as they become progressively more ill. Similar findings have been made in other types of heart disease. People with class I obesity and heart disease do not have greater rates of further heart problems than people of normal weight who also have heart disease. In people with greater degrees of obesity, however, risk of further events is increased. Even after cardiac bypass surgery, no increase in mortality is seen in the overweight and obese. One study found that the improved survival could be explained by the more aggressive treatment obese people receive after a cardiac event. Another found that if one takes into account chronic obstructive pulmonary disease (COPD) in those with PAD the benefit of obesity no longer exists.

Causes

At an individual level, a combination of excessive caloric intake and a lack of physical activity is thought to explain most cases of obesity. A limited number of cases are due primarily to genetics, medical reasons, or psychiatric illness. In contrast at a societal level increasing rates of obesity are felt to be due to an easily accessible and palatable diet, increased reliance on cars, and mechanized manufacturing.

A 2006 review identified ten other possible contributors to the recent increase of obesity: (1) insufficient sleep, (2) endocrine disruptors (environmental pollutants that interfere with lipid metabolism), (3) decreased variability in ambient temperature, (4) decreased rates of smoking, because smoking suppresses appetite, (5) increased use of medications that can cause weight gain (e.g., atypical antipsychotics), (6) proportional increases in ethnic and age groups that tend to be heavier, (7) pregnancy at a later age (which may cause susceptibility to obesity in children), (8) epigenetic risk factors passed on generationally, (9) natural selection for higher BMI, and (10) assortative mating leading to increased concentration of obesity risk factors (this would not necessarily increase the number of obese people, but would increase the average population weight). There is substantial but not conclusive evidence for these mechanisms, and the authors specify that they are probably less influential than the ones discussed in the previous paragraph (but still important).

Diet

The per capita dietary energy supply varies markedly between different regions and countries. It has also changed significantly over time. From the early 1970s to the late 1990s the average calories available per person per day (the amount of food bought) has increased in all parts of the world except Eastern Europe. The United States had the highest availability with 3,654 calories per person in 1996. This increased further in 2003 to 3,754. During the late 1990s Europeans had 3394 calories per person, in the developing areas of Asia there were 2,648 calories per person, and in sub-Sahara Africa people had 2,176 calories per person.

The widespread availability of nutritional guidelines has done little to address the problems of overeating and poor dietary choice. From 1971 to 2000, obesity rates in the United States increased from 14.5 per cent to 30.9 per cent. During the same period, an increase occurred in the average amount of calories consumed. For women, the average increase was 335 calories per day (1,542 calories in 1971 and 1,877 calories in 2004), while for men the average increase was 168 calories per day (2,450 calories in 1971 and 2,618 calories in 2004). Most of these extra calories came from an increase in carbohydrate consumption rather than fat consumption. The primary source of these extra carbohydrates is sweetened beverages, which now account for almost 25 per cent of daily calories in young adults in America. Consumption of sweetened drinks is believed to be contributing to the rising rates of obesity.

As societies become increasingly reliant on energy-dense, big-portion, fast-food meals, the association between fast-food consumption and obesity becomes more concerning. In the United States consumption of fast-food meals tripled and calorie intake from these meals quadrupled between 1977 and 1995.

Agricultural policy and techniques in the United States and Europe have led to lower food prices. In the United States, subsidization of corn, soy, wheat, and rice through the U.S. farm bill has made the main sources of processed food cheap compared to fruits and vegetables.

Obese people consistently under-report their food consumption as compared to people of normal weight. This is supported both by test of people carried out in a calorimeter rooms and by direct observation.

Sedentary Lifestyle

A sedentary lifestyle plays a significant role in obesity. Worldwide there has been a large shift towards less physically demanding work, and currently at least 60 per cent of the world's population gets insufficient exercise. This is primarily due to increasing use of mechanized transportation and a greater prevalence of labour-saving technology in the home. In children there appears to be declines in levels of physical activity due to less walking and physical education. World trends in active leisure time physical activity are less clear. The World Health Organization indicates that people worldwide are taking up less active recreational pursuits, while a study from Finland found an increase and a study from the United States found leisure-time physical activity has not changed significantly.

In both children and adults there is an association between television viewing time and the risk of obesity. A 2008 meta-analysis found that 63 of 73 studies (86%) showed an increased rate of childhood obesity with increased media exposure, with rates increasing proportionally to time spent watching television.

Genetics

Like many other medical conditions, obesity is the result of interplay between genetic and environmental factors. Polymorphisms in various genes controlling appetite and metabolism predispose to obesity when sufficient calories are present. As of 2006 more than 41 of these sites have been linked to the development of obesity when a favourable environment is present. The percentage of obesity that can be attributed to genetics varies, depending on the population examined, from 6 per cent to 85 per cent.

Obesity is a major feature in several syndromes, such as Prader-Willi syndrome, Bardet-Biedl syndrome, Cohen syndrome, and MOMO syndrome. (The term "non-syndromic obesity" is sometimes used to exclude these conditions.) In people with early-onset severe obesity (defined by an onset before 10 years of age and body mass index over three standard deviations above normal), 7 per cent harbor a single point DNA mutation.

Studies that have focused upon inheritance patterns rather than upon specific genes have found that 80 per cent of the offspring of two obese parents were obese, in contrast to less than 10 per cent of the offspring of two parents who were of normal weight.

The thrifty gene hypothesis postulates that certain ethnic groups may be more prone to obesity in an equivalent environment. Their ability to take advantage of rare periods of abundance by storing energy as fat would be advantageous during times of varying food availability, and individuals with greater adipose reserves would be more likely survive famine. This tendency to store fat, however, would be maladaptive in societies with stable food supplies. This is the presumed reason that Pima Indians, who evolved in a desert ecosystem, developed some of the highest rates of obesity when exposed to a Western lifestyle.

Medical and Psychiatric Illness

Certain physical and mental illnesses and the pharmaceutical substances used to treat them can increase risk of obesity. Medical illnesses that increase obesity risk include several rare genetic syndromes (listed above) as well as some congenital or acquired conditions: hypothyroidism, Cushing's syndrome, growth hormone deficiency, and the eating disorders: binge eating disorder and night eating syndrome. However, obesity is not regarded as a psychiatric disorder, and therefore is not listed in the DSM-IVR as a psychiatric illness.

Certain medications may cause weight gain or changes in body composition; these include insulin, sulfonylureas, thiazolidinediones, atypical antipsychotics, antidepressants, steroids, certain anticonvulsants (phenytoin and valproate), pizotifen, and some forms of hormonal contraception.

Social Determinants

While genetic influences are important to understanding obesity, they cannot explain the current dramatic increase seen within specific countries or globally. Though it is accepted that calorie consumption in excess of calorie expenditure leads to obesity on an individual basis, the cause of the shifts in these two factors on the societal scale is much debated. There are a number of theories as to the cause but most believe it is a combination of various factors.

The correlation between social class and BMI varies globally. A review in 1989 found that in developed countries women of a high social class were less likely to be obese. No significant differences were seen among men of different social classes. In the developing world, women, men, and children from high social classes had greater rates of obesity. An update of this review carried out in 2007 found the same relationships, but they were weaker. The decrease in strength of correlation was felt to be due to the effects of globalization.

Many explanations have been put forth for associations between BMI and social class. It is thought that in developed countries, the wealthy are able to afford more nutritious food, they are under greater social pressure to remain slim, and have more opportunities along with greater expectations for physical fitness. In undeveloped countries the ability to afford food, high energy expenditure with physical labour, and cultural values favouring a larger body size are believed to contribute to the observed patterns. Attitudes toward body mass held by people in one's life may also play a role in obesity. A correlation in BMI changes over time has been found between friends, siblings, and spouses.

Smoking has a significant effect on an individual's weight. Those who quit smoking gain an average of 4.4 kilograms (9.7 lb) for men and 5.0 kilograms (11.0 lb) for women over ten years. Changing rates of smoking however have had little effect on the overall rates of obesity.

In the United States the number of children a person has is related to their risk of obesity. A woman's risk increases by 7 per cent per child, while a man's risk increases by 4 per cent per child. This could be partly explained by the fact that having dependent children decreases physical activity in Western parents.

In the developing world urbanization is playing a role in increasing rate of obesity. In China overall rates of obesity are below 5 per cent however in some cities rates of obesity are greater than 20 per cent.

Malnutrition in early life is believed to play a role in the rising rates of obesity in the developing world. Endocrine changes that occur during periods of malnutrition may promote the storage of fat once more calories become available.

Infectious Agents

The study of the effect of infectious agents on metabolism is still in its early stages. Gut flora has been shown to differ between lean and obese humans. There is an indication that gut flora in obese and lean individuals can affect the metabolic potential. This apparent alteration of the metabolic potential is believed to confer a greater capacity to harvest energy contributing to obesity. Whether these differences are the direct cause or the result of obesity has yet to be determined unequivocally.

An association between viruses and obesity has been found in humans and several different animal species. The amount that these associations may have contributed to the rising rate of obesity is yet to be determined.

Pathophysiology

Flier summarizes the many possible pathophysiological mechanisms involved in the development and maintenance of obesity. This field of research had been almost unapproached until leptin was discovered in 1994. Since this discovery, many other hormonal mechanisms have been elucidated that participate in the regulation of appetite and food intake, storage patterns of adipose tissue, and development of insulin resistance. Since leptin's discovery, ghrelin, insulin, orexin, PYY 3-36, cholecystokinin, adiponectin, as well as many other mediators have been studied. The adipokines are mediators produced by adipose tissue; their action is thought to modify many obesity-related diseases.

Leptin and ghrelin are considered to be complementary in their influence on appetite, with ghrelin produced by the stomach modulating short-term appetitive control (i.e. to eat when the stomach is empty and to stop when the stomach is stretched). Leptin is produced by adipose tissue to signal fat storage reserves in the body, and mediates long-term appetitive controls (i.e. to eat more when fat storages are low and less when fat storages are high). Although administration of leptin may be effective in a small subset of obese individuals who are leptin deficient, most obese individuals are thought to be leptin resistant and have been found to have high levels of leptin. This resistance is thought to explain in part why administration of leptin has not been shown to be effective in suppressing appetite in most obese people.

While leptin and ghrelin are produced peripherally, they control appetite through their actions on the central nervous system. In particular, they and other appetite-related hormones act on the hypothalamus, a region of the brain central to the regulation of food intake and energy expenditure. There are several circuits within the hypothalamus that contribute to its role in integrating appetite, the melanocortin pathway being the best understood. The circuit begins with an area of the hypothalamus, the arcuate nucleus, that has outputs to the lateral hypothalamus (LH) and ventromedial hypothalamus (VMH), the brain's feeding and satiety centers, respectively.

The arcuate nucleus contains two distinct groups of neurons. The first group coexpresses neuropeptide Y (NPY) and agouti-related peptide (AgRP) and has stimulatory inputs to the LH and inhibitory inputs to the VMH. The second group coexpresses pro-opiomelanocortin (POMC) and cocaine-and amphetamine-regulated transcript (CART) and has stimulatory inputs to the VMH and inhibitory inputs to the LH. Consequently, NPY/AgRP neurons stimulate feeding and inhibit satiety, while POMC/CART neurons stimulate satiety and inhibit feeding. Both groups of arcuate nucleus neurons are regulated in part by leptin. Leptin inhibits the NPY/AgRP group while stimulating the POMC/CART group. Thus a deficiency in leptin signaling, either via leptin deficiency or leptin resistance, leads to overfeeding or may account for some genetic and acquired forms of obesity.

Management

The main treatment for obesity consists of dieting and physical exercise. Diet programmes may produce weight loss over the short term, but keeping this weight off can be a problem and often requires making exercise and a lower calorie diet a permanent part of a person's lifestyle. Success rates of long-term weight loss maintenance are low and range from 2-20 per cent. In a more structured setting, however, 67 per cent of people who lost greater than 10 per cent of their body mass maintained or continued to lose weight one year later. An average maintained weight loss of more than 3 kg (6.6 lb) or 3 per cent of total body mass could be sustained for five years. Some studies have found significant benefits in mortality in certain populations with weight loss. In a prospective study of obese women with weight related diseases, intentional weight loss of any amount was associated with a 20 per cent reduction in mortality. In obese women without obesity related illnesses a weight loss of greater than 9 kg (20 lb) was associated with a 25 per cent reduction in mortality. A recent review concluded that certain subgroups such as those with type 2 diabetes and women show long term benefits in all cause mortality well outcomes for men do not seem to be improved with weight loss. A subsequent study has found benefits in mortality from intentional weight loss in those who have severe obesity.

The most effective treatment for obesity is bariatric surgery however due to its cost and the risk of complications researchers are searching for less invasive yet effective treatments.

Dieting

Diets to promote weight loss are generally divided into four categories: low-fat, low-carbohydrate, low-calorie, and very low calorie. A meta-analysis of six randomized controlled trials found no difference between three of the main diet types (low calorie, low carbohydrate, and low fat), with a 2-4 kilogram (4.4-8.8 lb) weight loss in all studies. At two years these three methods resulted in similar weight loss irrespective of the macronutrients emphasized.

Very low calorie diets provide 200-800 kcal/day, maintaining protein intake but limiting calories from both fat and carbohydrates.

They subject the body to starvation and produce an average weekly weight loss of 1.5-2.5 kilograms (3.3-5.5 lb). These diets are not recommended for general use as they are associated with adverse side effects such as loss of lean muscle mass, increased risks of gout, and electrolyte imbalances. People attempting these diets must be monitored closely by a physician to prevent complications.

Exercise

With use, muscles consume energy derived from both fat and glycogen. Due to the large size of leg muscles, walking, running, and cycling are the most effective means of exercise to reduce body fat. Exercise affects macronutrient balance. During moderate exercise, equivalent to a brisk walk, there is a shift to greater use of fat as a fuel. To maintain health the American Heart Association recommends a minimum of 30 minutes of moderate exercise at least 5 days a week.

A meta-analysis of 43 randomized controlled trials by the Cochrane Collaboration found that exercising alone led to limited weight loss. In combination with diet, however, it resulted in a 1 kilogram weight loss over dieting alone. A 1.5 kilogram (3.3 lb) loss was observed with a greater degree of exercise. Even though exercise as carried out in the general population has only modest effects, a dose response curve is found, and very intense exercise can lead to substantial weight loss. During 20 weeks of basic military training with no dietary restriction, obese military recruits lost 12.5 kg (27.6 lb). High levels of physical activity seem to be necessary to maintain weight loss. A pedometer appears useful for motivation. Over an average of 18-weeks of use physical activity increased by 27 per cent resulting in a 0.38 decreased in BMI.

Signs that encourage the use of stairs as well as community campaigns has been shown to be effective in increasing exercise in a population. The city of Bogota, Colombia for example blocks off 113 kilometers (70 miles) of roads every Sunday and on holidays to make it easier for it citizens to get exercise. These pedestrian zones are part of an effort to combat chronic diseases, including obesity.

Weight Loss Programmes

Weight loss programmes often promote lifestyle changes and diet modification. This may involves eating smaller meals, by cutting down on certain types of food, and making a conscious effort to exercise more. These programmes enable people to connect with a group of others that are attempting to lose weight in the hopes that they will encourage and help each other out.

A number of different programmes exist including Weight Watchers, Overeaters Anonymous, and Jenny Craig. They appear to provide modest weight loss (2.9 kg, 6.4 lb) over dieting on one's own (0.2 kg, 0.4 lb) over a two year period. Internet based programmes appear to be ineffective. The Chinese government has introduced a number of fat farms where obese children go for reinforced exercise, and has passed a law which requires students to exercise or play sports for an hour a day at school.

Medication

Only two anti-obesity medications are currently approved by the FDA for long term use. One is orlistat (Xenical), which reduces intestinal fat absorption by inhibiting pancreatic lipase; the other is sibutramine (Meridia), which acts in the brain to inhibit deactivation of the neurotransmitters norepinephrine, serotonin, and dopamine (very similar to some anti-depressants), therefore decreasing appetite. Rimonabant (Acomplia), a third drug, works via a specific blockade of the endocannabinoid system. It has been

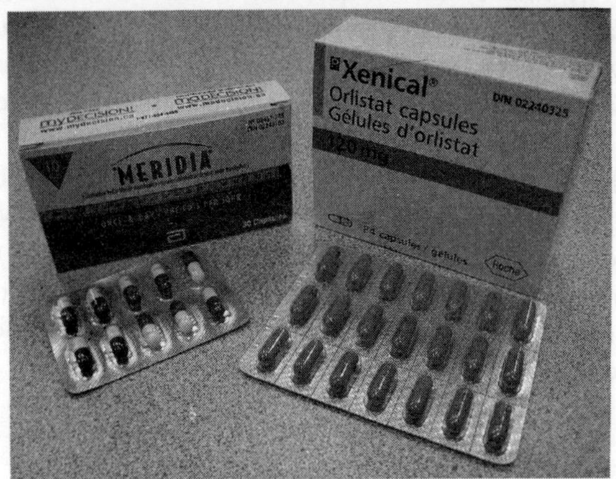

Fig. 2.4: The Two Most Commonly Used Medications to Treat Obesity: Orlistat (Xenical) and Sibutramine (Meridia)

developed from the knowledge that cannabis smokers often experience hunger, which is often referred to as "the munchies". It has been approved in Europe for the treatment of obesity but has not yet received approval in the United States or Canada due to safety concerns.

Weight loss with these drugs is modest; over the longer term, average weight loss on orlistat is 2.9 kg (6.4 lb), sibutramine is 4.2 kg (9.3 lb) and rimonabant is 4.7 kg (10.4 lb). Orlistat and rimonabant lead to a reduced incidence of diabetes, and all three drugs have some effect on cholesterol. There is however little data on how these drugs affect the longer-term complications or outcomes of obesity.

There are a number of less commonly used medication. Some are approved for only short term use, others are used off label, and still others are used illegally. Most are appetite suppressants that act on either one or more neurotransmitters. Phendimetrazine (Bontril), diethylpropion (Tenuate), and phentermine (Adipex-P) are approved by the FDA for short term use while bupropion (Wellbutrin), topiramate (Topamax), and zonisamide (Zonegran) are sometimes used off label.

Certain drugs are useful depending on the comorbities present. Metformin (Glucophage) is preferred in overweight diabetics as it may lead to mild weight loss in comparison to sulfonylureas or insulin. The thiazolidinediones, on the other hand, may cause weight gain, but decrease central obesity. Diabetics also achieve modest weight loss with fluoxetine (Prozac), orlistat and sibutramine over 12-57 weeks. The long-term health benefit of these treatments however remains unclear.

Fenfluramine and dexfenfluramine were withdrawn from the market in 1997, while ephedrine (Ma Huang) was removed from the market in 2004. Dexamphetamines are not approved by the FDA for the treatment of obesity due to concerns regarding addiction. These drugs are all not recommended due to potential side effects. People however do occasionally use these drugs illegally.

Surgery

Bariatric surgery ("weight loss surgery") is the use of surgical interventions in the treatment of obesity. As every operation may have complications, surgery is only recommended for severely obese people (BMI > 40) who have failed to lose weight with dietary modification and pharmacological treatment. Weight loss surgery relies on various principles; the most common approaches are reducing the volume of the stomach, producing an earlier sense of satiation (e.g. by adjustable gastric banding and vertical banded gastroplasty) and reduce the length of bowel that food will be in contact with, directly reducing absorption (gastric bypass surgery). Band surgery is reversible, while bowel shortening operations are not. Some procedures can be performed laparoscopically. Complications from weight loss surgery are frequent.

Surgery for severe obesity is associated with long-term weight loss and decreased overall mortality. One study found a weight loss of between 14 per cent and 25 per cent at 10 years depending on the type of procedure performed and a 29 per cent reduction in all cause mortality when compared to standard weight loss measures. A marked decrease in the risk of diabetes mellitus, cardiovascular disease and cancer has also been found after bariatric surgery. Weight loss is marked in the first few months after surgery and is sustained in the long term. In one study there was an unexplained increase in deaths from accidents and suicide but this did not outweigh the benefit in terms of disease prevention. When the two main techniques are compared gastric bypass procedures are found to lead to 30 per cent more weight loss than banding procedures one year after surgery.

The effects of liposuction on obesity are less well determined. Some small studies show benefits while others show none. A treatment involving the placement of an intragastric balloon via gastroscopy has shown promise. One type of balloon lead to a weight loss of 5.7 BMI units over 6 months or 14.7 kg (32.4 lb). Regaining of lost weight is however common after removal and 4.2 per cent of people were intolerant of the device.

Clinical Protocols

Much of the Western world has created clinical practice guidelines in an attempt to address rising rates of obesity. Australia, Canada, the European Union, and the United States have all published statements since 2004.

In a clinical practice guideline by the American College of Physicians, the following five recommendations are made:

1. People with a BMI of over 30 should be counseled on diet, exercise and other relevant behavioural interventions, and set a realistic goal for weight loss.
2. If these goals are not achieved, pharmacotherapy can be offered. The person needs to be informed of the possibility of side-effects and the unavailability of long-term safety and efficacy data.
3. Drug therapy may consist of sibutramine, orlistat, phentermine, diethylpropion, fluoxetine, and bupropion. For more severe cases of obesity, stronger drugs such as amphetamine and methamphetamine may be used on a selective basis. Evidence is not sufficient to recommend sertraline, topiramate, or zonisamide.
4. In people with a BMI over 40 who fail to achieve their weight loss goals (with or without medication) and who develop obesity-related complications, referral for bariatric surgery may be indicated. The person needs to be aware of the potential complications.
5. Those requiring bariatric surgery should be referred to high-volume referral centers, as the evidence suggests that surgeons who frequently perform these procedures have fewer complications.

A clinical practice guideline by the US Preventive Services Task Force (USPSTF) concluded that the evidence is insufficient to recommend for or against routine behavioural counseling to promote a healthy diet in unselected people in primary care settings, but that intensive behavioural dietary counseling is recommended in those with hyperlipidemia and other known risk factors for cardiovascular and diet-related chronic disease. Intensive counseling can be delivered by primary care clinicians or by referral to other specialists, such as nutritionists or dietitians.

Canada developed and published evidence based practice guidelines in 2006. They attempt to address the prevention and management of obesity at both the individual and population levels in both children and adults. The European Union published clinical practice guidelines in 2008 in an effort to address the rising rates of obesity in Europe. Australia came out with practice guidelines in 2004.

Epidemiology

Before the 20th century, obesity was rare; in 1997 the WHO formally recognized obesity as a global epidemic. As of 2005 the WHO estimates that at least 400 million adults (9.8%) are obese, with higher rates among women than men. The rate of obesity also increases with age at least up to 50 or 60 years old and severe obesity in the United States, Australia, and Canada is increasing faster than the overall rate of obesity. Once considered a problem only of high-income countries, obesity rates are raising worldwide and affecting both the developed and developing world. These increases have been felt most dramatically in urban settings. The only remaining region of the world where obesity is not common is sub-Saharan Africa.

Public Health

The World Health Organization (WHO) predicts that overweight and obesity may soon replace more traditional public health concerns such as undernutrition and infectious diseases as the most significant cause of poor health. Obesity is a public health and policy problem because of its prevalence, costs, and health effects. Public health efforts seek to understand and correct the environmental factors responsible for the increasing prevalence of obesity in the population. Solutions look at changing the factors that cause excess calorie consumption and inhibit physical activity. Efforts include federally reimbursed meal programmes in schools, limiting direct junk food marketing to children, and decreasing access to sweetened beverages in schools. When constructing urban environments, efforts have been made to increase access to parks and to develop pedestrian routes.

Many countries and groups have published reports pertaining to obesity. In 1998 the first US Federal guidelines were published, titled "Clinical Guidelines on the Identification, Evaluation, and Treatment of Overweight and Obesity in Adults: The Evidence Report". In 2006 the Canadian Obesity Network published the "Canadian Clinical Practice Guidelines (CPG) on the Management and Prevention of Obesity in Adults and Children". This is a comprehensive evidence-based guideline to address the management and prevention of overweight and obesity in adults and children. In 2004, the United Kingdom Royal College of Physicians, the Faculty of Public Health and the Royal College of Paediatrics and Child Health released the report "Storing up Problems", which highlighted the growing problem of obesity in the UK. The same year, the House of Commons Health Select Committee published its "most comprehensive inquiry [...] ever undertaken" into the impact of obesity on health and society in the UK and possible approaches to the problem. In 2006, the National Institute for Health and Clinical Excellence (NICE) issued a guideline on the diagnosis and management of obesity, as well as policy implications for non-healthcare organizations such as local councils. A 2007 report produced by Sir Derek Wanless for the King's Fund warned that unless further action was taken, obesity had the capacity to cripple the National Health Service financially.

Comprehensive approaches are being looked at to address the rising rates of obesity. The Obesity Policy Action (OPA) framework divides measure into 'upstream' policies, 'midstream' policies, and 'downstream' policies. 'Upstream' policies look at changing society, 'midstream' policies try to alter individual's behaviour to prevent obesity, and 'downstream' policies try to treat currently afflicted people.

Economic Impact

In addition to its health impacts, obesity leads to many problems including disadvantages in employment and increased business costs. These effects are felt by all levels of society from individuals, to corporations, to governments.

The estimate range for annual expenditures on diet products is $40 billion to $100 billion in the US alone. In 1998, the medical costs attributable to obesity in the US were $78.5 billion USD, or

9.1 per cent of all medical expenditures well the cost of obesity in Canada was estimated at $2 billion CAD in 1997 (2.4% of total health costs).

Obesity prevention programmes have been found to reduce the cost of treating obesity-related disease. However, the longer people live the more medical costs they incur. Researchers therefore conclude that reducing obesity may improve the public's health, but it is unlikely to reduce overall health spending.

Obesity can lead to social stigmatization and disadvantages in employment. Obese workers, on average when compared to their normal weight counterparts, have higher rates absenteeism from work and take more disability leave, thus increasing costs for employers and decreasing productivity. A study examining Duke University employees found that people with a BMI over 40 filed twice as many workers' compensation claims as those whose BMI was 18.5-24.9. They also had more than 12 times as many lost work days. The most common injuries in this group were due to falls and lifting, thus affecting the lower extremities, wrists or hands, and backs. The US state of Alabama Employees' Insurance Board approved a controversial plan to charge obese workers $25 per month if they do not take measures to reduce their weight and improve their health. These measures are set to start January 2010 and apply to those with a BMI of greater than 35 kg/m who fail to make improvements in their health after one year.

Some research shows that obese people are less likely to be hired for a job and are less likely to be promoted. Obese people are also paid less than their non-obese counterparts for an equivalent job. Obese women on average make 6 per cent less and obese men make 3 per cent less.

Specific industries, such as the airline and food industries, have special concerns. Due to rising rates of obesity, airlines face higher fuel costs and pressures to increase seating width. In 2000, the extra weight of obese passengers cost airlines US$275 million. Costs for restaurants are increased by litigation accusing them of causing obesity. In 2005 the US Congress discussed legislation to prevent civil law suits against the food industry in relation to obesity; however it did not become law.

History and Culture

Etymology

Obesity is from the Latin obesitas, which means "stout, fat, or plump." *Ēsus* is the past participle of edere (to eat), with ob (over) added to it. *The Oxford English Dictionary* documents its first usage in 1611 by Randle Cotgrave in *A Dictionarie of the French and English Tongues*.

Historical Trends

The Greeks were the first to recognize obesity as a medical disorder. Hippocrates states that "Corpulence is not only a disease itself, but the harbinger of others". It was known to the Indian surgeon Sushruta (6th century BCE), who related obesity to diabetes and heart disorder. He recommended physical work to help cure it and its side effects. For most of human history mankind struggled with food scarcity. Obesity has thus historically been viewed as a sign of wealth and prosperity. It was common among high officials in Europe in the Middle Ages and the Renaissance as well as in Ancient East Asian civilizations. With the onset of the industrial revolution it was realized that the military and economic might of nations were dependent on both the body size and strength of their soldiers and workers. Increasing the average body mass index from underweight to the normal range played a significant role in the development of industrialized societies. Height and weight thus both increased through the 19th century in the developed world. During the 20th century, as populations reached their genetic potential for height, weight began increasing much more than height, resulting in obesity. In the 1950s increasing wealth in the developed world decreased child mortality, but as body weight increased heart and kidney disease became more common. During this time period insurance companies realized the connection between weight and life expectancy and increased premiums for the obese.

Many cultures throughout history have viewed obesity as a flaw. The obesus or fat character in Greek comedy was a glutton and figure of mockery. During Christian times food was viewed as a gateway to the sins of sloth and lust. In modern Western culture, excess weight is often regarded as unattractive, and obesity is commonly associated with various negative stereotypes. All ages can face social stigmatization and may be targeted by bullies or shunned by their peers. In Western culture obesity is once again a reason for discrimination.

How weight is viewed has changed since the beginning of the 20th century. The weight that is viewed as an ideal has become lower since the 1920s. This is illustrated by the fact that the average height of Miss America pageant winners increased by 2 per cent from 1922 to 1999, while their average weight decreased by 12 per cent. People's perceptions of what is a healthy weight however have changed in the opposite direction. In Britain the weight at which people considered themselves to be overweight was significantly higher in 2007 than in 1999. These changes are believed to be due to increasing rates of adiposity leading to increased acceptance of extra body fat as being normal.

In many part of Africa obesity is still seen as a sign of wealth and well being. This has become particularly common since the HIV epidemic began.

The Arts

The first sculptural representations of the human body 20,000-35,000 years ago depict obese females. Some attribute the Venus figurines to the tendency to emphasize fertility while others feel they representation "fatness" in the people of the time. Corpulence is, however, absent in both Greek and Roman art, probably fitting with their ideals of moderation. This continued through much of Christian European history, with only those of low socioeconomic status being depicted as obese. During the Renaissance some of the upper class began flaunting their large size. This can be seen in portraits of Henry the VIII and Alessandro del Borro. Rubens (1577-1640) regularly depicted full-bodied women in his pictures, from which derives the term Rubenesque. These women, however, still maintained the "hourglass" shape with its relationship to fertility. During the 19th century, views on obesity changed in the Western world. After centuries of obesity being synonymous with wealth and social status, slimness began to be seen as the desirable standard.

Size Acceptance and the Obesity Controversy

The main effort of the fat acceptance movement is to decrease discrimination against people who are overweight and obese. However some in the movement are also attempting to challenge the established relationship between obesity and negative health outcomes.

A number of organizations exist that promote the acceptance of obesity. They have increased in prominence in the latter half of the 20th century. The US based National Association to Advance Fat Acceptance (NAAFA) was formed in 1969 and describes itself as a civil rights organization dedicated to ending size discrimination. The International Size Acceptance Association (ISAA) is an NGO which was founded in 1997. It has more of a global orientation and describes its mission as promoting size acceptance and helping to end weight-based discrimination. These groups often argue for the recognition of obesity as a disability under the US Americans With Disabilities Act (ADA). The American legal system however has decided that the potential public health costs exceed the benefits of extending this anti-discrimination law to cover obesity.

Multiple books such as *The Diet Myth* by Paul Campos argue that the health risks of obesity are mostly unproven and the real problem is the social stigma facing the obese. Similarly, The Obesity Epidemic by Michael Gard argues that obesity is a moral and ideological construct, rather than a health problem. Other groups are also trying to challenge obesity's connection to poor health. The Center for Consumer Freedom, an organization partly supported by the restaurant and food industry, has run ads saying that obesity is not an epidemic but "hype".

People are known to select potential partners based on a similar body mass. The rising rates of obesity have therefore provided greater opportunities for overweight people to find partners. Certain subcultures also label themselves as particularly attracted to the obese. Chubby culture and fat admirers are examples.

Childhood Obesity

The healthy BMI range varies with the age and sex of the child. Obesity in children and adolescents is defined as a BMI greater than the 95th percentile. The reference data that these percentiles

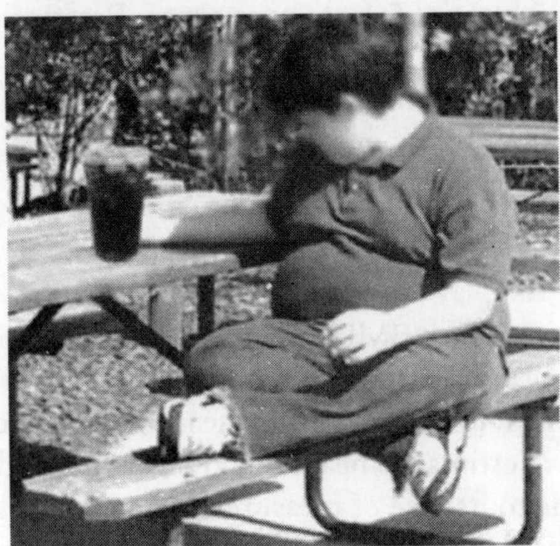

Fig. 2.5: An Overweight Child

are based on is from 1963 to 1994 and thus has not been affected by the recent increases in rates of obesity.

Childhood obesity has reached epidemic proportions in 21st century with rising rates in both the developed and developing world. Rates of obesity in Canadian boys have increased from 11 per cent in 1980s to over 30 per cent in 1990s, while during this same time period rates increased from 4 to 14 per cent in Brazilian children.

As with obesity in adults many different factors contribute to the rising rates of childhood obesity. Changing diet and decreasing physical activity are believed to be the two most important in causing the recent increase in the rate of obesity.

Because childhood obesity often persists into adulthood, and is associated with numerous chronic illnesses, children who are obese are often tested for hypertension, diabetes, hyperlipidemia, and fatty liver.

Treatments used in children are primarily lifestyle interventions and behavioural techniques. Medications are not FDA approved for use in this age group.

In Other Animals

Obesity in pets is common in many countries. Rates of overweight and obesity in dogs in the United States range from 23 per cent to

41 per cent with about 5.1 per cent obese. Rates of obesity in cats were slightly higher at 6.4 per cent. In Australia the rate of obesity among dogs in a veterinary setting has been found to be 7.6 per cent. The risk of obesity in dogs but not cats is related to whether or not their owners are obese.

BODY MASS INDEX

The body mass index (BMI), or Quetelet index, is a controversial statistical measurement which compares a person's weight and height. Though it does not actually measure the percentage of body fat, it is used to estimate a healthy body weight based on how tall a person is. Due to its ease of measurement and calculation, it is the most widely used diagnostic tool to identify weight problems within

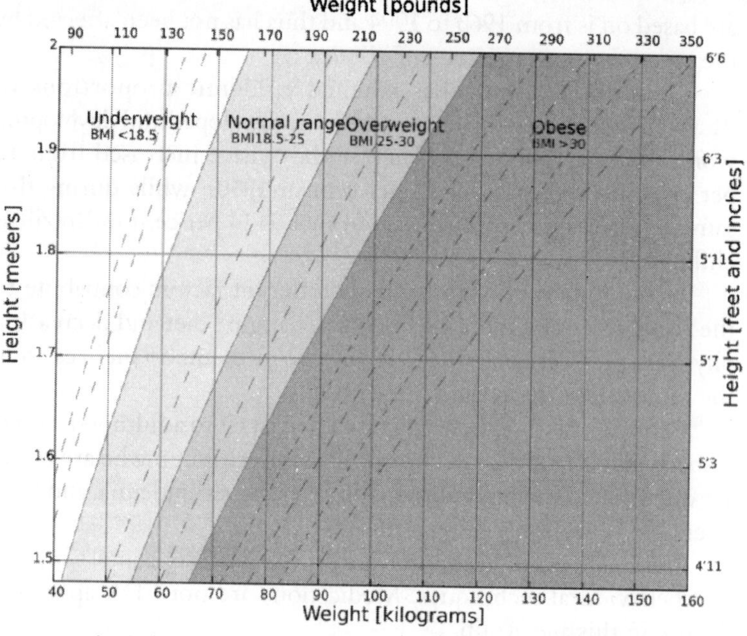

Fig. 2.6: A Graph of Body Mass Index is Shown Above. The Dashed Lines Represent Subdivisions within a Major Class. For Instance the "Underweight" Classification is Further Divided into "Severe," "Moderate," and "Mild" Subclasses Based on World Health Organization data here.

a population, usually whether individuals are underweight, overweight or obese. It was invented between 1830 and 1850 by the Belgian polymath Adolphe Quetelet during the course of developing "social physics". Body mass index is defined as the individual's body weight divided by the square of his or her height. The formulae universally used in medicine produce a unit of measure of kg/m^2. BMI can also be determined using a BMI chart, which displays BMI as a function of weight (horizontal axis) and height (vertical axis) using contour lines for different values of BMI or colours for different BMI categories.

Usage

While the formula for BMI dates to the 19th century, the term "body mass index" for the ratio and its popularity date to a 1972 paper by Ancel Keys, which found the BMI to be the best proxy for body fat percentage among ratios of weight and height; the interest in measuring body fat being due to obesity becoming a discernible issue in prosperous Western societies. BMI was explicitly cited by Keys as being appropriate for population studies, and inappropriate for individual diagnosis. Nevertheless, due to its simplicity, it came to be widely used for individual diagnosis, despite its inappropriateness.

BMI provided a simple numeric measure of a person's "fatness" or "thinness", allowing health professionals to discuss over-and under-weight problems more objectively with their patients. However, BMI has become controversial because many people, including physicians, have come to rely on its apparent numerical authority for medical diagnosis, but that was never the BMI's purpose; it is meant to be used as a simple means of classifying sedentary (physically inactive) individuals with an average body composition. For these individuals, the current value settings are as follows: a BMI of 18.5 to 25 may indicate optimal weight; a BMI lower than 18.5 suggests the person is underweight while a number above 25 may indicate the person is overweight; a BMI below 17.5 may indicate the person has anorexia nervosa or a related disorder; a number above 30 suggests the person is obese (over 40, morbidly obese).

For a given height, BMI is proportional to weight. However,

for a given weight, BMI is inversely proportional to the square of the height. So, if all body dimensions double, and weight scales naturally with the cube of the height, then BMI doubles instead of remaining the same. These results in taller people having a reported BMI that is uncharacteristically high compared to their actual body fat levels. This anomaly is partially offset by the fact that many taller people are not just "scaled up" short people, but tend to have narrower frames in proportion to their height. It has been suggested that instead of squaring the body height (as the BMI does) or cubing the body height (as seems natural and as the Ponderal index does), it would be more appropriate to use an exponent of between 2.3 to 2.7.

BMI Prime

BMI Prime, a simple modification of the BMI system, is the ratio of actual BMI to upper limit BMI (currently defined at BMI 25). As defined, BMI Prime is also the ratio of body weight to upper body weight limit, calculated at BMI 25. Since it is the ratio of two separate BMI values, BMI Prime is a dimensionless number, without associated units. Individuals with BMI Prime < 0.74 are underweight; those between 0.74 and 0.99 have optimal weight; and those at 1.00 or greater are overweight. BMI Prime is useful clinically because individuals can tell, at a glance, by what percentage they deviate from their upper weight limits. For instance, a person with BMI 34 has a BMI Prime of 34/25 = 1.36, and is 36 per cent over his or her upper mass limit. In Asian populations BMI Prime should be calculated using an upper limit BMI of 23 in the denominator instead of 25. Nonetheless, BMI Prime allows easy comparison between populations whose upper limit BMI values differ.

Categories

A frequent use of the BMI is to assess how much an individual's body weight departs from what is normal or desirable for a person of his or her height. The weight excess or deficiency may, in part, be accounted for by body fat (adipose tissue) although other factors such as muscularity also affect BMI significantly. The WHO regard a BMI of less than 18.5 as underweight and may indicate malnutrition, an eating disorder, or other health problems, while a BMI greater than 25 is considered overweight and above 30 is considered obese. These ranges of BMI values are valid only as statistical categories when applied to adults, and do not predict health.

Category	*BMI Range—kg/m2*	*BMI Prime*	*Mass (Weight) of a 1.8 Metres (5 ft 11 in) Person with this BMI*
Severely underweight	less than 16.5	less than 0.66	under 53.5 kilograms (8.42 st; 118 lb)
Underweight	from 16.5 to 18.4	from 0.66 to 0.73	between 53.5 and 60 kilograms (8.42 and 9.45 st; 118 and 132 lb)
Normal	from 18.5 to 24.9	from 0.74 to 0.99	between 60 and 81 kilograms (9.4 and 13 st; 130 and 180 lb)
Overweight	from 25 to 30	from 1.0 to 1.2	between 81 and 97 kilograms (12.8 and 15.3 st; 180 and 210 lb)
Obese Class I	from 30.1 to 34.9	from 1.21 to 1.4	between 97 and 113 kilograms (15.3 and 17.8 st; 210 and 250 lb)
Obese Class II	from 35 to 40	from 1.41 to 1.6	between 113 and 130 kilograms (17.8 and 20.5 st; 250 and 290 lb)
Obese Class III	over 40	over 1.6	over 130 kilograms (20 st; 290 lb)

The U.S. National Health and Nutrition Examination Survey of 1994 indicates that 59 per cent of American men and 49 per cent of women have BMIs over 25. Morbid obesity — a BMI of 40 or more — was found in 2 per cent of the men and 4 per cent of the women. The newest survey in 2007 indicates a continuation of the increase in BMI: 63 per cent of Americans are overweight, with 26 per cent now in the obese category (a BMI of 30 or more). There are differing opinions on the threshold for being underweight in females; doctors quote anything from 18.5 to 20 as being the lowest weight, the most frequently stated being 19. A BMI nearing 15 is usually used as an indicator for starvation and the health risks involved, with a BMI <17.5 being an informal criterion for the diagnosis of anorexia nervosa.

BMI-for-age

BMI is used differently for children. It is calculated the same way as for adults, but then compared to typical values for other children of the same age. Instead of set thresholds for underweight and overweight, then, the BMI percentile allows comparison with children of the same sex and age. A BMI that is less than the 5th percentile is considered underweight and above the 95th percentile is considered obese. Children with a BMI between the 85th and 95th percentile are considered to be overweight.

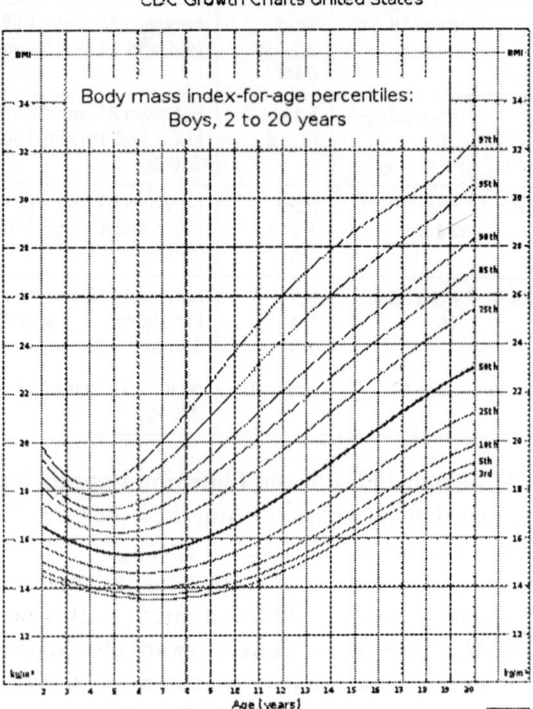

Fig. 2.7: BMI for Age Percentiles for Boys 2 to 20 Years of Age

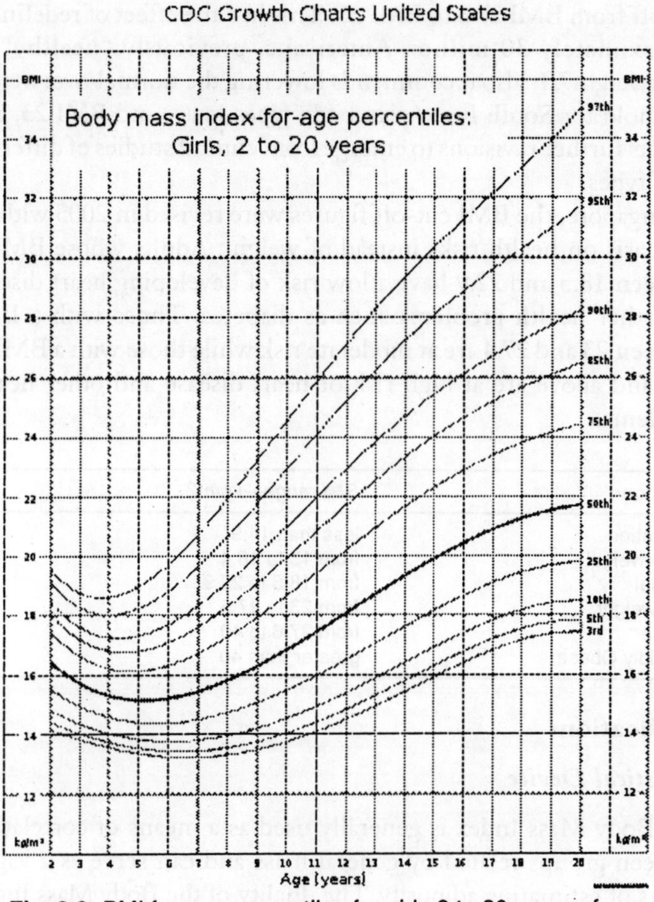

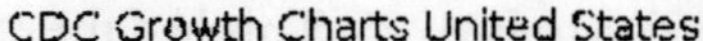

Fig. 2.8: BMI for age percentiles for girls 2 to 20 years of age

Recent studies in Britain have indicated those females between the ages 12 and 16 have a higher BMI than males of the same age by 1.0 kg/m^2 on average.

International Variations

These recommended distinctions along the linear scale may vary from time to time and country to country, making global, longitudinal surveys problematic. In 1998, the U.S. National Institutes of Health brought U.S. definitions into line with World Health Organization guidelines, lowering the normal/overweight cut-off from BMI 27.8 to BMI 25. This had the effect of redefining approximately 30 million Americans, previously "healthy" to "overweight". It also recommends lowering the normal/overweight threshold for South East Asian body types to around BMI 23, and expects further revisions to emerge from clinical studies of different body types.

In Singapore, the BMI cut-off figures were revised in 2005 with an emphasis on health risks instead of weight. Adults whose BMI is between 18.5 and 22.9 have a low risk of developing heart disease and other health problems such as diabetes. Those with a BMI between 23 and 27.4 are at moderate risk while those with a BMI of 27.5 and above are at high risk of heart disease and other health problems.

Category	*BMI range—kg/m2*
Starvation	less than 14.9
Underweight	from 15 to 18.4
Normal	from 18.5 to 22.9
Overweight	from 23 to 27.5
Obese	from 27.6 to 40
Morbidly Obese	greater than 40

Applications

Statistical Device

The Body Mass Index is generally used as a means of correlation between groups related by general mass and can serve as a vague means of estimating adiposity. The duality of the Body Mass Index is that, whilst easy-to-use as a general calculation, it is limited in how accurate and pertinent the data obtained from it can be. Generally, the Index is suitable for recognising trends within sedentary or overweight individuals because there is a smaller margin for errors.

This general correlation is particularly useful for consensus data regarding obesity or various other conditions because it can be used to build a semi-accurate representation from which a solution can be stipulated, or the RDA for a group can be calculated. Similarly, this is becoming more and more pertinent to the growth of children, due to the majority of their exercise habits.

The growth of children is usually documented against a BMI-measured growth chart. Obesity trends can be calculated from the difference between the child's BMI and the BMI on the chart. However, this method again falls prey to the obstacle of body composition: many children who primarily grow as endomorphs would be classed as obese despite body composition. Clinical professionals should take into account the child's body composition and defer to an appropriate technique such as densitometry e.g. Dual energy X-ray absorptiometry, also known as DEXA or DXA.

Clinical Practice

BMI has been used by the WHO as the standard for recording obesity statistics since the early 1980s. In the United States, BMI is also used as a measure of underweight, owing to advocacy on behalf of those suffering with eating disorders, such as anorexia nervosa and bulimia nervosa.

BMI can be calculated quickly and without expensive equipment. However, BMI categories do not take into account many factors such as frame size and muscularity. The categories also fail to account for varying proportions of fat, bone, cartilage, water weight, and more.

Despite this, BMI categories are regularly regarded as a satisfactory tool for measuring whether sedentary individuals are "underweight," "overweight" or "obese" with various qualifications, such as: Individuals who are not sedentary being exempt — athletes, children, the elderly, the infirm, and individuals who are naturally endomorphic or ectomorphic (i.e., people who don't have a medium frame).

One basic problem, especially in athletes, is that muscle is denser than fat. Some professional athletes are "overweight" or "obese" according to their BMI — unless the number at which they are considered "overweight" or "obese" is adjusted upward in some modified version of the calculation. In children and the elderly, differences in bone density and, thus, in the proportion of bone to total weight can mean the number at which these people are considered underweight should be adjusted downward.

Medical Underwriting

In the United States, where medical underwriting of private health insurance plans is widespread, most private health insurance providers will use a particular high BMI as a cut-off point in order to raise insurance rates for or deny insurance to higher-risk patients, thereby ostensibly reducing the cost of insurance coverage to all other subscribers in a 'normal' BMI range. The cutoff point is determined differently for every health insurance provider and different providers will have vastly different ranges of acceptability. Many will implement phased surcharges, in which the subscriber will pay an additional penalty, usually as a percentage of the monthly premium, for each arbitrary range of BMI points above a certain acceptable limit, up to a maximum BMI past which the individual will simply be denied admissibility regardless of price. This can be contrasted with group insurance policies which do not require medical underwriting and where insurance admissibility is guaranteed by virtue of being a member of the insured group, regardless of BMI or other risk factors that would likely render the individual inadmissible to an individual health plan.

Limitations and Shortcomings

Some argue that the error in the BMI is significant and so pervasive that it is not generally useful in evaluation of health. University of Chicago political science professor Eric Oliver says BMI is an inaccurate measure of weight and that academics and doctors have taken the easy way out and that at a minimum the standards of who is overweight and who is not need to be changed and that the US population has been forced to fit into these standards.

The medical establishment has generally acknowledged some shortcomings of BMI. Because the BMI is dependent only upon weight and height, it makes simplistic assumptions about distribution of muscle and bone mass, and thus may overestimate adiposity on those with more lean body mass (e.g. athletes) while underestimating adiposity on those with less lean body mass (e.g. the elderly).

A 2005 study in America showed that overweight people actually had a lower death rate than normal weight people as defined by BMI.

In an analysis of 40 studies involving 250,000 people, heart patients with normal BMIs were at higher risk of death from cardiovascular disease than people whose BMIs put them in the "overweight" range (BMI 25-29.9). In the intermediate range of BMI (25-29.9), BMI failed to discriminate between bodyfat percentage and lean mass. The study concluded that "the accuracy of BMI in diagnosing obesity is limited, particularly for individuals in the intermediate BMI ranges, in men and in the elderly... These results may help to explain the unexpected better survival in overweight/mild obese patients." Patients who were underweight (BMI <20) or severely obese (BMI =35) did, however, show an increased risk of death from cardiovascular disease.

Body composition for athletes is often better calculated using measures of body fat, as determined by such techniques as skinfold measurements or underwater weighing and the limitations of manual measurement have also led to new, alternative methods to measure obesity, such as the body volume index. However, recent studies of American football linemen who undergo intensive weight training to increase their muscle mass show that they frequently suffer many of the same problems as people ordinarily considered obese, notably sleep apnea.

A further limitation relates to loss of height through aging. In this situation, BMI will increase without any corresponding increase in weight.

A study by Romero-Corral et al., using data representing noninstitutionalized civilians in the United States, found that BMI-defined obesity was present in 19.1 per cent of men and 24.7 per cent of women, but that obesity as measured by bodyfat percentage was present in 43.9 per cent of men and 52.3 per cent of women.

The exponent of 2 in the denominator of the formula for BMI is arbitrary. It is meant to reduce variability in the BMI associated only with a difference in size, rather than with differences in weight relative to one's ideal weight. If taller people were simply scaled-up versions of shorter people, the appropriate exponent would be 3, as weight would increase with the cube of height. However, on average, taller people have a slimmer build relative to their height than do shorter people, and the exponent who matches the variation best is between 2 and 3. An analysis based on data gathered in the USA suggested an exponent of 2.6 would yield the best fit for children aged 2 to 19 years old. The exponent 2 is used instead by convention and for simplicity.

As a possible alternative to BMI, the concepts fat-free mass index (FFMI) and fat mass index (FMI) were introduced in the early 1990s.

MALNUTRITION

Malnutrition is a general term for a medical condition caused by an improper or insufficient diet. It most often refers to undernutrition resulting from inadequate consumption, poor absorption, or excessive loss of nutrients, but the term can also encompass overnutrition, resulting from overeating or excessive intake of specific nutrients. An individual will experience malnutrition if the appropriate amount of, or quality of nutrients comprising a healthy diet are not consumed for an extended period of time. An extended period of malnutrition can result in starvation, disease, and infection.

Malnutrition is the lack of sufficient nutrients to maintain healthy bodily functions and is typically associated with extreme poverty in economically developing countries. It is a common cause of reduced intelligence in parts of the world affected by famine. Malnutrition as the result of inappropriate dieting, overeating or the absence of a "balanced diet" is often observed in economically developed countries (eg. as indicated by increasing levels of obesity).

Most commonly, malnourished people either do not have enough calories in their diet, or are eating a diet that lacks protein, vitamins, or trace minerals. Medical problems arising from malnutrition are commonly referred to as deficiency diseases. Scurvy is a well-known and now rare form of malnutrition, in which the victim is deficient in vitamin C.

Common forms of malnutrition include protein-energy malnutrition (PEM) and micronutrient malnutrition. PEM refers to inadequate availability or absorption of energy and proteins in the body. Micronutrient malnutrition refers to inadequate availability of some essential nutrients such as vitamins and trace elements that are required by the body in small quantities. Micronutrient deficiencies lead to a variety of diseases and impair normal functioning of the body. Deficiency in micronutrients such as Vitamin A reduces the capacity of the body to resist diseases. Deficiency in iron, iodine and vitamin A is widely prevalent and represent a major public health challenge. An array of afflictions ranging from stunted growth, reduced intelligence and various cognitive abilities, reduced sociability, reduced leadership and assertiveness, reduced activity and energy, reduced muscle growth and strength, and poorer health overall are directly implicated to nutrient deficiencies. Also, another, although rare, effect of malnutrition is black spots appearing on the skin.

Hunger is the normal psychological response brought on by the physiological condition of needing food. Hunger can also affect the mental state of a person, and is often used as a metonym for general undernourishment.

According to the World Health Organization, hunger and malnutrition is the gravest single threat to the world's public health and malnutrition is by far the biggest contributor to child mortality, present in half of all cases.

Politics

As of 2008, malnutrition continues to be a worldwide problem, particularly in lesser developed countries. According to the Food and Agriculture Organization of the United Nations, "850 million people worldwide were undernourished in 1999 to 2005, the most recent years for which figures are available" and the number of malnourished people has recently been increasing. An orange awareness ribbon is used to raise awareness of malnutrition in the world. The FAO calculates undernourishment by comparing the amount of food available in a country at national level with how many people live in the country.

Some environmentalists claim that the fundamental issue causing malnutrition is that the human population exceeds the Earth's carrying capacity; however, Food First raises the issue of food sovereignty and claims that every country (with the possible minor exceptions of some city-states) has sufficient agricultural capacity to feed its own people, but that the "free trade" economic order associated with such institutions as the International Monetary Fund (IMF) and the World Bank prevent this from happening. At the other end of the spectrum, the World Bank itself claims to be part of the solution to malnutrition, asserting that the best way for countries to succeed in breaking the cycle of poverty and malnutrition is to build export-led economies that will give them the financial means to buy foodstuffs on the world market.

Amartya Sen won a 1998 Nobel Prize in part for his work suggesting that famine is not typically the product of a lack of food; rather, famine may arise from problems in food distribution networks or from governmental policies in the developing world.

The politics of food trade and food security are often difficult to grasp. Many people believe that sending food aid to the poor of the world is a worthy idea, but that each country should produce its own food.

Countries that have become more open to international trade in recent years (e.g. China, Vietnam or Peru) have greatly reduced the prevalence of undernourishment as measured by the FAO (food energy consumption below acceptable minimum) or as measured by the World Health Organization by the percentage of children under five who are stunted, wasted or underweight. Countries that remained closed to external trade (e.g. North Korea) have not improved or have worsened their food situation.

Some anti-globalization groups advocate "food sovereignty", stating that each country should be physically self sufficient in every food item consumed by their people; by this measure the United States, United Kingdom, Sweden, Belgium, and in fact almost all other countries in the world would be food insecure, and a desert nation like Saudi Arabia (with its current population) would not be viable as a country at all.

One policy adopted in recent decades to alleviate world malnutrition is food aid, i.e. the physical donation of food from rich to poor countries. From the rich donor countries' point of view, this is a suitable way to reduce excess supply created by domestic agricultural subsidies, stabilizing farm prices in rich countries, even if the cost of supplying the food to its final beneficiaries is often disproportionately high. Food aid may be provided for short-term emergencies (natural disasters like earthquakes, tsunamis, droughts and floods, or human-made like war and refugee flows) or in the form of a long-term programme for an extended period. From the viewpoint of recipient countries, the value of food-aid depends on the form it takes. Emergency food aid is welcome, though aid in cash may also be welcome because the food may often be purchased locally in zones not affected by the emergency, thus benefitting local farmers. Long-term foreign food aid has been criticized as discouraging local production and distorting markets. Instead, population control has been advocated as a much better approach to solve malnutrition/famine than merely providing food.

Effects

Mortality Due to Malnutrition

According to the World Health Organization, hunger is the gravest single threat to the world's public health. According to Jean Ziegler (the United Nations Special Rapporteur on the Right to Food for 2000 to March 2008), mortality due to malnutrition accounted for 58 per cent of the total mortality in 2006: "In the world, approximately 62 millions people, all causes of death combined, die each year. One in twelve people worldwide are malnourished. In 2006, more than 36 millions died of hunger or diseases due to deficiencies in micronutrients". The World Health Organization estimates that one-third of the world is well-fed, one-third is under-fed and one-third is starving. Every 3.6 seconds someone dies of hunger.

Hunger and malnutrition have an even bigger impact on children's health than was previously thought. According to the World Health Organization, malnutrition is by far the biggest contributor to child mortality, present in half of all cases. Underweight births and inter-uterine growth restrictions cause 2.2 million child deaths a year. Poor or non-existent breastfeeding causes another 1.4 million. Other deficiencies, such as lack of vitamin A or zinc, for example, account for 1 million. According to The Lancet, malnutrition in the first two years is irreversible. Malnourished children grow up with worse health and lower educational achievements. Their own children also tend to be smaller. Hunger was previously seen as something that exacerbates the problems of diseases such as measles, pneumonia and diarrhea. But malnutrition actually causes diseases as well, and can be fatal in its own right. This is the impact The Lancet seeks to identify.

Biological Effects

An extended period of malnutrition can result in starvation or deficiency diseases such as scurvy. Malnutrition increases the risk of infection and infectious disease; for example, it is a major risk factor in the onset of active tuberculosis.

Malnutrition appears to increase activity and movement in many animals—for example an experiment on spiders showed increased activity and predation in starved spiders, resulting in larger weight gain. This pattern is seen in many animals, including humans while sleeping. It even occurs in rats with their cerebral cortex or stomachs completely removed. Increased activity on hamster wheels occurred when rats were deprived not only of food, but also water or B vitamins such as thiamine This response may increase the animal's chance of finding food, though it has also been speculated the emigration response relieves pressure on the home population.

Action on Malnutrition

In recent years many foods, such as Spirulina and peanut butter, have been developed or refined for mass-production in hopes of combatting malnutrition and its effects.

Breast-feeding advice, food supplements and better hygiene all make a big difference. Most countries know what to do and run pilot programmes that work. But they rarely find the money for full-scale national efforts; the international outfits that might help are, in the words of the medical journal, The Lancet, fragmented and dysfunctional.

According to The Lancet's research, money for improving nutrition would be the most effective sort of aid. At the moment, roughly $300 million of aid goes to basic nutrition each year, less than $2 for each child below two in the 20 worst affected countries. In contrast, HIV/AIDS, which causes fewer deaths than child malnutrition, received $2.2 billion—$67 per person with HIV in all countries, including rich ones.

Statistics

Number of undernourished people (million) in 2001-2003, according to the FAO, the following countries had 5 million or more undernourished people:

Country	*Number of Undernourished (million)*
India	217.00
China	150.0
Bangladesh	43.1
Democratic Republic of Congo	37.0
Pakistan	35.2
Ethiopia	31.5
Tanzania	16.1
Philippines	15.2
Brazil	14.4
Indonesia	13.8
Vietnam	13.8
Thailand	13.4
Nigeria	11.5
Kenya	9.7
Sudan	8.8
Mozambique	8.3
North Korea	7.9
Yemen	7.1
Madagascar	7.1
Colombia	5.9
Zimbabwe	5.7
México	5.1
Zambia	5.1
Angola	5.0

Note: This table measures "undernourishment", as defined by FAO, and represents the number of people consuming (on average for years 2001 to 2003) less than the minimum amount of food energy (measured in kilocalories per capita per day) necessary for the average person to stay in good health while performing light physical activity. It is a conservative indicator that does not take into account the extra needs of people performing extraneous physical activity, nor seasonal variations in food consumption or other sources of variability such as inter-individual differences in energy requirements.

Malnutrition and undernourishment are cumulative or average situations, and not the work of a single day's food intake (or lack thereof). This table does not represent the number of people who "went to bed hungry today."

The U.S. Department of Agriculture reported that in 2003, only 1 out of 200 U.S. households with children became so severely food insecure that any of the children went hungry even once during the year. A substantially larger proportion of these same households (3.8%) had adult members who were hungry at least one day during the year because of their households' inability to afford enough food.

Overnourished vs Undernourished

In 2006, Professor Popkin from the University of North Carolina, said there were now more overweight people across the world than undernourished people. He told the International Association of Agricultural Economists the number of overweight people had topped one billion (of which 300 million are obese), compared with 800 million undernourished. He added this transition from a starving world to an obese one was accelerating.

PROTEIN-ENERGY MALNUTRITION

Protein-energy malnutrition refers to a form of malnutrition where there is inadequate protein intake.

Types include:

- Kwashiorkor
- Marasmus

Note that this may also be secondary to other conditions such as chronic renal disease or cancer cachexia in which protein energy wasting may occur.

KWASHIORKOR

Kwashiorkor is a virulent form of childhood malnutrition characterized by edema, irritability, anorexia, ulcerating dermatoses, and an enlarged liver with fatty infiltrates. The presence of edema caused by poor nutrition defines kwashiorkor. The cause of kwashiorkor was thought to be due to insufficient protein consumption alone, however micronutrient and antioxidant deficiencies are now believed to play important roles.

Jamaican pediatrician Cicely D. Williams introduced the name into the medical community in her 1935 Lancet article. The name is derived from the Ga language of coastal Ghana, translated literally "first-second", and reflecting the development of the condition in an older child who has been weaned from the breast when a younger sibling comes. Breast milk contains proteins and amino acids vital to a child's growth. In at-risk populations, kwashiorkor may develop after a mother weans her child from breast milk and replaces the diet with foods high in starches and carbohydrates and deficient in protein.

Signs and Symptoms

The defining sign of kwashiorkor in a malnourished child is pedal edema (swelling of the feet). Other signs include a distended abdomen, an enlarged liver with fatty infiltrates, thinning hair, and loss of teeth, skin depigmentation and dermatitis. Children with kwashiorkor often develop irritability and anorexia.

Victims of kwashiorkor fail to produce antibodies following vaccination against diseases, including diphtheria and typhoid. Generally, the disease can be treated by adding food energy and protein to the diet; however, it can have a long-term impact on a child's physical and mental development, and in severe cases may lead to death.

Possible Causes

There are various explanations for the development of kwashiorkor, and the topic remains controversial. It is now accepted that protein deficiency, in combination with energy and micronutrient deficiency, is necessary but not sufficient to cause kwashiorkor. The condition is likely due to deficiency of one of several types of nutrients (e.g., iron, folic acid, iodine, selenium, vitamin C), particularly those involved with anti-oxidant protection. Important anti-oxidants in the body that are reduced in children with kwashiorkor include glutathione, albumin, vitamin E and polyunsaturated fatty acids. Therefore, if a child with reduced type one nutrients or anti-oxidants is exposed to stress (e.g. an infection or toxin) he/she is more liable to develop kwashiorkor.

Ignorance of nutrition can be a cause. Dr. Latham, director of the Programme in International Nutrition at Cornell University cited a case where parents who fed their child cassava failed to recognize malnutrition because of the edema caused by the syndrome and insisted the child was well-nourished despite the lack of dietary protein.

One important factor in the development of kwashiorkor is aflatoxin poisoning. Aflatoxins are produced by molds and ingested with moldy foods. They are toxified by the cytochrome P450 system in the liver, the resulting epoxides damage liver DNA. Since many serum proteins, in particular albumin, are produced in the liver, the symptoms of kwashiorkor are easily explained. It is noteworthy that kwashiorkor occurs mostly in warm, humid climates that encourage mold growth. In dry climates, marasmus is the more frequent disease associated with malnutrition. This has important consequences for treatment of the patients. Protein should be supplied only for anabolic purposes. The catabolic needs should be satisfied with carbohydrate and fat. Protein catabolism involves the urea cycle, which is located in the liver and can easily overwhelm the capacity of an already damaged organ. The resulting liver failure can be fatal.

Other malnutrition syndromes include marasmus and cachexia, although the latter is often caused by underlying illnesses.

MARASMUS

Marasmus is a form of severe protein-energy malnutrition characterized by energy deficiency.

A child with marasmus looks emaciated. Body weight may be reduced to less than 80 per cent of the normal weight for that height. Marasmus occurrence increases prior to age 1, whereas kwashiorkor occurrence increases after 18 months.

The prognosis is better than it is in kwashiorkor.

Signs and Symptoms

The malnutrition associated with marasmus leads to extensive tissue and muscle wasting, as well as variable edema. Other common characteristics include dry skin, loose skin folds hanging over the glutei, axillae, etc. There is also drastic loss of adipose tissue from normal areas of fat deposits like buttocks and thighs. The afflicted are often fretful, irritable, and voraciously hungry.

Treatment

It is necessary to treat not only the symptoms but also the complications of the disorder, including infections, dehydration, and circulation disorders, which are frequently lethal and lead to high mortality if ignored.

Ultimately, marasmus can progress to the point of no return when the body's machinery for protein synthesis, itself made of protein, has been degraded to the point that it cannot handle any protein. At this point, attempts to correct the disorder by giving food or protein are futile.

Causes

Marasmus is caused by a severe deficiency of nearly all nutrients, especially protein and calories.

STARVATION

Starvation is a severe reduction in vitamin, nutrient, and energy intake. It is the most extreme form of malnutrition. In humans, prolonged starvation can cause permanent organ damage, and eventually death. The term *inanition* refers to the symptoms and effects of starvation.

According to the World Health Organization, hunger is the gravest single threat to the world's public health. The WHO also states that malnutrition is by far the biggest contributor to child mortality, present in half of all cases. According to the FAO, starvation currently affects more than one billion people or 1 of 6 people.

Common Causes

The basic cause of starvation is imbalance between energy intake and energy expenditure. In other words: the body spends more energy than it takes in as food. This imbalance can arise from a medical condition or circumstantial situation, some of which include:

Medical Causes

- Anorexia nervosa
- Bulimia nervosa
- Coma
- Depression
- Diabetes mellitus
- Digestive disease

Circumstantial Causes

- Famine for any reason, including overpopulation and war.
- Fasting, when done without proper medical supervision and lasting more than a month.
- Poverty
- Deprivation

Signs and Symptoms

Individuals experiencing starvation lose substantial fat (adipose) and muscle mass as the body breaks down these tissues for energy. *Catabolysis* is the process of a body breaking down its own muscles and other tissues in order to keep vital systems such as the nervous system and heart muscle (myocardium) functioning. Vitamin deficiency is a common result of starvation, often leading to anemia, beriberi, pellagra, and scurvy. These diseases collectively can also cause diarrhoea, skin rashes, edema, and heart failure. Individuals are often irritable and lethargic as a result.

Atrophy (wasting away) of the stomach weakens the perception of hunger, since the perception is controlled by the percentage of the stomach that is empty. Victims of starvation are often too weak to sense thirst, and therefore become dehydrated.

All movements become painful due to atrophy of the muscles, and due to dry, cracked skin caused by severe dehydration. With a weakened body, diseases are commonplace. Fungi, for example, often grow under the esophagus, making swallowing unbearably painful.

The energy deficiency inherent in starvation causes fatigue and renders the victim more apathetic over time. Interaction with one's surroundings diminishes as the starving person becomes too weak to move or even eat.

Biochemistry

The body's glycogen stores are used up in about 24 hours. The level of insulin in circulation is low and the level of glucagon is very high. The main means of energy production is lipolysis. Gluconeogenesis converts glycerol into glucose and the Cori cycle converts lactate into usable glucose. Two systems of energy enter the gluconeogenesis; proteolysis provides alanine and lactate produced from pyruvate. Acetyl CoA produces dissolved nutrients (Ketone bodies), which can be detected in urine and are used by the brain as a source of energy.

In terms of insulin resistance, a starvation condition makes more glucose available to the brain.

Efforts

Treatment

Starving patients can be treated, but this must be done cautiously to avoid refeeding syndrome.

Prevention

Supporting farmers in areas of food insecurity, through such measures as free or subsidized fertilizers and seeds, increases food harvest and reduces food prices. For example, in Malawi, almost five million of its 13 million people needed emergency food aid. Then, however, deep fertilizer subsidies and lesser ones for seed abetted by good rains, helped farmers produce record-breaking corn harvests in 2006 and 2007, according to government crop estimates. Corn production leapt to 2.7 million metric tons in 2006 and 3.4 million in 2007 from 1.2 million in 2005, the government reported. The harvest also helped the poor by lowering food prices and increasing wages for farm workers. Malawi became a major food exporter, selling more corn to the World Food Programme and the United Nations than any other country in Southern Africa. Over the 20 years prior to this change in policy by the World Bank and some rich nations Malawi depended on for aid have periodically pressed it to cut back or eliminate fertilizer subsidies, in the name of free market policies even as the United States and Europe extensively subsidized their own farmers. However, many, if not most, of its farmers are too poor to afford fertilizer at market prices. Proponents for helping the farmers include the economist Jeffrey Sachs, who has championed the idea that wealthy countries should invest in fertilizer and seed for Africa's farmers. He also conceived the Millennium Villages Project (MVP), which good seeds, fertilizers, and trains farmers how to use them. In a Kenyan village, where this was experimented, the project resulted in a tripling of its corn harvest, even though the village had previously had a cycle of hunger.

Organizations

Many organizations have been highly effective at reducing starvation in different regions. Aid agencies give direct assistance to individuals, while political organizations pressure political leaders to enact policies that will reduce famine and provide aid.

Hunger Statistics

In 2007, 923 million people were reported as being undernourished, an increase of 80 million since 1990-92.. It has also been recorded that the world already produces enough food support the world's population—6 billion people—and could support double—12 billion people.

Year	*Share of Hungry People in the Developing World*
1970	37 %
1980	28 %
1990	20 %
2005	16 %
2007	17 %

Hunger Mortality Statistics

- On the average, 1 person dies every second as a result of hunger—4000 every hour—100 000 each day—36 million each year—58 per cent of all deaths (2001-2004 estimates).
- On the average, 1 child dies every 5 seconds as a result of hunger—700 every hour—16 000 each day—6 million each year—60 per cent of all child deaths (2002-2008 estimates).

As Capital Punishment

Historically, starvation has been used as a death sentence. From the beginning of civilization to the Middle Ages, people were immured, or walled in, and would die for want of food.

In ancient Greco-Roman societies, starvation was sometimes used to dispose of guilty upper class citizens, especially erring female members of patrician families. For instance, in the year 31, Livilla, the niece and daughter-in-law of Tiberius, was discreetly starved to death by her mother for her adulterous relationship with Sejanus and for her complicity in the murder of her own husband, Drusus the Younger.

Another daughter-in-law of Tiberius, named Agrippina the Elder (a granddaughter of Augustus and the mother of Caligula), also died of starvation, in 33 AD. (However, it is not clear whether her starvation was self inflicted.)

A son and daughter of Agrippina were also executed by starvation for political reasons; Drusus Caesar, her second son, was put in prison in 33 AD, and starved to death by orders of Tiberius (he managed to stay alive for nine days by chewing the stuffing of his bed); Agrippina's youngest daughter, Julia Livilla, was exiled on an island in 41 by her uncle, Emperor Claudius, and not much later, her death by starvation was arranged by the empress Messalina.

It is also possible that Vestal Virgins were starved when found guilty of breaking their vows of celibacy.

Maximilian Kolbe, a Polish friar, offered his life to save another inmate sentenced to death in the Auschwitz concentration camp.

He was starved, along with another nine inmates. After two weeks of starvation, only Kolbe and three other inmates were still alive, and were executed with phenol injection.

Ugolino della Gherardesca, his sons and other members of his family were immured in the Muda, a tower of Pisa, and starved to death in the thirteenth century. Dante, his contemporary, wrote about Gherardesca in his masterpiece *The Divine Comedy.*

In Sweden in 1317, King Birger of Sweden imprisoned his two brothers for a coup they had staged several years earlier (Nyköping Banquet). A few weeks later, they died of starvation.

In Cornwall in 1671, John Trehenban from St Columb Major was condemned to be starved to death in a cage at Castle An Dinas for the murder of two girls.

HYPERALIMENTATION

Hyperalimentation refers to a state where quantities consumed are greater than appropriate. It includes overeating, as well as other routes of administration such as in parenteral nutrition. This term can also be used to describe ingestion to compensate for past deficiencies. In this context, it can refer to parenteral nutrition, though this has been described as incorrect. This is a procedure in which nutrients and vitamins are given to a person in liquid form through a vein. It is a medical procedure used for individuals who cannot get nutrients from food. This is done mainly due to impaired gastrointestinal (GI) conditions such as severe malabsorption, progressed eating disorders, etc, (since tube feeding is often preferred for non-GI related conditions).

It is a frequent iatrogenic cause of normal anion gap metabolic acidosis.

Hyperalimentation can also cause an osmotic diuresis due to an increased load of urea from protein catabolism. Frequently, it is also associated with opportunistic infections by Candida albicans.

FOOD INTOLERANCE

Food intolerance or non-allergic food hypersensitivity is a delayed, negative reaction to a food, beverage or food additive. It can involve symptoms in one or more body organs and systems, but is not a true allergy.

Intolerance can result from the absence of specific chemicals or enzymes needed to digest a food substance, or from reactions to naturally occurring chemicals in foods.

The precise distinction between food intolerance and a food allergy is often missed. A true food allergy requires the presence of IgE antibodies against the food. All other hypersensitivities or negative pharmacological reactions to foods can be considered food intolerances.

Definitions

Non-allergic food hypersensitivity is the medical name for food intolerance, loosely referred to as food hypersensitivity, or previously as pseudo-allergic reactions. Non-allergic food hypersensitivity should not be confused with allergic responses to foods as occurs with a food allergy.

A food allergy is an immunological hypersensitivity which occurs most commonly in response to food proteins such as those found in egg, milk, seafood, shellfish, tree nuts, soya, wheat and peanuts. True allergies are associated with a fast-acting immunoglobulin E (IgE) antibody response.

A non-allergic food hypersensitivity is an abnormal physiological response to food that does not involve an actual allergy. It can be difficult to determine the offending food causing an intolerance reaction because if the immune system is involved, the response is likely to be IgG-mediated and takes place slowly. Thus the causative agent and the response are separated in time, and may not be obviously related. Food intolerance reactions can include pharmacologic, metabolic, and toxic responses to foods or food components. Food intolerance does not include psychological responses.

- *Metabolic food reactions* are due to inborn or acquired errors of metabolism of nutrients, such as in diabetes melitus, lactase deficiency, phenylketonuria and favism. Toxic food reactions are caused by the direct action of a food or additive without immune involvement.

- *Pharmacological reactions* are generally due to low-molecular-weight chemicals which occur either as natural compounds, such as salicylates and amines, or to artificially added substances, such as preservatives, colouring, emulsifiers and taste enhancers (including glutamate [MSG]). These chemicals are capable of causing drug-like (biochemical) side effects in susceptible individuals.
- *Toxins* may either be present naturally in food, be released by bacteria, or be due to contamination of food products.
- *Psychological reactions* involve manifestation of clinical symptoms caused not by food but by emotions associated with food. These symptoms do not occur when the food is given in an unrecognisable form.

Elimination diets are useful to assist in the diagnosis of food allergies and pharmacological food intolerance. Metabolic, toxic and psychological reactions can be diagnosed by other means.

Signs and Symptoms

Non-IgE-mediated food hypersensitivity (food intolerance) is more chronic, less acute, less obvious in its presentation, and often more difficult to diagnose than a food allergy. Symptoms of food intolerance vary greatly, and can be mistaken for the symptoms of a food allergy. While true allergies are associated with fast-acting immunoglobulin IgE responses, it can be difficult to determine the offending food causing food intolerance because the response generally takes place over a prolonged period of time. Thus the causative agent and the response are separated in time, and may not be obviously related. Food intolerance symptoms usually begin about half an hour after eating or drinking the food in question, but sometimes symptoms may delay up to 48 h.

Food intolerance can present with symptoms affecting the skin, respiratory tract, gastrointestinal tract (GIT) either individually or in combination. On the skin may include skin rashes, urticaria (hives), angioedema, dermatitis , eczema. Respiratory tract symptoms can include nasal congestion, sinusitis, pharyngeal irritations, asthma and an unproductive cough. GIT symptoms include mouth ulcers, abdominal cramp, nausea, gas, intermittent diarrhea, constipation, and irritable bowel syndrome., and may include anaphylaxis

Food intolerance has been found associated with; irritable bowel syndrome and inflammatory bowel disease, chronic constipation, chronic hepatitis C infection , eczema , NSAID intolerance and respiratory complaints including asthma., rhinitis and headache, functional dyspepsia, eosinophilic esophagitis and ENT illnesses.

Causes

Reactions to chemical components of the diet are more common than true food allergies. They are caused by various organic chemicals occurring naturally in a wide variety of foods, both of animal and vegetable origin more often than to food additives, preservatives, colourings and flavourings, such as sulfites or dyes. Both natural and artificial ingredients may cause adverse reactions in sensitive people if consumed in sufficient amount, the degree of sensitivity varying between individuals.

Chemical intolerance can occur in individuals from both allergic and non-allergic family backgrounds. Symptoms may begin at any age, and may develop quickly or slowly. Triggers may range from a viral infection or illness to environmental chemical exposure. It occurs more commonly in women and may be because of hormone differences, as many food chemicals mimic hormones.

A deficiency in digestive enzymes can also cause some types of food intolerances. Dietary carbohydrate intolerances include, Lactose intolerance is a result of the body not producing sufficient lactase to digest the lactose in milk; dairy foods which are lower in lactose, such as cheese, are less likely to trigger a reaction in this case. Coeliac disease (gluten intolerance) results in damage to villi in the small intestine, which makes it difficult for the body to absorb water and nutrients from foods, and fructose intolerance.

The most widely distributed naturally occurring food chemical capable of provoking reactions is salicylate, although tartrazine and benzoic acid are well recognised in susceptable individuals.. Benzoates and salicylates occur naturally in many different foods, including fruits, juices, vegetables, spices, herbs, nuts, tea, wines, and coffee. Salicylate sensitivity causes reactions to not only aspirin and NSAID's but also foods in which salicylates naturally occur, such as cherries.

Other natural chemicals which commonly cause reactions and cross reactivity include amines, nitrates, sulphites and some anti-oxidants. Chemicals involved in aroma and flavour are often suspected.

The classification or avoidance of foods based on botanical families bears no relationship to their chemical content and is not relevant in the management of food intolerance.

Salicylate-containing foods include apples, citrus fruits, strawberries, tomatoes, and wine, while reactions to chocolate, cheese, bananas, avocado, tomato or wine point to amines as the likely food chemical. Thus exclusion of single foods does not necessarily identify the chemical responsible as several chemicals can be present in a food; the patient may be sensitive to multiple food chemicals and reaction more likely to occur when foods containing the triggering substance are eaten in a combined quantity that exceeds the patient's sensitivity thresholds. People with food sensitivities have different sensitivity thresholds, and so more sensitive people will react to much smaller amounts of the substance.

Pathogenesis

The term food allergy is widely misused for all sorts of symptoms and diseases caused by food. Food allergy (FA) is an adverse reaction to food (food hypersensitivity) occurring in susceptible individuals, which is mediated by a classical immune mechanism specific for the food itself. The best established mechanism in FA is due to the presence of IgE antibodies against the offending food. Food intolerance (FI) is all non-immune-mediated adverse reactions to food. The subgroups of FI are enzymatic (e.g. lactose intolerance due to lactase deficiency), pharmacological (e.g. reactions against biogenic amines, histamine intolerance), and undefined food intolerance (e.g. against some food additives).

Food intolerances are mainly caused by enzymatic defects in the digestive system, (e.g. lactose (milk sugar) intolerance), but may also result from pharmacological effects of vasoactive amines present in foods (e.g. Histamine).

A frequent misconception among the general public is confusion between cow's milk allergy (CMA) and cow's milk intolerance, which is mainly intolerance to lactose. There are at least two, and possibly more, distinct pathologies. Hypersensitivity to milk is often broadly classified into immunoglobulin E (IgE)-mediated allergy and non-IgE-mediated allergy/intolerance. The immunopathological mechanisms of non-IgE-mediated allergy/intolerance in particular remain poorly understood, and this has hindered the development of simple and reliable diagnostics. Adults with non-IgE-mediated allergy/intolerance to milk tend to suffer ongoing allergy without the development of milk tolerance. The precise immunopathological mechanisms of non-IgE-mediated intolerance remain unclear. A number of mechanisms have been implicated, including type-1 T helper cell (Th1) mediated reactions, the formation of immune complexes leading to the activation of Complement, or T-cell/mast cell/neuron interactions inducing functional changes in smooth muscle action and intestinal motility. Food antigens contact the immune system throughout the intestinal tract via the gut associated lymphoid system (GALT), where interactions between antigen presenting cells and T cells direct the type of immune response mounted. Unresponsiveness of the immune system to dietary antigens is termed "oral tolerance" and is believed to involve the deletion or switching off of reactive antigen-specific T cells and the production of regulatory T cells (T reg) that quell inflammatory responses to benign antigens. In the case of IgE-mediated allergies, a deficiency in regulation and a polarisation of specific effector T cells towards type-2 T helper cells (Th2) lead to signalling of B-cells to produce milk protein-specific IgE. Where as non-IgE-mediated reactions (intolerances) may be due to Th1 mediated inflammation. Dysfunctional T reg cell activity has been identified as a factor in both allergy/intolerance mechanisms.

Diagnosis

Diagnosis is made using medical history and cutaneous and serological tests to exclude other causes, but to obtain final confirmation a Double Blind Controlled Food Challenge must be performed. It is important to be able to distinguish between food allergy, food intolerance, and autoimmune disease in the management of these disorders. Non-IgE-mediated food hypersensitivity (food intolerance) is more chronic, less acute, less obvious in its clinical presentation, and often more difficult to diagnose than allergy, skin tests and immunological studies are not helpful.

Diagnosis can include an elimination diet and challenge testing. The antigen leukocyte cellular antibody test (ALCAT) has been commercially promoted as an alternative, but has not been reliably shown to be of clinical value. Clinical investigation is generally undertaken only for more serious cases, as for minor complaints which do not significantly limit the person's lifestyle the cure may be more inconvenient than the problem. Treatment can involve avoidance, and re-establishing a level of tolerance.

Testing of IgG4 to foods is considered irrelevant in the laboratory work-up of food intolerance and should not be performed in case of food-related complaints. In contrast to the disputed beliefs, IgG4 against foods indicates that the person has been repeatedly exposed to food components, recognized as foreign proteins by the immune system. Its presence should not be considered as a factor which induces hypersensitivity, but rather as an indicator for immunological tolerance, linked to the activity of T cells. In conclusion, food-specific IgG4 does not indicate (imminent) food allergy or intolerance, but rather a physiological response of the immune system after exposure to food components.

Prevention

There is emerging evidence from studies of cord bloods that both sensitization and the acquisition of tolerance can begin in pregnancy, however the window of main danger for sensitization to foods extends prenatally, remaining most critical during early infancy when the immune system and intestinal tract are still maturing. There is no conclusive evidence to support the restriction of dairy intake in the maternal diet during pregnancy in order to prevent. This is generally not recommended since the drawbacks in terms of loss of nutrition can out-weigh the benefits. However, further randomised, controlled trials are required to examine if dietary exclusion by lactating mothers can truly minimize risk to a significant degree and if any reduction in risk is out-weighed by deleterious impacts on maternal nutrition.

A Cochrane review has concluded feeding with a soy formula cannot be recommended for prevention of allergy or food intolerance in infants. Further research may be warranted to determine the role of soy formulas for prevention of allergy or food intolerance in infants unable to be breast fed with a strong family history of allergy or cow's milk protein intolerance. In the case of allergy and celiac disease others recommend a dietary regimen is effective in the prevention of allergic diseases in high-risk infants, particularly in early infancy regarding food allergy and eczema. The most effective dietary regimen is exclusively breastfeeding for at least 4-6 months or, in absence of breast milk, formulas with documented reduced allergenicity for at least the first 4 months, combined with avoidance of solid food and cow's milk for the first 4 months.

Treatment or Management

Individuals can try minor changes of diet to exclude foods causing obvious reactions, and for many this may be adequate without the need for professional assistance. For reasons mentioned above foods causing problems may not be so obvious since food sensitivities may not be noticed for hours or even days after one has digested food. Persons unable to isolate foods and those more sensitive or with disabling symptoms should seek expert medical and dietitian help. The dietetic department of a teaching hospital is a good start.

Guidance can also be given to your general practitioner to assist in diagnosis and management. Food elimination diets have been designed to exclude food chemicals likely to cause reactions and foods commonly causing true allergies and those foods where enzyme deficiency causes symptoms. These elimination diets are not every-day diets but intended to isolate problem foods and chemicals. Avoidance of foods with additives is also essential in this process.

Individuals and practitioners need to be aware that during the elimination process patients can display aspects of food addiction, masking, withdrawals, and further sensitization and intolerance. Those foods that an individual considers as 'must have every day' are suspect addictions; this includes tea, coffee, chocolate and health foods and drinks, as they all contain food chemicals. Individuals are also unlikely to associate foods causing problems because of masking or where separation of time between eating and symptoms occur. The elimination process can overcome addiction and unmask problem foods so that the patients can associate cause and effect.

It takes around five days of total abstinence to unmask a food or chemical, during the first week on an elimination diet withdrawal symptoms can occur but it takes at least two weeks to remove residual traces. If symptoms have not subsided after six weeks, food intolerance is unlikely involved and a normal diet should be restarted. Withdrawals are often associated with a lowering of the threshold for sensitivity which assists in challenge testing, but in this period individuals can be ultra-sensitive even to food smells so care must be taken to avoid all exposures.

After two or more weeks if the symptoms have reduced considerably or gone for at least five days then challenge testing can begin. This can be carried out with selected foods containing only one food chemical, so as to isolate it if reactions occur. In Australia, purified food chemicals in capsule form are available to doctors for patient testing. These are often combined with placebo capsules for control purposes. This type of challenge is more definitive. New challenges should only be given after 48 hours if no reactions occur or after five days of no symptoms if reactions occur.

Once all food chemical sensitivities are identified a dietitian can prescribe an appropriate diet for the individual to avoid foods with those chemicals. Lists of suitable foods are available from various hospitals and patient support groups can give local food brand advice. A dietitian will ensure adequate nutrition is achieved with safe foods and supplements if need be.

Over a period of time it is possible for individuals avoiding food chemicals to build up a level of resistance by regular exposure to small amounts in a controlled way, but care must be taken, the aim being to build up a varied diet with adequate composition.

Prognosis

The prognosis of children diagnosed with intolerance to milk is good: patients respond to diet which excludes cow's milk protein and the majority of patients succeed in forming tolerance. Children with non-IgE-mediated cows milk intolerance have a good prognosis, whereas children with IgE-mediated cows milk allergy in early childhood have a significantly increased risk for persistent allergy, development of other food allergies, asthma and rhinoconjunctivitis.

A study has demonstrated that identifying and appropriately addressing food sensit in IBS patients not previously responding to standard therapy results in a sustained clinical improvement and increased overall well being and quality of life.

Epidemiology

Estimates of the prevalence of food intolerance vary widely from 2 per cent to over 20 per cent of the population. So far only three prevalence studies in Dutch and English adults have been based on double-blind, placebo-controlled food challenges. The reported prevalence's of food allergy/intolerance (by questionnaires) were 12 per cent to 19 per cent, whereas the confirmed prevalence varied from 0.8 per cent to 2.4 per cent. For intolerance to food additives the prevalence varied between 0.01 to 0.23 per cent.

Food intolerance rates were found to be similar in the population in Norway. Out of 4,622 subjects with adequately filled-in questionnaires, 84 were included in the study (1.8%) Perceived food intolerance is a common problem with significant nutritional consequences in a population with IBS. Of these 59 (70%) had symptoms related to intake of food, 62 per cent limited or excluded food items from the diet. Tests were performed for food allergy and malabsorption, but not for intolerance. There were no associations between the tests for food allergy and malabsorption and perceived food intolerance, among those with IBS. Perceived food intolerance was unrelated to musculoskeletal pain and mood disorders.

According to the RACP working group, "Though not considered a "cause" of CFS, some patients with chronic fatigue report food intolerances that can exacerbate symptoms."

History

In 1978 Australian researchers published details of an 'exclusion diet' to exclude specific food chemicals from the diet of patients. This provided a basis for challenge with these additives and natural chemicals. Using this approach the role played by dietary chemical factors in the pathogenesis of chronic idiopathic urticaria (CIU) was first established and set the stage for future DBPCT trials of such substances in food intolerance studies.

In 1995 the European Academy of Allergology and Clinical Immunology suggested a classification on the basis of the responsible pathogenetic mechanism; according to this classification, non-toxic reactions can be divided into 'food allergies' when they recognize immunological mechanisms, and 'food intolerances' when there are no immunological implications. Reactions secondary to food ingestion are defined generally as 'adverse reactions to food'.

In year 2003 the Nomenclature Review Committee of the World Allergy Organization issued a report of revised nomenclature for global use on food allergy and food intolerance, that has had general acceptance. Food intolerance is described as a 'non allergic hypersensitivity' to food.

Society and Culture

In the UK, scepticism about food intolerance as a specific condition influenced doctors' (GPs') perceptions of patients and of the patients' underlying problems. However, rather than risk damaging the doctor-patient relationship, when GPs chose, despite their scepticism, and tempered by an element of awareness of the limitations of modern medicine, to negotiate mutually acceptable ground with patients and with patients' beliefs. That as a result, whether due to a placebo effect, secondary benefit, or as a biophysical result of excluding a food from the diet, the GPs acknowledged benefit, both personal and therapeutic.

In the Netherlands, patients and their doctors (GPs) have different perceptions of the efficacy of diagnostic and dietary interventions in IBS. Patients consider food intolerance and GPs regard lack of fibre as the main etiologic dietary factor. GPs should explore the patients' expectations and incorporate these in their approach to IBS patients.

New food labeling regulations were introduced into the USA and Europe in 2006. Which are said to benefit people with intolerances? In general, food-allergic consumers were not satisfied with the current labelling practices. In the USA food companies propose distinguishing between food allergy and food intolerance and use a mechanism-based (i.e., immunoglobulin-E-mediated), acute life-threatening anaphylaxis that is standardized and measurable and reflects the severity of health risk, as the principal inclusion criterion for food allergen labeling. Symptoms due to, or exacerbated by, food additives usually involve non-IgE-mediated mechanisms (food intolerance) and are usually less severe than those induced by food allergy, but can include anaphylaxis.

Research Directions

A randomised controlled trial on IBS patients found relaxing the diet led to a 24 per cent greater deterioration in symptoms compared to those on the elimination diet and concluded food elimination based on IgG antibodies may be effective in reducing IBS symptoms and is worthy of further biomedical research.

Intestinal or bowel hyperpermeability so called leaky gut has been linked to food allergies and some food intolerances. Research is currently focussing on specific conditions and effects of certain food constituents. At present there are a number of ways to limit the increased permeability, but additional studies are required to assess if this approach reduces the prevalence and severity of specific conditions.

FOOD ALLERGY

A food allergy is an adverse immune response to a food protein. Food allergy is distinct from other adverse responses to food, such as food intolerance, pharmacologic reactions, and toxin-mediated reactions.

Food Allergy	*Pharmacologic*	*Toxins*	*Intolerance*
Adverse immune response to a food protein	Caffeine tremors, cheese/ wine (tyramine) migraine, scombroid (histamine) fish poisoning	Bacterial food poisoning, staphylotoxin	Lactose intolerance (lactase deficiency)

The food protein triggering the allergic response is termed a food allergen. It is estimated that up to 12 million Americans have food allergies, and the prevalence is rising. Six to eight per cent of children under the age of three have food allergies and nearly four per cent of adults have them. Food allergies cause roughly 30,000 emergency room visits and 100 to 200 deaths per year in the United States. The most common food allergies in adults are shellfish, peanuts, tree nuts, fish, and eggs, and the most common food allergies in children are milk, eggs, peanuts, and tree nuts.

Treatment consists of avoidance diets, in which the allergic person avoids all forms of the food to which they are allergic. For people who are extremely sensitive, this may involve the total avoidance of any exposure with the allergen, including touching or inhaling the problematic food as well as touching any surfaces that may have come into contact with it. Areas of research include anti-IgE antibody (omalizumab, or Xolair) and specific oral tolerance induction (SOTI), which have shown some promise for treatment of certain food allergies. People diagnosed with a food allergy may carry an autoinjector of epinephrine such as an EpiPen or Twinject, wear some form of medical alert jewelry, or develop an emergency action plan, in accordance with their doctor.

Signs and Symptoms

Classic immunoglobulin-E (IgE)-mediated food allergies are classified as type-I immediate hypersensitivity reactions. These allergic reactions have an acute onset (from seconds to one hour) and may include:

- Angioedema: soft tissue swelling, usually involving the eyelids, face, lips, and tongue. Angioedema may result in severe swelling of the tongue as well as the larynx (voice box) and trachea, resulting in upper airway obstruction and difficulty breathing.

- Hives
- Itching of the mouth, throat, eyes, skin
- Nausea, vomiting, diarrhea, stomach cramps, and/or abdominal pain. This group of symptoms is termed gastrointestinal hypersensitivity.
- Rhinorrhea, nasal congestion
- Wheezing, scratchy throat, shortness of breath, or difficulty swallowing
- Anaphylaxis: a severe, whole-body allergic reaction that can result in death.

The reaction may progress to anaphylactic shock: A systemic reaction involving several different bodily systems including hypotension (low blood pressure), loss of consciousness, and possibly death. Allergens most frequently associated with this type of reaction are peanuts, nuts, milk, egg, and seafood, though many food allergens have been reported as triggers for anaphylaxis.

Food allergy is thought to develop more easily in patients with the atopic syndrome, a very common combination of diseases: allergic rhinitis and conjunctivitis, eczema and asthma. The syndrome has a strong inherited component; a family history of allergic diseases can be indicative of the atopic syndrome.

Conditions caused by food allergies are classified into 3 groups according to the mechanism of the allergic response:

IgE-mediated (Classic)

- Type-I immediate hypersensitivity reaction (symptoms described above)
- Oral allergy syndrome

IgE and/or non-IgE-mediated

- Allergic eosinophilic esophagitis
- Allergic eosinophilic gastritis
- Allergic eosinophilic gastroenteritis

Non-IgE Mediated

- Food protein-induced Enterocolitis syndrome (FPIES)
- Food protein proctocolitis/proctitis
- Food protein-induced enteropathy. An important example is Coeliac disease, which is an adverse immune response to the protein gluten.
- Milk-soy protein intolerance (MSPI) is a non-medical term used to describe a non-IgE mediated allergic response to milk and/or soy protein during infancy and early childhood. Symptoms of MSPI are usually attributable to food protein proctocolitis or FPIES.
- Heiner syndrome—lung disease due to formation of milk protein/IgG antibody immune complexes (milk precipitins) in the blood stream after it is absorbed from the GI tract. The lung disease commonly causes bleeding into the lungs and results in pulmonary hemosiderosis.

The Big Eight

The most common food allergies are:

- Dairy allergy
- Egg allergy
- Peanut allergy
- Tree nut allergy
- Seafood allergy
- Shellfish allergy
- Soy allergy
- Wheat allergy

These are often referred to as "the big eight." They account for over 90 per cent of the food allergies in the United States.

The top allergens vary somewhat from country to country but milk, eggs, peanuts, treenuts, fish, shellfish, soy, wheat and sesame tend to be in the top 10 in many countries. Allergies to seeds—especially sesame—seem to be increasing in many countries.

More Rare Food Allergies

Likelihood of allergy can increase with exposure. For example, rice allergy is more common in East Asia where rice forms a large part of the diet.

In Central Europe, celery allergy is more common. In Japan, allergy to buckwheat flour, used for Soba noodles, is more common.

Red meat allergy is extremely rare in the general population, but a geographic cluster of people allergic to red meat has been observed in Sydney, Australia. There appears to be a possible association between localised reaction to tick bite and the development of red meat allergy.

Fruit allergies exist, such as to apples, pears, jackfruit, strawberries, etc.

Corn allergy may also be prevalent in many populations, although it may be difficult to recognize in areas such as the United States and Canada where corn derivatives are common in the food supply.

Diagnosis

The best method for diagnosing food allergy is to be assessed by an allergist. The allergist will review the patient's history and the symptoms or reactions that have been noted after food ingestion. If the allergist feels the symptoms or reactions are consistent with food allergy, he/she will perform allergy tests.

Examples of allergy testing include:

- Skin prick testing is easy to do and results are available in minutes. Different allergists may use different devices for skin prick testing. Some use a "bifurcated needle", which looks like a fork with 2 prongs. Others use a "multi-test", which may look like a small board with several pins sticking out of it. In these tests, a tiny amount of the suspected allergen is put onto the skin or into a testing device, and the device is placed on the skin to prick, or break through, the top layer of skin. This puts a small amount of the allergen under the skin. A hive will form at any spot where the person is allergic. This test generally yields a positive or negative result. It is good for quickly learning if a person is allergic to a particular food or not, because it detects allergic antibodies known as IgE. Skin tests cannot predict if a reaction would occur or what kind of reaction might occur if a person ingests that particular allergen. They can however confirm an allergy in light of a patient's history of reactions to a particular food. Non-IgE mediated allergies cannot be detected by this method.

- Blood tests are another useful diagnostic tool for evaluating IgE-mediated food allergies. For example, the RAST (RadioAllergoSorbent Test) detects the presence of IgE antibodies to a particular allergen. A CAP-RAST test is a specific type of RAST test with greater specificity: it can show the amount of IgE present to each allergen. Researchers have been able to determine "predictive values" for certain foods. These predictive values can be compared to the RAST blood test results. If a persons RAST score is higher than the predictive value for that food, then there is over a 95 per cent chance the person will have an allergic reaction (limited to rash and anaphylaxis reactions) if they ingest that food. Currently, predictive values are available for the following foods: milk, egg, peanut, fish, soy, and wheat. Blood tests allow for hundreds of allergens to be screened from a single sample, and cover food allergies as well as inhalants. However, non-IgE mediated allergies cannot be detected by this method.
- Food challenges, especially double-blind placebo-controlled food challenges (DBPCFC), are the gold standard for diagnosis of food allergies, including most non-IgE mediated reactions. Blind food challenges involve packaging the suspected allergen into a capsule, giving it to the patient, and observing the patient for signs or symptoms of an allergic reaction. Due to the risk of anaphylaxis, food challenges are usually conducted in a hospital environment in the presence of a doctor.
- Additional diagnostic tools for evaluation of eosinophilic or non-IgE mediated reactions include endoscopy, colonoscopy, and biopsy.

Important differential diagnoses are:

- Lactose intolerance; this generally develops later in life but can present in young patients in severe cases. This is due to an enzyme deficiency (lactase) and not allergy. It occurs in many non-Western people.
- Celiac disease; this is an autoimmune disorder triggered by gluten proteins such as gliadin (present in wheat, rye and barley). It is a non-IgE mediated food allergy by definition.
- Irritable bowel syndrome (IBS)
- C1 esterase inhibitor deficiency (hereditary angioedema); this rare disease generally causes attacks of angioedema, but can present solely with abdominal pain and occasional diarrhea.

Pathophysiology

Generally, introduction of allergens through the digestive tract is thought to induce immune tolerance. In individuals who are predisposed to developing allergies (atopic syndrome), the immune system produces IgE antibodies against protein epitopes on non-pathogenic substances, including dietary components. The IgE molecules are coated onto mast cells, which inhabit the mucosal lining of the digestive tract.

Upon ingesting an allergen, the IgE reacts with its protein epitopes and release (degranulate) a number of chemicals (including histamine), which lead to oedema of the intestinal wall, loss of fluid and altered motility. The product is diarrhea.

Any food allergy has the potential to cause anaphylaxis, which in rare cases may be fatal.

Causes

The immune system's eosinophils, once activated in a histamine reaction, will register any foreign proteins they see. One theory regarding the causes of food allergies focuses on proteins presented in the blood along with vaccines, which are designed to provoke an immune response. Influenza vaccines and the Yellow Fever vaccine are still egg-based, but the Measles-Mumps-Rubella vaccine stopped using eggs in 1994. However large scientific studies do not support this theory, especially as it applies to autoimmune disease.

Another theory focuses on whether an infant's immune system is ready for complex proteins in a new food when it is first introduced.

One hypothesis at this time is the Hygiene hypothesis. While there is no proof for the hygiene hypothesis, people speculate that in modern, industrialized nations, such as the United States, food allergies are more common due to the lack of early exposure to dirt and germs, in part due to the over-use of antibiotics and antibiotic cleansers. This hypothesis is based partly on studies showing less allergy in third world countries. Some research suggests that the body, with less dirt and germs to fight off, turns on itself and attacks food proteins as if they were foreign invaders.

Antibiotics have also been implicated in Leaky Gut Syndrome which is another possible cause of food allergies.

A lower incidence of food allergies in the developing world could also be due to differences in diet from the West and less exposure to food allergens.

Others have found that food allergies are due to widespread usage of baby skin-care products that contain allergens, such as lotions based upon peanut oil. These skin-care products are cheaper to manufacture than non-allergenic ones and using them sensitizes the baby, which later develops into a food allergy. This theory has yet to come with sufficient explanation as to why the occurrence of allergies has been on a steady rise in the last two decades.

Prevention

According to a report issued by the American Academy of Pediatrics, "There is evidence that breastfeeding for at least 4 months, compared with feeding infants formula made with intact cow milk protein, prevents or delays the occurrence of atopic dermatitis, cow milk allergy, and wheezing in early childhood."

Treatment

The mainstay of treatment for food allergy is avoidance of the foods that have been identified as allergens.

If the food is accidentally ingested and a systemic reaction (anaphylaxis) occurs, then epinephrine (best delivered with an autoinjector of epinephrine such as an Epipen or Twinject) should be used. It is possible that a second dose of epinephrine may be required for severe reactions. The patient should also seek medical care immediately.

At this time, there is no cure for food allergies. There are no allergy desensitization or allergy "shots" available for food allergies. Some doctors feel they do not work in food allergies because even minute amounts of the food in question or even food extracts (as in the case of allergy shots) can cause an allergic response in many sufferers.

Ronald van Ree of Amsterdam University expects that vaccines can in theory be created using genetic engineering to cure allergies. If this can be done, food allergies could be eradicated in about ten years.

Statistics

For reasons that are not entirely understood, the diagnosis of food allergies has apparently become more common in Western nations in recent times. In the United States food allergy affects as many as 5 per cent of infants less than three years of age and 3 per cent to 4 per cent of adults. There is a similar prevalence in Canada.

The most common food allergens include peanuts, milk, eggs, tree nuts, fish, shellfish, soy, and wheat—these foods account for about 90 per cent of all allergic reactions.

Differing Views

Various medical practitioners have differing views on food allergies. Irritable Bowel Syndrome (IBS) patients have been studied with regards to food allergies. Some studies have reported on the role of food allergy in IBS; only one epidemiological study on functional dyspepsia and food allergy has been published. However, since 2005 several studies have demonstrated strong correlation between IgG and/or IgE food allergy and IBS symptoms. The mechanisms by which food activates mucosal immune system are incompletely understood, but food specific IgE and IgG4 appeared to mediate the hypersensitivity reaction in a subgroup of IBS patients. Specific chemicals and receptors have been demonstrated to be critical in food allergy development in murine models. Exclusion diets based on skin prick test, RAST for IgE or IgG4, hypoallergic diet and clinical trials with oral disodium cromoglycate have been conducted, and some success has been reported in a subset of IBS patients.

Studies comparing skin prick testing and ELISA blood testing have found that the results of skin prick testing correlate poorly with symptoms of irritable bowel syndrome that correlate with food allergies demonstrated through ELISA testing and dietary challenge.

Extensive clinical experience has demonstrated significant improvement of patients with IBS whose ELISA-based food allergy testing is positive and where treatment includes a careful exclusion diet.

In addition, many practitioners of alternative medicine ascribe symptoms to food allergy where other doctors do not. The causal relationships between some of these conditions and food allergies have not been studied extensively enough to provide sufficient evidence to become authoritative. The interaction of histamine with the nervous system receptors has been demonstrated, but more study is needed. Other immune response effects are commonly known (swelling, irritation, etc.), but their relationships to some conditions has not been extensively studied. Examples are arthritis, fatigue, headaches, and hyperactivity. Nevertheless, hypoallergenic diets reportedly can be of benefit in these conditions, indicating that the current medical views on food allergy may be too narrow.

In Children

Milk and soy allergies in children can often go undiagnosed for many months, causing much worry for parents and health risks for infants and children. Many infants with milk and soy allergies can show signs of colic, blood in the stool, mucous in the stool, reflux, rashes and other harmful medical conditions. These conditions are often misdiagnosed as viruses or colic.

Some children who are allergic to cow's milk protein also show a cross sensitivity to soy-based products. There are infant formulas in which the milk and soy proteins are degraded so when taken by an infant, their immune system does not recognize the allergen and they can safely consume the product. Hypoallergenic infant formulas can be based on hydrolyzed proteins, which are proteins partially predigested in a less antigenic form. Other formulas, based on free amino acids, are the least antigenic and provide complete nutrition support in severe forms of milk allergy.

Seventy-five per cent of children who have allergies to milk protein are able to tolerate baked-in milk products, i.e., muffins, cookies, cake.

About 50 per cent of children with allergies to milk, egg, soy, and wheat will outgrow their allergy by the age of 6. Those that don't, and those that are still allergic by the age of 12 or so, have less than an 8 per cent chance of outgrowing the allergy.

Peanut and tree nut allergies are less likely to be outgrown, although evidence now shows that about 20 per cent of those with peanut allergies and 9 per cent of those with tree nut allergies will outgrow their allergies. In such a case, they need to consume nuts in some regular fashion to maintain the non-allergic status. This should be discussed with a doctor.

Those with other food allergies may or may not outgrow their allergies.

Labeling Laws

In response to the risk that certain foods pose to those with food allergies, countries have responded by instituting labeling laws that require food products to clearly inform consumers if their products contain major allergens or by-products of major allergens.

United States Law

Under the Food Allergen Labeling and Consumer Protection Act of 2004 (Public Law 108-282), companies are required to disclose on the label whether the product contains a major food allergen in clear, plain language. The allergens have to clearly be called out in the ingredient statement. Most companies list allergens in a statement separate from the ingredient statement.

DIET AND CANCER

Dietary patterns, foods, nutrients, and other dietary constituents are closely associated with the risk for several types of cancer. And while it is not yet possible to provide quantitative estimates of the overall risks, it has been estimated that 35 per cent of cancer deaths may be related to dietary factors.

Reducing-risk Factors

Increasing evidence suggests that diets high in foods containing fibre (or fiber) are associated with a reduced risk for cancer, especially cancer of the colon.

A few studies have also shown a reduced risk for cancers of the breast, rectum, oral cavity, pharynx, stomach, and other sites with diets rich in fruits, vegetables and grain products . Numerous studies have found evidence that carotenoids reduce the risk of some cancers. The evidence is particularly strong for lung cancer, even after taking smoking into account. Vitamin C is found in fruits, particularly citrus fruits and juices, and in green vegetables, as well as in some fortified foods. Of a group of epidemiologic studies investigating the role of vitamin C, three-quarters found that vitamin C, or fruit rich in vitamin C, provides significant protection.

A leaner diet is believed to lower cancer risk. Tomatoes, calcium, agaricus blazei mushrooms, other minerals, saponins, sausage tree, sea mat, cat's claw, and licorice are believed to prevent or suppress different kinds of cancerous tumors. Currently there is not enough evidence for using mushrooms or mushroom extracts in the treatment of cancer, but there is significant potential for research in the area and future clinical trials, due to the numerous scientific studies which have shown they may offer a beneficial effect.

Mushrooms

Some mushrooms offer an anti-cancer effect, which is thought to be linked to their ability to up-regulate the immune system. Some mushrooms known for this effect include, Reishi, Agaricus blazei, Maitake, and Trametes versicolor. Research suggests the compounds in medicinal mushrooms most responsible for up-regulating the immune system and providing an anti-cancer effect, are a diverse collection of polysaccharide compounds, particularly beta-glucans. Beta-glucans are known as "biological response modifiers", and their ability to activate the immune system is well documented. Specifically, beta-glucans stimulate the innate branch of the immune system. Research has shown beta-glucans have the ability to stimulate macrophage, NK cells, T cells, and immune system cytokines. The mechanisms in which beta-glucans stimulate the immune system is only partially understood. One mechanism in which beta-glucans are able to activate the immune system, is by interacting with the Macrophage-1 antigen (CD18) receptor on immune cells.

A highly purified compound isolated from the medicinal mushroom Trametes versicolor, known as Polysaccharide-K, has become incorporated into the health care system of a few countries, such as Japan. Japan's Ministry of Health, Labour and Welfare approved the use of Polysaccharide-K in the 1980s, to stimulate the immune systems of patients undergoing chemotherapy.

Risk Factors

Fast foods are said to raise cancer risk.

Alcohol

Alcohol is a risk factor for cancers of the mouth, esophagus, pharynx, and larynx, breast cancer, colorectal cancer, and liver cancer.

Contrary Evidence

More recent studies have cast doubt on the claim that dietary fiber reduces the risk of colon cancer. Regarding prostate cancer, a major 2002 study concluded that "A low-fat, high-fiber diet heavy in fruits and vegetables has no impact on PSA levels in men over a four-year period, and does not affect the incidence of prostate cancer."

The belief that dietary fiber prevents these cancers was based on epidemiological evidence showing a very low incidence in the developing world. Dr. Denis Burkitt was the main proponent of this theory, and his 1979 best-selling book, "Don't Forget Fibre in Your Diet," was translated into nine languages. Less well-known is his theory, mentioned in the book, that the squatting defecation posture used in the developing world where Ottoman toilets are more widespread than the Western world is also a preventative factor, especially for colon diseases.

Methionine Metabolism

Although numerous cellular mechanisms are involved in food intake, many investigations over the past decades have pointed out defections in the methionine metabolic pathway as cause of cancerogenesis. For instance, deficiencies of the main dietary sources of methyl donors, methionine and choline, lead to the formation of liver cancer in rodents. Methionine is an essential amino acid

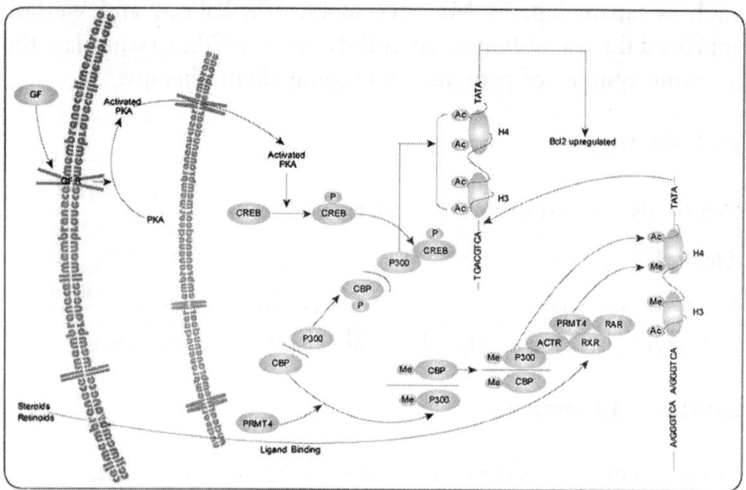

Fig. 2.9: Growth Factor (GF) and Steroid/retinoid Activation of PRMT4

that must be provided by dietary intake of proteins or methyl donors (choline and betaine found in beef, eggs and some vegetables). Assimilated methionine is transformed in S-adenosyl methionine (SAM) which is a key metabolite for polyamine synthesis, e.g. spermidine, and cysteine formation. Methionine breakdown products are also recycled back into methionine by homocysteine remethylation and methylthioadenosine (MTA) conversion. Vitamins B6, B12, folic acid and choline are essential cofactors for these reactions. SAM is the substrate for methylation reactions catalyzed by DNA, RNA and protein methyltransferases.

The products of these reactions are methylated DNA, RNA or proteins and S-adenosylhomocysteine (SAH). SAH has a negative feedback on its own production as an inhibitor of methyltransferase enzymes. Therefore SAM:SAH ratio directly regulates cellular methylation, whereas levels of vitamins B6, B12, folic acid and choline regulates indirectly the methylation state via the methionine metabolism cycle. A near ubiquitous feature of cancer is a maladaption of the methionine metabolic pathway in response to genetic or environmental conditions resulting in depletion of SAM and/or SAM-dependent methylation. Whether it is deficiency in enzymes such as methylthioadenosine phosphorylase, methionine-dependency of cancer cells, high levels of polyamine synthesis in cancer, or induction of cancer through a diet deprived of extrinsic methyl donors or enhanced in methylation inhibitors, tumor formation is strongly correlated with a decrease in levels of SAM in mice, rats and humans. Many indirect and thinly circumstantial theories have been put forth related to methylation status of DNA or attacks upon the capacity for DNA mutation and repair. The discovery that methyltransferases whose activity would be directly influenced by SAM levels also act as tumor suppressors potentially provides a more direct bridge. This has important ramifications for chemoprevention strategies as well as chemotherapy.

Arginine Methyltransferase

Protein arginine N-methyltransferase-4 (PRMT4) methylation of arginine residues within proteins plays a critical key role in transcriptional regulation. PRMT4 binds to the classes of transcriptional activators known as p160 and CBP/p300. The modified forms of these proteins are involved in stimulation of gene expression via steroid hormone receptors. Significantly, PRMT4 methylates core histones H3 and H4, which are also targets of the histone acetylase activity of CBP/p300 coactivators. PRMT4 recruitment chromatin by binding to coactivators increases histone methylation and enhances the accessibility of promoter regions for transcription. Methylation of the transcriptional coactivator CBP by PRMT4 inhibits binding to CREB and thereby partitions the limited cellular pool of CBP for steroid hormone receptor interaction.

DIET, CARDIOVASCULAR AND HEART DISEASE

Diet is a significant contributing factor to the presence (or absence) of heart disease, an umbrella term describing many heart ailments. For example, some claim a diet high in cholesterol may lead to coronary heart disease, a condition in which a buildup of plaque occurs in the arteries near the heart.

Alcohol and Cardiovascular Disease

Excessive alcohol intake is associated with elevated risk of liver disease, heart failure, cancer, and accidental injury, and is a leading cause of death in industrialized countries. However, considerable research suggests that moderate alcohol intake is associated with health benefits, among them a decreased risk of cardiovascular disease.

An early study of the relationship between alcohol consumption and atherosclerosis was published in 1904. Public awareness of the supposed French paradox in the early 1990s stimulated increased interest in the subject of alcohol and heart disease.

Processes whereby Alcohol Benefits Cardiovascular Health

Given the epidemiological evidence that moderate drinking reduces heart disease, it becomes important to examine how alcohol might confer its cardiovascular benefits. Research suggests that moderate consumption of alcohol improves cardiovascular health in a number of ways, including the following.

I. Alcohol improves blood lipid profile.
 A. It increases HDL ("good") cholesterol.
 B. It decreases LDL ("bad") cholesterol.
 C. It improves cholesterol (both HDL and LDL) particle size

(Mukamal, K.J. *et al*. Alcohol consumption and lipoprotein subclasses in older adults. Journal of Clinical Endocrinology and Metabolism, 2007, April. PMID: 17440017)

II. Alcohol decreases thrombosis (blood clotting). .
 A. It reduces platelet aggregation.
 B. It reduces fibrinogen (a blood clotter).
 C. It increases fibrinolysis (the process by which clots dissolve).

III. Alcohol acts through additional ways.
 A. It reduces coronary artery spasm in response to stress.
 B. It increases coronary blood flow.
 C. It reduces blood pressure.
 D. It reduces blood insulin level.
 E. It increases estrogen levels

There is a lack of medical consensus about whether moderate consumption of beer, wine, or distilled spirits has a stronger association with heart disease. Studies suggest that each is effective, with none having a clear advantage. Most researchers now believe that the most important ingredient is the alcohol itself

The American Heart Association has reported that "More than a dozen prospective studies have demonstrated a consistent, strong, dose-response relation between increasing alcohol consumption and decreasing incidence of CHD (coronary heart disease). The data are similar in men and women in a number of different geographic and ethnic groups. Consumption of one or two drinks per day is associated with a reduction in risk of approximately 30 per cent to 50 per cent".

Heart disease is the largest cause of mortality in the United States and many other countries. Therefore, some physicians have suggested that patients be informed of the potential health benefits of drinking alcohol in moderation, especially if they abstain and alcohol is not contraindicated. Others, however, argue against the practice in fear that it might lead to heavy or abusive alcohol consumption. Heavy drinking is associated with a number of health and safety problems.

Debate over Research Methods

Ex-drinkers versus Never-drinkers

A logical possibility is that some of the alcohol abstainers in research studies previously drank excessively and had undermined their health, thus explaining their high levels of risk. To test this hypothesis, some studies have excluded all but those who had avoided alcohol for their entire lives. The conclusion remained the same in some studies: moderate drinkers are less likely to suffer heart disease. A paper concludes, "In this population of light to moderate drinkers, alcohol consumption in general was associated with decreased MI [myocardial infarction] risk in women; however, episodic intoxication was related to a substantial increase in risk."

An analysis by sociologist Kaye Fillmore and colleagues failed to find significant support. Analyzing 54 prospective studies, the authors found that those studies which were free of the potential error (including former drinkers in the abstaining group) did not demonstrate significant cardiac protection from alcohol, although they continued to exhibit a J-shaped relationship in which moderate drinkers were less likely (but not at a statistically significantly level of confidence) to suffer cardiac disease than lifelong abstainers. The instructor of nursing says research is needed that looks at the reasons people abstain, which hers did not do.

Cardiologist Dr. Arthur Klatsky notes that Fillmore's study, which she freely acknowledges proves nothing but only raises questions, is itself seriously flawed. To overcome the inherent weaknesses of all epidemiological studies, even when properly conducted, he calls for a randomized trial in which some subjects are assigned to abstain while others are assigned to drink alcohol in moderation and the health of all is monitored for a period of years.

Lifestyle as a Possible Confounder

Another possibility is that moderate drinkers have more healthful lifestyles (making them healthier), higher economic status (giving them greater access to better foods or better healthcare), higher educational levels (causing them to be more aware of disease symptoms), etc. However, when these and other factors are considered, the conclusion again remains the same: moderate drinkers are less likely to suffer heart disease.

Tests of Alternative Hypotheses

A study concluded, "Even in men already at low risk on the basis of body mass index, physical activity, smoking, and diet, moderate alcohol intake is associated with lower risk for MI [myocardial infarction]." Other research also addresses this question.

Another study found that when men increased their alcohol intake from very low to moderate, they significantly reduced their risk of coronary heart disease. The study monitored the health of 18,455 males for a period of seven years.

These and similar studies reduce the possibility that it is not alcohol itself that reduces the risk of cardiovascular disease.

Understanding specifically how alcohol improves cardiovascular health and reduces disease also significantly increases scientific confidence in the health benefits of moderate drinking.

HEALTHY DIET

A healthy diet is one that is arrived at with the intent of improving or maintaining optimal health.

This usually involves consuming nutrients by eating the appropriate amounts from all of the food groups, including an adequate amount of water. Since human nutrition is complex, a healthy diet may vary widely, and is subject to an individual's genetic makeup, environment, and health. For around 20 per cent of the human population, lack of food and malnutrition are the main impediments to healthy eating. Conversely, people in developed countries have the opposite problem; they are more concerned about obesity.

Generally, a healthy diet is said to include:

1. Sufficient calories to maintain a person's metabolic and activity needs, but not so excessive as to result in fat storage greater than roughly 30 per cent of body mass. For most people the recommended daily allowance of energy is 2,000 calories, but it depends on age, sex, height, weight, and physical activity.
2. Sufficient quantities of fat, including monounsaturated fat, polyunsaturated fat and saturated fat, with a balance of omega-6 and long-chain omega-3 lipids. The recommended daily allowance of fat is 65-80 grams.
3. Maintenance of a good ratio between carbohydrates and lipids (4:1): four grams of the first for one gram of the second.
4. Avoidance of excessive saturated fat (20grams recommended limit, although the "evidence" for this claim is forever in debate after the testimony of results provided by the Framingham Heart Study of 1948-1998)
5. Avoidance of trans fat.
6. Sufficient essential amino acids ("complete protein") to provide cellular replenishment and transport proteins. All essential amino acids are present in animals. A select few plants (such as soy and hemp) give all the essential acids. A combination of other plants may also provide all essential amino acids (except rice and beans which have limitations).
7. Essential micronutrients such as vitamins and certain minerals.
8. Avoiding directly poisonous (e.g. heavy metals) and carcinogenic (e.g. benzene) substances;
9. Avoiding foods contaminated by human pathogens (e.g. E. coli, tapeworm eggs);
10. Avoiding chronic high doses of certain foods that are benign or beneficial in small or occasional doses, such as
    - foods that may burden or exhaust normal functions

(e.g. refined carbohydrates without adequate dietary fiber);

- foods that may interfere at high doses with other body processes (e.g. refined table salt);
- foods or substances with directly toxic properties at high chronic doses (e.g. ethyl alcohol).

11. Combination of foods eaten and timing of meals so that hunger is kept in check; for example, to meet calorie goal of 2000 calories to avoid gaining weight.

Detrimental Eating Habits

In specific individuals, ingesting foods containing natural allergens (e.g. peanuts, shell food) or drug-induced triggers (e.g. tyramine for a person taking an MAO inhibitor) may be life-threatening.

Some foods have low nutritional value, and if consumed on a regular basis will contribute to the decline of human health. This has been demonstrated by various epidemiological studies that have determined that foods such as processed and fast foods are linked to diabetes and various heart problems.

When improperly cut or prepared, a small number of foods (such as fugu) can result in death.

The ingredient usually cited as being most crucial to good health, water, has even been known to result in death when consumed in extraordinary quantities.

Cultural and Psychological Factors

From a psychological perspective, a new healthy diet may be difficult to achieve for a person with poor eating habits. This may be due to tastes acquired in early adolescence and preferences for fatty foods. It may be easier for such a person to transition to a healthy diet if treats such as chocolate are allowed; sweets may act as mood stabilizers, which could help reinforce correct nutrient intake.

It is known that the experiences we have in childhood relating to consumption of food affect our perspective on food consumption in later life. From this, we are able to determine ourselves our limits of how much we will eat, as well as foods we will not eat—which can develop into eating disorders, such as anorexia, bulimia, or orthorexia This is also true with how we perceive the sizes of the meals or amounts of food we consume daily; people have different interpretations of small and large meals based on upbringing.

While plants, vegetables, and fruits are known to help reduce the incidence of chronic disease, the benefits on health posed by plant-based foods, as well as the percentage of which a diet needs to be plant based in order to have health benefits is unknown. Nevertheless, plant-based food diets in society and between nutritionist circles are linked to health and longevity, as well as contributing to lowering cholesterol, weight loss, and in some cases, stress reduction.

Indeed, ideas of what counts as "healthy eating" have varied in different times and places, according to scientific advances in the field of nutrition, cultural fashions, religious proscriptions, or personal considerations.

Public Policy Issues

Fears of high cholesterol were frequently voiced up until the mid-1990s. However, more recent research has shown that the distinction between high-and low-density lipoprotein ('good' and 'bad' cholesterol, respectively) must be addressed when speaking of the potential ill effects of cholesterol. Low-density lipoprotein is often prevalent in animal products, such as bacon and egg yolks, whereas high-density lipoprotein is more common in plant and fish tissues, such as olive oil and salmon.

Media coverage of mass-produced, processed, "snack" or "sweet" products directly marketed at children has worked to undermine policy efforts to improve eating habits. The main problem with such advertisements for foods is that alcohol and fast food are portrayed as offering excitement, escape and instant gratification.

Particularly within the last five years government agencies have attempted to combat the amount and method of media coverage lavished upon "junk" foods. Governments also put pressure on businesses to promote healthy food options, consider limiting the availability of junk food in state-run schools, and tax foods that are high in fat. Most recently, the United Kingdom removed the rights for McDonald's to advertise its products as the majority of the foods that were seen to have low nutrient values were aimed at children under the guise of the "Happy Meal". The British Heart Foundation released its own government-funded advertisements, labeled "Food4Thought", which were targeted at children and adults displaying the gory nature of how fast food is generally constituted.

Food Additive Controversy

Some claim that food additives, such as artificial sweeteners, colourants, preserving agents, and flavorings may cause health problems such as increasing the risk of cancer or ADHD. Examples of fast food critics include Morgan Spurlock and Eric Schlosser.

HEALTH FOOD

The term Health food has been used in the United States since the 1920s to refer to specific foods claimed to be especially beneficial to health.

In contrast to a healthy diet, proponents of health foods claim that a specific food has good effects on health. Examples of healtn foods include alfalfa sprouts, wheat germ and yogurt. Natural foods and organic food are related concepts. Health foods are sold in health food stores or in the health/organic section of the supermarket.

DIETARY FIBER

Dietary fiber (fibre), sometimes called roughage, is the indigestible portion of plant foods that pushes food through the digestive system, absorbing water and easing defecation. It acts by changing the nature of the contents of the gastrointestinal tract, and by changing how other nutrients and chemicals are absorbed.

Dietary fiber can be soluble (able to dissolve in water) or insoluble (not able to dissolve in water). Soluble fiber, like all fiber, cannot be digested. But it does change as it passes through the digestive tract, being transformed (fermented) by bacteria there. Soluble fiber also absorbs water to become a gelatinous substance that passes through the body. Insoluble fiber has bulking action but is mostly unchanged by fermentation as it passes through the body.

Chemically, dietary fiber consists of non-starch polysaccharides such as cellulose and many other plant components such as dextrins, inulin, lignin, waxes, chitins, pectins, beta-glucans and oligosaccharides. The term "fiber" is somewhat of a misnomer, since many types of so-called dietary fiber are not fibers at all.

Food sources of dietary fiber are often divided according to whether they provide (predominantly) soluble or insoluble fiber. To be precise, both types of fiber are present in all plant foods, with varying degrees of each according to a plant's characteristics.

Potential advantages of consuming fiber are the production of health-promoting compounds during the fermentation of soluble fiber, and insoluble fiber's ability (via its passive water-attracting properties) to increase bulk, soften stool and shorten transit time through the intestinal tract.

Types of Fiber

Originally, fiber was defined to be the components of plants that resist human digestive enzyme, a definition that includes lignin and polysaccharides. The definition was later changed to also include resistant starches, along with inulin and other oligosaccharides.

Soluble fibers, such as pectin, are viscous and fermented in the colon; insoluble fibers, such as wheat bran, are fermented only to a limited extent, although they do have bulking action.

Sources of Fiber

Dietary fiber is found in plants. While all plants contain some fiber, plants with high fiber concentrations are generally the most practical source.

Fiber-rich plants can be eaten directly. Or, alternatively, they can be used to make supplements and fiber-rich processed foods.

The American Dietetic Association (ADA) recommends consuming a variety of fiber-rich foods.

Plant Sources of Fiber

Some plants contain significant amounts of soluble and insoluble fiber. For example plums (or prunes) have a thick skin covering a juicy pulp. The plum's skin is an example of an insoluble fiber source, whereas soluble fiber sources are inside the pulp.

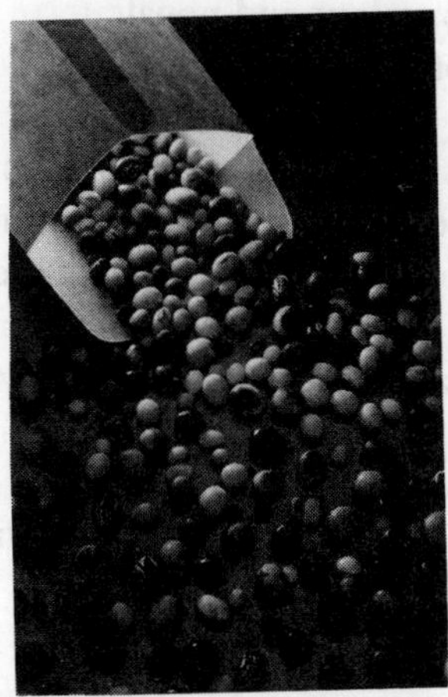

Fig. 2.10: Legumes such as Soybeans Contain Dietary Fibers

Soluble fiber is found in varying quantities in all plant foods, including:

- legumes (peas, soybeans, and other beans)
- oats, rye, chia, and barley
- some fruits and fruit juices (including prune juice, plums, berries, bananas, and the insides of apples and pears)
- certain vegetables such as broccoli, carrots and Jerusalem artichokes
- root vegetables such as potatoes, sweet potatoes, and onions (skins of these vegetables are sources of insoluble fiber)
- psyllium seed husk (a mucilage soluble fiber).

Sources of insoluble fiber include:

- whole grain foods

- wheat and corn bran
- nuts and seeds
- potato skins
- flax seed
- lignans
- vegetables such as green beans, cauliflower, zucchini (courgette), celery, and nopal
- the skins of some fruits, including tomatoes

The five most fiber-rich plant foods, according to the Micronutrient Center of the Linus Pauling Institute, are legumes (15-19 grams of fiber per US cup serving, including several types of beans, lentils and peas), wheat bran (17 grams per cup), prunes (12 grams), Asian pear (10 grams each, 3.6% by weight), and quinoa (9 grams).

Rubus fruits such as raspberry (8 grams of fiber per serving) and blackberry (7.4 grams of fiber per serving) are exceptional sources of fiber.

Fiber Supplements

These are a few example forms of fiber that have been sold as supplements or food additives. These may be marketed to consumers for nutritional purposes, treatment of various gastrointestinal disorders, and for such possible health benefits as lowering cholesterol levels, reducing risk of colon cancer, and losing weight.

Soluble fiber supplements may be beneficial for alleviating symptoms of irritable bowel syndrome, such as diarrhea and/or constipation and abdominal discomfort. Prebiotic soluble fiber products, like those containing inulin or oligosaccharides, may contribute to relief from inflammatory bowel disease, as in Crohn's disease, ulcerative colitis, and *Clostridium difficile*, due in part to the short-chain fatty acids produced with subsequent anti-inflammatory actions upon the bowel. Fiber supplements may be effective in an overall dietary plan for managing irritable bowel syndrome by modification of food choices.

Inulins

Chemically defined as oligosaccharides occurring naturally in most plants, inulins have nutritional value as carbohydrates, or more specifically as fructans, a polymer of the natural plant sugar, fructose. Inulin is typically extracted by manufacturers from enriched plant sources such as chicory roots or Jerusalem artichokes for use in prepared foods. Subtly sweet, it can be used to replace sugar, fat, and flour, is often used to improve the flow and mixing qualities of powdered nutritional supplements, and has significant potential health value as a prebiotic fermentable fiber.

Inulin is advantageous because it contains 25-30 per cent the food energy of sugar or other carbohydrates and 10-15 per cent the food energy of fat. As a prebiotic fermentable fiber, its metabolism by gut flora yields short-chain fatty acids (discussed above) which increase absorption of calcium, magnesium, and iron, resulting from upregulation of mineral-transporting genes and their membrane transport proteins within the colon wall. Among other potential beneficial effects noted above, inulin promotes an increase in the mass and health of intestinal *Lactobacillus* and *Bifidobacterium* populations.

Vegetable Gums

Vegetable gum fiber supplements are relatively new to the market. Often sold as a powder, vegetable gum fibers dissolve easily with no aftertaste. They are effective for the treatment of irritable bowel syndrome (Parisi, 2002). Examples of vegetable gum fibers are guar gum (e.g., the brand Benefiber reformulated to wheat dextrin in 2006) and acacia gum.

Mechanism

The main action of dietary fiber is to change the nature of the contents of the gastrointestinal tract, and to change how other nutrients and chemicals are absorbed. Soluble fiber binds to bile acids in the small intestine, making them less likely to enter the body; this in turn lowers cholesterol levels in the blood. Soluble fiber also inhibits the absorption of sugar and reduces sugar response after eating. Although insoluble fiber is associated with reduced diabetes risk, the mechanism by which this occurs is unknown.

Dietary fiber is has not been formally proposed or accepted as an essential nutrient. Like fluoride, fiber is a nutrient that acts against a harmful biological process; in fiber's case the harm comes from bile acids and sugars in the intestine.

Benefits of Fiber Intake

Eating fiber has many benefits for your health. The consumption of soluble fiber has been shown to protect you from developing heart disease by reducing your cholesterol levels. The consumption of insoluble fiber reduces your risk of developing constipation, colitis, colon cancer, and hemorrhoids.

Dietary Fiber Functions and Benefits

Functions	*Benefits*
Adds bulk to your diet, making you feel full faster	May reduce appetite
Attracts water and turns to gel during digestion, trapping carbohydrates and slowing absorption of glucose	Lowers variance in blood sugar levels
Lowers total and LDL cholesterol	Reduces risk of heart disease
Regulates blood sugar	May reduce onset risk or symptoms of metabolic syndrome and diabetes
Speed the passage of foods through the digestive system	Facilitates regularity
Adds bulk to the stool	Alleviates constipation
Balance intestinal pH and stimulates intestinal fermentation production of short-chain fatty acids	May reduce risk of colorectal cancer

Fiber does not bind to minerals and vitamins and therefore does not restrict their absorption, but rather evidence exists that fermentable fiber sources improve absorption of minerals, especially calcium. Some plant foods can reduce the absorption of minerals and vitamins like calcium, zinc, vitamin C and magnesium, but this is caused by the presence of phytate (which is also thought to have important health benefits), not by fiber.

Guidelines on Fiber Intake

Current recommendations from the United States National Academy of Sciences, Institute of Medicine, suggest that adults should consume 20-35 grams of dietary fiber per day, but the average American's daily intake of dietary fiber is only 12-18 grams.

The ADA recommends a minimum of 20-35 g/day for a healthy adult depending on calorie intake (e.g., a 2000 cal/8400 kJ diet should include 25 g of fiber per day). The ADA's recommendation for children is that intake should equal age in years plus 5 g/day (e.g., a 4 year old should consume 9 g/day). No guidelines have yet been established for the elderly or very ill. Patients with current constipation, vomiting, and abdominal pain should see a physician. Certain bulking agents are not commonly recommended with the prescription of opioids because the slow transit time mixed with larger stools may lead to severe constipation, pain, or obstruction.

The British Nutrition Foundation has recommended a minimum fiber intake of 12-24 g/day for healthy adults.

Fiber Recommendations in North America

On average, North Americans consume less than 50 per cent of the dietary fiber levels required for good health. In the preferred food choices of today's youth, this value may be as low as 20 per cent, a factor considered by experts as contributing to the obesity crisis seen in many developed countries.

Recognizing the growing scientific evidence for physiological benefits of increased fiber intake, regulatory agencies such as the Food and Drug Administration (FDA) of the United States have given approvals to food products making health claims for fiber.

In clinical trials to date, these fiber sources were shown to significantly reduce blood cholesterol levels, an important factor for general cardiovascular health, and to lower risk of onset for some types of cancer.

Soluble (fermentable) fiber sources gaining FDA approval are:

- Psyllium seed husk (7 grams per day)
- Beta-glucan from oat bran, whole oats, oatrim or rolled oats (3 grams per day)

- Beta-glucan from whole grain or dry-milled barley (3 grams per day)

Other examples of fermentable fiber sources (from plant foods or biotechnology) used in functional foods and supplements include inulin, resistant dextrins, fructans, xanthan gum, cellulose, guar gum, fructooligosaccharides (FOS) and oligo-or polysaccharides.

Consistent intake of fermentable fiber through foods like berries and other fresh fruit, vegetables, whole grains, seeds and nuts is now known to reduce risk of some of the world's most prevalent diseases — obesity, diabetes, high blood cholesterol, cardiovascular disease, and numerous gastrointestinal disorders. In this last category are constipation, inflammatory bowel disease, ulcerative colitis, hemorrhoids, Crohn's disease, diverticulitis, and colon cancer — all disorders of the intestinal tract where fermentable fiber can provide healthful benefits.

Insufficient fiber in the diet can complicate defecation. Low-fiber feces are dehydrated and hardened, making them difficult to evacuate — defining constipation and possibly leading to development of hemorrhoids or anal fissures.

Although many researchers believe that dietary fiber intake reduces risk of colon cancer, one study conducted by researchers at the Harvard School of Medicine of over 88,000 women did not show a statistically significant relationship between higher fiber consumption and lower rates of colorectal cancer or adenomas.

Fiber Recommendations in the UK

In June 2007, the British Nutrition Foundation issued a statement to define dietary fiber more concisely and list the potential health benefits established to date:

'Dietary fiber' has been used as a collective term for a complex mixture of substances with different chemical and physical properties which exert different types of physiological effects. The use of certain analytical methods to quantify 'dietary fiber' by nature of its indigestibility results in many other indigestible components being isolated along with the carbohydrate components of dietary fiber. These components include resistant starches and oligosaccharides along with other substances that exist within the plant cell structure and contribute to the material that passes through the digestive tract. Such components are likely to have physiological effects. Yet, some differentiation has to be made between these indigestible plant components and other partially digested material, such as protein, that appears in the large bowel. Thus, it is better to classify fiber as a group of compounds with different physiological characteristics, rather than to be constrained by defining it chemically. Diets naturally high in fiber can be considered to bring about several main physiological consequences:

- helps prevent constipation
- reduces the risk of colon cancer
- improvements in gastrointestinal health
- improvements in glucose tolerance and the insulin response
- reduction of hyperlipidemia, hypertension and other coronary heart disease risk factors
- reduction in the risk of developing some cancers
- increased satiety and hence some degree of weight management

Therefore, it is not appropriate to state that fiber has a single all encompassing physiological property as these effects are dependent on the type of fiber in the diet. The beneficial effects of high fiber diets are the summation of the effects of the different types of fiber present in the diet and also other components of such diets. Defining fiber physiologically allows recognition of indigestible carbohydrates with structures and physiological properties similar to those of naturally occurring dietary fibers.

Fiber and Calories

Calories or kilojoules (as used on nutrition labels) are intended to be a measure of how much energy is available from the food source. This energy can be used immediately, for example allowing the body to move during exercise, or to make the heart beat. Energy that is not used immediately is stored as sugars in the short term and later converted to fats, which act as energy reserves.

Energy is extracted from food in a chemical reaction. Because of the principle of conservation of energy, energy can only be extracted when the chemical structure of food particles is changed. Since insoluble fiber particles do not change inside the body, the body should not absorb any energy (or Calories/kilojoules) from them.

Because soluble fiber is changed during fermentation, it could provide energy (Calories/kilojoules) to the body. As of 2009 nutritionists have not reached a consensus on how much energy is actually absorbed, but some approximate around 2 Calories (8.5 kilojoules) per gram of soluble fiber.

Regardless of the type of fiber, the body absorbs less than 4 Calories (16.7 kilojoules) per gram of fiber, which can create inconsistencies for actual product nutrition labels. In some countries, fiber is not listed on nutrition labels, and is considered 0 Calories/gram when the food's total Calories are computed. In other countries all fiber must be listed, and is considered 4 Calories/gram when the food's total Calories are computed (because chemically fiber is a type of carbohydrate and other carbohydrates contribute 4 Calories per gram). In the US, soluble fiber must be counted as 4 Calories per gram, but insoluble fiber may be (and usually is) treated as 0 Calories per gram and not mentioned on the label.

Short-chain Fatty Acids

When soluble fiber is fermented, short-chain fatty acids (SCFA) are produced. SCFA are involved in numerous physiological processes promoting health, including:

- stabilize blood glucose levels by acting on pancreatic insulin release and liver control of glycogen breakdown
- stimulate gene expression of glucose transporters in the intestinal mucosa, regulating glucose absorption
- provide nourishment of colonocytes, particularly by the SCFA butyrate
- suppress cholesterol synthesis by the liver and reduce blood levels of LDL cholesterol and triglycerides responsible for atherosclerosis

- lower colonic pH (i.e., raises the acidity level in the colon) which protects the lining from formation of colonic polyps and increases absorption of dietary minerals
- stimulate production of T helper cells, antibodies, leukocytes, cytokines and lymph mechanisms having crucial roles in immune protection
- improve barrier properties of the colonic mucosal layer, inhibiting inflammatory and adhesion irritants, contributing to immune functions

SCFA that are not absorbed by the colonic mucosa pass through the colonic wall into the portal circulation (supplying the liver), and the liver transports them into the general circulatory system.

Overall, SCFA affect major regulatory systems, such as blood glucose and lipid levels, the colonic environment and intestinal immune functions.

The major SCFA in humans are butyrate, propionate and acetate where butyrate is the major energy source for colonocytes, propionate is destined for uptake by the liver, and acetate enters the peripheral circulation to be metabolized by peripheral tissues.

FDA-approved Health Claims

The FDA allows producers of foods containing 1.7 g per serving of psyllium husk soluble fiber or 0.75 g of oat or barley soluble fiber as beta-glucans to claim that reduced risk of heart disease can result from their regular consumption.

The FDA statement template for making this claim is: Soluble fiber from foods such as [name of soluble fiber source, and, if desired, name of food product], as part of a diet low in saturated fat and cholesterol, may reduce the risk of heart disease. A serving of [name of food product] supplies __ grams of the [necessary daily dietary intake for the benefit] soluble fiber from [name of soluble fiber source] necessary per day to have this effect..

Eligible sources of soluble fiber providing beta-glucan include:

1. Oat bran
2. Rolled oats

3. Whole oat flour
4. Oatrim
5. Whole grain barley and dry milled barley
6. Soluble fiber from psyllium husk with purity of no less than 95 per cent

The allowed label may state that diets low in saturated fat and cholesterol and that include soluble fiber from certain of the above foods "may" or "might" reduce the risk of heart disease.

As discussed in FDA regulation 21 CFR 101.81, the daily dietary intake levels of soluble fiber from sources listed above associated with reduced risk of coronary heart disease are:

- 3 g or more per day of beta-glucan soluble fiber from either whole oats or barley, or a combination of whole oats and barley
- 7 g or more per day of soluble fiber from psyllium seed husk.

Soluble fiber from consuming grains is included in other allowed health claims for lowering risk of some types of cancer and heart disease by consuming fruit and vegetables (21 CFR 101.76, 101.77 and 101.78).

Soluble Fiber Fermentation

The American Association of Cereal Chemists has Defined Soluble Fiber this Way: "the edible parts of plants or similar carbohydrates resistant to digestion and absorption in the human small intestine with complete or partial fermentation in the large intestine."

In this definition:

- *Edible Parts of Plants* — indicates that some parts of a plant we eat — skin, pulp, seeds, stems, leaves, roots — contain fiber. Both insoluble and soluble sources are in those plant components.
- *Carbohydrates* — complex carbohydrates, such as long-chained sugars also called starch, oligosaccharides or polysaccharides, are sources of soluble fermentable fiber.

- *Resistant to Digestion and Absorption in the Human Small Intestine* — foods providing nutrients are digested by gastric acid and digestive enzymes in the stomach and small intestine where the nutrients are released then absorbed through the intestinal wall for transport via the blood throughout the body. A food resistant to this process is undigested, as insoluble and soluble fibers are. They pass to the large intestine only affected by their absorption of water (insoluble fiber) or dissolution in water (soluble fiber).
- *Complete or Partial Fermentation in the Large Intestine* — The large intestine comprises a segment called the colon within which additional nutrient absorption occurs through the process of fermentation. Fermentation occurs by the action of colonic bacteria on the food mass, producing gases and short-chain fatty acids. It is these short-chain fatty acids — butyric, ethanoic (acetic), propionic, and valeric acids — that scientific evidence is revealing to have significant health properties.

As an example of fermentation, shorter-chain carbohydrates (a type of fiber found in legumes) cannot be digested, but are changed via fermentation in the colon into short-chain fatty acids and gases (which are typically expelled as flatulence).

According to a 2002 journal article, fibers compounds with partial or low fermentability include:

- cellulose, a polysaccharide
- hemicellulose, a polysaccharide
- lignans, a group of phytoestrogens
- plant waxes
- resistant starches

Fiber compounds with high fermentability include:

- beta-glucans, a group of polysaccharides
- pectins, a group of heteropolysaccharides
- natural gums, a group of polysaccharides

- inulins, a group of polysaccharides
- oligosaccharides, a group of short-chained or simple sugars
- resistant dextrins

F-PLAN

The F-plan is a high fibre diet designed to induce healthy weight loss, created in the 1980s by British author Audrey Eyton, founder of Slimming Magazine, and based on the work of Denis Burkitt. The *F-Plan diet* book was in the top ten best selling books in America in April and May of 1983. The diet works by restricting the daily intake of calories to less than 1,500 whilst consuming well-above the recommended level of dietary fibre. The fibre has a number of beneficial effects, such as making the dieter feel "full" for much longer than normal, reducing the urge to overeat, and promoting a healthy digestive system.

The disadvantages include excessive flatulence in the first few weeks and having to eat food that is harder work to chew and swallow. Some people also express a dislike of the texture of such a high fibre diet. The dieter will need to consume more water than usual to prevent constipation.

Nevertheless, the diet is very effective when followed faithfully and remains a popular choice of diet, with genuine health benefits.

In 2006 Audrey Eyton published "F2", a revised version of the F-plan written in the light of subsequent medical discoveries, which claims to be faster and more effective and campaigns against low-carbohydrate diets, particularly the Atkins Diet.

HIGH FIBER FAVOURITES

- High Fibre Food
- Plan Sample Day
- Dietary Sources
- Fibre and Digestion

Diet Reviews

- Atkins Diet

- Blood Group Diet
- Cabbage Soup
- Detox Diets
- GI Diets
- Grapefruit Diet
- Lighter Life Diet
- Low Carb Diets
- South Beach Diet
- Vegetarian Diet
- Weight Watchers Report
- Zone Diet

Diet Success Stories

- Colin
- Rob
- James
- Ann
- WLR Free Trial
- Site Map
- Weight Loss

High Fibre Diet Review

WLR's dietitian Juliette Kellow is a big fan of high fibre diets like the F Plan because they're great for both weight loss and good health.

HIGH FIBER DIETS

With the recent popularity of low-carb plans like Atkins and the South Beach diet, it's hard to remember a time when filling up on fibre was trendy. But back in the early 80's, wholemeal bread, bran cereals and jacket spuds were almost as popular as Spandau Ballet, Rubik's cubes and puffball skirts. Following huge amounts of scientific research, health professionals suddenly revealed that if you wanted to stay healthy and lose weight, you should eat more dietary fibre.

Enter Audrey Eyton's world-famous F-plan diet! In May 1982, copies of The F-Plan Diet went on sale, and even today it remains popular. Ultimately, it promoted a high-fibre, low-fat, calorie-controlled eating plan — in fact, pretty much what nutrition experts still recommend today if you want to lose weight.

What is Dietary Fibre?

Previously called 'roughage', dietary fibre is the term that describes the carbohydrates that human's can't digest. Dietary fibre is found in plant foods such as cereals, pulses, fruits and vegetables and occurs mainly in the plant cell wall where it provides structural support for the plant.

What's the Link with Weight Loss?

Most high-fibre plans for weight loss still come with a reduction in calories. The F-Plan diet, for example, recommended a calorie restriction of between 850-1,500 calories a day — and of course, it's this calorie restriction that helps you lose weight. However, there are many reasons why including more fibre in your diet can help boost weight loss and make slimming less painful.

To start with, unlike other carbohydrates, most dietary fibre doesn't provide any calories. This means fibre-rich foods are often lower in energy than foods containing no fibre or only small amounts, making them ideal for people who are trying to lose weight.

Secondly, high fibre foods generally take longer to chew. As well as helping you to feel more satisfied when you eat, this automatically slows down the speed at which you eat, giving your brain time to register feelings of fullness so that you're less like to overeat. But that's not the only way fibre-rich foods help to control appetite. Fibre acts like a sponge and absorbs and holds on to water as its chewed in the mouth and passes into the stomach. This means fibre-rich foods swell up in your stomach and this can help to fill you up. Better still, fibre stays in the stomach for longer as it's harder to digest and this helps to keep you feeling fuller for longer, so you're less likely to want to snack in between meals.

So How Much Fibre should I Eat a Day to Lose Weight and How Much can I Expect to Lose?

Regardless of whether you want to lose weight or maintain your weight, the Department of Health recommends adults eat an average of 18g of fibre a day with a range of 12-24g. If you want to lose weight, you'll still need to restrict your calorie intake as recommended by Weight Loss Resources and the amount you can expect to lose will depend entirely on the degree of this restriction. Weight Loss Resources recommends you aim to lose no more than 2lb a week, although you might lose slightly more in the first few weeks when your body loses water as well as fat. This follows the guidelines recommended by nutrition experts.

Has a High-Fibre Diet Got Any Other Health Benefits?

Definitely. Having spent a long time in the stomach, fibre moves through the large intestine relatively quickly and health experts believe this helps to keep the digestive system healthy, preventing bowel problems such as constipation, diverticular disease and haemorrhoids (piles), as well as reducing the risk of bowel cancer. Interestingly, all these conditions tend to be uncommon in undeveloped countries where intakes of fibre are high, compared to Western societies where these medical problems are widespread and fibre intakes are low.

Furthermore, most fibre-rich foods are also low in fat and packed with vitamins and minerals — and when it comes to preventing disease, it seems that it's this whole package of nutrients that's important. For example, wholegrains like wheat, barley, oats, rye and rice contain not just fibre, but a number of nutrients that may reduce the risk of heart disease, stroke, certain cancers and diabetes by as much as 30 per cent. These include antioxidant nutrients vitamin E, zinc and selenium and a range of plant compounds called phytochemicals.

I'd Heard that a High-fibre Intake was Good for my Heart. What's the link?

Several large studies in America, Finland and Norway have found that people who eat relatively large amounts of wholegrain cereals have significantly lower rates of heart disease and stroke. It's thought that a particular type of fibre called soluble fibre may be partly responsible as it helps to lower blood cholesterol levels.

Tell Me More about Soluble Fibre?

Dietary fibre can be divided into two main types — soluble and insoluble fibre. Soluble fibre is thought to bind with cholesterol and prevent it from being reabsorbed into the bloodstream. This lowers the amount of cholesterol in the blood, therefore reducing the risk of heart disease. But that's not all. Soluble fibre also forms a gel in the intestine, which is thought to slow down the digestion and absorption of carbohydrates, especially glucose. This means it can help to keep blood sugar levels steady, preventing feelings of hunger that leave you reaching for the biscuit tin. Foods rich in soluble fibre include fruits, vegetables, oats, barley, and pulses such as beans, lentils and peas.

In contrast, insoluble fibre helps to keep the digestive system in good working order by increasing the bulk and softness of the stools, which in turn assists the smooth passage of food through the body. It's this type of fibre that helps to prevent bowel complaints like constipation and cancer. Foods rich in insoluble fibre include wholemeal flour and bread, wholegrain breakfast cereals, bran, brown rice, wholemeal pasta, grains and some fruits and vegetables.

Eating a range of fibre-rich foods, rather than just one or two sources, is the best way to ensure you get a mixture of both soluble and insoluble fibre — and make the most of the health benefits offered by both.

So is a High-Fibre Diet Suitable for People with Diabetes?

Yes, health experts recommend that people with diabetes have a good intake of fibre in the same way as the rest of the population. But it's always wise to speak to your doctor or dietitian before making any changes to your diet, especially if you are on medication such as tablets or insulin.

What about High-Fibre Intakes for Children?

Although older children and teenagers will benefit from eating plenty of fibre-rich foods, very young children shouldn't be given large amounts. This is because they have small tummies and generally consume much smaller quantities of food than older children and adults. Because fibre-rich foods tend to be filling but reasonably low in energy, young children may not be able to satisfy their energy requirements and this may mean they don't grow as well as they should.

Is It Still Possible to Get Enough Fibre if I Follow a Wheat-Free Diet?

Yes, providing you include plenty of fruit, veg, pulses and brown rice. See the chart here to see how you can make up 18g of fibre a day using non-wheat foods.

Is There a Link with Fibre and the Glycaemic Index of a Food?

Yes. Generally speaking, the more fibre a food contains the lower its glycaemic index will be. This is because fibre acts as a physical barrier and slows down the absorption of carbohydrates into the blood.

Are There Any Cons to High Fibre Diets?

Wind is the main problem! Some fibre is fermented in the large intestine by bacteria that live there and this results in the production of gases like methane, hydrogen and carbon dioxide. The amount of gas produced depends on the type of fibre eaten and the gut bacteria present. But it explains why some slimmers find that excessive wind, discomfort and bloating occur if they suddenly boost their fibre intake to help them lose weight.

Fortunately, this is usually a short-lived problem as the large intestine and gut bacteria gradually adapt to an increased intake of fibre. That's why it's important to introduce fibre-rich foods into the diet gradually — and to persevere with them.

Constipation can also be a side effect of a high-fibre diet if fluid intake isn't also increased. This is because fibre acts like a sponge and absorbs water. The easiest way to avoid this, is to boost fluid intakes together with fibre intakes.

Juliette's Verdict

Like most nutritionists and dietitians, I'm a big fan of high-fibre diets, not just because they can help to reduce the risk of health problems ranging from constipation and piles to heart disease and cancer, but also because they help to fill us up. This is crucial if we want to lose weight, but it's also important in helping us to keep our weight steady, so that we avoid becoming overweight or obese in the future. I suggest people who worry that eating more fibre will give them wind, at least give it a go and continue to persevere. This really is a small price to pay for such major health and weight loss benefits and is only a temporary problem anyway. Once you see the pounds starting to drop off, you'll automatically reach for all things brown and ditch the white stuff from your daily diet.

LOW RESIDUE DIET

A low residue diet is a diet designed to reduce the frequency and volume of stools while prolonging intestinal transit time. It is similar to a low fiber diet, but typically includes restrictions on foods that increase bowel activity, such as milk and milk products and prune juice. A low residue diet typically contains less than 10-15 grams of fiber per day. Long term use of this diet, with its reduced intake of fruits and vegetables may not provide required amounts of vitamin C, calcium, and folic acid.

General Guidelines

Foods to Include

- White bread, refined pasta and cereals, and white rice
- Limited servings of canned or well-cooked vegetables that do not include skins
- Moderate fresh fruits without peels or seeds, certain canned or well-cooked fruits
- Tender, ground, and well cooked meat, fish, eggs, and poultry
- Milk and yogurt (usually limited to 2 cups per day), mild cheese, ricotta, cottage cheese

- Butter, mayonnaise, vegetable oils, margarine, plain gravies and dressings
- Broth and strained soups from allowed foods
- Pulp free, strained, or clear juices

Foods to Avoid

- Whole grain breads and pastas, corn bread or muffins, products made with whole grain products, or bran
- Strong cheeses, yogurt containing fruit skins or seeds
- Raw vegetables, except lettuce and other leaves
- Tough meat, meat with gristle
- Crunchy peanut butter
- Millet, buckwheat, flax, oatmeal
- Dried beans, peas, and legumes
- Dried fruits, berries, other fruits with skin or seeds
- Chocolate with Cocoa Powder (white chocolate has no fiber)
- Food containing whole coconut
- Juices with pulp
- Highly spiced food and dressings, pepper, hot sauces
- Caffeine
- Popcorn
- Nuts and Seeds

Conditions that may require a Low Residue Diet

- 1st and 2nd stages of labour
- Pre-and post-abdominal or intestinal surgery
- Bowel inflammation
- Crohn's disease
- Diverticulitis
- Ulcerative colitis
- Radiation therapy to the pelvis and lower bowel
- Chemotherapy
- Preparation for and participation in space flight (as per the Space toilet)
- Preparation for a colonoscopy

FOOD FORTIFICATION

Food fortification is the public health policy of adding micronutrients (essential trace elements and vitamins) to foodstuffs to ensure that minimum dietary requirements are met.

Simple diets based on staple foods with little variation are often deficient in certain nutrients, either because they are not present in sufficient amounts in the soil of a region, or because of the inherent inadequacy of the diet. Addition of micronutrients to staples and condiments can prevent large-scale deficiency diseases in these cases.

Rationale

Several ranges of food supplements are recognised:

- additives which repair a deficit to "normal" levels
- additives which appear to enhance a food
- supplements taken in addition to the normal diet

Many physicians today disagree with the premise that foodstuffs need supplementation, but accept that—for example—added calcium may provide benefit, or that adding folic acid may correct a nutritional deficiency especially in pregnant women.

On a more controversial level, but well founded in scientific basis, is the science of using foods and food supplements to achieve a defined health goal. A common example of this use of food supplements is the extent to which body builders will use amino acid mixtures, vitamins and phytochemicals to enhance natural hormone production, increase muscle and reduce fat.

Moving on from this reasonably accepted usage, there is increasing evidence for the use of food supplements in established medical conditions. This nutritional supplementation using foods as medicine (nutraceuticals) has been effectively used in treating disorders affecting the immune system up to and including cancers. This goes beyond the definition of "food supplement", but should be included for the sake of completeness.

Food Supplements

There are several main groups of food supplements which can be considered:

- Vitamins and co-vitamins
- Essential minerals
- Essential fatty acids
- Essential amino acids
- Glyconutrients
- Phytonutrients

Examples of Fortified Foods

Iodised salt has been used in the United States since before World War II.

Folic acid is added to flour in many industrialized countries, and has prevented a significant number of neural tube defects in infants. It is, however, not uniform in its application, with more intake of folic acid through fortified flour among those who were already receiving high amounts through their diet.

Niacin has been added to bread in the USA since 1938 (when voluntary addition started), a programme which substantially reduced the incidence of pellagra.

Vitamin D is added to a few foods (especially margarine).

Fluoride salts are added to water and toothpastes to prevent tooth decay. Water fluoridation is a controversial topic in some segments of the general public, although less so amongst established scientific bodies.

Calcium is frequently added to fruit juices, carbonated beverages and rice.

"Golden rice" is a variety of rice which has been genetically modified to produce beta carotene.

A wide range of iron compounds, including ferrous sulfate, ferrous fumarate and even elemental iron powder are added to food (usually cereal flours, but also table salt, milk and condiments) in a number of countries to prevent iron deficiency anemia. Although iron intake is often sufficient in developing countries, the bioavailability of the dietary iron is low, due to such factors as polyphenols and phytic acid binding the iron and preventing its absorption. Major challenges in iron fortification are to avoid undesirable changes in the appearance and taste of the food, and to target the population segment that needs the fortification the most.

DIETARY SUPPLEMENT

A dietary supplement, also known as food supplement or nutritional supplement, is a preparation intended to provide nutrients, such as vitamins, minerals, fiber, fatty acids or amino acids, that are missing or are not consumed in sufficient quantity in a person's diet. Some countries define dietary supplements as foods, while in others they are defined as drugs.

Supplements containing vitamins or dietary minerals are included in the Codex Alimentarius Commission, a guidebook on food safety sponsored by the United Nations.

Regulation

European Union

The Food Supplements Directive requires that supplements be demonstrated to be safe, both in quantity and quality. Some vitamins are essential in small quantities but dangerous in large quantities, notably Vitamin A. Consequently, only those supplements that have been proven to be safe may be sold without prescription. A survey conducted in Ireland in 2001, of adults aged 18-64 years, suggested that with the possible exception of niacin (flushing) and vitamin B6 (neuropathy), there appears to be little risk of the occurrence of adverse effects due to excessive consumption of vitamins in this population, based on current dietary practices.

As a category of food, food supplements cannot be labeled with drug claims in the bloc but can bear health claims and nutrition claims.

Legal Challenge

The dietary supplements industry in the UK, one of the 27 countries in the European Union, strongly opposed the Directive. In addition, a large number of consumers throughout Europe, including over one million in the UK, and many doctors and scientists, have signed petitions against what are viewed by the petitioners as unjustified restrictions of consumer choice. In 2004, along with two British trade associations, the Alliance for Natural Health had a legal challenge to the European Union's Food Supplements Directive referred to the European Court of Justice by the High Court in London. Although the European Court of Justice's Advocate General subsequently said that the EU's plan to tighten rules on the sale of vitamins and food supplements should be scrapped, he was eventually overruled by the European Court, which decided that the measures in question were necessary and appropriate for the purpose of protecting public health. ANH, however, interpreted the ban as applying only to synthetically produced supplements—and not to vitamins and minerals normally found in or consumed as part of the diet. Nevertheless, the European judges did acknowledge the Advocate General's concerns, stating that there must be clear procedures to allow substances to be added to the permitted list based on scientific evidence. They also said that any refusal to add a product to the list must be open to challenge in the courts.

Russia

Russian legislation, Ministry of Health's order number 117 dated as of 15 April 1997, under the title "Concerning the procedure for the examination and health certification of Biologically Active Dietary Supplements", provides the usage of the following terminology:

> As a rule, BADSs are foodstuffs with clinically proven effectiveness. BADSs are recommended not only for prophylactics, but can be included into a complex therapy for the prevention of pharmaceutical therapy's side effects and for the achievement of complete remission.

The development of BADSs and their applications has been very fast moving. They were originally considered as dietary supplements for people who had heightened requirements for some normal dietary components (for example, sportsmen). Later, they were employed as preventive medicines against chronic diseases.

United States

In the United States, a dietary supplement is defined under the Dietary Supplement Health and Education Act of 1994 (DSHEA) as a product that is intended to supplement the diet and contains any of the following dietary ingredients:

- a vitamin
- a mineral
- an herb or other botanical (excluding tobacco)
- an amino acid
- a dietary substance for use by people to supplement the diet by increasing the total dietary intake, or
- a concentrate, metabolite, constituent, extract, or combination of any of the above

Furthermore, it must also conform to the following criteria:

- intended for ingestion in pill, capsule, tablet, powder or liquid form
- not represented for use as a conventional food or as the sole item of a meal or diet
- labeled as a "dietary supplement"

The hormones DHEA (a steroid), pregnenolone (also a steroid) and the pineal hormone melatonin are marketed as dietary supplements in the US.

United States Regulation

Pursuant to the DSHEA, the Food and Drug Administration (FDA) regulates dietary supplements as foods, and not as drugs. While pharmaceutical companies are required to obtain FDA approval proving the safety or effectiveness of their products prior to their entry into the market, dietary supplements, like food, do not need to be pre-approved by FDA before they can enter the market.

The DSHEA gave the FDA the express responsibility to regulate the manufacturing processes of dietary supplements, and the FDA issued its first proposed rule in 2003. In June 2007 it issued its final rule, which requires all dietary supplement manufacturers to ensure by June 2010 that production of dietary supplements complies with *current good manufacturing practices*, and be manufactured with "controls that result in a consistent product free of contamination, with accurate labeling." In addition, the industry is now required to report to the FDA "all serious dietary supplement related adverse events." The new rules have been criticized, however, with skeptics arguing lack of FDA resources, loopholes, and an exception on quality assurance for raw material suppliers (with the burden placed on manufacturers) will lead to continued quality problems. There's also concern that supplement manufacturers and retailers will hide behind the new regulations. Prior to the rule supplements have had major quality problems, and the number of FDA investigators has declined.

The DSHEA, passed in 1994, was the subject of lobbying efforts by the manufacturers of dietary supplements. At the time of its passage DSHEA received strong support from consumer grassroots organizations, and Members of Congress. In recognition of this, President Bill Clinton, on signing DSHEA into law, stated that "After several years of intense efforts, manufacturers, experts in nutrition, and legislators, acting in a conscientious alliance with consumers at the grassroots level, have moved successfully to bring common sense to the treatment of dietary supplements under regulation and law." He also noted that the passage of DSHEA "speaks to the diligence with which an unofficial army of nutritionally conscious people worked democratically to change the laws in an area deeply important to them" and that "In an era of greater consciousness among people about the impact of what they eat on how they live, indeed, how long they live, it is appropriate that we have finally reformed the way Government treats consumers and these supplements in a way that encourages good health."

Popular support may have been based on a misunderstanding of the situation after the deregulation of the supplement industry. A large survey by the AARP, for example, found that 77 per cent of respondents (including both users and non-users of supplements) believed that the federal government should review the safety of dietary supplements and approve them before they can be marketed to consumers. In an October 2002 nationwide Harris poll, 59 per cent of respondents believed that supplements had to be approved by a government agency before they could be marketed; 68 per cent believed that supplements had to list potential side effects on their labels; and 55 per cent believed that supplement labels could not make claims of safety without scientific evidence. All of these beliefs were incorrect as a result of provisions of the DSHEA.

A 2001 study, published in *Archives of Internal Medicine,* found broad public support for greater governmental regulation of dietary supplements than was currently permitted by DSHEA. The researchers found that a majority of Americans supported pre-marketing approval by the FDA, increased oversight of harmful supplements, and greater scrutiny of the truthfulness of supplement label claims.

Quality

Under the FDA's final rule on good manufacturing practices, quality is defined as meaning "that the dietary supplement consistently meets the established specifications for identity, purity, strength, and composition and has been manufactured, packaged, labeled, and held under conditions to prevent adulteration under section 402(a)(1), (a)(2), (a)(3), and (a)(4) of the Federal Food, Drug, and Cosmetic Act". The new regulations allow FDA inspectors to look at a company's records upon request. However, enforcement could be difficult given the number of supplement manufacturers and the 16 per cent decline in FDA investigators from 2003 to 2006. Much of the contamination is due to poor raw ingredients. Suppliers provide certificates of analysis stating that they have tested the material. Under the 2003 proposed rule, manufacturers would have been required to retest the supplied ingredients. Under the final rule, testing for identity is always required. Other retesting is not required if the manufacturer has verified the reliability of the ingredient supplier.

In the U.S., contamination and false labeling are "not uncommon". Independent certification programmes exist, but these may have problems as well. United States Pharmacopeia manages the Dietary Supplement Verification Programme (DSVP). Its USP Verified Mark seal indicates that the product has been tested for integrity, purity, dissolution, and safe manufacturing, and it is the only certification programme which conducts random off-the-shelf testing. The USP programme will not certify products which contain ingredients that the USP's Dietary Supplement Information Expert Committee determines have a safety risk. ConsumerLab.com randomly tests some dietary supplements and makes the results available to subscribers. It has reported that 25 per cent of the supplements it tests have problems, and for multivitamins about half had problems. In 2008 ConsumerLab criticized the USP for proposing a 10 microgram perdaily serving limit on lead in dietary supplements and drugs. It noted that under the FDA's 2006 guidance on lead in candy, only 0.2 micrograms of lead per serving are allowed. NSF International, HFL Sport Science, and the Natural Products Association also have a dietary supplement certification programmes.

Permissible Claims

If a dietary supplement claims to cure, mitigate, or treat a disease, it would be considered to be an unauthorized new drug and in violation of the applicable regulations and statutes. As the FDA states it in a response to this question in a FAQ:

Is it legal to market a dietary supplement product as a treatment or cure for a specific disease or condition?

No, a product sold as a dietary supplement and promoted on its label or in labeling* as a treatment, prevention or cure for a specific disease or condition would be considered an unapproved—and thus illegal—drug. To maintain the product's status as a dietary supplement, the label and labeling must be consistent with the provisions in the Dietary Supplement Health and Education Act (DSHEA) of 1994.

Dietary supplements are permitted to make structure/function claims. These are broad claims that the product can support the

---

* Labeling refers to the label as well as accompanying material that is used by a manufacturer to promote and market a specific product.

structure or function of the body (e.g., "glucosamine helps support healthy joints", "the hormone melatonin helps establish normal sleep patterns"). The FDA must be notified of these claims within 30 days of their first use, and there is a requirement that these claims be substantiated. In reality, misleading claims about supplements are common, particularly on poorly-regulated commercial websites. For example, the compound hydrazine sulfate is sold as a dietary supplement in the USA and promoted as a treatment for cancer, despite little evidence that it is either safe or effective.

Other claims that required approval from FDA include health claims and qualified health claims. Health claims are permitted to be made if they meet the requirements for the claims found in the applicable regulations. Qualified health claims can be made through a petition process, including scientific information, if FDA has not approved a prior petition.

HEALTH RESORTS

Health resorts differ from recreational areas, because besides therapeutic resources they also have a system of technical, medical and organizational resources and that's why they can render medical assistance to patients with various diseases.

Baden-Baden is a town located in the state of Baden-Württemberg in Germany. It is situated on the western slopes of the Schwarzwald mountain. Its population is approximately 54 thousand people. It's famous all around the world as a heath resort location.

DIETOTHERAPY

An important part of a complex health resort therapy is dietotherapy or clinical nutrition. Its major goal is to satisfy the physiological demand of the human organism for nutrient materials and normalization of the functional state of various organs and metabolic processes that were impaired as a result of a specific disease or improper nutrition, stresses, etc. In case of health resort therapy clinical nutrition must be applied in compliance with all principles of balanced diet. This principle is applied not only in relation to the basic ingredients contained in food (like protein, fat, carbohydrates), but also to amino acids, vitamins and micro elements. Everything must be taken into account: the nutritive value of the whole meal, as well as the rational combination of dishes during every meal. The most appropriate eating pattern used most often in health resorts is four meals a day, although this pattern may be changed depending on the character of the disease, as well as on many other factors that are determined individually by the physician dealing with a particular patient. Thus, some patients with diseases of the digestive system and bad metabolism (like peptic ulcer, chronic gastritis, obesity, pancreatic diabetes) are prescribed to have 5 or even 6 meals a day. Of course, while staying in a health resort a patient should get not only clinical nutrition in order to get rid of his or her health problems, but various methods and techniques must be combined in a complex, so that the best result may be attained.

CASE STUDY: CHINESE DIETOTHERAPY

In China, the concept of medicinal foods, or ordinary food that can be used to treat illness, is not new. In his book *Eating Your Way to Health*, Cai Jingfeng explains that food and medicine had a common origin, since during prehistoric times, man must have eaten plants and fruits that had therapeutic effect on the body as well as providing nutrition.

The legendary Shen Nong, who is credited with introducing agriculture to China, was said to have tasted all the plants and waters to know which was poisonous or beneficial. In the course of his experiments, he was poisoned at least seventy times.

As early as the Warring States period, the effect that food could have on health has been chronicled in Chinese writing. Cai cites a quotation from the *Book of Han Fei* (280-233 BC) that mentioned how people got sick after eating food that had an adverse affect on the body. In the 11th century, a king named Tang from the Shang dynasty was reputed to have a cook named Yi Yin, who cooked soups for the king when he was ill. The soups were credited with bringing the king back to health.

In Traditional Chinese Medicine, according to Cai, the body is considered healthy when it is in a harmonious state. Traditional Chinese Medicine uses many common food as medicine, taking into account both the nature and flavor of food to achieve this. Food can be cool, cold, warm or hot. It can be salty, sour, sweet, bitter and pungent. In Traditional Chinese Medicine, disease is cured by applying the opposite nature and flavor to that of the illness.

Illnesses with symptoms such as high fever, thirst, headache, deep-coloured urine and yellow fur on the tongue surface are said to be of a hot and excessive nature, Cai explains. Diseases with symptoms such as cold extremities, chills and shortness of breath are of a cold and deficient nature. In severe cases of hot illnesses, cold remedies should be used; in milder ones, cool remedies. Cold diseases, then, are treated with hot or warm remedies.

Here's a brief list of medicinal foods and what they are used for:

Neutral Food

- black beans—to blacken hair and to ease post-partum pain
- soybeans—for anemia, asthma and to promote lactation
- carrots—to prevent night blindness and promotes digestive function
- chrysanthemum—for fever, also relieves dizziness

Cold Food

- banana—for constipation and hemorrhoids
- freshwater clams—for fever and detoxifying
- cucumber—for fever, sore throat and red eyes
- pear—for thirst and constipation

Cool Food

- bitter almond—for chronic bronchitis
- celery—for hypertension
- duck—hypertension with dizziness
- watermelon—for sore throat and to relieve summer heat

Hot Food

- chili—to stimulate the appetite
- black and white pepper—warms up the body

- clove—warms the spleen and stomach, stops vomiting

Warm Food

- aniseed—relieves intestinal spasm
- beef—for the tendons and bones
- garlic—for dysentery
- coriander—for skin rashes

DIETOTHERAPY FOR COMMON GASTROINTESTINAL AILMENTS

In general, gastrointestinal ailments involve different degrees of upper abdominal pain. Chinese medicine categories this as part of stomach disease, and reckoned that gastrointestinal ailments are caused by exposure to cold air on the stomach, eating and drinking habits, as well as energy from liver damaging gastric functions. From this diagnosis, they would prescreen the appropriate treatment.

(A) Liver Energy that Hurts the Stomach

It is usually manifested as dilation of the stomach, and can be caused by emotional reasons. Sini Powder is used to soothe the liver and regulates energy.

(B) Exposure to Cold that Harms the Stomach

It is usually seen as cold pains on the upper abdomen, and the pain subsides as temperature rises, and increase as temperature drops. Treatment is focused on gaining warmth and expelling cold. Galangale soup is prescribed to treat this ailment.

(C) Harm to the Stomach Gue to Eating and Drinking Habits

Symptoms displayed are swelling of the stomach cavity, belching of stomach acids, or vomiting undigested food. Baohe pills are prescribed to aid digestion and clear stagnation.

(D) There is not enough Stomach-yin for Nourishment

Long-term illness hurts the spleen and stomach. Displayed symptoms include blistering pain of stomach cavity, dryness of mouth and throat, little intake of food, dry stools. Yangyin-yiwei decoction is prescribed to reduce the symptoms.

(E) Cold Deficiency of the Spleen and Stomach

Recurrence of gastritis, vomiting of clear fluids, lack of strength and energy, infrequency of excretory stolls. Treatment is focused on strengthening the spleen and reducing pain in a warm setting. Astragalus soup is prescribed to heal this ailment.

(F) Stagnation and Stasis of Blood

When having gastrointestinal ailments, the pain is sustained at a fixed location. If it is as prickling pain, then it is classified as stagnation of blood. Treatment is focused on reducing pain, invigorating blood to remove extraverted blood. Shixiao powder is prescribed to this condition.

(G) Damp Heat Obstructing the Middle Passage

Displayed symptoms include burning sensation of stomach cavity, sticky and bitter mouth, and yellowish urine. Qingzhong decoction is prescribed to clear heat and expel dampness, as well as regulate stomach function and energy.

Dietotherapy For Gastrointestinal Ailments

(I) 3-5 slices of fresh ginger, moderate amounts of brown sugar; immerse ingredients in hot water ans consume. This is useful in treating gastrointestinal ailments caused by exposure to colds.

(II) 1g of pepper, 3 stalks of fiveleaf gynostemma herb, 3-5slices of ginger. Boil the fiveleaf gynowstemma herb and ginger for a while then add pepper to the concoction and consume the soup when warm. This is useful in treating gastrointestinal ailments caused by colds.

(III) Add water to 65g of honey, stir and consumes with an empty stomach. This is useful in treating gastrointestinal ailments due to secretion of too much gastric acid.

(IV) Prepare 250g of fresh mutton, cut them into cubes and cook till soft; then add polished round-grained rice and make porridge. Consume 2 servings a day, it can treat gastrointestinal ailments related to cold vacuity of the stomach. (V) 100g of polished round-grained rice, 25g of pork floss; cook polished rice into porridge form, add pork floss and stir evenly. Consume when it's hot. Useful treating gastrointestinal ailments related to cold vacuity of the spleen and stomach.

(VI) Boil 20g of bergamot orange and remove residue, place 100g of polished rice in water and cook into porridge form. Add the Bergamot orange extract and cook for a while before consumptions. It is useful in treating gastrointestinal ailments related to liver energy that hurts the stomach.

(VII) 30-60g of cactus, 1 pig's stomach. Stuff cactus into pig's stomach, and put all ingredients in a pot with appropriate amounts of water. Cook with a slow fire till contents are mashed form. Drinking the soup and eating the pig's stomach helps to treat patients who experience stagnation of vital energy flow and blood stasis, as well as those who suffer from chronic gastrointestinal ailments.

MEGAVITAMIN THERAPY

Megavitamin therapy is the use of large doses of vitamins, often many times greater than the recommended dietary allowance (RDA) in the attempt to prevent or treat diseases. It is typically used in complementary and alternative medicine by practitioners who call their approach "orthomolecular medicine", but also used in mainstream medicine for "exceedingly rare" genetic conditions which respond to megadoses of vitamins. In 2002, a review of these conditions identified about 50 which respond to "high-dose vitamin therapy". Further understanding of these conditions is expected to play a part in the emerging field of nutrigenomics.

Nutrients may be useful in preventing and treating some illnesses, but the conclusions of medical research are that the broad claims of disease treatment by advocates of megavitamin therapy are unsubstantiated by the available evidence. Critics have described some aspects of orthomolecular medicine as food faddism or even quackery. Research on nutrient supplementation in general suggests that some nutritional supplements might be beneficial, and that others might be harmful; several specific nutritional therapies are associated with an increased likelihood of the condition they are meant to prevent. A study of 161,000 individuals (post-menopausal women) provided, in the words of the authors, "convincing evidence that multivitamin use has little or no influence on the risk of common cancers, cardiovascular disease, or total mortality in postmenopausal women".

History

In the 1930s and 1940s, some scientific and clinical evidence suggested that there might be beneficial uses of vitamins C, E and B-3 in large doses. Beginning in the 1930s, the Shutes in Canada developed a megadose vitamin E therapy for cardiovascular and circulatory complaints, naming it the "Shute protocol". Tentative experiments in the 1930s with larger doses of vitamin C were superseded by Fred R. Klenner's development of megadose intravenous vitamin C treatments in the 1940s. William Kaufman published articles in the 1940s that detailed his treatment of arthritis with frequent, high doses of niacinamide.

In 1954, R. Altschul and Abram Hoffer applied large doses of the immediate release form of niacin (Vitamin B-3) to treat hypercholesterolemia (high cholesterol). The 1956 publication of Roger J. Williams Biochemical Individuality introduced concepts for individualized megavitamins and nutrients. In the 1960s, biochemist Irwin Stone, author of The Healing Factor, observed that vitamin C's utility in the megadose treatments of human disease parallels the amounts of vitamin C physiologically produced in most animals and postulated humans' evolutionary loss of this capability.

Megavitamin therapies were also publicly advocated by Linus Pauling in the late 1960s.

Several orthomolecular megavitamin protocols have been publicized. While formal medical recognition of niacin therapy for hypercholesterolemia followed confirmation by William Parsons of the Mayo Clinic (1956) and the Canner study (1986), the success of several popular books since the 1980s has made the public more aware of niacin's role in combination with other medications, for dyslipidemias (abnormal lipid levels in the blood). Pauling's advocacy of megadoses of vitamin C for colds, beginning in the 1960s, and later for cancer, made millions aware of the concept of megavitamin treatment in disease. Pauling's vitamin C recommendations are lower than some modern recommendations.

Other treatments include orthomolecular oral dosing schedules for an early treatment of colds, and for bowel tolerance for more established colds.

Usage of Therapy

An American cottage industry in the late 20th century, the evolving megavitamin therapy are integrated with orthomolecular and naturopathic medicine. Although megavitamin therapy still largely remains outside of the structure of evidence-based medicine, they are increasingly used by patients, with or without the approval of their treating physicians. In the 21st century, proposed megavitamin therapies with vitamin C are being evaluated for their possible use in cancer, but clinical results have shown no effect on treating or reducing the risk of cancer.

In 2008 researchers established that higher vitamin C intake reduces serum uric acid levels, and is associated with lower incidence of gout. The effect is more pronounced as intake increases into the megavitamin range

Criticism

The proposed efficacy of various megavitamin therapies has been contradicted by results of numerous clinical trials. For example, a thorough review of clinical trials in the treatment of colds with small and large doses of Vitamin C has established that there is no evidence for its efficacy.

Toxic effects of high doses of vitamin A, and vitamin D are well-established. Some vitamins such as vitamin B12 have no recommended maximum dosage, or tolerable upper intake level. A 1986 article argued that although "it is not known whether maintaining a prolonged high level of vitamin B12 is harmful", megadoses of vitamin B12 should not be used in dialysis patients because there are no "demonstrable benefits" and a possible risk of toxicity based on epidemiological and animal evidence. In 1998 the group which set the U.S. Dietary Reference Intakes stated that "there appear to be no risks associated with intakes of supplemental B12 that are more than two orders of magnitude higher than the ninety-fifth percentile of intake".

MULTIVITAMIN

A multivitamin is a preparation intended to supplement a human diet with vitamins, dietary minerals and other nutritional elements. Such preparations are available in the form of tablets, capsules, pastilles, powders, liquids and injectable formulations. Other than injectable formulations, which are only available and administered under medical supervision, multivitamins are recognized by the Codex Alimentarius Commission (the United Nations' authority on food standards) as a category of food. Multivitamin supplements are commonly provided in combination with minerals. A multivitamin/mineral supplement is defined in the United States as a supplement containing 3 or more vitamins and minerals but does not include herbs, hormones, or drugs, with each nutrient at a dose below the tolerable upper level determined by the Food and Drug Board and the maximum daily intake to not cause a risk for adverse health effects.

The terms multivitamin and multimineral are often used interchangeably. There is no scientific definition for either. Linguistically, the terms are compounded words of which meaning can be derived in that capacity.

History

Multivitamin-multimineral products providing more than vitamins

A and D became available in pharmacies and grocery stores in the mid-1930s. In 1934 Nutrilite Company introduced the first multivitamin-multimineral tablets. These supplements were made from natural dried and compressed vegetable and fruit concentrates. In the early 1940s other brands started to produce synthetic tablets.

Multivitamin Products and Components

Many multivitamins are formulated and/or labeled to differentiate consumer sectors e.g. prenatal, children, mature or 50+, men's, women's, diabetic, stress or megavitamin. Consumer multivitamin formulas are available as tablets, capsules, bulk powder, or liquid. Once and twice per day multivitamin formulas dominate common usage, although some formulas are designed for consumption 3-7 times per day or even allow hourly use.

Compositional variation amongst brands and lines allows substantial consumer choices. Modern multivitamin products roughly classify into RDA centric multivitamins with or without iron, RDA centric multivitamin/multimineral formulas with or without iron, higher potency formulas with mostly above RDA components with or without iron, and more specialized formulas by condition, such as for diabetics or by less common components, such as diversified antioxidants, herbal extracts or premium vitamin and mineral forms. Legally, the United States Food and Drug Administration allows a multivitamin to be called "high potency" if at least two-thirds of its nutrients have at least 100 per cent of the DV. In practice, "high potency" usually means substantially increased vitamin C and Bs with some other enhanced vitamin and mineral levels, but some minerals may still be much less than DV.

Some components are typically much lower than RDA amounts, often for cost reasons, e.g. biotin, usually the most expensive vitamin component, at over $4000 per active pound, is typically added in at only 5 per cent-30 per cent of RDA in many one per day formulations. Sometimes low content composition is for population subgroups, where the RDA would be inappropriate, such often occurs with iron, where the original population intake calculation was ca 12-13 mg iron per day by including menstruating females but some percentage of HFE variant gene bearing males with high iron retention, and others, may only need as little as ~1 mg iron per day including the normal dietary contribution.

Basic commercial multivitamin supplement products often contain the following ingredients: vitamin C, B_1, B_2, B_3, B_6, folic acid (B_9), B_{12}, B_5 (pantothenate), H (biotin), A, E, D_3, K_1, potassium iodide, cupric (sulfate anhydrous, picolinate, sulfate monohydrate, trioxide), selenomethionine, borate(s), zinc, calcium, magnesium, chromium, manganese, molybdenum, betacarotene, and iron. Other formulas may include additional ingredients such as other carotenes (e.g. lutein, lycopene), higher than RDA amounts of B, C or E vitamins including gamma-tocopherol, "near" B vitamins (inositol, choline, PABA), trimethylglycine (anhydrous betaine), betaine hydrochloride, vitamin K_2 as menaquinone-7, lecithin, citrus bioflavinoids or nutrient forms variously described as more easily absorbable.

Uses

By supplementing the diet with additional vitamins and minerals, multivitamins can be a valuable tool for those with dietary imbalances or different nutritional needs. People with dietary imbalances may include those on restrictive diets and those who can't or won't eat a nutritious diet. Pregnant women and elderly adults have different nutritional needs than other adults, and a multivitamin may be indicated by their physicians.

The proponents of orthomolecular medicine recommend individually optimized vitamin intakes, usually at higher doses than standard recommendations (such as the US RDA). They also recommend more absorbable forms of vitamins and minerals, in inexpensive but higher potency formulas, spread across the day.

Precautions

While multivitamins can be a valuable tool to correct dietary imbalances, it is worth exercising basic caution before taking them, especially if any medical conditions exist. In particular, pregnant women should generally consult their doctors before taking any multivitamins: for example, either an excess or deficiency of vitamin

A can cause birth defects. Some analyses have suggested that long-term use of beta-carotene, vitamin A, and vitamin E supplements may shorten life rather than extend it, with the additional risk being particularly large in smokers.

Severe vitamin and mineral deficiencies require medical treatment and can be very difficult to treat with common over-the-counter multivitamins. In such situations, special vitamin or mineral forms with much higher potencies are available, either as individual components or as specialized formulations, sometimes requiring a prescription.

Multivitamins in large quantities may pose a risk of an acute overdose, due to the toxicity of some components, principally iron. However, in contrast to iron tablets, which can be lethal to children, toxicity from overdoses of multivitamins are very rare. There appears to be little risk to supplement users of experiencing acute side effects due to excessive intakes of micronutrients. There also are strict limits on the retinol content for vitamin A during pregnancies that are specifically addressed by prenatal formulas. Additionally, various medical conditions and medications may adversely interact with multivitamins.

For normal adults taking a multivitamin for general health purposes, it is recommend that a multivitamin should contain 100 per cent DRI/RDA or less for each ingredient. However, many common brand supplements in the United States contain above-DRI amounts for some vitamins or minerals. Many brands offer low iron or iron-free versions of their multivitamin supplements.

Scientific Assessment

Evidence in Favour

In 2002, the Journal of the American Medical Association stated that "it appears prudent for all adults to take vitamin supplements." In this article, which examined the clinical applications of vitamins for the prevention of chronic diseases in adults, the authors, Robert H. Fletcher and Kathleen M. Fairfield from the Harvard School of Medicine, examined English-language articles about vitamins in relation to chronic diseases published between 1966 and 2002, and concluded that inadequate intake of several vitamins has been linked to the development of diseases including coronary heart disease, cancer, and osteoporosis.

Similarly, the April 9, 1998 issue of the New England Journal of Medicine featured an editorial entitled "Eat Right and Take a Multivitamin" that was based on studies that showed health benefits resulting from the consumption of supplemental folate to prevent birth defects and possibly decrease the incidence of cardiovascular disease.

Bruce Ames, professor of Biochemistry and Molecular Biology at the University of California, Berkeley, and a senior scientist at Children's Hospital Oakland Research Institute (CHORI), suggests that "to maximize human health and lifespan, scientists must abandon outdated models of micronutrients" and that "a metabolic tune-up through an improved supply of micronutrients is likely to have great health benefits."

Evidence Against

In 2006 the National Institutes of Health convened an expert panel to examine the available evidence on nutrient supplements. This review concluded that "Most of the studies we examined do not provide strong evidence for beneficial health-related effects of supplements taken singly, in pairs, or in combinations of three or more." They noted that multivitamins could provide health benefits to some groups of people, such as postmenopausal women, but that there was "disturbing evidence of risk" in other groups, such as smokers. The panel's report concluded that the "present evidence is insufficient to recommend either for or against the use of Multivitamin/Mineral Supplements by the American public to prevent chronic disease."

Similarly, a 2006 report for the United States Department of Health and Human Services concluded that "regular supplementation with a single nutrient or a mixture of nutrients for years has no significant benefits in the primary prevention of cancer, cardiovascular disease, cataract, age-related macular degeneration or cognitive decline." However, the report noted that multivitamins have beneficial effects in people with poor nutritional status, vitamin D and calcium can help prevent fractures in older people, and that zinc and antioxidants can help prevent age-related macular degeneration in people at a high risk of developing this disease.

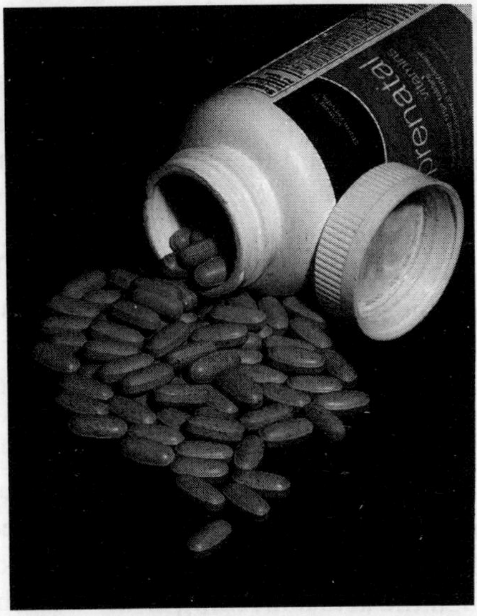

Fig. 2.11: Prenatal Vitamins Contain Higher Levels of Iron and Folic Acid, Compared with Typical Multivitamins

In 2007 the United Kingdom Food Standards Agency published an updated set of recommendations for eating a healthy diet. The recommendations stated that pregnant women should take extra folic acid and iron and that older people might need extra vitamin D and iron. However, the report advised that "Vitamin and mineral supplements are not a replacement for good eating habits" and stated that supplements are unnecessary for healthy adults who eat a balanced diet.

In February 2009, a study conducted in\161,808 postmenopausal women from the Women's Health Initiative clinical trials concluded that after 8 years of follow-up "multivitamin use has little or no influence on the risk of common cancers, cardiovascular disease, or total mortality". ·

Regulations by Governmental Agencies

United States

Because of their categorization as a dietary supplement by the Food and Drug Administration (FDA), most multivitamins sold in the

U.S. are not required to undergo the rigorous testing procedures typical of pharmaceutical drugs.

However, some multivitamins contain very high doses of one or several vitamins or minerals, or are specifically intended to treat, cure, or prevent disease, and therefore require a prescription or medicinal license in the U.S. Since such drugs contain no new substances, they do not require the same testing as would be required by a New Drug Application, but were allowed on the market as drugs due to the Drug Efficacy Study Implementation programme.

VITAMIN

A vitamin is an organic compound required as a nutrient in tiny amounts by an organism. The term 'vitamin' first became popular in the early 1800's as a contraction of the words 'vital' and 'mineral', though the actual meaning of the word has developed somewhat since that time. A compound is called a vitamin when it cannot be synthesized in sufficient quantities by an organism, and must be obtained from the diet. Thus, the term is conditional both on the circumstances and the particular organism. For example, ascorbic acid functions as vitamin C for some animals but not others, and vitamins D and K are required in the human diet only in certain circumstances. The term vitamin does not include other essential nutrients such as dietary minerals, essential fatty acids, or essential amino acids, nor does it encompass the large number of other nutrients that promote health but are otherwise required less often.

Vitamins are classified by their biological and chemical activity, not their structure. Thus, each "vitamin" may refer to several vitamer compounds that all show the biological activity associated with a particular vitamin. Such a set of chemicals are grouped under an alphabetized vitamin "generic descriptor" title, such as "vitamin A", which includes the compounds retinal, retinol, and many carotenoids. Vitamers are often inter-converted in the body.

Vitamins have diverse biochemical functions, including function as hormones (e.g. vitamin D), antioxidants (e.g. vitamin

E), and mediators of cell signaling and regulators of cell and tissue growth and differentiation (e.g. vitamin A). The largest number of vitamins (e.g. B complex vitamins) function as precursors for enzyme cofactor bio-molecules (coenzymes), that help act as catalysts and substrates in metabolism. When acting as part of a catalyst, vitamins are bound to enzymes and are called prosthetic groups. For example, biotin is part of enzymes involved in making fatty acids. Vitamins also act as coenzymes to carry chemical groups between enzymes. For example, folic acid carries various forms of carbon group — methyl, formyl and methylene—in the cell. Although these roles in assisting enzyme reactions are vitamins' best-known function, the other vitamin functions are equally important.

Until the 1900s, vitamins were obtained solely through food intake, and changes in diet (which, for example, could occur during a particular growing season) can alter the types and amounts of vitamins ingested. Vitamins have been produced as commodity chemicals and made widely available as inexpensive pills for several decades, allowing supplementation of the dietary intake.

History

Discovery of Vitamins and their Sources

Year of Discovery	*Vitamin*	*Source*
1909	Vitamin A (Retinol)	Cod liver oil
1912	Vitamin B1 (Thiamine)	Rice bran
1912	Vitamin C (Ascorbic acid)	Lemons
1918	Vitamin D (Calciferol)	Cod liver oil
1920	Vitamin B2 (Riboflavin)	Eggs
1922	Vitamin E (Tocopherol)	Wheat germ oil, Cosmetics and Liver
1926	Vitamin B12 (Cyanocobalamin)	Liver
1929	Vitamin K (Phylloquinone)	Alfalfa
1931	Vitamin B5 (Pantothenic acid)	Liver
1931	Vitamin B7 (Biotin)	Liver
1934	Vitamin B6 (Pyridoxine)	Rice bran
1936	Vitamin B3 (Niacin)	Liver
1941	Vitamin B9 (Folic acid)	Liver

The value of eating a certain food to maintain health was

recognized long before vitamins were identified. The ancient Egyptians knew that feeding liver to a patient would help cure night blindness, an illness now known to be caused by a vitamin A deficiency. The advancement of ocean voyage during the Renaissance resulted in prolonged periods without access to fresh fruits and vegetables, and made illnesses from vitamin deficiency common among ships' crews.

In 1749, the Scottish surgeon James Lind discovered that citrus foods helped prevent scurvy, a particularly deadly disease in which collagen is not properly formed, causing poor wound healing, bleeding of the gums, severe pain, and death. In 1753, Lind published his *Treatise on the Scurvy,* which recommended using lemons and limes to avoid scurvy, which was adopted by the British Royal Navy. This led to the nickname Limey for sailors of that organization. Lind's discovery, however, was not widely accepted by individuals in the Royal Navy's Arctic expeditions in the 19th century, where it was widely believed that scurvy could be prevented by practicing good hygiene, regular exercise, and by maintaining the morale of the crew while on board, rather than by a diet of fresh food. As a result, Arctic expeditions continued to be plagued by scurvy and other deficiency diseases. In the early 20th century, when Robert Falcon Scott made his two expeditions to the Antarctic, the prevailing medical theory was that scurvy was caused by "tainted" canned food.

During the late 18th and early 19th centuries, the use of deprivation studies allowed scientists to isolate and identify a number of vitamins. Initially, lipid from fish oil was used to cure rickets in rats, and the fat-soluble nutrient was called "antirachitic A". Thus, the first "vitamin" bioactivity ever isolated, which cured rickets, was initially called "vitamin A", although confusingly the bioactivity of this compound is now called vitamin D. In 1881, Russian surgeon Nikolai Lunin studied the effects of scurvy while at the University of Tartu in present-day Estonia. He fed mice an artificial mixture of all the separate constituents of milk known at that time, namely the proteins, fats, carbohydrates, and salts. The mice that received only the individual constituents died, while the mice fed by milk itself developed normally. He made a conclusion that "a natural food such as milk must therefore contain, besides these known principal ingredients, small quantities of unknown substances essential to life." However, his conclusions were rejected by other researchers when they were unable to reproduce his results. One difference was that he had used table sugar (sucrose), while other researchers had used milk sugar (lactose) that still contained small amounts of vitamin B.

In east Asia, where polished white rice was the common staple food of the middle class, beriberi resulting from lack of vitamin B1 was endemic. In 1884, Takaki Kanehiro, a British trained medical doctor of the Imperial Japanese Navy, observed that beriberi was endemic among low-ranking crew who often ate nothing but rice, but not among crews of Western navies and officers who consumed a Western-style diet. With the support of the Japanese navy, he experimented using crews of two battleships; one crew was fed only white rice, while the other was fed a diet of meat, fish, barley, rice, and beans. The group that ate only white rice documented 161 crew members with beriberi and 25 deaths, while the latter group had only 14 cases of beriberi and no deaths. This convinced Kanehiro and the Japanese Navy that diet was the cause of beriberi, but mistakenly believed that sufficient amounts of protein prevented it. That diseases could result from some dietary deficiencies was further investigated by Christiaan Eijkman, who in 1897 discovered that feeding unpolished rice instead of the polished variety to chickens helped to prevent beriberi in the chickens. The following year, Frederick Hopkins postulated that some foods contained "accessory factors"—in addition to proteins, carbohydrates, fats, et cetera—that were necessary for the functions of the human body. Hopkins and Eijkman were awarded the Nobel Prize for Physiology or Medicine in 1929 for their discovery of several vitamins.

In 1910, Japanese scientist Umetaro Suzuki succeeded in extracting a water-soluble complex of micronutrients from rice bran and named it aberic acid. He published this discovery in a Japanese scientific journal. When the article was translated into German, the translation failed to state that it was a newly discovered nutrient, a claim made in the original Japanese article, and hence his discovery failed to gain publicity. In 1912 Polish biochemist Kazimierz Funk isolated the same complex of micronutrients and proposed the complex be named “Vitamine” (a portmanteau of “vital amine”). The name soon became synonymous with Hopkins’ “accessory factors”, and by the time it was shown that not all vitamins were amines, the word was already ubiquitous. In 1920, Jack Cecil Drummond proposed that the final “e” be dropped to deemphasize the “amine” reference after the discovery that vitamin C had no amine component.

In 1931, Albert Szent-Györgyi and a fellow researcher Joseph Svirbely determined that “hexuronic acid” was actually vitamin C and noted its anti-scorbutic activity. In 1937, Szent-Györgyi was awarded the Nobel Prize in Physiology or Medicine for his discovery. In 1943 Edward Adelbert Doisy and Henrik Dam were awarded the Nobel Prize in Physiology or Medicine for their discovery of vitamin K and its chemical structure. In 1967, George Wald was awarded the Nobel Prize (along with Ragnar Granit and Haldan Keffer Hartline) for his discovery that vitamin A could participate directly in a physiological process.

In Humans

Vitamins are classified as either water-soluble or fat soluble. In humans there are 13 vitamins: 4 fat-soluble (A, D, E and K) and 9 water-soluble (8 B vitamins and vitamin C). Water-soluble vitamins dissolve easily in water, and in general, are readily excreted from the body, to the degree that urinary output is a strong predictor of vitamin consumption. Because they are not readily stored, consistent daily intake is important. Many types of water-soluble vitamins are synthesized by bacteria. Fat-soluble vitamins are absorbed through the intestinal tract with the help of lipids (fats). Because they are more likely to accumulate in the body, they are more likely to lead to hypervitaminosis than are water-soluble vitamins. Fat-soluble vitamin regulation is of particular significance in cystic fibrosis.

List of Vitamins

Each vitamin is typically used in multiple reactions and, therefore, most have multiple functions.

Vitamin Generic Descriptor Name	*Vitamer Chemical Name(s) (List not Complete)*	*Solubility*	*Recommended Dietary Allowances (Male, age 19-70)*	*Deficiency Disease*	*Upper Intake Level (UL/day)*	*Overdose Disease*
Vitamin A	Retinoids (retinol, retinoids and carotenoids)	Fat	900 µg	Night-blindness and Keratomalacia	3,000 µg	Hypervitaminosis A
Vitamin B1	Thiamine	Water	1.2 mg	Beriberi, Wernicke-Korsakoff syndrome	N/D	Drowsiness or muscle relaxation with large doses.
Vitamin B2	Riboflavin	Water	1.3 mg	Ariboflavinosis	N/D	
Vitamin B3	Niacin, niacinamide	Water	16.0 mg	Pellagra	35.0 mg	Liver damage (doses > 2g/day) and other problems
Vitamin B5	Pantothenic acid	Water	5.0 mg	Paresthesia	N/D	Diarrhea; possibly nausea and heartburn.
Vitamin B6	Pyridoxine, pyridoxamine, pyridoxal	Water	1.3-1.7 mg	Anemia peripheral neuropathy.	100 mg	Impairment of proprioception, nerve damage (doses > 100 mg/day)
Vitamin B7	Biotin	Water	30.0 µg	Dermatitis, enteritis	N/D	

(Contd.)

Vitamin Generic Descriptor Name	*Vitamer Chemical Name(s) (List not Complete)*	*Solubility*	*Recommended Dietary Allowances (Male, age 19-70)*	*Deficiency Disease*	*Upper Intake Level (UL/day)*	*Overdose Disease*
Vitamin B9	Folic acid, folinic acid	Water	400 μg	Deficiency during pregnancy is associated with birth defects, such as neural tube defects	1,000 μg	May mask symptoms of vitamin B12 deficiency; other effects.
Vitamin B12	Cyanocobalamin, hydroxycobalamin, methylcobalamin	Water	2.4 μg	Megaloblastic anemia	N/D	No known toxicity
Vitamin C	Ascorbic acid	Water	90.0 mg	Scurvy	2,000 mg	Vitamin C megadosage
Vitamin D	Ergocalciferol, cholecalciferol	Fat	5.0 μg-10 μg	Rickets and Osteomalacia	50 μg	Hypervitaminosis D
Vitamin E	Tocopherols, tocotrienols	Fat	15.0 mg	Deficiency is very rare; mild hemolytic anemia in newborn infants.	1,000 mg	Increased congestive heart failure seen in one large randomized study.
Vitamin K	phylloquinone, menaquinones	Fat	120 μg	Bleeding diathesis	N/D	Increases coagulation in patients taking warfarin.

In Nutrition and Diseases

Vitamins are essential for the normal growth and development of a multicellular organism. Using the genetic blueprint inherited from its parents, a fetus begins to develop, at the moment of conception, from the nutrients it absorbs. It requires certain vitamins and minerals to be present at certain times. These nutrients facilitate the chemical reactions that produce among other things, skin, bone, and muscle. If there is serious deficiency in one or more of these nutrients, a child may develop a deficiency disease. Even minor deficiencies may cause permanent damage.

For the most part, vitamins are obtained with food, but a few are obtained by other means. For example, microorganisms in the intestine—commonly known as "gut flora"—produce vitamin K and biotin, while one form of vitamin D is synthesized in the skin with the help of the natural ultraviolet wavelength of sunlight. Humans can produce some vitamins from precursors they consume. Examples include vitamin A, produced from beta carotene, and niacin, from the amino acid tryptophan.

Once growth and development are completed, vitamins remain essential nutrients for the healthy maintenance of the cells, tissues, and organs that make up a multicellular organism; they also enable a multicellular life form to efficiently use chemical energy provided by food it eats, and to help process the proteins, carbohydrates, and fats required for respiration.

Deficiencies

Because human bodies do not store most vitamins, humans must consume them regularly to avoid deficiency. Human bodily stores for different vitamins vary widely; vitamins A, D, and B_{12} are stored in significant amounts in the human body, mainly in the liver, and an adult human's diet may be deficient in vitamins A and B_{12} for many months before developing a deficiency condition. Vitamin B_3 is not stored in the human body in significant amounts, so stores may only last a couple of weeks. Deficiencies of vitamins are classified as either primary or secondary. A primary deficiency occurs when an organism does not get enough of the vitamin in its food. A secondary deficiency may be due to an underlying disorder that prevents or limits the absorption or use of the vitamin, due to a "lifestyle factor", such as smoking, excessive alcohol consumption, or the use of medications that interfere with the absorption or use of the vitamin. People who eat a varied diet are unlikely to develop a severe primary vitamin deficiency. In contrast, restrictive diets have the potential to cause prolonged vitamin deficits, which may result in often painful and potentially deadly diseases.

Well-known human vitamin deficiencies involve thiamine (beriberi), niacin (pellagra), vitamin C (scurvy) and vitamin D (rickets). In much of the developed world, such deficiencies are rare; this is due to (1) an adequate supply of food; and (2) the addition of vitamins and minerals to common foods, often called fortification. In addition to these classical vitamin deficiency diseases, some evidence has also suggested links between vitamin deficiency and a number of different disorders.

Side Effects and Overdose

In large doses, some vitamins have documented side effects that tend to be more severe with a larger dosage. The likelihood of consuming too much of any vitamin from food is remote, but overdosing from vitamin supplementation does occur. At high enough dosages some vitamins cause side effects such as nausea, diarrhea, and vomiting.

When side effects emerge, recovery is often accomplished by reducing the dosage. The concentrations of vitamins an individual can tolerate vary widely, and appear to be related to age and state of health. In the United States, overdose exposure to all formulations of vitamins was reported by 62,562 individuals in 2004 (nearly 80% of these exposures were in children under the age of 6), leading to 53 "major" life-threatening outcomes and 3 deaths; a small number in comparison to the 19,250 people who died of unintentional poisoning of all kinds in the U.S. in the same year (2004).

Supplements

Dietary supplements, often containing vitamins, are used to ensure that adequate amounts of nutrients are obtained on a daily basis, if optimal amounts of the nutrients cannot be obtained through a varied diet. Scientific evidence supporting the benefits of some vitamin supplements is well established for certain health conditions, but others need further study. In some cases, vitamin supplements may have unwanted effects, especially if taken before surgery, with other dietary supplements or medicines, or if the person taking them has certain health conditions. Dietary supplements may also contain levels of vitamins many times higher, and in different forms, than one may ingest through food.

A meta-analysis published in 2006 suggested that Vitamin A and E supplements not only provide no tangible health benefits for generally healthy individuals, but may actually increase mortality, although two large studies included in the analysis involved smokers, for which it was already known that beta-carotene supplements can be harmful. Another study released in May 2009 found that antioxidants such as vitamins C and E may actually curb some benefits of exercise.

Governmental Regulation of Vitamin Supplements

Most countries place dietary supplements in a special category under the general umbrella of foods, not drugs. This necessitates that the manufacturer, and not the government, be responsible for ensuring that its dietary supplement products are safe before they are marketed. Unlike drug products, which must explicitly be proven safe and effective for their intended use before marketing, there are often no provisions to "approve" dietary supplements for safety or effectiveness before they reach the consumer. Also unlike drug products, manufacturers and distributors of dietary supplements are not generally required to report any claims of injuries or illnesses that may be related to the use of their products.

Names in Current and Previous Nomenclatures

The reason the set of vitamins seems to skip directly from E to K is that the vitamins corresponding to "letters" F-J were either reclassified over time, discarded as false leads, or renamed because of their relationship to "vitamin B", which became a "complex" of vitamins. The German-speaking scientists who isolated and described vitamin K (in addition to naming it as such) did so because

Nomenclature of Reclassified Vitamins

Previous Name	*Chemical Name*	*Reason for Name Change*
Vitamin B4	Adenine	DNA metabolite
Vitamin B8	Adenylic acid	DNA metabolite
Vitamin F	Essential fatty acids	Needed in large quantities (does not fit the definition of a vitamin)
Vitamin G	Riboflavin	Reclassified as Vitamin B2
Vitamin H	Biotin	Reclassified as Vitamin B7
Vitamin J	Catechol, Flavin	Protein metabolite
Vitamin L1	Anthranilic acid	Protein metabolite
Vitamin L2	Adenylthiomethylpentose	RNA metabolite
Vitamin M	Folic acid	Reclassified as Vitamin B9
Vitamin O	Carnitine	Protein metabolite
Vitamin P	Flavonoids	No longer classified as a vitamin
Vitamin PP	Niacin	Reclassified as Vitamin B3
Vitamin U	S-Methylmethionine	Protein metabolite

the vitamin is intimately involved in the *Koagulation* of blood following wounding. At the time, most (but not all) of the letters from F through to J were already designated, so the use of the letter K was considered quite reasonable. The table on the right lists chemicals that had previously been classified as vitamins, as well as the earlier names of vitamins that later became part of the B-complex.

VITAMIN POISONING

Vitamin poisoning, hypervitaminosis or vitamin overdose refers to a condition of high storage levels of vitamins, which can lead to toxic symptoms. The medical names of the different conditions are derived from the vitamin involved: an excess of vitamin A, for example, is called hypervitaminosis A.

With few exceptions, like some vitamins from B complex, hypervitaminosis usually occurs more with fat-soluble vitamins, which are stored in the liver and fatty tissues of the body. Because of this, these vitamins build up and remain for a longer time in the body than water soluble vitamins.

High dosage vitamin A; high dosage, slow release vitamin B_3; and very high dosage vitamin B_6 alone (i.e. without vitamin B complex) are sometimes associated with vitamin side effects that usually rapidly cease with supplement reduction or cessation.

Vitamin C has a brief, pronounced laxative effect when taken in large amounts, typically in the range of 5-20 grams per day in divided doses for a person in normal "good health," although seriously ill people, may take 100-200 grams without inducing vitamin poisoning.

High doses of mineral supplements can also lead to side effects and toxicity. Mineral-supplement poisoning does occur occasionally due to excessive and unusual intake of iron-containing supplements, including some multivitamins, but is not common.

Generally, toxic levels of vitamins are achieved through high supplement intake and not from dietary sources. Toxicities of fat-soluble vitamins result also can be caused by a large intake of highly fortified foods, but foods never deliver dangerous levels of water-soluble vitamins.

The Dietary Reference Intake recommendations from the United States Department of Agriculture define a "tolerable upper intake level" for most vitamins.

Comparative Safety Statistics

Death by vitamin poisoning appears to be quite uncommon in the US, typically none in a given year.

Before 1998, several deaths per year were associated with pharmaceutical iron-containing supplements, especially brightly-coloured, sugar-coated, high-potency iron supplements, and most deaths were children. Unit packaging restrictions on supplements with more than 30 mg of iron have since reduced deaths to 0 or 1 per year. These statistics compare with 59 deaths due to aspirin poisoning in 2003 and 147 deaths associated with acetaminophen-containing products in 2003.

3

Food Industry Trade Groups, Institutes, Guilds, Associations, Councils and Research Centres: Select Case Studies

FOOD INDUSTRY TRADE GROUPS

- American Frozen Food Institute
- American Meat Institute
- American Mushroom Institute
- Bread Bakers Guild of America
- British Potato Council
- British Sandwich Association
- Canadian Meat Council
- Canadian Restaurant and Foodservices Association
- Dairy Farmers of Manitoba
- Efficient Consumer Response
- FEFANA
- Florida Citrus Mutual
- Food Products Association
- Food and Drink Federation
- Freshfel Europe
- Grain and Feed Trade Association
- Grocery Manufacturers Association
- Idaho Potato Commission
- International Bottled Water Association
- International Food Information Council
- International Life Sciences Institute
- Juice Products Association
- Melton Mowbray Pork Pie Association
- Mutton Renaissance Campaign
- NBWA

- National Association for the Specialty Food Trade
- National Chicken Council
- National Confectioners Association
- National Frozen and Refrigerated Foods Association
- National Meat Association
- National Restaurant Association
- National Turkey Federation
- Natural Products Association
- North American Meat Processors Association
- Produce Marketing Association
- Southern Hemisphere Association of Fresh Fruit Exporters
- Specialty Coffee Association of Indonesia
- The Washington Restaurant Association
- U.S. Poultry and Egg Association
- United States Brewers' Association
- Wine and Spirits Wholesalers of America
- Wisconsin Restaurant Association
- Wisconsin Restaurant Association Education Foundation
- World Apple and Pear Association
- Worldwide Food Expo

CASE STUDY: AMERICAN MEAT INSTITUTE

The American Meat Institute is an organization composed primarily of US meat producers. It was founded in 1906 and is today located in Washington, DC. AMI provides assistance and representation for member organizations. It also sponsors several large conferences for the meat industry.

Information

The American Meat Institute (AMI) is an industry trade group that serves the meat packing industry. AMI serves several roles for the industry such as providing resources and information to member companies, providing opportunities for interaction between industry members, and engaging in public relations on behalf of the meat industry. AMI is headquartered in Washington, DC and claims to represent through membership nearly three quarters of the meat and poultry industries. Meat industry organizations become AMI members through an application process and yearly dues based primarily on the size of the member organization with larger organizations paying larger membership fees.

AMI is run by a board of officers elected each year. The current officers are as follows: AMI president and CEO: J. Patrick Boyle, Chairman: Robert Manley, Vice Chairman: Richard Bond, Tresurer: David Miniat, and Secretary: Rod Brenneman.

Another organization founded by AMI is the American Meat Institute Foundation which conducts scientific research on AMI's behalf.

AMI celebrated its organizational centennial in 2006 after being founded in 1906 in Chicago as the American Meat Packers Association. The organization was created only shortly after the passage of the Federal Meat Inspection Act and spent much its early years helping meat packers adjust to new inspection requirements. The name was changed in 1919 to the Institute of American Meat Packers (IAMP), and finally again in 1940 to the current American Meat Institute. AMI moved its headquarters in 1979 to Washington, DC, where it remains as of 2006. AMI established its research branch, the AMI Foundation, in 1991.

AMI operates several websites with information for both industry members and consumers. In addition to the organization's own website, AMI operates www.meatsafety.org which provides consumers with food safety information regarding cooking, handling, and storage of meat products.

Events

AMI sponsors or cosponsors a number of industry meetings and conferences each year. In March 2006 AMI sponsored the 13th Annual Meat Conference. Some of the notable events at the 2006 conference were presentations on consumer trends, a seminar on leadership strategies, and a product tasting fair.

Additionally, AMI cosponsors the biennial Worldwide Food Expo. This conference has grown in popularity as in 2005 more than 25,000 people from more than 100 nations attended and visited the 1,100 exhibitors. The AMI Foundation also hosts a more research focused conference, the Meat Industry Research Conference, immediately preceding the Worldwide Food Expo.

CASE STUDY: BREAD BAKERS GUILD OF AMERICA

The Bread Bakers Guild of America is a non-profit alliance of professional bakers, farmers, millers, suppliers, educators, students, home bakers, technical experts, bakery owners, and managers. Founded in 1993 by Pittsburgh bakery owner, Thomas McMahon, The Guild is now based in Sonoma, California, and has a diverse membership from across the United States and around the world.

The mission of The Bread Bakers Guild of America is to shape the knowledge and skills of the artisan baking community through education. In support of this mission, The Guild is committed to:

1. Providing educational resources to artisan bakers
2. Supporting and fostering the growth of the artisan baking community
3. Defining and upholding the highest professional standards
4. Celebrating the craft of the passion of the artisan baker

Besides holding bread baking classes, other regional events, and publishing a quarterly newsletter, The Bread Bakers Guild of America also sponsors Bread Bakers Guild Team USA, which has competed in every Coupe du Monde de la Boulangerie since 1994. Bread Bakers Guild Team USA won a gold medal in the Baguette and Specialty Breads category and overall medals in 1999 (gold), 2002 (silver), and 2005 (gold).

CASE STUDY: BRITISH POTATO COUNCIL

The Potato Council is a non-departmental public body whose mission is to develop and promote Britain's potato industry. The Potato Council promotes the health benefits of potatoes to the general public, showing how potatoes are low in both fat and calories and packed full of vitamins and minerals. The industry invests significant amounts of effort in teaching children about healthy eating and showing how potatoes are grown. Many of the industry's farmers work hard to re-connect children to their food, by spending time working with children in schools and on their farms, showing how they plant, grow and harvest their crops. The Potato Council, which has 56 employees, raises all of its money from a compulsory levy on potato growers and seed merchants and receives no funding from the government. It is based in Cowley in Oxfordshire. There is a Scottish office in Newbridge in Midlothian and an experimental station in Sutton Bridge in Lincolnshire. It was set up by the *Potato Industry Development Council Order 1997.*

Campaigns

The potato council runs a number of campaigns throughout the year, among these are *National Chip Week,* a campaign to expand coverage and knowledge of chips and chip shops.

Love Potatoes is another, to encourage people to eat more of the potato, due to health benefits of eating the skins along with the flesh.

CASE STUDY: BRITISH SANDWICH ASSOCIATION

The British Sandwich Association (BSA) was founded in January 1990. Its aim is to set technical standards for sandwich making and encourage improvement in the industry.

Activities

The British Sandwich Association is a non-commercial organisation run on behalf of its members by J&M Group Ltd. It is based in Chepstow.

Awards

The BSA also host the Sammies annual awards for sandwich manufacturers and retailers.

CASE STUDY: CANADIAN MEAT COUNCIL

The Canadian Meat Council (CMC) is Canada's national trade association for the federally inspected red meat packers and processors. It is an industry trade group associated with the meat packing industry. Federally inspected plants account for over 90 per cent of all the meat processed in Canada.

As a key component of Canada's agriculture sector, the red meat industry is the largest sector of Canada's food processing industry, representing 15 per cent of Canada's agri-food exports and employing more than 45,000 Canadians. It is also one of Canada's leading manufacturing sectors with annual sales of over $15 billion.

History

A group of Ontario meat packers met in Toronto in August, 1919 to decide if an association is needed to represent the industry which underwent tremendous growth during and after the WWI. With overwhelming support for the idea, Samuel E. "Sam" Todd was appointed to head the Council (then called as "The Industrial and Development Council of Canadian Meat Packers") on September 1, 1919. J.S. McLean was elected as the first president of the Council. E.B. Roberts, a journalist by profession was hired by beginning of 1920 to take care of the Councils media and publicity relations.

The first office of the organization was located at 186 King St. W., Toronto. Membership included Harris Abattoir Lts., William Davies Co. Ltd., Swift Canadian Co. Ltd., Gunns Ltd., Canadian Packing Co Ltd., Puddys Ltd., F.W. Fearman Co., Ingersoll Packaging Co. Ltd., Whyte Packing Co. Ltd., Gallagher-Holman and Lafrance Co. Ltd., Gordon-Ironside & Fares Packers Ltd., Wilson Canadian Co. Ltd., and Armour and Company.

Presidents—Past and Present

Jack S. Whyte President, Whyte Packing Co. of Stratford ON. Jack is a very important person because he was our President 50 years ago, in February 1958. Jack has the distinction of being the only living past president to have chaired meetings of the Meat Packers

Council of Canada in its boardroom at 200 Bay St., at the corner of Bay and Wellington, in Toronto.

Graeme R. Bieman President, Coleman Packing Company, London ON. Graeme became Council president in 1965. Graeme is the only past president here who chaired meetings at the Council Board Room in the Six Points Plaza. In 1971, the Council office was completely destroyed in a fire. Gone were many irreplaceable pieces of Council history.

Kenneth R. Murray President J.M. Schneider Inc., Kitchener ON. Ken assumed the Council presidency from Art Mill at the Council Annual Meeting in Winnipeg in 1973. In 1984, at the Council meeting in Quebec City he received the president's gavel from Jean Bienvenue.

Ed J. Roberts VP Packinghouse Div. Canada Packers Limited, Toronto. Ed Roberts was named President at the Quebec City Annual Meeting in 1975, following Joe Rapoport's term.

Allan K. Beswick VP Meat Division, Swift Canadian Company, Etobicoke. At the 1976 Convention in Edmonton, Al received the gravel from Ed Roberts. He stepped into the fray again in 1980, following Nigel Goodall. The Council got a new name — the former Meat Packers Council of Canada became the CMC/CVC.

Henry G. Beben President J.M. Schneider Inc., Kitchener. When John Nielsen resigned late in 1977, Henry assumed the presidency and continued through 1978. I

Nigel L. Goodall VP, Marketing, Hygrade Foods Inc., Montreal PQ. Nigel received the gavel of office from Henry Beben at the 1979 An. Mtg. in Calgary. The Council hosted 60th Anniversary Receptions in: Edmonton, Winnipeg, Ottawa and Montreal with an average attendance of 70 consumer, press, government and industry representatives at each event.

Jean Bienvenue Managing Director, Salaisons Olympia, St. Simon, PQ. Jean Bienvenue took over the presidency from Bob Nadeau at the Toronto meeting in 1983 and presided over the 1984 Convention in Quebec City.

Lloyd W. Macleod VP & GM, Fresh Meat Div. Canada Packers Inc. Toronto. At the Council Convention in Toronto in 1986, Lloyd succeeded Fred Mitchell as President.

Russell W.r. Baker VP of Operations, Intercontinental Packers,

Saskatoon, SK. Russ became President at the Quebec City Convention in 1988, taking over from Yvon Mercier.

Frank Powell General Manager, Quality Meat Packers, Toronto ON. Frank received the gavel of office from Russ Baker at the annual meeting in Vancouver in 1989.

Max R. Dingle President, Shopsy Foods Inc., Toronto (Unox Meats). Max moved up to the Council Presidency at the Quebec Convention in 1991, succeeding Yvon Mercier.

Wayne Urbonas Burns Meats. Wayne received the gavel from Yves Lalonde at the 1995 Convention in Vancouver and presided at the 1996 Convention in Toronto.

Don Davidson — Maple Leaf Foods President in 1996. Next, in 1999, *Laurent Brochu* of Olymel. David Schwartz of Quality Meat Packers was Council President in 2002. He was followed in 2003 by *Brian Read* of Levinoff Meat Products Ltd. *Willie Van Solkema*, then of Cargill Foods, took over for part of 2004 and for the balance of 2004, *Brain Read* returned to the presidency. The Council president for 2005 was *Arie Nuys* of Delft Blue Inc. Then for 2006, there is our immediate past president, *Conrad Huber* of Piller Sausages & Deli Ltd.

Meat Packers Council of Canada

The Industrial and Development Council of Canadian Meat Packers was considered lengthy by many members and an alternate name "Meat Packers Council of Canada" was proposed. It was not until Sam Todd retired in 1952 that the name was officially changed to Meat Packers Council of Canada. The council was "incorporated" as an association in 1961 after serving as a voluntary, unincorporated association for nearly 40 years.

Publications

Two booklets, Canadian Livestock Future and Better Livestock—The Nation's Welfare were published in the early 1920's.

A monthly series called "A letter on Canadian Livestock Products" was published since 1921.

Three editions of Food Service Meat Manual was published so far. Third Edition is available currently from the Council.

A series of position papers on issues facing the Canadian Meat Industry are available only for the members of the Council.

Proceedings of the Technical Symposium of the Canadian Meat Science Association.

CASE STUDY: MYPYRAMID

MyPyramid, released by the United States Department of Agriculture (USDA) on April 19, 2005, is an update on the American food guide pyramid. The new icon stresses activity and moderation along with a proper mix of food groups in one's diet. As part of the MyPyramid food guidance system, consumers are asked to visit the MyPyramid website for personalized nutrition information. Significant changes from the previous food pyramid include:

- Inclusion of a new symbol—a person on the stairs—representing physical activity.
- Measuring quantities in cups and ounces instead of servings.

MyPyramid was designed to educate consumers about a lifestyle consistent with the January 2005 *Dietary Guidelines for Americans*, an 80-page document. The guidelines, produced jointly by the USDA and Department of Health and Human Services (HHS), represented the official position of the U.S. government and served as the foundation of Federal nutrition policy. Currently published every five years, an update is expected in 2010.

Overview

Mypyramid contains eight divisions. From left to right on the pyramid are a person and six food groups:

- Physical activity, represented by a person climbing steps on the pyramid, to illustrate moderate physical activity every day, in addition to usual activity. The key recommendations for 2005 (other specific recommendations are provided for children and adolescents, pregnant and breastfeeding women, for older adults and for weight maintenance) are:

- ▪ Engage in regular physical activity and reduce sedentary activities to promote health, psychological well-being, and a healthy body weight. (At least 30 minutes on most, and if possible, every day for adults and at least 60 minutes each day for children and teenagers, and for most people increasing to more vigorous-intensity or a longer duration will bring greater benefits.)
- ▪ Achieve physical fitness by including cardiovascular conditioning, stretching exercises for flexibility, and resistance exercises or calisthenics for muscle strength and endurance.

- Grains, recommending that at least half of grains consumed be as whole grains
- Vegetables, emphasizing dark green vegetables, orange vegetables, and dry beans and peas
- Fruits, emphasizing variety and deemphasizing fruit juices
- Oils, recommending fish, nut, and vegetables sources
- Milk, a category that includes fluid milk and many other milk-based products
- Meat and beans, emphasizing low-fat and lean meats such as fish as well as more beans, peas, nuts, and seeds

There is one other category:

- Discretionary calories, represented by the narrow tip of each coloured band, including items such as candy, alcohol, or additional food from any other group.

Themes

The USDA encoded several themes into the design of the MyPyramid icon. According to the USDA, MyPyramid incorporated:

- *Personalization*, demonstrated by the MyPyramid website.

To find a personalized recommendation of the kinds and amounts of food to eat each day, individuals must visit MyPyramid.gov.

- *Gradual improvement,* represented by the slogan *Steps to a Healthier You.* It suggests that individuals can benefit from taking small steps to improve their diet and lifestyle each day.
- *Physical activity*, represented by the steps and the person climbing them, as a reminder of the importance of daily physical activity.
- *Variety*, symbolized by the six colour bands representing the five food groups of MyPyramid and oils. Suggests that foods from all groups are needed each day for good health.
- *Moderation*, represented by the narrowing of each food group from bottom to top. The wider base stands for foods with little or no solid fats, added sugars, or caloric sweeteners. Suggests these should be selected more often to get the most nutrition from calories consumed.
- *Proportionality*, shown by the different widths of the food group bands. The widths suggest how much food a person should choose from each group. The widths are just a general guide.

Differences from the Food Guide Pyramid

In a departure from the food guide pyramid, which was launched in 1992, no foods are pictured on the MyPyramid logo itself. Instead, coloured vertical bands represent different food groups. Additionally, the logo emphasizes physical activity by showing a person climbing steps on the side of the pyramid. MyPyramid was intentionally made simpler than the food guide pyramid after several USDA studies indicated that consumers widely misunderstood the original design. Consumers are asked to visit the MyPyramid.gov website for personalized nutrition information.

The food guide pyramid gave recommendations measured in serving sizes, which some people found confusing. MyPyramid gives its recommendations in common household measures, such as cups, ounces, and other measures that may be easier to understand.

The food guide pyramid gave a single set of specific recommendations for all people. In contrast, MyPyramid has 12 sets of possible recommendations, with the appropriate guide for an individual selected based on sex, age group, and activity level.

Controversy

Some claim that the USDA was and is unduly influenced by political pressure exerted by lobbyists for food production associations, in particular dairy and meat. Some of the recommended portion sizes are up to eight times the size of portions recommended in other countries, although the number of portions recommended are the same.

Development

In September 2005, a "child-friendly version" of the food pyramid graphic and food guidance system launched. Three of five meetings had been held as of May 2009 towards the publication of 2010 dietary guidelines.

The research process and results used to create the MyPyramid Food Guidance System was documented in a supplemental issue of the *Journal of Nutrition Education and Behaviour* published in November/December 2006 that included the following articles:

- Britten P, Marcoe K, Yamini S, Davis, C., "Development of Food Intake Patterns for the MyPyramid Food Guidance System"
- Marcoe K, Juan WY, Yamini S, Carlson A, Britten P., "Development of Food Group Composite and Nutrient Profiles for MyPyramid Food Guidance System"
- Britten P, Haven J, Davis C., "Consumer Research for Development of Educational Messages for the MyPyramid Food Guidance System"
- Haven J, Burns A, Britten P, Davis C., "Developing the Consumer Interface for the MyPyramid Food Guidance System"
- Yamimi S, Juan WY, Marcoe K, Britten P. "Impact of Using

Updated Food Consumption and Composition data on Selected MyPyramid Food Group Nutrient Profiles"

- Britten P, Lyon J, Weaver C, Kris-Etherton P, Nicklas T, Weber J, Davis C. "MyPyramid Food Intake pattern Modeling for the Dietary Guidelines Advisory Committee
- Haven J, Burns A, Herring D, Britten P., Great Educational Materials (GEM) No. 426, "MyPyramid.gov Provides Consumers with Practical Nutrition Information at their Fingertips"
- Juan WY, Gerrior S, Hiza H., GEM No. 427, "MyPyramid Tracker Assesses Food Consumption, Activity, and Energy Balance Status Interactively"
- French L, Howell G, Haven J, Britten P., GEM No. 428, "Designing MyPyramid for Kids materials to help Children Eat Right, Exercise, Have Fun"

CASE STUDY: CENTER FOR NUTRITION POLICY AND PROMOTION

The Center for Nutrition Policy and Promotion (CNPP) is an agency of the U.S. Department of Agriculture created on December 1, 1994, and is the focal point within the USDA where scientific research is linked with the nutritional needs of the American public.

The creation of the Center came at a time when the American public was becoming increasingly aware of the importance of diet, yet was receiving conflicting nutrition messages. The Center, therefore, serves as a touchstone where the public is assured that the nutrition guidance they receive is based on sound research and analysis.

The Center reports to the Office of the Under Secretary of Agriculture for Food, Nutrition, and Consumer Services. The staff of the Center is composed primarily of nutritionists, nutrition scientists, dietitians, economists, and policy experts, all of whom were chosen for their expertise. Dr. Rajen Anand is the current Executive Director of the Center. The Deputy Director is Dr. Robert C. Post.

CNPP carries out its mission by (1) advancing and promoting food and nutrition guidance for all Americans; (2) assessing diet quality; and (3) advancing consumer, nutrition, and food economic knowledge.

Major Projects Administered by CNPP are

- Dietary Guidelines for Americans
- MyPyramid Food Guidance System
- Healthy Eating Index
- U.S. Food Plans
- Nutrient Content of the U.S. Food Supply
- Expenditures on Children by Families

Dietary Guidelines for Americans

The Center serves as the administrative agency within U.S. Department of Agriculture (USDA) for the issuance of the Dietary Guidelines for Americans, which are the cornerstone of Federal nutrition policy and nutrition education activities. The Guidelines are jointly issued and updated every 5 years by USDA and the U.S. Department of Health and Human Services (HHS).

The Dietary Guidelines provide authoritative advice for people 2 years and older about how good dietary habits can promote health and reduce risk for major chronic diseases.

MyPyramid

The MyPyramid Food Guidance System translates nutritional recommendations into the kinds and amounts of food to eat each day. MyPyramid was released in April 2005 and replaces the Food Guide Pyramid (1992). The MyPyramid.gov website provides information and personalized interactive tools for consumers. MyPyramid is also available in Spanish at MiPirámide.gov.

Healthy Eating Index

The Healthy Eating Index (HEI) is a measure of diet quality that assesses conformance to federal dietary guidance. The original HEI was created by the U.S. Department of Agriculture in 1995. The

HEI was revised in 2006 to reflect the 2005 Dietary Guidelines for Americans. A fact sheet and a technical report describing development and evaluation of the HEI-2005 can be accessed.

U.S. Food Plans

CNPP also maintains and updates the Thrifty, Low-Cost, Moderate-Cost, and Liberal Food Plans. Each food plan represents a nutritious diet at a different cost. The Thrifty Food Plan serves as the nutritional basis for determination of Food Stamp Programme benefits.

Nutrient Content of the U.S. Food Supply

The Nutrient Content of the U.S. Food Supply is a historical data series, beginning in 1909, on the amounts of nutrients per capita per day in food available for consumption. An interactive version of this series allows users to query nutrient and pyramid servings information online.

Expenditures on Children by Families

Expenditures on Children by Families provides estimates of the cost of raising children from birth through age 17 for major budgetary components.

Evidence Analysis Library Division

The Evidence Analysis Library Division (EALD) monitors, assesses, gathers, analyzes, and consults on the scientific evidence in support of nutrition, food, dietary guidance, nutrition education, and nutrition research policies and outreach programmes. The EALD designs and leads a wide range of scientific review projects that inform and support nutrition policy and guidance and serve as the basis for nutrition promotion and education activities. The Nutrition Evidence Library, a major function of the Division, supports the Dietary Guidelines 2010 process. EALD was formed to provide a broader—based evidence library to support Federal and external organizations as a repository of the most up-to-date credible literature available in the areas relative to the Dietary Guidelines for Americans: obesity, food groups, weight management, physical activity, food safety, methods of consumer nutrition education programme development, risk analysis and nutrients, and social marketing. EALD serves as the USDA model upon which USDA agencies approach science review to support the policies for which they have responsibility.

There has been some controversy regarding the Center's impartiality due to its being a part of the USDA. The oversight of the Dietary Guidelines is controlled jointly by CNPP (a center within the USDA) and the Department of Health and Human Services (specifically, the Office of Disease Prevention and Health Promotion). Every five years, the Departments charter a committee of 13 nutrition experts to review the peer-reviewed, published science on diet and health and develop a report of its recommendations for the next edition of the Guidelines.

Executive Directors of the Center for Nutrition Policy and Promotion

Sl. No.	*Executive Directors*	*Education*	*Term of Office*	*President(s) Served under*
1.	Eileen Kennedy	D.Sc.	1994-1997	Bill Clinton
2.	Rajen Anand	D.V.M., Ph.D.	1997-2001	
3.	Eric Hentges	Ph.D.	2003-2007	George W. Bush
4.	Brian Wansink	Ph.D.	2007-2009	
5.	Rajen Anand	D.V.M., Ph.D.	2009-present	Barack Obama

CASE STUDY: WAGENINGEN UNIVERSITY AND RESEARCH CENTRE

Wageningen University and Research Centre (also known as Wageningen UR; abbreviation: WUR) is a research and higher education concern which consistis of Wageningen University, the

Van Hall-Larenstein School of Higher Professional Education, and the former agricultural research institutes (Dienst Landbouwkundig Onderzoek) from the Dutch Ministry of Agriculture. With its combination of knowledge and experience in higher eduction and research Wageningen UR aims to train specialists (BSc, MSc and PhD) in life sciences and through its research contribute actively to solving scientific, social and commercial problems in the field of life sciences and natural resources. Wageningen UR approaches national and international research topics from the perspectives of various disciplines, with an integrated approach and in close collaboration with governments, companies, stakeholder organisations, citizens, and other knowledge institutions. The research should pay attention to the balance between three priorities in society: *economics, culture and nature.*

It is based in the Dutch city of Wageningen.

Wageningen University

Wageningen University was established in 1918 and was the successor of the Agricultural School founded in 1876.

Wageningen University provides education and generates knowledge in the field of life sciences and natural resources. Wageningen UR aims to make a real contribution to our quality of life. Quality of life means to the university both an adequate supply of safe and healthy food and drink, on the one hand, and the chance to live, work and play in a balanced ecosystem with a large variety of plants and animals.

The university has about 6,000 students from 98 countries. Its core business are life and agricultural sciences.

ECTS-Label

Wageningen University was the first Dutch University or school that was allowed to use the ECTS label. This label is awarded by the European Commission and guarantees the quality of the study programme. An important consideration is that the University consequently applies the European Credit Transfer System; this promotes the mobility of students within Europe and prevents study delay. The label is a prestigious acknowledgment of the international character of the University. Out of 56 European applications in 2005, only 3 ECTS labels were awarded.

BSc Programmes

Wageningen University offers 18 BSc programmes (2005-2006). The language of instruction is partly Dutch, partly English. For some BSc programmes the language of instruction is English. The programmes start each year in September, they last three years and consist of 180 ECTS credits. The programmes are in the field of economy and society, health, life sciences and technology, nature and environment, animals and plants.

Economy and Society

- Business and consumer studies
- Economics and policy
- International development studies

Health

- Health and society
- Nutrition and health

Technology

- Agro technology
- Biotechnology
- Food technology
- Molecular life sciences

Nature and Environment

- Soil, water and air
- Forest and nature conservation
- International land and water conservation
- Landscape architecture and spatial planning
- Environmental studies

Animals and Plants

- Biology
- Biological Production Sciences
- Animal sciences
- Plant sciences

MSc Programmes

Wageningen University offers a wide range of MSc programmes (2005-2006). The language of instruction is English. The programmes start each year in September, they last two years and consist of 120 ECTS credits. Most programmes offer various specialisations and possibilities for majors.

- Agricultural and Bioresource Engineering
- Animal Sciences and Aquaculture
- Aquaculture and Fisheries
- Bioinformatics
- Biology
- Biotechnology
- Communication Science
- Earth System Science
- Environmental Sciences
- European Masters Degree in Food Studies
- Food Quality Management
- Food Safety
- Food Technology
- Forest and Nature Conservation
- Geo-information Science
- Hydrology and Water Quality
- International Development Studies
- International Land and Water Management
- Landscape Architecture and Planning
- Leisure, Tourism and Environment
- Management of Agro-ecological Knowledge and Social Change
- Management, Economics and Consumer Studies
- Meteorology and Air Quality
- Molecular Life Sciences
- Nutrition and Health
- Organic Agriculture
- Plant Biotechnology
- Plant Sciences
- Soil Science
- Urban Environmental Management

PhD Programme

The PhD programme is a four-year programme which consists of a research component and a smaller education component. To apply for a PhD position, the applicant must contact one of the Graduate Schools of Wageningen University. In order to guarantee adequate supervision, the research subject must fit in the research programme of a Graduate School. The four-year PhD programme consists of a research component (conducting research under supervision and writing a thesis) and a smaller education component (up to 15 per cent of the total PhD time) Upon completion of PhD programme, the PhD student is expected to be:

- Able to function as an independent scientist.
- Able to integrate his/her own work in the theoretical framework of his/her discipline(s) in a broader area of research and able to communicate this in a scientific or general setting.
- Competent in identifying priority areas of research and in formulating questions and experimental hypotheses pertinent to this research.

Research Institutes

The following research institutes are part of Wageningen UR:

- Agricultural Economics Research Institute (LEI)
- Agrotechnology and Food Sciences Group (AFSG)
- Alterra—Research Institute for the Green World (ALTERRA)
- International Institute for Land Reclamation and Improvement (ILRI)
- Animal Sciences Group (ASG)
- Applied Plant Research (PPO)
- Central Institute for Animal Disease Control (CIDC-Lelystad)
- International Agricultural Centre (IAC)
- Plant Research International (PRI)
- RIKILT-Institute of Food Safety

Van Hall-Larenstein School of Higher Professional Education

The Van Hall-Larenstein School was formed out of a merger of the Van Hall Instituut and Larenstein, School of Professional Education.

Van Hall Larenstein offers 14 bachelor's degree programmes and 6 professional master's degree programmes to a total of 4,400 students of 20 nationalities. The study programmes are mainly in Dutch.

Student Activities and Associations

M.S.V. Alchimica is a study association for students of Molecular Life Sciences. For over 35 years it has been organising many different activities for its members.

CODON is a study association for students of Biotechnology and Bioinformatics established by the first students of *Bioprocesstechnology* on 16 September 1991. At that time the association carried the name "BiPS" which was later changed to CODON. The association's main language is English.

Nicolas Appert (study association) is the study association for the students of Food technology and Food Safety of both the University and the Van Hall Larenstein College. It was founded on September 6, 1962, and was named after the French food scientist Nicolas Appert.

Heeren XVII is the study association for the students of Agrotechnology and Agricultural and Bioresource Engineering. It was founded on April 1, 1965.

Genius Loci is the study association for the students of Landscape architecture and spatial planning. The name reflects the atmosphere of a certain place. It was founded on February 15, 1990 after the merger of two older study programmes.

Licere is the study association for the students of the MSc Leisure, Tourism and Environment. It was founded in 2006 and its name means 'Leisure time' in Latin.

Mercurius is the study association for the students of the BSc's Business and Consumer Studies and Economics and Policy and for the students of the MSc Management, Economics and Consumer Studies.

De Veetelers is the study association of students Animal Sciences (both BSc and MSc). The name means literally Animal Breeders and was founded in 1962.

Notable Alumni

- Reinier van den Berg
- Jan Just Bos
- Gerrit Braks
- Staf Depla
- Jeroen Dijsselbloem
- Willem Hilbrand van Dobben
- Louise Fresco
- Volkert van der Graaf
- Wilbert Hetterscheid
- Gerrit Hiemstra
- Martijn Katan
- Ruud Koopmans
- Ferdinand Antoon Langguth Oliviera
- Joan Leemhuis-Stout
- Helga van Leur
- Jan Odink
- Theo Quené
- Rudy Rabbinge
- Ramsewak Shankar
- Bernard Slicher van Bath
- Harry Snelders
- Katja Staartjes, first Dutch woman on Mount Everest
- Onno van de Stolpe, CEO of Galapagos Genomics.
- Rob Urgert
- Jan Valckenier Suringar
- Cees Veerman
- Joris Voorhoeve
- Anne Vondeling
- Marijke Vos
- Henk Vredeling
- Simon Vroemen
- Karel Vuursteen, CEO of Heineken

- Clive West
- Onno Wijnands
- Mamoudou H. DICKO

University Pages

- WUR Homepage
- Wageningen University
- RIKILT institute of Food Safety
- Van Hall-Larenstein

4

Aerobic and Anaerobic Organisms, Saturated and Unsaturated Fats and Food Groups

AEROBIC ORGANISM

An aerobic organism or *aerobe* is an organism that can survive and grow in an oxygenated environment.

Types

- Obligate aerobes require oxygen for aerobic cellular respiration. In a process known as cellular respiration, these organisms use oxygen to oxidize substrates (for example sugars and fats) in order to obtain energy.
- Facultative anaerobes can use oxygen, but also have anaerobic methods of energy production.
- Microaerophiles are organisms that may use oxygen, but only at low concentrations.
- Aerotolerant organisms can survive in the presence of oxygen, but they are anaerobic because they do not use it as a terminal electron acceptor.

Glucose

A good example would be the oxidation of glucose (a monosaccharide) in aerobic respiration.

$$C_6H_{12}O_6 + 6\ O_2 + 38\ ADP + 38\ phosphate \rightarrow 6\ CO_2 + 6\ H_2O + 38\ ATP$$

Notice that oxygen is used during the oxidation of glucose and water is produced.

This equation is a summary of what actually happens in three series of biochemical reactions: glycolysis, the Krebs cycle, and oxidative phosphorylation.

Diversity

Almost all animals, most fungi, and several bacteria are obligate aerobes. Most anaerobic organisms are bacteria. Being an obligate aerobe—although advantageous from the energetical point of view, also means obligatory exposure to high levels of oxidative stress.

Yeast is an example of a facultative aerobe. Individual human cells are also facultative aerobes: they switch to lactic acid fermentation if oxygen is not available. However, for the whole organism this cannot be sustained for long, and humans are therefore obligate aerobes.

YEAST

Yeasts are eukaryotic micro-organisms classified in the kingdom Fungi, with about 1,500 species currently described; they dominate fungal diversity in the oceans. Most reproduce asexually by budding, although a few do so by binary fission. Yeasts are unicellular, although some species with yeast forms may become multicellular through the formation of a string of connected budding cells known as pseudohyphae, or *false hyphae* as seen in most molds. Yeast size can vary greatly depending on the species, typically measuring 3-4 μm in diameter, although some yeasts can reach over 40 μm.

The yeast open species *Saccharomyces cerevisiae* has been used in baking and fermenting alcoholic beverages for thousands of years. It is also extremely important as a model organism in modern cell biology research, and is one of the most thoroughly researched eukaryotic microorganisms. Researchers have used it to gather information about the biology of the eukaryotic cell and ultimately human biology. Other species of yeast, such as *Candida albicans*, are opportunistic pathogens and can cause infections in humans. Yeasts have recently been used to generate electricity in microbial fuel cells, and produce ethanol for the biofuel industry.

Yeasts do not form a specific taxonomic or phylogenetic grouping. At present it is estimated that only 1 per cent of all yeast species have been described. The term *"yeast"* is often taken as a synonym for S. cerevisiae, but the phylogenetic diversity of yeasts is shown by their placement in both divisions Ascomycota and Basidiomycota. The budding yeasts ("true yeasts") are classified in the order Saccharomycetales.

History

The word "yeast" comes from Old English gist, gyst, and from the Indo-European root yes-, meaning boil, foam, or bubble. Yeast microbes are probably one of the earliest domesticated organisms. People have used yeast for fermentation and baking throughout history. Archaeologists digging in Egyptian ruins found early grinding stones and baking chambers for yeasted bread, as well as drawings of 4,000-year-old bakeries and breweries. In 1680 the Dutch naturalist Antonie van Leeuwenhoek first microscopically observed yeast, but at the time did not consider them to be living organisms but rather globular structures. In 1857 French microbiologist Louis Pasteur proved in the paper *"Mémoire sur la fermentation alcoolique"* that alcoholic fermentation was conducted by living yeasts and not by a chemical catalyst. Pasteur showed that by bubbling oxygen into the yeast broth, cell growth could be increased, but the fermentation inhibited—an observation later called the *Pasteur effect.*

In the United States, naturally occurring airborne yeasts were used almost exclusively until commercial yeast was marketed at the Centennial Exposition in 1876 in Philadelphia, where Charles L. Fleischmann exhibited the product and a process to use it, as well as serving the resultant baked bread.

Growth and Nutrition

Yeasts are chemoorganotrophs as they use organic compounds as a source of energy and do not require sunlight to grow. Carbon is obtained mostly from hexose sugars such as glucose and fructose, or disaccharides such as sucrose and maltose. Some species can metabolize pentose sugars like ribose, alcohols, and organic acids. Yeast species either require oxygen for aerobic cellular respiration (obligate aerobes), or are anaerobic but also have aerobic methods of energy production (facultative anaerobes). Unlike bacteria, there are no known yeast species that grow only anaerobically (obligate anaerobes). Yeasts grow best in a neutral or slightly acidic pH environment.

Yeasts will grow over a temperature range of 10°C (50°F) to 37°C (99°F), with an optimal temperature range of 30°C (86°F) to 37°C (99°F), depending on the type of species (*S. cerevisiae* works best at about 30°C (86°F). Above 37°C (99°F) yeast cells become stressed and will not divide properly. Most yeast cells die above 50°C (122°F). If the solution reaches 105°C (221°F) the yeast will disintegrate. There is little activity in the range of 0°C (32°F)-10°C (50°F). The cells can survive freezing under certain conditions, with viability decreasing over time.

Yeasts are very common in the environment, but are usually isolated from sugar-rich material. Some good examples include naturally occurring yeasts on the skins of fruits and berries (such as grapes, apples or peaches), and exudates from plants (such as plant saps or cacti). Some yeasts are found in association with soil and insects. Yeast are generally grown in the laboratory on solid growth media or liquid broths. Common media used for the cultivation of yeasts include; potato dextrose agar (PDA) or potato dextrose broth, Wallerstein Laboratories Nutrient (WLN) agar, Yeast Peptone Dextrose agar (YPD), and Yeast Mould agar or broth (YM). The antibiotic cycloheximide is sometimes added to yeast growth media to inhibit the growth of *Saccharomyces* yeasts and select for wild/ indigenous yeast species. This will change the yeast process.

Reproduction

Yeasts have asexual and sexual reproductive cycles, however the most common mode of vegetative growth in yeast is asexual reproduction by budding or fission. Here a small bud, or daughter cell, is formed on the parent cell. The nucleus of the parent cell splits into a daughter nucleus and migrates into the daughter cell. The bud continues to grow until it separates from the parent cell, forming a new cell.

Under high stress conditions haploid cells will generally die, however under the same conditions diploid cells can undergo sporulation, entering sexual reproduction (meiosis) and producing a variety of haploid spores, which can go on to mate (conjugate), reforming the diploid.

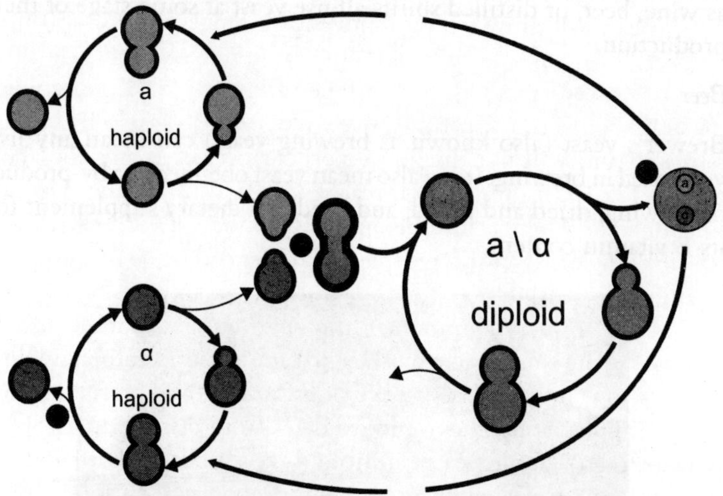

Fig. 4.1: The Yeast Cell's Life Cycle: 1. Budding, 2. Conjugation, 3. Spore

Yeast of the species Schizosaccharomyces pombe reproduce by binary fission instead of budding.

Uses

The useful physiological properties of yeast have led to their use in the field of biotechnology. Fermentation of sugars by yeast is the oldest and largest application of this technology. Many types of yeasts are used for making many foods: Baker's yeast in bread production, brewer's yeast in beer fermentation, yeast in wine fermentation and for xylitol production. Yeasts are also one of the most widely used model organisms for genetics and cell biology.

Alcoholic Beverages

Alcoholic beverages are defined as beverages that contain ethanol (C_2H_5OH). This ethanol is almost always produced by fermentation—the metabolism of carbohydrates by certain species of yeast under anaerobic or low-oxygen conditions. Beverages such as wine, beer, or distilled spirits all use yeast at some stage of their production.

Beer

Brewer's yeast (also known as brewing yeast) can mean any live yeast used in brewing. It can also mean yeast obtained as a by-product of brewing, dried and killed, and used as a dietary supplement for its B vitamin content.

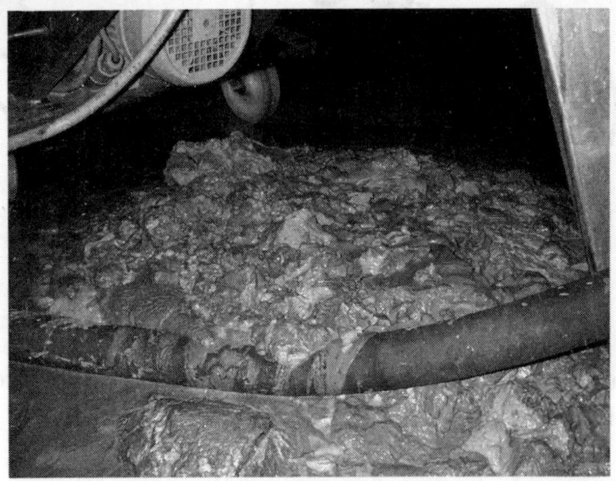

Fig. 4.2: A Mixture of Diatomaceous Earth and Yeast after Filtering Beer

Brewers classify yeasts as top-fermenting and bottom-fermenting. This distinction was introduced by the Dane Emil Christian Hansen. "Top-fermenting yeasts" are so called because they form a foam at the top of the wort during fermentation. They can produce higher alcohol concentrations and prefer higher temperatures, typically 16°C (61°F)-24°C (75°F), producing fruitier, sweeter, ale-type beers. An example of top-fermenting yeast is Saccharomyces cerevisiae, known to brewers as ale yeast. "Bottom-fermenting yeasts" are typically used to produce lager-type beers, though can also produce ale-type beers. These yeasts ferment more sugars, leaving a crisper taste, and grow well at low temperatures. An example of bottom fermenting yeast is Saccharomyces pastorianus, formerly known as *Saccharomyces carlsbergensis.*

For both types, yeast is fully distributed through the beer while it is fermenting, and both equally flocculate (clump together and precipitate to the bottom of the vessel) when it is finished. By no means do all top-fermenting yeasts demonstrate this behaviour, but it features strongly in many English ale yeasts which may also exhibit chain forming (the failure of budded cells to break from the mother cell) which is technically different from true flocculation.

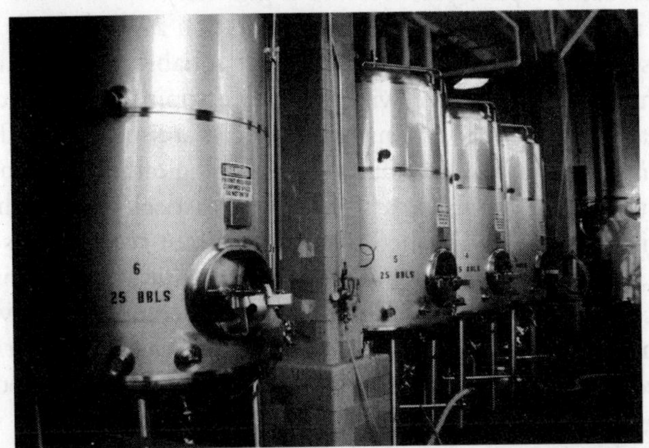

Fig. 4.3: Fermenting Tanks with Yeast being Used to Brew Beer

In industrial brewing, to ensure purity of strain, a 'clean' sample of the yeast is stored refrigerated in a laboratory. After a certain number of fermentation cycles, a full scale propagation is produced from this laboratory sample. Typically, it is grown up in about three or four stages using sterile brewing wort and oxygen.

Brettanomyces: A genus of "wild" yeast used in brewing lambic. There are three main species: Brettanomyces lambicus; Brettanomyces bruxellensis; and Brettanomyces claussenii, which is found in Britain.

Distilled Beverages

A distilled beverage is a beverage that contains ethanol that has been purified by distillation. Carbohydrate-containing plant material is fermented by yeast, producing a dilute solution of ethanol in the process. Spirits such as whiskey and rum are prepared by distilling these dilute solutions of ethanol. Components other than ethanol are collected in the condensate, including water, esters, and other alcohols which account for the flavor of the beverage.

Yeast is used in winemaking where it converts the sugars present in grape juice or must into alcohol. Yeast is normally already invisibly present on the grapes. The fermentation can be done with this endogenous (or *wild*) yeast; however, this may give unpredictable results depending on the exact types of yeast species that are present. For this reason a pure yeast culture is generally added to the must, which rapidly predominates the fermentation as it proceeds. This represses the wild yeasts and ensures a reliable and predictable fermentation. Most added wine yeasts are strains of *Saccharomyces cerevisiae*, though not all strains of the species are suitable. Different *S. cerevisiae* yeast strains have differing physiological and fermentative properties, therefore the actual strain of yeast selected can have a direct impact on the finished wine. Significant research has been undertaken into the development of novel wine yeast strains that produce atypical flavour profiles or increased complexity in wines.

The growth of some yeasts such as *Zygosaccharomyces* and *Brettanomyces* in wine can result in wine faults and subsequent spoilage. Brettanomyces produces an array of metabolites when growing in wine, some of which are volatile phenolic compounds. Together these compounds are often referred to as *"Brettanomyces character"*, and are often described as antiseptic or *"barnyard"* type aromas. Brettanomyces is a significant contributor to wine faults within the wine industry.

Baking

Yeast, most commonly *Saccharomyces cerevisiae*, is used in baking as a leavening agent, where it converts the fermentable sugars present in the dough into carbon dioxide. This causes the dough to expand or rise as the carbon dioxide forms pockets or bubbles. When the dough is baked the yeast dies off and the air pockets "sets", giving the baked product a soft and spongy texture. The use of potatoes, water from potato boiling, eggs, or sugar in a bread dough accelerates the growth of yeasts. Salt and fats such as butter slow down yeast growth. The majority of the yeast used in baking is of the same species common in alcoholic fermentation. Additionally, *Saccharomyces exiguus* (also known as S. minor) is a wild yeast found on plants, fruits, and grains that is occasionally used for baking. Sugar and vinegar are the best conditions for yeast to ferment. In bread making the yeast respires aerobically at first producing carbon dioxide and water. When the oxygen is used up anaerobic respiration is used producing ethanol as a waste product; however, this is evaporated during the baking process.

It is not known when yeast was first used to bake bread. The first records that show this use came from Ancient Egypt. Researchers speculate that a mixture of flour meal and water was left longer than usual on a warm day and the yeasts that occur in natural contaminants of the flour caused it to ferment before baking. The resulting bread would have been lighter and tastier than the normal flat, hard cake.

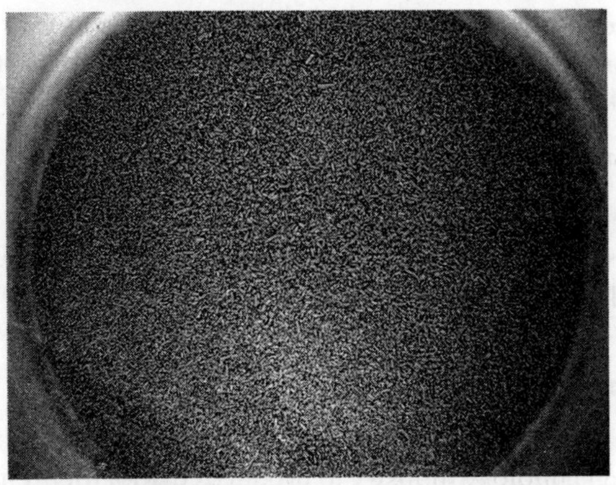

Fig. 4.4: Active Dried Yeast, a Granulated Form in Which Yeast is Commercially Sold

Today there are several retailers of baker's yeast; one of the best-known in North America is Fleischmann's Yeast, which was developed in 1868. During World War II Fleischmann's developed a granulated active dry yeast, which did not require refrigeration and had a longer shelf life than fresh yeast. The company created yeast that would rise twice as fast, cutting down on baking time. Baker's yeast is also sold as a fresh yeast compressed into a square "cake". This form perishes quickly, and must be used soon after production in order to maintain viability. A weak solution of water and sugar can be used to determine if yeast is expired. When dissolved in the solution, active yeast will foam and bubble as it ferments the sugar into ethanol and carbon dioxide. Some recipes refer to this as proofing the yeast as it 'proves' [tests] the viability of the yeast before the other ingredients are added. When using a sourdough starter, flour and water are added instead of sugar and this is referred to as proofing the sponge.

When yeast is used for making bread, it is mixed with flour, salt, and warm water (or milk). The dough is kneaded until it is smooth, and then left to rise, sometimes until it has doubled in size. Some bread doughs are knocked back after one rising and left to rise again. A longer rising time gives a better flavour, but the yeast can fail to raise the bread in the final stages if it is left for too long initially. The dough is then shaped into loaves, left to rise until it is the correct size, and then baked. Dried yeast is usually specified for use in a bread machine, however a (wet) sourdough starter can also work.

Bioremediation

Some yeasts can find potential application in the field of bioremediation. One such yeast *Yarrowia lipolytica* is known to degrade palm oil mill effluent, TNT (an explosive material), and other hydrocarbons such as alkanes, fatty acids, fats and oils.

Industrial Ethanol Production

The ability of yeast to convert sugar into ethanol has been harnessed by the biotechnology industry to produce ethanol fuel. The process starts by milling a feedstock, such as sugar cane, field corn, or cheap cereal grains, and then adding dilute sulfuric acid, or fungal alpha amylase enzymes, to break down the starches into complex sugars. A gluco amylase is then added to break the complex sugars down into simple sugars. After this, yeasts are added to convert the simple sugars to ethanol, which is then distilled off to obtain ethanol up to 96 per cent in concentration.

Saccharomyces yeasts have been genetically engineered to ferment xylose, one of the major fermentable sugars present in cellulosic biomasses, such as agriculture residues, paper wastes, and wood chips. Such a development means that ethanol can be efficiently produced from more inexpensive feedstocks, making cellulosic ethanol fuel a more competitively priced alternative to gasoline fuels.

Kombucha

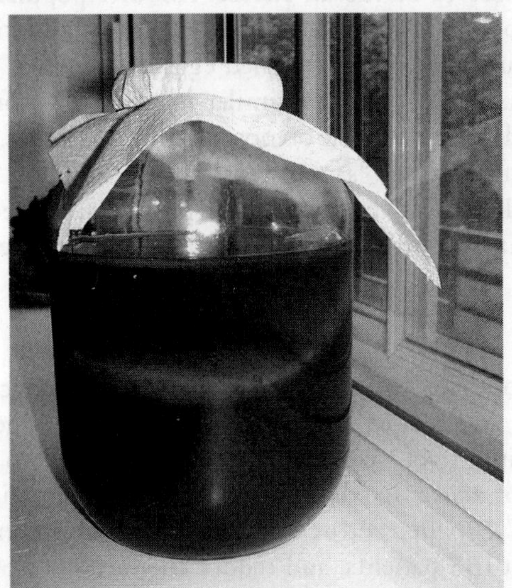

Fig. 4.5: A Kombucha Culture Fermenting in a Jar

Yeast in symbiosis with acetic acid bacteria is used in the preparation of Kombucha, a fermented sweetened tea. Species of yeast found in the tea can vary, and may include: *Brettanomyces bruxellensis, Candida stellata, Schizosaccharomyces pombe, Torulaspora delbrueckii and Zygosaccharomyces bailii.*

Nutritional Supplements

Yeast is used in nutritional supplements popular with vegans and the health conscious, where it is often referred to as "nutritional yeast". It is a deactivated yeast, usually *Saccharomyces cerevisiae*. It is an excellent source of protein and vitamins, especially the B-complex vitamins, whose functions are related to metabolism as well as other minerals and cofactors required for growth. It is also naturally low in fat and sodium. Some brands of nutritional yeast, though not all, are fortified with vitamin B12, which is produced separately from bacteria. Nutritional yeast, though it has a similar appearance to brewer's yeast, is very different and has a very different taste.

Nutritional yeast has a nutty, cheesy, creamy flavor which makes it popular as an ingredient in cheese substitutes. It is often used by vegans in place of Parmesan cheese. Another popular use is as a topping for popcorn. It can also be used in mashed and fried potatoes, as well as putting it into scrambled eggs. It comes in the form of flakes, or as a yellow powder similar in texture to cornmeal, and can be found in the bulk aisle of most natural food stores. In Australia it is sometimes sold as "savory yeast flakes". Though "nutritional yeast" usually refers to commercial products, inadequately fed prisoners have used "home-grown" yeast to prevent vitamin deficiency.

Probiotics

Some probiotic supplements use the yeast Saccharomyces boulardii to maintain and restore the natural flora in the large and small gastrointestinal tract. *S. boulardii* has been shown to reduce the symptoms of acute diarrhea in children, prevent reinfection of *Clostridium difficile*, reduce bowel movements in diarrhea predominant IBS patients, and reduce the incidence of antibiotic, traveler's, and HIV/AIDS associated diarrheas.

Root Beer and Sodas

Root beer and other sweet carbonated beverages can be produced using the same methods as beer, except that fermentation is stopped sooner, producing carbon dioxide, but only trace amounts of alcohol, and a significant amount of sugar is left in the drink.

Aquarium Hobby

Yeast is often used by aquarium hobbyists to generate carbon dioxide (CO_2) to fertilize plants in planted aquariums. A homemade setup is widely used as a cheap and simple alternative to pressurized CO_2 systems. While not as effective as these, the homemade setup is considerably cheaper for less demanding hobbyists.

There are several recipes for homemade CO_2, but they are variations of the basic recipe: Baking yeast is inserted in a plastic bottle together with sugar, baking soda and water. This produces CO_2 for about 2 or 3 weeks. The CO_2 is injected in the aquarium via a narrow hose and released through a CO_2 diffuser that helps dissolve the gas in the water. The CO_2 is used by plants in the photosynthesis process.

CO_2 injection is very important to plant growth in planted aquariums.

Science

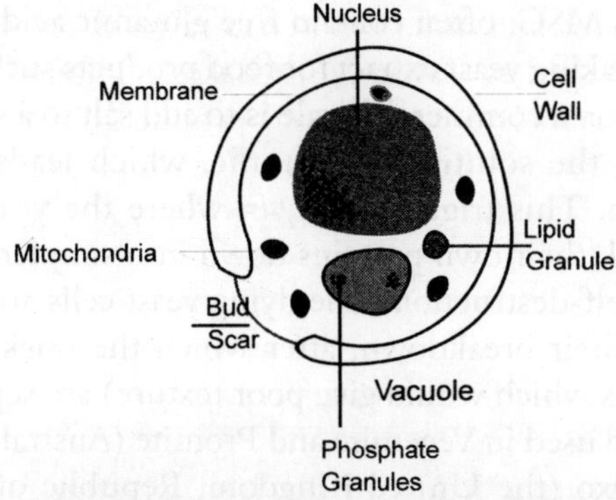

Fig. 4.6: Diagram Showing a Yeast Cell

Several yeasts, particularly *Saccharomyces cerevisiae*, have been widely used in genetics and cell biology. This is largely because the cell cycle in a yeast cell is very similar to the cell cycle in humans, and therefore the basic cellular mechanics of DNA replication, recombination, cell division and metabolism are comparable. Also yeasts are easily manipulated and cultured in the lab which has allowed for the development of powerful standard techniques, such as Yeast two-hybrid, Synthetic genetic array analysis and tetrad analysis. Many proteins important in human biology were first discovered by studying their homologs in yeast; these proteins include cell cycle proteins, signaling proteins, and protein-processing enzymes.

On 24 April 1996 S. cerevisiae was announced to be the first eukaryote to have its genome, consisting of 12 million base pairs, fully sequenced as part of the Genome project. At the time it was the most complex organism to have its full genome sequenced and took 7 years and the involvement of more than 100 laboratories to accomplish. The second yeast species to have its genome sequenced was *Schizosaccharomyces pombe*, which was completed in 2002. It was the 6th eukaryotic genome sequenced and consists of 13.8 million base pairs.

Yeast Extract

Yeast extract is the common name for various forms of processed yeast products that are used as food additives or flavours. They are often used in the same way that monosodium glutamate (MSG) is used, and like MSG, often contain free glutamic acid. The general method for making yeast extract for food products such as Vegemite and Marmite on a commercial scale is to add salt to a suspension of yeast making the solution hypertonic, which leads to the cells shrivelling up. This triggers *autolysis*, where the yeast's digestive enzymes break their own proteins down into simpler compounds, a process of self-destruction. The dying yeast cells are then heated to complete their breakdown, after which the husks (yeast with thick cell walls which would give poor texture) are separated. Yeast autolysates are used in Vegemite and Promite (Australia); Marmite, Bovril and Oxo (the United Kingdom, Republic of Ireland and South Africa); and Cenovis (Switzerland).

Pathogenic Yeasts

Some species of yeast are opportunistic pathogens where they can cause infection in people with compromised immune systems.

Cryptococcus neoformans is a significant pathogen of immunocompromised people causing the disease termed Cryptococcosis. This disease occurs in about 7-9 per cent of AIDS patients in the USA, and a slightly smaller percentage (3-6%) in western Europe. The cells of the yeast are surrounded by a rigid polysaccharide capsule, which helps to prevent them from being recognised and engulfed by white blood cells in the human body.

Yeasts of the *Candida* genus are another group of opportunistic pathogens which causes oral and vaginal infections in humans, known as Candidiasis. Candida is commonly found as a commensal

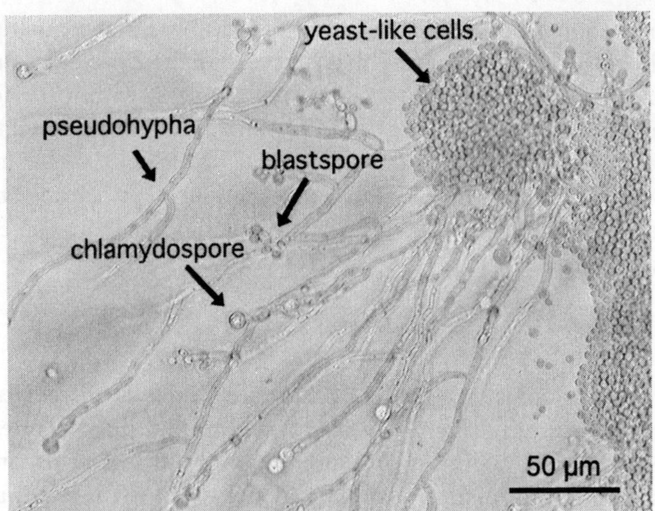

Fig. 4.7: A Photomicrograph of Candida Albicans Showing Hyphal Outgrowth and Other Morphological Characteristics

yeast in the mucus membranes of humans and other warm-blooded animals. However, sometimes these same strains can become pathogenic. Here the yeast cells sprout a hyphal outgrowth, which locally penetrates the mucosal membrane, causing irritation and shedding of the tissues. The pathogenic yeasts of candidiasis in probable descending order of virulence for humans are: *C. albicans, C. tropicalis, C. stellatoidea, C. glabrata, C. krusei, C. parapsilosis, C. guilliermondii, C. viswanathii, C. lusitaniae and Rhodotorula mucilaginosa. Candida glabrata* is the second most common *Candida* pathogen after *C. albicans*, causing infections of the urogenital tract, and of the bloodstream (Candidemia).

Food Spoilage

Yeasts are able to grow in foods with a low pH, (5.0 or lower) and in the presence of sugars, organic acids and other easily metabolized carbon sources. During their growth, yeasts metabolize some food components and produce metabolic end products. This causes the physical, chemical, and sensory properties of a food to change, and the food is spoiled. The growth of yeast within food products is often seen on their surface, as in cheeses or meats, or by the fermentation of sugars in beverages, such as juices, and semi-liquid products, such as syrups and jams. The yeast of the *Zygosaccharomyces* genus have had a long history as a spoilage yeast within the food industry. This is mainly due to the fact that these species can grow in the presence of high sucrose, ethanol, acetic acid, sorbic acid, benzoic acid, and sulfur dioxide concentrations, representing some of the commonly used food preservation methods. Methylene Blue is used to test for the presence of live yeast cells.

MOLD

Molds (or moulds; see spelling differences) include all species of microscopic fungi that grow in the form of multicellular filaments, called hyphae. In contrast, microscopic fungi that grow as single cells are called yeasts. A connected network of these tubular branching hyphae has multiple, genetically identical nuclei and is considered a single organism, referred to as a colony or in more technical terms a mycelium.

Molds do not form a specific taxonomic or phylogenetic grouping, but can be found in the divisions *Zygomycota, Deuteromycota and Ascomycota*. Although some molds cause disease or food spoilage, others are useful for their role in biodegradation or in the production of various foods, beverages, antibiotics and enzymes.

Biology

There are thousands of known species of molds, which include opportunistic pathogens, saprotrophs, aquatic species, calders and thermophiles. Like all fungi, molds derive energy not through photosynthesis but from the organic matter in which they live. Typically, molds secrete hydrolytic enzymes, mainly from the hyphal tips. These enzymes degrade complex biopolymers such as starch, cellulose and lignin into simpler substances which can be absorbed by the hyphae. In this way, molds play a major role in causing decomposition of organic material, enabling the recycling of nutrients throughout ecosystems. Many molds also secrete mycotoxins which, together with hydrolytic enzymes, inhibit the growth of competing microorganisms.

Molds reproduce through small spores, which may contain a single nucleus or be multinucleate. Mold spores can be asexual (the products of mitosis) or sexual (the products of meiosis); many species can produce both types. Some can remain airborne indefinitely, and many are able to survive extremes of temperature and pressure.

Although molds grow on dead organic matter everywhere in nature, their presence is only visible to the unaided eye when mold colonies grow. A mold colony does not comprise discrete organisms, but an interconnected network of hyphae called a mycelium. Nutrients and in some cases organelles may be transported throughout the mycelium. In artificial environments like buildings, humidity and temperature are often stable enough to foster the growth of mold colonies, commonly seen as a downy or furry coating growing on food or other surfaces.

Some molds can begin growing at temperatures as low as 2°C. When conditions do not enable growth, molds may remain alive in a dormant state depending on the species, within a large range of temperatures before they die. The many different mold species vary enormously in their tolerance to temperature and humidity extremes. Certain molds can survive harsh conditions such as the snow-covered soils of Antarctica, refrigeration, highly acidic solvents, and even petroleum products such as jet fuel.

Xerophilic molds use the humidity in the air as their only water source; other molds need more moisture.

Common Molds

- Acremonium
- Aspergillus
- Cladosporium
- Fusarium
- Mucor
- Penicillium
- Rhizopus
- Stachybotrys
- Trichoderma

Uses

Food Production

Cultured molds are used in the production of foods, including:

- cheese *(Penicillium spp.)*
- tempeh *(Rhizopus oligosporus)*
- oncom *(Neurospora sitophila)*
- Quorn *(Fusarium venenatum)*
- bread
- sausages
- soy sauce

The koji molds are a group of *Aspergillus* species, notably *Aspergillus oryzae,* that have been cultured in eastern Asia for many centuries. They are used to ferment a soybean and wheat mixture to make soybean paste and soy sauce. They are also used to break down the starch in rice (saccharification) in the production of sake and other distilled spirits.

Drug Creation

Alexander Fleming's famous discovery of the antibiotic penicillin involved the mold *Penicillium chrysogenum.*

Several cholesterol-lowering drugs (such as Lovastatin, from *Aspergillus terreus*) are derived from molds.

The immunosuppressant drug cyclosporine, used to suppress the rejection of transplanted organs, is derived from the mold *Tolypocladium inflatum.*

Health Effects

Molds are ubiquitous in nature, and mold spores are a common component of household and workplace dust. However, when mold spores are present in large quantities, they can present a health hazard to humans, potentially causing allergic reactions and respiratory problems.

Some molds also produce mycotoxins that can pose serious health risks to humans and animals. Exposure to high levels of mycotoxins can lead to neurological problems and in some cases death. Prolonged exposure, e.g. daily workplace exposure, can be particularly harmful. The term toxic mold refers to molds that produce mycotoxins, such as Stachybotrys chartarum, and not to all molds in general.

Growth in Buildings and Homes

Mold growth in buildings can lead to a variety of health issues. Various practices can be followed to mitigate mold issues in buildings, the most important of which is to reduce moisture levels that can facilitate mold growth. Removal of affected materials after the source of moisture has been reduced and/or eliminated may be necessary for remediation.

ANAEROBIC ORGANISM

An anaerobic organism or anaerobe is any organism that does not require oxygen for growth and may even die in its presence. There are three types: obligate anaerobes, which cannot use oxygen for growth and are even harmed by it; aerotolerant organisms, which cannot use oxygen for growth, but tolerate the presence of it; and facultative anaerobes, which can grow without oxygen, but if present can utilize it.

Metabolism

Obligate anaerobes may use fermentation or anaerobic respiration. Aerotolerant organisms are strictly fermentative. In the presence of oxygen, facultative anaerobes use aerobic respiration; without oxygen some of them ferment, some use anaerobic respiration.

Fermentation

There are many anaerobic fermentative reactions.

Fermentative anaerobic organisms mostly use the lactic acid fermentation pathway:

$$C_6H_{12}O_6 + 2\,ADP + 2\,phosphate \rightarrow 2\,lactic\ acid + 2\,ATP$$

The energy released in this equation is approximately 150 kJ per mol, which is conserved in regenerating two ATP from ADP per glucose. This is only 5 per cent of the energy per sugar molecule that the typical aerobic reaction generates.

Plants and fungi (e.g., yeasts) generally use alcohol (ethanol) fermentation when oxygen becomes limiting:

$$C_6H_{12}O_6 + 2\,ADP + 2\text{ phosphate} \rightarrow 2\,C_2H_5OH + 2\,CO_2 + 2\,ATP$$

The energy released is about 180 kJ per mol, which is conserved in regenerating two ATP from ADP per glucose.

Anaerobic bacteria and archaea use these and many other fermentative pathways, e.g., propionic acid fermentation, butyric acid fermentation, solvent fermentation, mixed acid fermentation, butanediol fermentation, Stickland fermentation, acetogenesis or methanogenesis.

Some anaerobic bacteria produce toxins (e.g., tetanus or botulinum toxins) that are highly dangerous to higher organisms, including humans.

Culturing Anaerobes

Given that normal microbial culturing is undertaken in an aerobic environment, the culturing of anaerobes poses a problem. To overcome this, a number of techniques are employed by microbiologists. One way required the injection of the bacteria into a Dicot. The Dicot would then provide an environment without oxygen thus ensuring the survival of the anaerobes. The GasPak System is an isolated container which achieves an anaerobic environment by the reaction of water with sodium borohydride and sodium bicarbonate tablets to produce hydrogen gas and carbon dioxide. Hydrogen then reacts with oxygen gas on a palladium catalyst to produce more water, thereby removing oxygen gas. The issue with the Gaspak method is that an adverse reaction can take place where the bacteria may die which is why a thioglycollate medium should be used. The Thioglycollate supplied a medium mimicking that of a Dicot thus providing not only an anaerobic environment but all the nutrients needed for the bacteria to thrive.

SATURATED FAT

Saturated fat is fat that consists of triglycerides containing only saturated fatty acid radicals. There are several kinds of naturally occurring saturated fatty acids, which differ by the number of carbon atoms, ranging from 3 carbons (Propionic Acid) to 36 (Hexatriacontanoic acid). *Saturated* fatty acids have no double bonds between the carbon atoms of the fatty acid chain and are thus fully saturated with hydrogen atoms.

Fat that occurs naturally in living matter contains varying proportions of saturated and unsaturated fat. Examples of foods containing a high proportion of saturated fat include dairy products (especially cream and cheese but also butter and ghee), animal fats such as suet, tallow, lard and fatty meat, coconut oil, cottonseed oil, palm kernel oil, chocolate, and some prepared foods.

Serum saturated fatty acid is generally higher in smokers, alcohol drinkers and obese people.

Fat Profiles

While nutrition labels usually combine them, the saturated fatty acids appear in different proportions among food groups. Lauric and myristic acid radicals are most commonly found in "tropical" oils (e.g. palm kernel, coconut) and dairy products. The saturated fat in meat, eggs, chocolate, and nuts is primarily the triglycerides of palmitic and stearic acid.

Saturated Fat Profile of Common Foods (Esterified Fatty Acids as Percentage of Total Fat)

Food	*Lauric Acid*	*Myristic Acid*	*Palmitic Acid*	*Stearic Acid*
Coconut oil	47%	18%	9%	3%
Butter	3%	11%	29%	13%
Ground beef	0%	4%	26%	15%
Dark chocolate	0%	0%	34%	43%
Salmon	0%	1%	29%	3%
Eggs	0%	0%	27%	10%
Cashews	2%	1%	10%	7%
Soybean oil	0%	0%	11%	4%

Fat Composition in Different Foods

Food	Saturated	Mono-unsaturated	Poly-unsaturated
	As Weight Percent (%) of Total Fat		
Cooking Oils			
Canola oil	7	59	29
Corn oil	13	24	59
Olive oil	13	74	8
Soybean oil	15	24	58
Dairy Products			
Cheese, regular	64	29	3
Cheese, light	60	30	0
Milk, whole	62	28	4
Milk, 2%	62	30	0
Ice cream, gourmet	62	29	4
Ice cream, light	62	29	4
Meats			
Beef	33	38	5
Ground sirloin	38	44	4
Pork chop	35	44	8
Ham	35	49	16
Chicken breast	29	34	21
Chicken	34	23	30
Turkey breast	30	20	30
Turkey drumstick	32	22	30
Fish, orange roughy	23	15	46
Salmon	28	33	28
Hot dog, beef	42	48	5
Hot dog, turkey	28	40	22
Burger, fast food	36	44	6
Cheeseburger, fast food	43	40	7
Breaded chicken sandwich	20	39	32
Grilled chicken sandwich	26	42	20
Sausage, Polish	37	46	11
Sausage, turkey	28	40	22
Pizza, sausage	41	32	20
Pizza, cheese	60	28	5
Nuts			
Almonds dry roasted	9	65	1
Cashews dry roasted	20	59	17
Macadamia dry roasted	15	79	2
Peanuts dry roasted	14	50	31
Pecans dry roasted	8	62	25
Flaxseeds, ground	8	23	65
Sesame seeds	14	38	44
Soybeans	14	22	57
Sunflower seeds	11	19	66
Walnuts dry roasted	9	23	63

(Contd.)

Food	*Saturated*	*Mono-unsaturated*	*Poly-unsaturated*
	As Weight Percent (%) of Total Fat		
Sweets and Baked Goods			
Candy, chocolate bar	59	33	3
Candy, fruit chews	14	44	38
Cookie, oatmeal raisin	22	47	27
Cookie, chocolate chip	35	42	18
Cake, yellow	60	25	10
Pastry, Danish	50	31	14
Fats Added during Cooking or at the Table			
Butter, stick	63	29	3
Butter, whipped	62	29	4
Margarine, stick	18	39	39
Margarine, tub	16	33	49
Margarine, light tub	19	46	33
Lard	39	45	11
Shortening	25	45	26
Chicken fat	30	45	21
Beef fat	41	43	3
Dressing, blue cheese	16	54	25
Dressing, light Italian	14	24	58
Other			
Egg yolk fat	36	44	16

Unless else specified in boxes, then reference is:

Examples of Saturated Fatty Acids

Some common examples of fatty acids:

- Lauric acid with 12 carbon atoms (contained in coconut oil, palm oil, and breast milk)
- Myristic acid with 14 carbon atoms (contained in cow's milk and dairy products)
- Palmitic acid with 16 carbon atoms (contained in palm oil and meat)
- Stearic acid with 18 carbon atoms (also contained in meat and cocoa butter)

Stable Deepfry and Baking Medium

Deepfry oils and baking fats that are high in saturated fats, like palm oil, tallow or lard, can withstand extreme heat (of 180-200 degrees

Celsius) and is resistant to oxidation. A 2001 parallel review of 20-year dietary fat studies in the United Kingdom, the United States of America and Spain concluded that polyunsaturated oils like soya, canola, sunflower and corn degrade easily to toxic compounds and trans fat when heated up. Prolonged consumption of trans fat-laden oxidized oils can lead to atherosclerosis, inflammatory joint disease and development of birth defects. The scientists also questioned global health authories' wilful recommendation of large amounts of polyunsaturated fats into the human diet without accompanying measures to ensure the protection of these fatty acids against heat- and oxidative-degradation.

Diseases with Ties to Saturated Fat Intake

Cardiovascular Diseases

Diets high in saturated fat have been correlated with an increased incidence of atherosclerosis and coronary heart disease.

Combined cholesterol and saturated fat feeding has shown an increase in cholesterol levels of African green monkeys, while one study with baboons showed the opposite effect on LDL cholesterol. Rudel (1995). "Dietary polyunsaturated fat modifies low-density lipoproteins and reduces atherosclerosis of nonhuman primates with high and low diet responsiveness"..

An increase in cholesterol levels has been observed in humans with an increase in saturated fat intake, such as a study of 22 hypercholesterolemic men. Some studies have suggested that diets high in saturated fat increase the risk of heart disease and stroke. Epidemiological studies have found that those whose diets are high in saturated fats, including lauric, myristic, palmitic, and stearic acid, had a higher prevalence of coronary heart disease. Additionally, controlled experimental studies have found that people consuming high saturated fat diets experience negative cholesterol profile changes.

In 1999, volunteers were randomly assigned to either Mediterranean (which replaces saturated fat with mono and polyunsaturated fat) or a control diet showed that subjects assigned to a Mediterranean diet exhibited a significantly decreased likelihood of suffering a second heart attack, cardiac death, heart failure or stroke.

An evaluation of data from Harvard Nurses' Health Study found that "diets lower in carbohydrate and higher in protein and fat are not associated with increased risk of coronary heart disease in women. When vegetable sources of fat and protein are chosen, these diets may moderately reduce the risk of coronary heart disease."

Meta-studies conducted by scientists in 1997 and 2003 found high corelation between excessive amounts of saturated fats and coronary heart disease. Mayo Clinic highlighted oils that are high in saturated fats include coconut, palm oil and palm kernel oil. Those of lower amounts of saturated fats, and higher levels of unsaturated (preferably monounsaturated) fats like olive oil, peanut oil, canola oil, avocados, safflower, corn, sunflower, soy and cottonseed oils are generally healthier. The National Heart, Lung and Blood Institute, and other health authorities like World Heart Federation have urged saturated fats be replaced with polyunsaturated and monounsaturated fats. The health body list olive and canola oils as sources of monosaturated oils while soybean and sunflower oils are rich with polyunsaturated fat. A 2005 research in Costa Rica suggests consumption of non-hydrogenated unsaturated oils like soybean and sunflower over palm oil.

The Cochrane Collaboration published a meta-analyses of fat modification trials finding no significant effect on total mortality, but with significant reductions in the rate of cardiovascular events that was statistically significant in the high risk group.

Fatty Acid Specificity

Epidemiological studies of heart disease have implicated the four major saturated fatty acids to varying degrees. The World Health Organization has determined that there is "convincing" evidence that myristic and palmitic acid intake increases the probability, "possible" risk from lauric acid, and no increased risk at all from stearic acid consumption.

In 2005, Dutch scientists at Department of Human Biology, Maastricht University compared the effects of stearic acid with oleic and linoleic acids. Forty five subjects (27 women and 18 men) consumed, in random order, three experimental diets, each for five weeks. The results suggest stearic acid is not highly thrombogenic compared with oleic and linoleic acids.

Cancer

Breast Cancer

There is one theorized association between saturated fatty acids intake and increased breast cancer risk.

Prostate Cancer

Myristic and palmitic saturated fatty acids are associated with prostate cancer.

Small Intestine Cancer

A prospective study of data from the NIH-AARP Diet and Health Study correlated saturated fat intake with cancer of the small intestine"

Dietary Recommendations

A 2004 statement released by the Centers for Disease Control (CDC) determined that "Americans need to continue working to reduce saturated fat intake..." Additionally, reviews by the American Heart Association led the Association to recommend reducing saturated fat intake to less than 7 per cent of total calories according to its 2006 recommendations. This concurs with similar conclusions made by the World Health Organization (WHO) and the US Department of Health and Human Services, both of which determined that reduction in saturated fat consumption would positively affect health and reduce the prevalence of heart disease.

The World Health Organization (WHO) has concluded that saturated fats negatively affect cholesterol profiles, predisposing individuals to heart disease, and recommends avoiding saturated fats in order to reduce the risk of a cardiovascular disease.

Dr German and Dr Dillard of University of California and Nestle Research Center in Switzerland, in their 2004 review, pointed out that "no lower safe limit of specific saturated fatty acid intakes has been identified". No randomized clinical trials of low-fat diets or low-saturated fat diets of sufficient duration have been carried out. The influence of varying saturated fatty acid intakes against a background of different individual lifestyles and genetic backgrounds should be the focus in future studies.

Contrary Research

One confounding issue in studies may be the formation of exogenous (outside the body) advanced glycation endproducts (AGEs) and oxidation products generated during cooking, which it appears some of the studies have not controlled for. It has been suggested that, "given the prominence of this type of food in the human diet, the deleterious effects of high-(saturated) fat foods may be in part due to the high content in glycotoxins, above and beyond those due to oxidized fatty acid derivatives." The glycotoxins, as he called them, are more commonly called AGEs

- A 3-year study conducted of 235 postmenopausal women with established coronary artery disease, many also having metabolic syndrome concluded that "in postmenopausal women with relatively low total fat intake, a greater saturated fat intake is associated with less progression of coronary atherosclerosis." Nevertheless, the authors deemed that "the findings do not establish causality."
- A study of 297 Portuguese males with acute myocardial infarction (MI), found that "total fat intake, lauric acid, palmitic acid [two common saturated fats] and oleic acid [a monoinsaturated fat] were inversely associated with acute MI" and concluded that "low intake of total fat and lauric acid from dairy products was related to acute MI". The authors suggest that "recommendations on fatty acid intake should aim for both an upper and lower limit".
- Fulani of northern Nigeria get around 25 per cent of energy from saturated fat, yet their lipid profile is indicative of a low risk of cardiovascular disease. This finding is likely due to their high activity level and their low total energy intake.
- A 2004 article in *The American Journal of Clinical Nutrition* raised the possibility that the supposed causal relationship between saturated fats and heart disease may actually be a statistical bias. The authors take the example of the "Finnish mental hospital study" in which saturated fat

intakes were monitored more closely than were total fat intakes, therefore ignoring the possibility that simply a larger fat intake may lead to a higher risk of coronary diseases. It also suggests that other parameters were overlooked, such as carbohydrates intakes.

Molecular Description

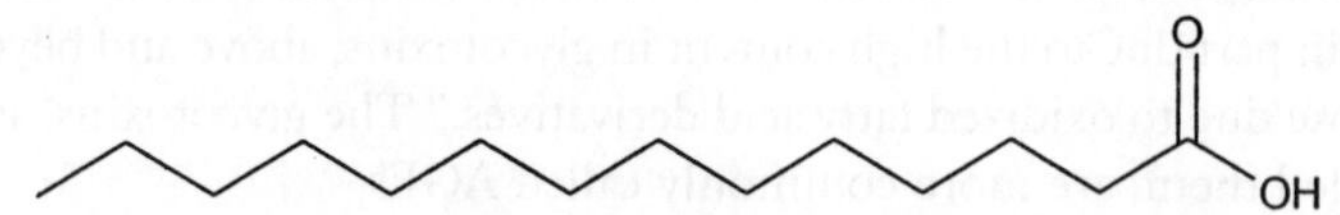

Fig. 4.8: Two-dimensional Representation of the Saturated Fatty Acid Myristic Acid

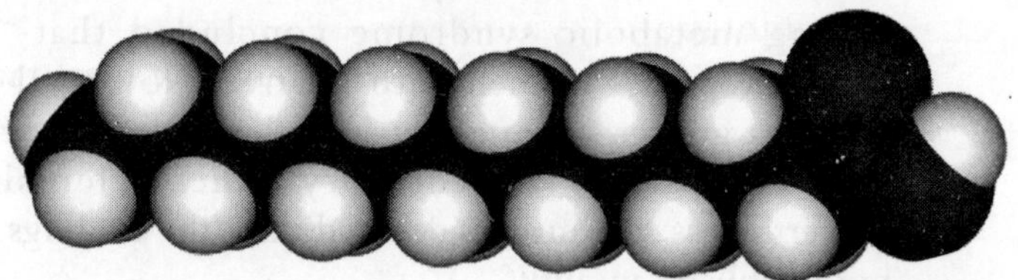

Fig.4.9: A Space-Filling Model of the Saturated Fatty Acid Myristic Acid

UNSATURATED FAT

An unsaturated fat is a fat or fatty acid in which there are one or more double bonds in the fatty acid chain. A fat molecule is monounsaturated if it contains one double bond, and polyunsaturated if it contains more than one double bond. Where double bonds are formed, hydrogen atoms are eliminated. Thus, a saturated fat is "saturated" with hydrogen atoms. In cellular metabolism hydrogen-carbon bonds are broken down — or oxidized — to produce energy, thus an unsaturated fat molecule contains somewhat less energy (i.e. fewer calories) than a comparable sized saturated fat. The greater the degree of unsaturation in a fatty acid (ie, the more double bonds in the fatty acid), the more vulnerable it is to lipid peroxidation (rancidity). Antioxidants can protect unsaturated fat from lipid peroxidation.

Chemistry and Nutrition

Double bonds may be in either a cis or a trans isomer, depending on the geometry of the double bond. In the cis conformation hydrogen atoms are on the same side of the double bond, whereas in the trans conformation they are on opposite sides. Saturated fats are popular with manufacturers of processed foods because they are less vulnerable to rancidity and are generally more solid at room temperature than *unsaturated* fats. Unsaturated chains have a lower melting point, hence increasing fluidity of the cell membranes.

Although both monounsaturated and polyunsaturated fats can replace saturated fat in the diet, trans unsaturated fats should be avoided. Substituting (replacing) saturated fats with unsaturated fats helps to lower levels of total cholesterol and LDL cholesterol in the blood. Trans unsaturated fats are particularly risky because the double bond stereochemistry allows the fat molecules to assume a linear conformation which leads to efficient packing (i.e., plaque formation). The geometry of the cis double bond introduces a bend in the molecule precluding stable formations. Natural sources of fatty acids are rich in the cis isomer.

Although polyunsaturated fats are protective against cardiac arrhythmias, a study of post-menopauseal women with a relatively low fat intake showed that polyunsaturated fat was positively associated with progression of coronary atherosclerosis, whereas monounsaturated fat was not. This probably is an indication of the greater vulnerability of polyunsaturated fats to lipid peroxidation, against which Vitamin E has been shown to be protective.

Examples of unsaturated fats are palmitoleic acid, oleic acid, myristoleic acid, linoleic acid, and arachidonic acid. Foods containing unsaturated fats include avocado, nuts, and vegetable oils such as canola, and olive oils. Meat products contain both saturated and unsaturated fats.

Although unsaturated fats are healthier than saturated fats, the Food and Drug Administration (FDA) recommendation stated that the amount of unsaturated fat consumed should not exceed 30 per cent of one's daily caloric intake (or 67 grams given a 2000 Calorie diet). The new dietary guidelines have eliminated this recommendation. Most food contain both unsaturated and saturated fats. Marketers only advertise one or the other, depending on which one makes up the majority. Thus, various unsaturated fat vegetable oils, such as olive oils, also contain saturated fat.

Role of Dietary Fats in the Prevention of Prostate Cancer

Insulin resistance correlates positively with monounsaturated fat (especially oleic acid) and negatively with polyunsaturated fat (especially arachidonic acid) in the phospholipids of human skeletal muscle.

Membrane Composition as a Metabolic Pacemaker

Cell membranes of mammals have a higher composition of polyunsaturated fat (DHA, omega-3 fatty acid) and a lower composition of monounsaturated fat than do reptiles. Higher polyunsaturated membrane content gives greater membrane fluidity (and functionality), commensurate with the higher metabolic rate of the warm-blooded species. In fish, however, increasingly cold environments lead to increasingly high cell membrane content of both monounsaturated and polyunsaturated fatty acids, presumably to maintain greater membrane fluidity (and functionality) at the lower temperatures.

Component in Different Foods

Fat Composition in Different Foods

Food	*Saturated*	*Monounsaturated*	*Polyunsaturated*
	As Weight Percent (%) of Total Fat		
Cooking Oils			
Canola oil	7	59	29
Corn oil	13	24	59
Olive oil	13	74	8
Soybean oil	15	24	58
Dairy Products			
Cheese, regular	64	29	3
Cheese, light	60	30	0
Milk, whole	62	28	4
Milk, 2%	62	30	0

(Contd.)

Food	Saturated	Monounsaturated	Polyunsaturated
	As Weight Percent (%) of Total Fat		
Ice cream, gourmet	62	29	4
Ice cream, light	62	29	4
Meats			
Beef	33	38	5
Ground sirloin	38	44	4
Pork chop	35	44	8
Ham	35	49	16
Chicken breast	29	34	21
Chicken	34	23	30
Turkey breast	30	20	30
Turkey drumstick	32	22	30
Fish, orange roughy	23	15	46
Salmon	28	33	28
Hot dog, beef	42	48	5
Hot dog, turkey	28	40	22
Burger, fast food	36	44	6
Cheeseburger, fast food	43	40	7
Breaded chicken sandwich	20	39	32
Grilled chicken sandwich	26	42	20
Sausage, Polish	37	46	11
Sausage, turkey	28	40	22
Pizza, sausage	41	32	20
Pizza, cheese	60	28	5
Nuts			
Almonds dry roasted	9	65	1
Cashews dry roasted	20	59	17
Macadamia dry roasted	15	79	2
Peanuts dry roasted	14	50	31
Pecans dry roasted	8	62	25
Flaxseeds, ground	8	23	65
Sesame seeds	14	38	44
Soybeans	14	22	57
Sunflower seeds	11	19	66
Walnuts dry roasted	9	23	63
Sweets and Baked Goods			
Candy, chocolate bar	59	33	3
Candy, fruit chews	14	44	38
Cookie, oatmeal raisin	22	47	27
Cookie, chocolate chip	35	42	18
Cake, yellow	60	25	10
Pastry, Danish	50	31	14

(Contd.)

Food	Saturated	Monounsaturated	Polyunsaturated
	As Weight Percent (%) of Total Fat		
Fats Added during Cooking or at the Table			
Butter, stick	63	29	3
Butter, whipped	62	29	4
Margarine, stick	18	39	39
Margarine, tub	16	33	49
Margarine, light tub	19	46	33
Lard	39	45	11
Shortening	25	45	26
Chicken fat	30	45	21
Beef fat	41	43	3
Dressing, blue cheese	16	54	25
Dressing, light Italian	14	24	58
Other			
Egg yolk fat	36	44	16

Unless else specified in boxes, then reference is:

LIST OF SATURATED FATTY ACIDS

Common Name	Systematic Name	Structural Formula	Lipid Numbers
Propionic acid	Propanoic acid	CH_3CH_2COOH	C3:0
Butyric acid	Butanoic acid	$CH_3(CH_2)_2COOH$	C4:0
Valeric acid	Pentanoic acid	$CH_3(CH_2)_3COOH$	C5:0
Caproic acid	Hexanoic acid	$CH_3(CH_2)_4COOH$	C6:0
Enanthic acid	Heptanoic acid	$CH_3(CH_2)_5)COOH$	C7:0
Caprylic acid	Octanoic acid	$CH_3(CH_2)_6COOH$	C8:0
Pelargonic acid	Nonanoic acid	$CH_3(CH_2)_7COOH$	C9:0
Capric acid	Decanoic acid	$CH_3(CH2)_8COOH$	C10:0
Undecylic acid	Undecanoic acid	$CH_3(CH2)_9COOH$	C11:0
Lauric acid	Dodecanoic acid	$CH_3(CH_2)_{10}COOH$	C12:0
Tridecylic acid	Tridecanoic acid	$CH_3(CH_2)_{11}COOH$	C13:0
Myristic acid	Tetradecanoic acid	$CH_3(CH_2)_{12}COOH$	C14:0
Pentadecylic acid	Pentadecanoic acid	$CH_3(CH_2)_{13}COOH$	C15:0
Palmitic acid	Hexadecanoic acid	$CH_3(CH_2)_{14}COOH$	C16:0
Margaric acid	Heptadecanoic acid	$CH_3(CH_2)_{15}COOH$	C17:0
Stearic acid	Octadecanoic acid	$CH_3(CH_2)_{16}COOH$	C18:0
Nonadecylic acid	Nonadecanoic acid	$CH_3(CH_2)_{17}COOH$	C19:0
Arachidic acid	Eicosanoic acid	$CH_3(CH_2)_{18}COOH$	C20:0
Heneicosylic acid	Heneicosanoic acid	$CH_3(CH_2)_{19}COOH$	C21:0
Behenic acid	Docosanoic acid	$CH_3(CH_2)_{20}COOH$	C22:0
Tricosylic acid	Tricosanoic acid	$CH_3(CH_2)_{21}COOH$	C23:0
Lignoceric acid	Tetracosanoic acid	$CH_3(CH_2)_{22}COOH$	C24:0

(*Contd.*)

Common Name	*Systematic Name*	*Structural Formula*	*Lipid Numbers*
Pentacosylic acid	Pentacosanoic acid	$CH_3(CH_2)_{23}COOH$	C25:0
Cerotic acid	Hexacosanoic acid	$CH_3(CH_2)_{24}COOH$	C26:0
Heptacosylic acid	Heptacosanoic acid	$CH_3(CH_2)_{25}COOH$	C27:0
Montanic acid	Octacosanoic acid	$CH_3(CH_2)_{26}COOH$	C28:0
Nonacosylic acid	Nonacosanoic acid	$CH_3(CH_2)_{27}COOH$	C29:0
Melissic acid	Triacontanoic acid	$CH_3(CH_2)_{28}COOH$	C30:0
Henatriacontylic acid	Henatriacontanoic acid	$CH_3(CH_2)_{29}COOH$	C31:0
Lacceroic acid	Dotriacontanoic acid	$CH_3(CH_2)_{30}COOH$	C32:0
Psyllic acid	Tritriacontanoic acid	$CH_3(CH_2)_{31}COOH$	C33:0
Geddic acid	Tetratriacontanoic acid	$CH_3(CH_2)_{32}COOH$	C34:0
Ceroplastic acid	Pentatriacontanoic acid	$CH_3(CH_2)_{33}COOH$	C35:0
Hexatriacontylic acid	Hexatriacontanoic acid	$CH_3(CH_2)_{34}COOH$	C36:0

LIST OF VEGETABLE OILS

There are three methods for extracting vegetable oils from plants. The relevant part of the plant may be placed under pressure to "extract" the oil, giving an expressed oil. Oils may also be extracted from plants by dissolving parts of plants in water or another solvent. The solution may be separated from the plant material and concentrated, giving an extracted or leached oil. The mixture may also be separated by distilling the oil away from the plant material. Oils extracted by this latter method are called essential oils. Essential oils often have different properties and uses than pressed or leached vegetable oils. Macerated oils are made by infusing parts of plants in a base oil a process known as maceration.

Although most plants contain some oil, only the oil from certain major oil crops complemented by a few dozen minor oil crops is widely used and traded. These oils are one of several types of plant oils.

Vegetable oils can be classified in several ways, for example:

- By source: most, but not all vegetable oils are extracted from the fruits or seeds of plants, and the oils may be classified by grouping oils from similar plants, such as "nut oils".
- By use: oils from plants are used in cooking, for fuel, for

cosmetics, for medical purposes, and for other industrial purposes.

The vegetable oils are grouped below in common classes of use.

Edible Oils

Major Oils

These oils account for a significant fraction of worldwide edible oil production. All are also used as fuel oils.

- Coconut oil, a cooking oil, high in saturated fat, particularly used in baking and cosmetics.
- Corn oil, a common cooking oil with little odor or taste.
- Cottonseed oil, used in manufacturing potato chips and other snack foods. Very low in trans fats.
- Olive oil, used in cooking, cosmetics, soaps, and as a fuel for traditional oil lamps.
- Palm oil, the most widely produced tropical oil. Popular in West African and Brazilian cuisine. Also used to make biofuel.
- Peanut oil (Ground nut oil), a clear oil used for dressing salads and, due to its high smoke point, especially used for frying.
- Rapeseed oil, including Canola oil, one of the most widely used cooking oils.
- Safflower oil, produced for export for over 50 years, first for use in paint industry, now mostly as a cooking oil.
- Sesame oil, cold pressed as light cooking oil, hot pressed for a darker and stronger flavor.
- Soybean oil, produced as a byproduct of processing soy meal.
- Sunflower oil, a common cooking oil, also used to make biodiesel.

Nut Oils

Nut oils are generally used in cooking, for their flavor. They are also quite costly, because of the difficulty of extracting the oil.

- Almond oil, used as an edible oil, but primarily in the manufacture of pharmaceutical drugs.
- Cashew oil, somewhat comparable to olive oil. May have value for fighting dental cavities.
- Hazelnut oil, mainly used for its flavor. Also used in skin care, because of its slight astringent nature.
- Macadamia oil, strongly flavored, contains no trans fat, and a good balance of omega-3 and omega-6 fatty acids.
- *Mongongo nut oil (or* manketti oil*), from the seeds of the* Schinziophyton rautanenii, *a tree which grows in South Africa. High in vitamin E. Also used in skin care.*
- Pecan oil, valued as a food oil, but requiring fresh pecans for good quality oil.
- Pine nut oil usually added to foods as a flavoring agent.
- Pistachio oil, strongly flavored oil, particularly for use in salads.
- Walnut oil, used for its flavor, also used by Renaissance painters in oil paints.

Oils from Melon and Gourd Seeds

Members of the cucurbitaceae include gourds, melons, pumpkins, and squashes. Seeds from these plants are noted for their oil content, but little information is available on methods of extracting the oil. In most cases, the plants are grown as food, with dietary use of the oils as a byproduct of using the seeds as food.

- Bottle gourd oil, extracted from the seeds of the *Lagenaria siceraria*, widely grown in tropical regions throughout the world. Used medicinally and as an edible oil.
- Buffalo gourd oil, from the seeds of the *Cucurbita foetidissima*, a vine with a rank odor, native to southwest North America.
- Pumpkin seed oil, a specialty cooking oil, produced in Austria and Slovenia. Poor tolerance for high temperatures.
- Watermelon seed oil, pressed from the seeds of *Citrullus vulgaris.* Traditionally used in cooking in West Africa.

Food Supplements

A number of oils are used as food supplements, for their nutrient content or medical effect.

- Acai oil, from the fruit of several species of the Açaí Palm (*Euterpe*). Grown in the Amazon region. Similar to grape seed oil. They are used in cosmetics and as a food supplement.
- Blackcurrant seed oil, used as a food supplement, because of high content of omega-3 and omega-6 fatty acids.
- Borage seed oil, similar to blackcurrant seed oil, used primarily medicinally.
- Evening primrose oil, used as a food supplement for its purported medicinal properties.

Other Edible Oils

- Amaranth oil, high in squalene and unsaturated fatty acids, used in food and cosmetic industries.
- Apricot oil, similar to, but much cheaper than almond oil, which it resembles. Only obtained from certain cultivars.
- Apple seed oil, used in cosmetics and shampoos. Also used as an edible oil.
- Argan oil, a food oil from Morocco that has also attracted recent attention in Europe.
- Artichoke oil, extracted from the seeds of the *Cynara cardunculus.* Similar in use and composition to safflower and sunflower oil.
- Avocado oil, a nutty-flavored culinary oil, also used as a base for infusions. Also used in cosmetics. Unusually high smoke point of 510°F.
- Babassu oil, similar to, and used as a substitute for, coconut oil.
- Ben oil, extracted from the seeds of the *Moringa oleifera.* High in behenic acid. Extremely stable edible oil. Also suitable for biofuel.
- Borneo tallow nut oil, extracted from the fruit of species of genus *Shorea.* Used as a substitute for cocoa butter, and to make soap, candles, cosmetics and medicines.

- Cape Chestnut oil, otherwise known as Yangu oil, is a popular oil in African skin care.
- Cocoa butter, from the cacao plant. Used in the manufacture of chocolate, as well as in some cosmetics.
- Carob pod oil (Algaroba oil), from carob, used medicinally.
- Cocklebur oil, from species of genus *Xanthium*, with similar properties to poppyseed oil, similar in taste and smell to sunflower oil.
- Cohune oil, from the Attalea *cohune* (cohune palm), similar to coconut oil in makeup and usage.
- Coriander seed oil, from coriander seeds, used medicinally. Also used as a flavoring agent in pharmaceutical and food industries.
- Dika oil, from *Irvingia gabonensis* seeds, native to West Africa. Used to make margarine, soap and pharmaceuticals, where is it being examined as a tablet lubricant. Largely underdeveloped.
- False flax oil made of the seeds of *Camelina sativa*, available in Russia as ryjhikovoye maslo (рыжиковое масло). Considered promising as a food or fuel oil.
- Flax seed oil (called linseed oil when used as a drying oil). High in omega 3 and lignans, which can be used medicinally. Easily turns rancid.
- Grape seed oil, suitable for cooking at high temperatures. Also used as a salad oil, and in cosmetics.
- Hemp oil, a high quality food oil.
- Kapok seed oil, used as an edible oil, and in soap production.
- Lallemantia oil, from the seeds of *Lallemantia iberica*, discovered at archaeological sites in northern Greece.
- Marula oil, extracted from the kernel of *Sclerocarya birrea.* Used in the food and cosmetic industry, it has strong antioxidant and moisturising properties.
- Meadowfoam seed oil, highly stable oil, with over 98 per cent long-chain fatty acids. Competes with rapeseed oil for industrial applications.
- Mustard oil (pressed), used in India as a cooking oil. Also used as a massage oil.

- Nutmeg butter, extracted by expression from the fruit of cogeners of genus *Myristica*. Nutmeg butter has a large amount of trimyristin. Nutmeg oil, by contrast, is an essential oil, extracted by steam distillation.
- Okra seed oil (Hibiscus seed oil), from the seed of the *Hibiscus esculentus.* Composed predominantly of oleic and linoleic acids. The greenish yellow edible oil has a pleasant taste and odor.
- Papaya seed oil.
- Perilla seed oil, high in omega-3 fatty acids. Used as an edible oil, for medicinal purposes, in skin care products and as a drying oil.
- Pequi oil, extracted from the seeds of *Caryocar brasiliense.* Used in Brazil as a highly prized cooking oil.
- Pine nut oil. An expensive food oil, from pine nuts, used in salads and as a condiment.
- Poppyseed oil, used for cooking, moisturizing skin, in paints and varnishes, and in soaps.
- Prune kernel oil, marketed as a gourmet cooking oil.
- Quinoa oil, similar in composition and use to corn oil.
- Ramtil oil, pressed from the seeds of the one of several species of genus *Guizotia abyssinica* (Niger pea) in India and Ethiopia. Used for both cooking and lighting.
- Rice bran oil, suitable for high temperature cooking. Widely used in Asia.
- Royle oil, pressed from the seeds of *Prinsepia utilis*, a wild, edible oil shrub that grows in the higher Himalayas. Used medicinally in Nepal.
- Sacha Inchi oil, from the Peruvian Amazon. High in omega-3 and omega-6 fatty acids.
- Tea seed oil (Camellia oil), widely used in southern China as a cooking oil. Also used in making soaps, hair oils and a variety of other products.
- Thistle oil, pressed from the seeds of *Silybum marianum.* Relatively unstable. Also used for skin care products.
- Tomato seed oil. High in unsaturated fats and lysine. Potentially useful as a protein supplement.

- Wheat germ oil, used as a dietary supplement, and for its "grainy" flavor. Also used medicinally. Highly unstable.

Oils Used for Biofuel

A number of the oils listed above are used for biofuel (biodiesel and Straight Vegetable Oil) in addition to having other uses. A number of oils are used only as biofuel.

Although diesel engines were invented, in part, with vegetable oil in mind, diesel fuel is almost exclusively petroleum-based. Vegetable oils are evaluated for use as a biofuel based on:

1. Suitability as a fuel, based on flash point, energy content, viscosity, combustion products and other factors
2. Cost, based in part on yield, effort required to grow and harvest, and post-harvest processing cost

Multipurpose Oils also Used as Biofuel

The oils listed immediately below are all (primarily) used for other purposes—all but tung oil are edible—but have been considered for use as biofuel.

- Castor oil, lower cost than many candidates. Kinematic viscosity may be an issue.
- Coconut oil (copra oil), promising for local use in places that produce coconuts.
- Corn oil, appealing because of the abundance of maize as a crop.
- Cottonseed oil, shown in one study not to be cost effective when compared with standard diesel.
- *False flax oil, from* Camelina sativa, *used in Europe in oil lamps until the 18th century.*
- Hemp oil, relatively low in emissions. High flash point. Production is problematic in some countries because of its association with marijuana.
- Mustard oil, shown to be comparable to Canola oil as a biofuel.
- Palm oil, very popular for biofuel, but the environmental

impact from growing large quantities of oil palms has recently called the use of palm oil into question.

- Peanut oil, used in one of the first demonstrations of the Diesel engine in 1900.
- Radish oil. Wild radish contains up to 48 per cent oil, making it appealing as a fuel.
- Rapeseed oil, the most common base oil used in Europe in biodiesel production.
- Ramtil oil, used for lighting in India.
- Rice bran oil, appealing because of lower cost than many other vegetable oils. Widely grown in Asia.
- Safflower oil, explored recently as a biofuel in Montana.
- Salicornia oil, from the seeds of *Salicornia bigelovii*, a halophyte (salt-loving plant) native to Mexico.
- Soybean oil, not economical as a fuel crop, but appealing as a byproduct of soybean crops for other uses.
- Sunflower oil, suitable as a fuel, but not necessarily cost effective.
- Tung oil, referenced in several lists of vegetable oils that are suitable for biodiesel.

Inedible Oils Used Only or Primarily as Biofuel

These oils are extracted from plants that are cultivated solely for producing oil-based biofuel. These, plus the major oils described above, have received much more attention as fuel oils than other plant oils.

- Algae oil, recently developed by MIT scientist Isaac Berzin. Byproduct of a smokestack emission reduction system.
- Copaiba, an oleoresin tapped from species of genus Copaifera. Used in Brazil as a cosmetic product and a major source of biodiesel.
- Honge oil, pioneered as a biofuel by Udipi Shrinivasa in Bangalore, India.
- Jatropha oil, widely used in India as a fuel oil. Has attracted strong proponents for use as a biofuel.
- Jojoba oil, from the Simmondsia chinensis, a desert shrub.
- Milk bush, popularized by chemist Melvin Calvin in the

1950s. Researched in the 1980s by Petrobras, the Brazilian national petroleum company.

- Petroleum nut oil, from the Petroleum nut (Pittosporum resiniferum) native to the Philippines. The Philippine government once explored the use of the petroleum nut as a biofuel.

Drying Oils

Drying oils are vegetable oils that dry to a hard finish at normal room temperature. Such oils are used as the basis of oil paints, and in other paint and wood finishing applications. In addition to the oils listed here, walnut, sunflower and safflower oil are also considered to be drying oils.

- Dammar oil, from the Canarium strictum, used in paint as an oil drying agent. Can also be used as in oil lamps.
- Linseed oil, used in paints, also suitable for human consumption.
- Poppyseed oil, similar in usage to linseed oil but with better colour stability.
- Stillingia oil (also called Chinese vegetable tallow oil), obtained by solvent from the seeds of Sapium sebiferum. Used as a drying agent in paints and varnishes.
- Tung oil, used in wood finishing.
- Vernonia oil is produced from the seeds of the Vernonia galamensis. It is composed of 73-80 per cent vernolic acid, which can be used to make epoxies for manufacturing adhesives, varnishes and paints, and industrial coatings.

Other Oils

A number of pressed vegetable oils are either not edible, or not used as an edible oil.

- Amur cork tree fruit oil, pressed from the fruit of the Phellodendron amurense, used medicinally and as an insecticide.

- Balanos oil, pressed from the seeds of Balanites aegyptiaca, was used in ancient Egypt as the base for perfumes.
- Bladderpod oil; pressed from the seeds of Lesquerella fendleri, native to North America. Rich in lesquerolic acid, which is chemically similar to the ricinoleic acid found in castor oil. Many industrial uses. Possible substitute for castor oil as it requires much less moisture than castor beans.
- Brucea javanica oil, extracted from the seeds of the Brucea javanica. Used medicinally.
- Burdock oil (Bur oil) extracted from the root of the burdock. Used medicinally in scalp treatment.
- Candlenut oil (Kukui nut oil), produced in Hawai'i, used primarily for skin care products.
- Carrot seed oil (pressed), from carrot seeds, used in skin care products.
- Castor oil, with many industrial and medicinal uses. Castor beans are also a source of the toxin ricin.
- Chaulmoogra oil, from the seeds of Taraktogenos kurzii, used for many centuries, internally and externally, to treat leprosy. Also used to treat secondary syphilis, rheumatism, scrofula, and in phthisis.
- Crambe oil, extracted from the seeds of the Crambe abyssinica, is used as an industrial lubricant, a corrosion inhibitor, and as an ingredient in the manufacture of synthetic rubber.
- Cuphea oil, from a number of species of genre Cuphea. Of interest as sources of medium chain triglycerides.
- Illipe butter, from the nuts of the Shorea stenoptera. Similar to cocoa butter, but with a higher melting point. Used in cosmetics.
- Jojoba oil, used in cosmetics as an alternative to whale oil spermaceti.
- Lemon oil, similar in fragrance to the fruit. One of a small number of cold pressed essential oils. Used medicinally, as an antiseptic, and in cosmetics.
- Mango oil, pressed from the stones of the mango fruit, is high in stearic acid, and can be used for making soap.
- Mowrah butter, from the seeds of the Madhuca latifolia

and Madhuca longifolia, both native to India. Crude Mowrah butter is used as a fat for spinning wool, for making candles and soap. The refined fat is used as an edible fat and vegetable ghee in India.

- Neem oil, used in cosmetics, for medicinal purposes, and as an insecticide.
- Ojon oil, extracted from the nut of the American palm (Elaeis oleifera). Used as a skin and hair treatment. Oil extracted from both the nut and husk is also used as an edible oil in Central and South America.
- Orange oil, like lemon oil, cold pressed rather than distilled. Consists of 90 per cent d-Limonene. Used as a fragrance, in cleaning products and in flavoring foods.
- Rose hip seed oil, used primarily in skin care products, particularly for aging or damaged skin. Produced in Chile.
- Rubber seed oil, pressed from the seeds of the Rubber tree (Hevea brasiliensis), has received attention as a potential use of what otherwise would be a waste product from making rubber. It has been explored as a drying oil in Nigeria as a diesel fuel in India and as food for livestock in Cambodia and Vietnam
- Sea buckthorn oil, derived from Hippophae rhamnoides, produced in northern China, used primarily medicinally.
- Shea butter, used primarily in skin care products.
- Snowball seed oil (Viburnum oil), from Viburnum opulus seeds. High in tocopherol, carotenoides and unsaturated fatty acids. Used medicinally.
- Tall oil, produced as a byproduct of wood pulp manufacture. A further byproduct called tall oil fatty acid (TOFA) is a cheap source of oleic acid.
- Tamanu oil, originates in Tahiti, from the Calophyllum tacamahaca, used for skin care and medicinally.
- Tonka bean oil (Cumaru oil), used for flavoring tobacco and snuff.

TRANS FAT

Trans fat is the common name for unsaturated fat with trans-isomer fatty acid(s). Trans fats may be monounsaturated or polyunsaturated but never saturated.

Unsaturated fat is a fat molecule, containing one or more double bonds between the carbon atoms. Since the carbons are double-bonded to each other, there are fewer bonds connected to hydrogen, so there are fewer hydrogen atoms, hence "unsaturated". Cis and trans are terms that refer to the arrangement of chains of carbon atoms across the double bond. In the cis arrangement, the chains are on the same side of the double bond, resulting in a kink. In the trans arrangement, the chains are on opposite sides of the double bond, and the chain is straight.

The process of hydrogenation adds hydrogen atoms to cis-unsaturated fats, eliminating a double bond and making them more saturated. These saturated fats have a higher melting point, which makes them attractive for baking and extends shelf-life. However, the process frequently has a side effect that turns some cis-isomers into trans-unsaturated fats instead of hydrogenating them completely.

There is another class of trans fats, vaccenic acid, which occurs naturally in trace amounts in meat and dairy products from ruminants.

Unlike other dietary fats, trans fats are not essential, and they do not promote good health. The consumption of trans fats increases one's risk of coronary heart disease by raising levels of "bad" LDL cholesterol and lowering levels of "good" HDL cholesterol. Health authorities worldwide recommend that consumption of trans fat be reduced to trace amounts. Trans fats from partially hydrogenated oils are more harmful than naturally occurring oils.

History

Nobel laureate Paul Sabatier worked in the late 1890s to develop the chemistry of hydrogenation which enabled the margarine, oil hydrogenation, and synthetic methanol industries. While Sabatier only considered hydrogenation of vapors, the German chemist Wilhelm Normann showed in 1901 that liquid oils could be hydrogenated, and patented the process in 1902. During the years 1905-1910 Normann built a fat hardening facility in the Herford company. At the same time the invention was extended to a large scale plant in Warrington, England, at Joseph Crosfield and Sons, Limited. It took only two years until the hardened fat could be successfully produced in the plant in Warrington, commencing production in the autumn of 1909. The initial year's production totalled nearly 3,000 tonnes. In 1909, Procter and Gamble acquired the US rights to the Normann patent; in 1911, they began marketing the first hydrogenated shortening, Crisco (composed largely of partially hydrogenated cottonseed oil). Further success came from the marketing technique of giving away free cookbooks in which every recipe called for Crisco.

Normann's hydrogenation process made it possible to stabilize affordable whale oil or fish oil for human consumption, a practice kept secret to avoid consumer distaste.

Prior to 1910, dietary fats primarily consisted of butterfat, beef tallow, and lard. During Napoleon's reign in France in the early 1800s, a type of margarine was invented to feed the troops using tallow and buttermilk; it did not gain acceptance in the U.S. In the early 1900s, soybeans began to be imported into the U.S. as a source of protein; soybean oil was a by-product. What to do with that oil became an issue. At the same time, there was not enough butterfat available for consumers. The method of hydrogenating fat and turning a liquid fat into a solid one had been discovered, and now the ingredients (soybeans) and the "need" (shortage of butter) were there. Later, the means for storage, the refrigerator, was a factor in trans fat development. The fat industry found that hydrogenated fats provided some special features to margarines, which unlike butter, allowed margarine to be taken out of the refrigerator and immediately spread on a slice of bread. By some minor changes to the chemical composition of hydrogenated fat, they also found such hydrogenated fat provided superior baking properties compared to lard. Margarine made from hydrogenated soybean oil began to replace butterfat. Hydrogenated fat such as Crisco and Spry, sold in England, began to replace lard in the baking of bread, pies, cookies, and cakes in 1920.

In the 1940s Dr Catherine Kousmine researched the effects of trans fats on cancer.

Production of hydrogenated fats increased steadily until the

1960s as processed vegetable fats replaced animal fats in the US and other western countries. At first, the argument was a financial one due to lower costs; however, advocates also said that the unsaturated trans fats of margarine were healthier than the saturated fats of butter.

There were suggestions in the scientific literature as early as 1988 that trans fats could be a cause of the large increase in coronary artery disease. In 1994, it was estimated that trans fats caused 30,000 deaths annually in the US from heart disease.

In January 2007, faced with the prospect of an outright ban on the sale of their product, Crisco was reformulated to meet the United States Food and Drug Administration definition of "zero grams trans fats per serving" (that is less than one gram per tablespoon) by boosting the saturation and then cutting the resulting solid with oils. A University of Guelph research group has found a way to mix oils (such as olive, soybean and canola), water, monoglycerides and fatty acids to form a "cooking fat" that acts the same way as trans and saturated fats.

Chemistry

Chemically, trans fat refers to a lipid molecule that contains one or more double bonds in trans geometric configuration. A double bond may exhibit one of two possible configurations; trans or cis. In trans configuration, the carbon chain extends from opposite sides of the double bond, rendering a straighter molecule, whereas in cis configuration, the carbon chain extends from the same side of thedouble bond, rendering a bent molecule.

Trans (Elaidic Acid)	*Cis (Oleic Acid)*	*Saturated (Stearic Acid)*
Elaidic acid is the principal trans unsatu-rated fatty acid often found in partially hydrogena-ted vegetable oils.	Oleic acid is a cis unsaturated fatty acid that comp-rises 55-80 per cent of olive oil.	Stearic acid is a saturated fatty acid found in animal fats and is the intended product in full hydrogenation. Stearic acid is neither cis nor trans because it has no double bonds.
These fatty acids are geometric isomers (structurally identical except for the arrangement of the double bond).		This fatty acid contains no double bond and is not isomeric with the previous two.

Fatty acids are characterized as either saturated or unsaturated based on the presence of double bonds in its structure. If the molecule contains no double bonds, it is said to be saturated; otherwise, it is unsaturated to some degree.

Only unsaturated fats can be trans fats. Saturated fatty acids are never trans fats because they have no double bonds, and therefore cannot display a trans-configuration. Moreover, lipids containing a triple bond (but no double bonds) cannot be trans fats because a triple bond can only assume one configuration.

Carbon atoms are tetravalent, forming four covalent bonds with other atoms, while hydrogen atoms bond with only one other atom. In saturated fatty acids, each carbon atom is connected to its two neighbour carbon atoms as well as two hydrogen atoms. In unsaturated fatty acids the carbon atoms that are missing a hydrogen atom are joined by double bonds rather than single bonds so that each carbon atom participates in four bonds.

Hydrogenation of an unsaturated fatty acid refers to the addition of hydrogen atoms to the acid, causing double bonds to become single ones as carbon atoms acquire new hydrogen partners (to maintain four bonds per carbon atom). Full hydrogenation results in a molecule containing the maximum amount of hydrogen (in other words the conversion of an unsaturated fatty acid into a saturated one). Partial hydrogenation results in the addition of hydrogen atoms at some of the empty positions, with a corresponding reduction in the number of double bonds. Commercial hydrogenation is typically partial in order to obtain a malleable mixture of fats that is solid at room temperature, but melts upon baking (or consumption).

In most naturally occurring unsaturated fatty acids, the hydrogen atoms are on the same side of the double bonds of the carbon chain (cis configuration — meaning "on the same side" in Latin). However, partial hydrogenation reconfigures most of the double bonds that do not become chemically saturated, twisting them so that the hydrogen atoms end up on different sides of the chain. This type of configuration is called trans, which means "across" in Latin. The trans conformation is the lower energy form, and is favoured when catalytically equilibriated as a side reaction in hydrogenation.

The same molecule, containing the same number of atoms, with a double bond in the same location, can be either a trans or a cis fatty acid depending on the conformation of the double bond. For example, oleic acid and elaidic acid are both unsaturated fatty acids with the chemical formula $C_9H_{17}C_9H_{17}O_2$. They both have a double bond located midway along the carbon chain. It is the conformation of this bond that sets them apart. The conformation has implications for the physical-chemical properties of the molecule. The trans configuration is straighter, while the cis configuration is noticeably kinked as can be seen from the following three-dimensional representation.

The trans fatty acid elaidic acid has different chemical and physical properties owing to the slightly different bond configuration. Notably, it has a much higher melting point, 45°C rather than oleic acid's 13.4°C, due to the ability of the trans molecules to pack more tightly, forming a solid that is more difficult to break apart. This notably means that it is a solid at human body temperatures.

In food production, the goal is not to simply change the configuration of double bonds while maintaining the same ratios of hydrogen to carbon. Instead, the goal is to decrease the number of double bonds and increase the amount of hydrogen in the fatty acid. This changes the consistency of the fatty acid and makes it less prone to rancidity (in which free radicals attack double bonds). Production of trans fatty acids is therefore a side-effect of partial hydrogenation.

Catalytic partial hydrogenation necessarily produces trans-fats, because of the reaction mechanism. In the first reaction step, one hydrogen is added, with the other, coordinatively unsaturated, carbon being attached to the catalyst. The second step is the addition of hydrogen to the remaining carbon, producing a saturated fatty acid. The first step is reversible, such that the hydrogen is readsorbed on the catalyst and the double bond is re-formed. Unfortunately, the intermediate with only one hydrogen added contains no double bond, and can freely rotate. Thus, the double bond can re-form as either cis and trans, of which trans is favoured, regardless the starting material. Complete hydrogenation also hydrogenates any produced trans fats to give saturated fats.

Researchers at the United States Department of Agriculture have investigated whether hydrogenation can be achieved without the side effect of trans fat production. They varied the pressure under which the chemical reaction was conducted — applying 1400 kPa (200 psi) of pressure to soybean oil in a 2 litre vessel while heating it to between 140°C and 170°C. The standard 140 kPa (20 psi) process of hydrogenation produces a product of about 40 per cent trans fatty acid by weight, compared to about 17 per cent using the high pressure method. Blended with unhydrogenated liquid soybean oil, the high pressure processed oil produced margarine containing 5 to 6 per cent trans fat. Based on current U.S. labelling requirements the manufacturer could claim the product was free of trans fat. The level of trans fat may also be altered by modification of the temperature and the length of time during hydrogenation.

Trans fat levels may be measured. Measurement techniques include chromatography (by silver ion chromatography on thin layer chromatography plates, or small high performance liquid chromatography columns of silica gel with bonded phenylsulfonic acid groups whose hydrogen atoms have been exchanged for silver ions). The role of silver lies in its ability to form complexes with unsaturated compounds. Gas chromatography and mid-infrared spectroscopy are other methods in use.

Presence in Food

A type of trans fat occurs naturally in the milk and body fat of ruminants (such as cattle and sheep) at a level of 2-5 per cent of total fat. Natural trans fats, which include conjugated linoleic acid (CLA) and vaccenic acid, originate in the rumen of these animals. However, CLA is also a cis fat.

Animal-based fats were once the only trans fats consumed, but by far the largest amount of trans fat consumed today is created by the processed food industry as a side-effect of partially hydrogenating unsaturated plant fats (generally vegetable oils). These partially hydrogenated fats have displaced natural solid fats and liquid oils in many areas, notably in the fast food, snack food, fried food and baked good industries.

Partially hydrogenated oils have been used in food for many reasons. Partial hydrogenation increases product shelf life and decreases refrigeration requirements. Because baking often requires semi-solid fats to suspend solids at room temperature, partially hydrogenated oils can replace the animal fats traditionally used by bakers (such as butter and lard). They are also an inexpensive alternative to other semi-solid oils such as palm oil. Because partially hydrogenated plant oils can replace animal fats, the resulting products can be consumed (barring other ingredient and preparation violations) by adherents to Kashrut (kosher) and Halal, as well as by adherents to vegetarianism in Buddhism, vegetarianism in Hinduism, veganism, and other forms of vegetarianism. However, the same can be said of non-hydrogenated plant shortenings made from naturally saturated, Palm oil, Coconut oil and Palm Kernel oil which have the added benefit of being trans-fat free.

Foods containing artificial trans fats formed by partially hydrogenating plant fats may contain up to 45 per cent trans fat compared to their total fat. Baking shortenings generally contain 30 per cent trans fats compared to their total fats, while animal fats from ruminants such as butter contain up to 4 per cent. Those margarines not reformulated to reduce trans fats may contain up to 15 per cent trans fat by weight.

It has been established that trans fats in human milk fluctuate with maternal consumption of trans fat, and that the amount of trans fats in the bloodstream of breastfed infants fluctuates with the amounts found in their milk. Reported percentages of trans fats (compared to total fats) in human milk range from 1 per cent in Spain, 2 per cent in France, 4 per cent in Germany, and 7 per cent in Canada.

Trans fats are also found in shortenings commonly used for deep frying in restaurants. In the past, the decreased rancidity of partially hydrogenated oils meant that they could be reused for a longer time than conventional oils. Recently, however, non-hydrogenated vegetable oils have become available that have lifespans exceeding that of the frying shortenings. As fast food chains routinely use different fats in different locations, trans fat levels in products can have large variation. For example, an analysis of samples of McDonald's french fries collected in 2004 and 2005 found that fries served in New York City contained twice as much trans fat as in Hungary, and 28 times as much trans fat as in Denmark (where trans fats are restricted). At KFC, the pattern was reversed with Hungary's product containing twice the trans fat of the New York product. Even within the US there was variation, with fries in New York containing 30 per cent more trans fat than those from Atlanta.

Nutritional Guidelines

The National Academy of Sciences (NAS) advises the United States and Canadian governments on nutritional science for use in Public policy and product labeling programmes. Their 2002 Dietary Reference Intakes for Energy, Carbohydrate, Fiber, Fat, Fatty Acids, Cholesterol, Protein, and Amino Acids contains their findings and recommendations regarding consumption of trans fat (summary).

Their recommendations are based on two key facts. First, "trans fatty acids are not essential and provide no known benefit to human health", whether of animal or plant origin. Second, while both saturated and trans fats increase levels of LDL cholesterol (so-called bad cholesterol), trans fats also lower levels of HDL cholesterol (good cholesterol); thus increasing the risk of coronary heart disease. The NAS is concerned "that dietary trans fatty acids are more deleterious with respect to coronary heart disease than saturated fatty acids". This analysis is supported by a 2006 New England Journal of Medicine (NEJM) scientific review that states "from a nutritional standpoint, the consumption of trans fatty acids results in considerable potential harm but no apparent benefit."

Because of these facts and concerns, the NAS has concluded there is no safe level of trans fat consumption. There is no adequate level, recommended daily amount or tolerable upper limit for trans fats. This is because any incremental increase in trans fat intake increases the risk of coronary heart disease.

Despite this concern, the NAS dietary recommendations have not recommended the elimination of trans fat from the diet. This is because trans fat is naturally present in many animal foods in trace quantities, and therefore its removal from ordinary diets might introduce undesirable side effects and nutritional imbalances if proper nutritional planning is not undertaken. The NAS has therefore "recommended that trans fatty acid consumption be as low as possible while consuming a nutritionally adequate diet". Like the NAS, the World Health Organization has tried to balance public health goals with a practical level of trans fat consumption, recommending in 2003 that trans fats be limited to less than 1 per cent of overall energy intake.

The US National Dairy Council has asserted that the trans fats present in animal foods are of a different type than those in partially hydrogenated oils, and do not appear to exhibit the same negative effects. While a recent scientific review agrees with the conclusion (stating that "the sum of the current evidence suggests that the Public health implications of consuming trans fats from ruminant products are relatively limited") it cautions that this may be due to the low consumption of trans fats from animal sources compared to artificial ones.

Health Risks

Partially hydrogenated vegetable oils have been an increasingly significant part of the human diet for about 100 years (particularly so in the latter half of the 20th century and in the West where more processed foods are consumed), and some deleterious effects of trans fat consumption are scientifically accepted, forming the basis of the health guidelines discussed above.

The exact biochemical methods by which trans fats produce specific health problems are a topic of continuing research. The most prevalent theory is that the human lipase enzyme is specific to the cis configuration, rendering the human body unable to metabolize or remove trans fat. A lipase is a water-soluble enzyme that catalyzes the hydrolysis of ester bonds in water-insoluble, lipid substrates. Lipases thus comprise a subclass of the esterases. Lipases perform essential roles in the digestion, transport and processing of dietary lipids (e.g. triglycerides, fats, oils) in most — if not all — living organisms. The human lipase enzyme is ineffective with the trans configuration, so trans fat remains in the blood stream for a much longer period of time and is more prone to arterial deposition and subsequent plaque formation. While the mechanisms through which trans fats contribute to coronary heart disease are fairly well understood, the mechanism for trans fat's effect on diabetes is still under investigation.

Coronary Heart Disease

The primary health risk identified for trans fat consumption is an elevated risk of coronary heart disease (CHD). A comprehensive review of studies of trans fats was published in 2006 in the New England Journal of Medicine reports a strong and reliable connection between trans fat consumption and CHD, concluding that "On a per-calorie basis, trans fats appear to increase the risk of CHD more than any other macronutrient, conferring a substantially increased risk at low levels of consumption (1 to 3% of total energy intake)". This study estimates that between 30,000 and 100,000 cardiac deaths per year in the United States are attributable to the consumption of trans fats.

The major evidence for the effect of trans fat on CHD comes from the Nurses' Health Study (NHS) — a cohort study that has been following 120,000 female nurses since its inception in 1976. In this study, Hu and colleagues analyzed data from 900 coronary events from the NHS population during 14 years of followup. He determined that a nurse's CHD risk roughly doubled (relative risk of 1.94, CI: 1.43 to 2.61) for each 2 per cent increase in trans fat calories consumed (instead of carbohydrate calories). By contrast, it takes more than a 15 per cent increase in saturated fat calories (instead of carbohydrate calories) to produce a similar increase in risk. Eating non-trans unsaturated fats instead of carbohydrates reduces the risk of CHD rather than increasing it. Hu also reports on the benefits of reducing trans fat consumption. Replacing 2 per cent of food energy from trans fat with non-trans unsaturated fats more than halves the risk of CHD (53%). By comparison, replacing a larger 5 per cent of food energy from saturated fat with non-trans unsaturated fats reduces the risk of CHD by 43 per cent.

Another study considered deaths due to CHD, with consumption of trans fats being linked to an increase in mortality, and consumption of polyunsaturated fats being linked to a decrease in mortality.

There are two accepted tests that measure an individual's risk for coronary heart disease, both blood tests. The first considers ratios of two types of cholesterol, the other the amount of a cell-signalling cytokine called C-reactive protein. The ratio test is more accepted, while the cytokine test may be more powerful but is still being studied. The effect of trans fat consumption has been documented on each as follows:

- *Cholesterol Ratio*: This ratio compares the levels of LDL (so-called "bad" cholesterol) to HDL (so-called "good" cholesterol). Trans fat behaves like saturated fat by raising the level of LDL, but unlike saturated fat it has the additional effect of decreasing levels of HDL. The net increase in LDL/HDL ratio with trans fat is approximately double that due to saturated fat. (Higher ratios are worse.) One randomized crossover study published in 2003 comparing the postprandial effect on blood lipids of (relatively) cis and trans fat rich meals showed that cholesteryl ester transfer (CET) was 28 per cent higher after the trans meal than after the cis meal and that lipoprotein concentrations were enriched in apolipoprotein(a) after the trans meals.
- *C-reactive Protein (CRP)*: A study of over 700 nurses showed that those in the highest quartile of trans fat consumption had blood levels of CRP that were 73 per cent higher than those in the lowest quartile.

Other Effects

There are suggestions that the negative consequences of trans fat consumption go beyond the cardiovascular risk. In general, there is much less scientific consensus that eating trans fat specifically increases the risk of other chronic health problems:

- *Alzheimer's Disease*: A study published in Archives of Neurology in February 2003 suggested that the intake of both trans fats and saturated fats promote the development of Alzheimer disease.
- *Cancer*: There is no scientific consensus that consumption of trans fats significantly increases cancer risks across the board. The American Cancer Society states that a

relationship between trans fats and cancer "has not been determined." However, one recent study has found connections between trans fat and prostate cancer. An increased intake of trans-fatty acids may raise the risk of breast cancer by 75 per cent, suggest the results from the French part of the European Prospective Investigation into Cancer and Nutrition.

- *Diabetes*: There is a growing concern that the risk of type 2 diabetes increases with trans fat consumption. However, consensus has not been reached. For example, one study found that risk is higher for those in the highest quartile of trans fat consumption. Another study has found no diabetes risk once other factors such as total fat intake and BMI were accounted for.
- *Obesity*: Research indicates that trans fat may increase weight gain and abdominal fat, despite a similar caloric intake. A 6-year experiment revealed that monkeys fed a trans-fat diet gained 7.2 per cent of their body weight, as compared to 1.8 per cent for monkeys on a mono-unsaturated fat diet. Although obesity is frequently linked to trans fat in the popular media, this is generally in the context of eating too many calories; there is no scientific consensus connecting trans fat and obesity.
- *Liver Dysfunction*: Trans fats are metabolized differently by the liver than other fats and interfere with delta 6 desaturase. Delta 6 desaturase is an enzyme involved in converting essential fatty acids to arachidonic acid and prostaglandins, both of which are important to the functioning of cells.
- *Infertility*: One 2007 study found, "Each 2 per cent increase in the intake of energy from trans unsaturated fats, as opposed to that from carbohydrates, was associated with a 73 per cent greater risk of ovulatory infertility...".

Public Response and Regulation

International

The international trade in food is standardized in the Codex

Alimentarius. Hydrogenated oils and fats come under the scope of Codex Stan 19. Non-dairy fat spreads are covered by Codex Stan 256-2007.. In the Codex Alimentarius, trans fat to be labelled as such is defined as the geometrical isomers of monounsaturated and polyunsaturated fatty acids having non-conjugated [interrupted by at least one methylene group (-CH2-CH2-)] carbon-carbon double bonds in the trans configuration. This definition excludes specifically the healthy 'trans fats' (vaccenic acid and conjugated linoleic acid) which are present especially in human milk, dairy products, and beef.

Australia

The Australian federal government has indicated that it wants to actively pursue a policy of reducing trans fats from fast foods. The former federal assistant health minister, Christopher Pyne, asked fast food outlets to reduce their trans fat usage. A draft plan was proposed, with a September 2007 timetable, in order to reduce reliance on trans fats and saturated fats. Currently, Australia's food labeling laws do not require.trans fats to be shown separately from the total fat content. However, margarine in Australia has been free of trans fat since 1996.. In spite of the efforts mentioned above, Australia has chosen to define trans fats strictly as any fat containing a trans bond. In this sense Australia is diverting from codex (although having agreed on codex definition for trans fats), and also from the regulatory definitions implemented in the US, and EU member states regulations. Considering this, the present Australian/New Zealand food act is positioning human milk as rich (3-6%) in trans fat, and as such unacceptable for human use. Both scientifically and politically seen, this is an isolated position implicitly considering human milk as unhealthy. How the act positions beef meat and dairy products is another story altogether.

Canada

In November 2004, an opposition day motion seeking a ban similar to Denmark's was introduced by Jack Layton of the New Democratic Party, and passed through the House of Commons by an overwhelming 193-73 vote. Like all Commons motions, it served as an expression of the views of the House but was not binding on the government and has no force under the law.

Since December 2005, Health Canada has required that food labels list the amount of trans fat in the nutrition facts section for most foods. Products with less than 0.2 grams of trans fat per serving may be labeled as free of trans fats. These labelling allowances are not widely known, but as an awareness of them develops, controversy over truthful labelling is growing. In Canada, trans fat quantities on labels include naturally occurring trans fats from animal sources.

In June 2006, a task force co-chaired by Health Canada and the Heart and Stroke Foundation of Canada recommended a limit of 5 per cent trans fat (of total fat) in all products sold to consumers in Canada (2% for tub margarines and spreads). The amount was selected such that "most of the industrially produced trans fats would be removed from the Canadian diet, and about half of the remaining trans fat intake would be of naturally occurring trans fats". This recommendation has been endorsed by the Canadian Restaurant and Foodservices Association and Food and Consumer Products of Canada has congratulated the task force on the report, although it did not recommend delaying implementation to 2010 as they had previously advocated.

Ten months after submitting their report the Heart and Stroke Foundation of Canada and Toronto Public Health issued a plea to the government of Canada: "to act immediately on the task force's recommendations and to eliminate harmful trans fat from Canada's food supply."

On June 20, 2007, the federal government announced its intention to regulate trans fats to the June 2006 standard unless the food industry voluntarily complied with these limits within two years.

On January 1, 2008, Calgary became the first city in Canada to ban trans fats from restaurants and fast food chains. Trans fats present in cooking oils may not exceed 2 per cent of the total fat content. However, the replacement of local health regions with the Alberta Health Services Board in 2009 has temporarily eliminated all enforcement of the ban.

Effective September 30, 2009, British Columbia became the first province in Canada to mandate the June 2006 recommendation in provincially regulated food services establishments.

Denmark

Denmark became the first country to introduce laws strictly regulating the sale of many foods containing trans fats in March 2003, a move which effectively bans partially hydrogenated oils. The limit is 2 per cent of fats and oils destined for human consumption. It should be noted that this restriction is on the *ingredients* rather than the final products. This regulatory approach has made Denmark the only country in which it is possible to eat "far less" than 1 g of industrially produced trans fats on a daily basis, even with a diet including prepared foods. It is hypothesized that the Danish government's efforts to decrease trans fat intake from 6g to 1g per day over 20 years is related to a 50 per cent decrease in deaths from ischemic heart disease.

Switzerland

Switzerland followed Denmark's trans fats ban, and implemented its own beginning in April 2008.

European Union

On request the European Food Safety Authority produced a scientific opinion on trans fatty acids.

United Kingdom

In October 2005, the Food Standards Agency (FSA) asked for better labelling in the UK. In the July 29, 2006 edition of the British Medical Journal, an editorial also called for better labelling. In January 2007, the British Retail Consortium announced that major UK retailers, including Asda, Boots, Co-op, Iceland, Marks and Spencer, Sainsbury's, Tesco and Waitrose intend to cease adding trans fatty acids to their own products by the end of 2007.

Sainsbury's became the first UK major retailer to ban all trans fat from all their own brand foods.

On 13 December 2007, the Food Standards Agency issued news releases stating that voluntary measures to reduce trans fats in food had already resulted in safe levels of consumer intake.

United States

Before 2006, consumers in the United States could not directly determine the presence (or quantity) of trans fats in food products. This information could only be inferred from the ingredient list, notably from the partially hydrogenated ingredients. According to the FDA, the average American consumes 5.8 grams of trans fat per day (2.6% of calories.)

On July 11, 2003, the Food and Drug Administration (FDA) issued a regulation requiring manufacturers to list trans fat on the Nutrition Facts panel of foods and some dietary supplements. The new labeling rule became mandatory across the board, even for companies that petitioned for extensions, on January 1, 2008. However, unlike in many other countries, trans fat levels of less than 0.5 grams per serving can be listed as 0 grams trans fat on the food label. According to a study published in the Journal of Public Policy and Marketing, without an interpretive footnote or further information on recommended daily value, many consumers do not know how to interpret the meaning of trans-fat content on the Nutrition Facts panel. In fact, without specific prior knowledge about trans fat and its negative health effects, consumers, including those at risk for heart disease, may misinterpret nutrient information provided on the panel. The FDA did not approve nutrient content claims such as "trans fat free" or "low trans fat", as they could not determine a "recommended daily value". Nevertheless, the agency is planning a consumer study to evaluate the consumer understanding of such claims and perhaps consider a regulation allowing their use on packaged foods. However, there is no requirement to list trans fats on institutional food packaging; thus bulk purchasers such as schools, hospitals, and cafeterias are unable to evaluate the trans fat content of commercial food items. The FDA defines trans fats as containing one or more trans linkage that are not in a conjugated system. This is an important distinction, as it distinguishes non-conjugated synthetic trans fats from naturally occurring fatty acids with conjugated trans double bonds, such as conjugated linoleic acid.

Critics of the plan, including FDA advisor Dr. Carlos Camargo, have expressed concern that the 0.5 gram per serving threshold is too high to refer to a food as free of trans fat. This is because a person eating many servings of a product, or eating multiple products over the course of the day may still consume a significant amount of trans fat. Despite this, the FDA estimates that by 2009, trans fat labeling will have prevented from 600 to 1,200 cases of coronary heart disease and 250 to 500 deaths each year. This benefit is expected to result from consumers choosing alternative foods lower in trans fats as well as manufacturers reducing the amount of trans fats in their products.

The American Medical Association supports any state and federal efforts to ban the use of artificial trans fats in U.S. restaurants and bakeries.

The American Public Health Association adopted a new policy statement regarding trans fats in 2007. These new guidelines, entitled Restricting Trans Fatty Acids in the Food Supply, recommend that the government require nutrition facts labeling of trans fats on all commercial food products. They also urge federal, state, and local governments to ban and monitor use of trans fats in restaurants. Furthermore, the APHA recommends barring the sales and availability of foods containing significant amounts of trans fat in public facilities including universities, prisons, and day care facilities etc.

Local Regulation in the United States

Some US cities are acting to reduce consumption of trans fats. In May 2005, Tiburon, California, became the first American city wherein all restaurants voluntarily cook with trans fat-free oils. Montgomery County, Maryland approved a ban on partially hydrogenated oils, becoming the first county in the nation to restrict trans fats.

New York City embarked on a campaign in 2005 to reduce consumption of trans fats, noting that heart disease is the primary cause of resident deaths. This has included a Public education campaign and a request to restaurant owners to eliminate trans fat from their offerings voluntarily. Finding that the voluntary programme was not successful, New York City's Board of Health in 2006 solicited public comments on a proposal to ban artificial trans fats in restaurants. The board voted to ban trans fat in restaurant food on December 5, 2006. New York was the first large US city to strictly limit trans fats in restaurants. Restaurants were barred from using most frying and spreading fats containing artificial trans fats above 0.5 g per serving on July 1, 2007, and were supposed to have met the same target in all of their foods by July 1, 2008.

Philadelphia also recently passed a ban on trans fats. Philadelphia's City Council voted unanimously to pass a ban on February 8, 2007, which was signed into law on February 15, 2007, by Mayor John F. Street. By September 1, 2007, eateries must cease frying food in trans fats. A year later, trans fat must not be used as an ingredient in commercial kitchens. The law does not apply to prepackaged foods sold in the city. On October 10, 2007, the Philadelphia City Council approved the use of trans-fats by small bakeries throughout the city.

Albany County of New York passed a ban on trans fats. The ban was adopted after a unanimous vote by the county legislature on May 14, 2007. The decision was made after New York City's decision, but no plan has been put into place. Legislators received a letter from Rick J. Sampson, president and CEO of the New York State Restaurant Association, calling on them to "delay any action on this issue until the full impact of the New York City ban is known."

San Francisco officially asked its restaurants to stop using trans fat in January 2008. The voluntary programme will grant a city decal to restaurants that comply and apply for the decal. Legislators say the next step will be a mandatory ban.

Chicago also considered a ban on oils containing trans fats for large chain restaurants, and finally settled on a partial ban on oils and posting requirements for fast food restaurants.

On December 19, 2006, Massachusetts state representative Peter Koutoujian filed the first state level legislation that would ban restaurants from preparing foods with trans fats. The statewide legislation has not yet passed. However, the city of Boston did ban the sale of fooas containing artificial trans fats at more than 0.5 grams per serving, which is similar to the New York City regulation; there are some exceptions for clearly labeled packaged foods and charitable bake sales.

Maryland and Vermont were considering statewide bans of trans fats as of March 2007.

King County of Washington passed a ban on artificial trans fats effective February 1, 2009.

On July 25, 2008, California became the first state to ban trans fats in restaurants. Effective January 1, 2010, Californian restaurants will be prohibited from using oil, shortening, and margarine containing artificial trans fats in spreads or for frying, with the exception of deep frying donuts. Donuts and other baked goods will be prohibited from containing artificial trans fats as of January 1, 2011. Packaged foods, however, are not covered by the ban and will continue to be permitted to contain trans fats.

Food Industry Response

Manufacturer Response

Palm oil, a natural oil extracted from the fruit of oil palm trees that is semi-solid at room temperature (15-25 degrees Celsius), is increasingly being used as an alternative to partially hydrogenated fats in baking and processed food applications.

The J.M. Smucker Company, American manufacturer of Crisco (the original partially hydrogenated vegetable shortening), in 2004 released a new formulation made from solid saturated palm oil cut with soybean oil and sunflower oil. This blend yielded an equivalent shortening much like the previous partially hydrogenated Crisco, and was labelled zero grams of trans fat per 1 tablespoon serving (as compared with 1.5 grams per tablespoon of original Crisco). As of January 24, 2007, Smucker claims that all Crisco shortening products in the US have been reformulated to contain less than one gram of trans fat per serving while keeping saturated fat content less than butter. The separately marketed trans-fat free version introduced in 2004 was discontinued.

On May 22, 2004, Unilever, the corporate descendant of Joseph Crosfield and Sons (the original producer of Wilhelm Normann's hydrogenation hardened oils) announced that they have eliminated transfats from all their margarine products in Canada, including their flagship Becel brand.

Agribusiness giant Bunge Limited, through their Bunge Oils division, are now producing and marketing an NT product line of non-hydrogenated oils, margarines and shortenings, made from corn, canola, and soy oils.

Since 2003, Loders Croklaan, a wholly-owned subsidiary of

Malaysia's IOI Group has been providing trans fat free bakery and confectionery fats, made from palm oil, for giant food companies in the United States to make more heart healthy margarine.

Major Users' Response

Some major food chains have chosen to remove or reduce trans fats in their products. In some cases these changes have been voluntary. In other cases, however, food vendors have been targeted by legal action that has generated a lot of media attention. In May 2003, BanTransFats.com Inc., a U.S. non-profit corporation, filed a lawsuit against the food manufacturer Kraft Foods in an attempt to force Kraft to remove trans fats from the Oreo cookie. The lawsuit was withdrawn when Kraft agreed to work on ways to find a substitute for the trans fat in the Oreo. In November 2006, Arby's announced that by May 2007, it would be eliminating trans fat from its french fries and reducing it in other products.

Similarly, in 2006, the Center for Science in the Public Interest sued KFC over its use of trans fats in fried foods. Concerning their class action complaint. KFC reviewed alternative oil options, saying "there are a number of factors to consider including maintaining KFC's unique taste and flavor of Colonel Sanders' Original Recipe". On October 30, 2006, KFC announced that it will replace the partially hydrogenated soybean oil it currently uses with a zero-trans-fat low linoleic soybean oil in all restaurants in the US by April 2007, although its biscuits will still contain trans-fats. Despite the US-specific nature of the lawsuit, KFC is making changes outside of the US as well; in Canada, KFC's brand owner is switching to trans-fat free Canadian canola oil by early 2007. Wendy's announced in June 2006 plans to eliminate trans-fats from 6,300 restaurants in the United States and Canada, starting in August 2006. In November 2006, Taco Bell made a similar announcement, pledging to remove Trans Fat from many of their menu items by switching to canola oil. By April 2007, 15 Taco Bell menu items were completely free of Trans Fat. In January 2007, McDonald's announced they will start phasing out the trans fat in their fries after years of testing and several delays. This can be partially attributed to New York's recent ban, with the company stating they would not be selling a unique oil just for New York customers but would implement a nationwide change. Chick-fil-A's menu is

Trans Fat free as of October 9, 2007. Raising Canes fast food chicken restaurant recently tested a trans-fat free chicken strip, but there is no plan to reduce their current menu due to the new strip being considered tasting "unsatisfactory."

In response to a May 2007 law suit from the Center for Science in the Public Interest, Burger King announced that its 7,100 US restaurants will begin the switch to zero trans-fat oil by the end of 2007.

The Walt Disney Company announced that they will begin getting rid of trans fats in meals at US theme parks by the end of 2007, and will stop the inclusion of trans fats in licensed or promotional products by 2008.

The Girl Scouts of America announced in November 2006 that all of their cookies will contain less than 0.5g trans fats per serving, thus meeting or exceeding the FDA guidelines for the "zero trans fat" designation.

Health Canada's monitoring programme, which tracks the changing amounts of TFA and SFA in fast and prepared foods shows considerable progress in TFA reduction by some industrial users while others lag behind. In many cases, SFAs are being substituted for the TFAs.

ADVANCED GLYCATION END PRODUCT

- *Nutritional Supplements*: Applied Nutrition Concepts offers only the very best assortment of nutritional supplements available only through health care providers. These high-quality formulas are all-natural and allergen free. We carry many products in our office and we are able to special order products for our clients. We welcome you to come by to pick up your products, or we can mail them to your home or business.
- *Herbal Products*: ANC carries only the highest quality herbal products, favouring the Medi-Herb line. This herbal line originates in Australia under the direction of Kerry Bone, Master Herbalist. They are then shipped to Standard Process in Wisconsin. They can be purchased in either tablet, capsule of tincture for your specific need.

- *Homeopathic Products*: Pekana, Heel/BHI, Sanum Pleomorphic and SanPharma are some of the lines that ANC feels are the highest quality homeopathic products. These are all German brands which give the most variety to serve our patient's needs.
- *Pet Nutrition*: We offer whole food nutritional supplements for dogs and cats, puppies and kittens. You can prevent a lot of health problems by changing your pet's diet and adding whole food nutrition to their daily food intake. Call us for a free brochure or to order your supplements today.
- *Tapes*: Dr. Lois has created a one-hour audio tape entitled 10 Tips To Living a Longer, Stronger Life. The tape covers the 10 hottest topics in nutrition, such as Detoxification, Vitamins and Minerals, Water, and others that can help you enhance your health and longevity. Call to order yours today. Cost: $10 per tape + shipping and handling $4
- *Products we like*:
  - *EDAP*: We feel this is one of the best hand/face/body creams on the market. It has vitamins E, D, and A in a base of Panthenol (hence the name). We have given this to people with sunburn, windburn, cuts, abrasions, and any and all types of skin problems. The results seem too good to be true. For flaky, itchy, dry skin or protection after a day in the sun to help return anti-oxidants back to the skin. This is one of the longest-used products in my practice (over 20 years).
  - *2 oz.* tube $10.00 4 oz. jar $18.00
  - *Sombra*: An alcohol-free natural pain relieving gel. This gel comes highly recommended by our clients who participate in lots of sports. They find it to be a great help in treating aches, pains, swelling, inflammation, and soreness of muscles and joints. Arthritic clients find it helps as well. All natural ingredients. It has six botanical extracts to help counteract pain. Cruelty free.
  - 4 oz. jar $10.00

- *Inflamyar*: By Pekana. A spagyric homeopathic ointment used for sprins, strins, joint problems or inflammation. It is effective for treating bursitis, sciatica, or sports injuries. Supported by a multi-center clinical study conducted by German medical doctors. 3.5 oz. tube $25.00.

IODINE VALUE

The iodine value (or "iodine adsorption value" or "iodine number" or "iodine index") in chemistry is the mass of iodine in grams that is consumed by 100 grams of a chemical substance. An iodine solution is yellow/brown in colour and any chemical group in the substance that reacts with iodine will make the colour disappear at a precise concentration. The amount of iodine solution thus required to keep the solution yellow/brown is a measure of the amount of iodine sensitive reactive groups.

One application of the iodine number is the determination of the amount of unsaturation contained in fatty acids. This unsaturation is in the form of double bonds which react with iodine compounds. The higher the iodine number, the more unsaturated fatty acid bonds are present in a fat. In a typical procedure the acid is treated with an excess of the Hanus solution which is a solution of iodobromine (BrI) (or Wij's iodine solution which a solution of iodine monochloride (ICl) in glacial acetic acid). Unreacted iodobromine (or iodine monochloride) is reacted with potassium iodide which converts it to iodine. The iodine concentration is then determined by titration with sodium thiosulfate.

Standard methods for analysis are for example ASTM D5768-02(2006) and DIN 53241.

For a simple analysis, 0.2 grams of the fat is mixed with 20 ml Wij's solution and 10 ml 1,1,1-trichloroethane. It is then left in the dark for 30 minutes. Next, 15 ml of 10 per cent potassium iodide solution and 10 ml of deionized water is added. This is then titrated against 0.1 M sodium thiosulfate (VI) solution. 1 ml of 0.1 M sodium thiosulfate solution = 0.01269 g of iodine. The difference between a control titration and the titration with the fat present multiplied by this factor gives the mass of iodine absorbed by the oil.

FOOD GROUP

Food groups refers to a method of classification for the various foods that animals consume in their everyday lives, based on the nutritional properties of these types of foods and their location in a hierarchy of nutrition. Eating certain amounts and proportions of foods from the different categories is recommended by most guides to healthy eating as one of the most important ways to achieve a healthy lifestyle through diet.

There are various systems of dividing foods into groups to develop models of optimum nutrition for humans. Among these systems are the USDA's programme titled MyPyramid, the Healthy eating pyramid published by the Harvard School of Public Health, the Canadian Government's Canada's Food Guide, the United Kingdom Food Standards Agency's "Balance of Good Health" guide, the Portuguese food wheel, and others.

SOUP KITCHEN

A soup kitchen, a bread line, or a meal center is a place where food is offered to the hungry for free or at a reasonably low price. Frequently located in lower-income neighborhoods, they are often staffed by volunteer organizations, such as church groups or community groups. Soup kitchens sometimes obtain food from a food bank for free or at a low price, because they are considered a charity.

History

The concept of soup kitchens hit the mainstream of U.S. consciousness during the Great Depression. One soup kitchen in Chicago was even sponsored by Italian mobster Al Capone in an effort to clean up his image. Inventor Benjamin Thompson, contemporary to the Founding Fathers of the United States, is said to have invented the soup kitchen.

Issues

Besides the obvious social/political issues of community acceptance, there is much involved in setting up a soup kitchen.

The Society of St. Vincent de Paul in Pontiac, Michigan, cites the following considerations and issues for their "Nutritional Center":

- Volunteers
- Paid employees
- Food Sources
- Food Transportation
- Other kitchens in the area
- Inventory of kitchen supplies
- Check the dishwasher, freezers, coolers, grease traps, etc.
- Check the city codes and food handler certificates
- Liability insurance
- Tax status
- Rodent control
- Supplies
- Set goals and objectives
  - Type of meals to be served.
  - How and where will they be prepared?
  - Who will be served?
  - Will there be any eligibility requirements?
  - When will the meals be served?
  - Support
  - Funding
  - Other goals besides supplying meals

And this list is only to set up a soup kitchen and get prepared to operate one. Once the operation is started, there are ongoing needs to manage the operation and to adhere to strict health and food safety rules and regulations. It is advisable to develop a set of operational objectives in terms of meal nutrition as well as service standards so that both volunteers and paid staff alike work by an accepted set of goals.

A 1985 pilot study found that 95 per cent of homeless men served by a soup kitchen had vitamin deficiencies. This shows the need for emphasis on selecting menu ingredients containing appropriate vitamins including Vitamin C and B-9.

And reporting key statistics is important in determining trends as well as meeting accepted goals of the kitchen. For example, St. Luke's Episcopal Church in Eastport (Annapolis, Maryland), reports serving (all services including food bank distributions) as many needy families and individuals in the first calendar quarter of 2009 as in all of 2008.

MEAT SPOILAGE

The spoilage of meat occurs, if the meat is untreated, in a matter of hours or days and results in the meat becoming unappetizing, poisonous or infectious. Spoilage is caused by the practically unavoidable infection and subsequent decomposition of meat by bacteria and fungi, which are borne by the animal itself, by the people handling the meat, and by their implements. Meat can be kept edible for a much longer time — though not indefinitely — if proper hygiene is observed during production and processing, and if appropriate food safety, food preservation and food storage procedures are applied.

Infection

The organisms spoiling meat may infect the animal either while still alive ("endogenous disease") or may contaminate the meat after its slaughter ("exogenous disease"). There are numerous diseases that humans may contract from endogenously infected meat, such as anthrax, bovine tuberculosis, brucellosis, salmonellosis, listeriosis, trichinosis or taeniasis.

Infected meat, however, should be eliminated through systematic meat inspection in production, and consequently, consumers will more often encounter meat exogenously spoiled by bacteria or fungi after the death of the animal. One source of infectious organisms is bacteraemia, the presence of bacteria in the blood of slaughtered animals. The large intestine of animals contains some 3.3×10^{13} viable bacteria, which may infect the flesh after death if the carcass is improperly dressed. Contamination can also occur at the slaughterhouse through the use of improperly cleaned slaughter or dressing implements, such as powered knives, on which bacteria persist. A captive bolt pistol's bolt alone may carry about

400,000 bacteria per square centimeter. After slaughter, care must be taken not to infect the meat through contact with any of the various sources of infection in the abattoir, notably the hides and soil adhering to them, water used for washing and cleaning, the dressing implements and the slaughterhouse personnel.

Bacterial genera commonly infecting meat while it is being processed, cut, packaged, transported, sold and handled include Salmonella spp., Shigella spp., E. coli, B. proteus, Staph. albus and Staph. aureus, Cl. welchii, B. cereus and faecal streptococci. These bacteria are all commonly carried by humans; infectious bacteria from the soil include Cl. botulinum. Among the molds commonly infecting meat are Penicillium, Mucor, Cladosporium, Alternaria, Sporotrichium and Thamnidium.

As these microorganisms colonize a piece of meat, they begin to break it down, leaving behind toxins that can cause enteritis or food poisoning, potentially lethal in the rare case of botulism. The microorganisms do not survive a thorough cooking of the meat, but several of their toxins and microbial spores do. The microbes may also infect the person eating the meat, although against this the microflora of the human gut is normally an effective barrier.

Testing

The presence of infectious agents can be detected with a number of tests during the production and processing of meat, but testing by itself is not sufficient to ensure adequate food safety. The industry-standard Hazard Analysis Critical Control Points (HACCP) system provides for a comprehensive quality management framework as a part of which such tests can be conducted. Testing methods applied include phage and serological typing, direct epifluorescence filter techniques (DEFT) and plasmid profiling.

Symptoms

Microbial Spoilage

Depending on ogygen availability, meat spoilage by micro-organisms can manifest itself as follows:

Oxygen	*Microbial agent*	*Symptoms*
Present	Aerobic bacteria	• Surface slime • Discolouration • Gas production • Change in odor • Fat decomposition
Present	Yeasts	• Surface slime • Discolouration • Change in odor and taste • Fat decomposition
Present	Molds	• Sticky and "whiskery" surface • Discolouration • Change in odor • Fat decomposition
Absent	Anaerobic bacteria	• Putrefaction and foul odors • Gas production • Souring

5

Applied Nutrition: Concepts, Services and Tests

APPLIED NUTRITION

Nutrition science is defined globally as the study of food systems, foods and drinks, and their nutrients and other constituents; and of their interactions within and between all relevant biological, social and environmental systems.(1) Outside the biological sciences, which are core to practice in nutritional therapy, applied nutritionists have knowledge, skills and understanding which underpin competence in areas which may include inter alia epidemiology, public health practice, food technology and development, food safety, food law, ecological and environmental sustainability, economics, catering, journalism, politics and social science. The National Occupational Standards (NOS) for Nutritional Therapy cover clinical practice only. Practitioners working in applied nutrition have qualifications, training and experience additional to those required to meet the NOS for clinical practice.

Membership

- Benefits of Joining
- Membership Classes
- Admissions Policy
- Membership Forms
- Insurance
- Yellow Pages

Training

- Training
- Nutritional Therapy Council—NTC
- First Aid

General Information

- Nutrition Titles
- Applied Nutrition
- About BANT
- BANT Council
- Ethics Committee
- CPD Committee
- Regional Coordinators

APPLIED NUTRITION CONCEPTS

Applied Nutrition Concepts is committed to helping you achieve the highest health goals you have for yourself and your family, using all-natural methods. At ANC, we want to fully understand your specific needs. We ask questions and take detailed inventories. We may perform functional tests to determine your biochemistry. Then we find the safest and most natural way for you to achieve your health goals. We recommend dietary and lifestyle changes based on your specific biochemistry and provide the targeted nutrients to correct any imbalances. This correction often leads to a healthier and happier you.

Information in this site is not intended to countermand any advice given by your health professional. Please check with them before starting any health programme.

About Applied Nutrition Concepts

ANC is a private consulting practice that helps people learn more about health, healing and natural remedies. Dr. Lois M. Vanderhoof provides personal counseling services for individuals and families. She helps them with their health goals, incorporating natural health and wellness principles into their lifestyles.

Dr. Lois offers classes, lectures, and presentations to groups, clubs, businesses and corporations, which assists them in learning about and achieving healthy principles. She has helped many employers to decrease employee illness and sick days, thereby reducing costly expense.

ANC performs functional testing using blood, hair, saliva, stool and urine samples to determine biochemical imbalances which my be contributing to your health concerns and symptoms.

ANC supplies nutrients recommended for specific problems, health enhancement and prevention strategies. We offer an assortment of vitamins, minerals, herbal and homeopathic products to supplement your diet and support your vital organs. Whole food nutrition is vital in achieving and maintaining a healthy, balanced lifestyle.

SERVICES

Applied Nutrition Concepts offers complete nutritional and biochemical analysis for our clients. Then we design a specific protocol designed to meet their personal needs and health goals. We have several service offerings available to our clients.

- *Consulting*: Nutritional consultations for individuals and families are offered as a single comprehensive visit to get you started on the right track. Many of our clients elect to continue counseling with on-going support and encouragement. We are available as often as you need by appointment.
- *SCENAR Energy Medicine*: A remarkable new energetic healing device from Russia. Russian research has shown that the SCENAR device can help reduce and remove pain. It has helped both acute and chronic injuries, as well as many other physical problems including sinusitis, pneumonia, swelling, wounds that won't heal, bones that are slow to mend, and many others. Ask us if SCENAR is right for your type of pain or injury.

The SCENAR machine is rubbed lightly over the affected areas. It is non-invasive and painless. SCENAR is completely safe for adults and children.

- *Body Composition Analysis*: This analysis will reveal information about your lean muscle mass, your per cent body fat and your hydration or water level. This non-invasive test provides numerical scores about your cell health and the degree of toxicity in your body.
- Red Blood Cell Analysis: Using a drop of your blood from a finger stick, we can observe the size and shape of your red and white blood cells. This test can reveal nutritional deficiencies based on those changes in your cells. Using this test we can monitor progress of your nutritional status over time.

PRODUCTS

- *Nutritional Supplements*: Applied Nutrition Concepts offers only the very best assortment of nutritional supplements available only through health care providers. These high-quality formulas are all-natural and allergen free. We carry many products in our office and we are able to special order products for our clients. We welcome you to come by to pick up your products, or we can mail them to your home or business.
- *Herbal Products*: ANC carries only the highest quality herbal products, favouring the Medi-Herb line. This herbal line originates in Australia under the direction of Kerry Bone, Master Herbalist. They are then shipped to Standard Process in Wisconsin. They can be purchased in either tablet, capsule of tincture for your specific need.
- *Homeopathic Products*: Pekana, Heel/BHI, Sanum Pleomorphic and SanPharma are some of the lines that ANC feels are the highest quality homeopathic products. These are all German brands which give the most variety to serve our patient's needs.
- *Pet Nutrition*: We offer whole food nutritional supplements for dogs and cats, puppies and kittens. You can prevent a

lot of health problems by changing your pet's diet and adding whole food nutrition to their daily food intake. Call us for a free brochure or to order your supplements today.

- Tapes: Dr. Lois has created a one-hour audio tape entitled 10 Tips To Living a Longer, Stronger Life. The tape covers the 10 hottest topics in nutrition, such as Detoxification, Vitamins and Minerals, Water, and others that can help you enhance your health and longevity. Call to order yours today. Cost: $10 per tape + shipping and handling $4
- Products we like:
    - *EDAP*: We feel this is one of the best hand/face/body creams on the market. It has vitamins E, D, and A in a base of Panthenol (hence the name). We have given this to people with sunburn, windburn, cuts, abrasions, and any and all types of skin problems. The results seem too good to be true. For flaky, itchy, dry skin or protection after a day in the sun to help return anti-oxidants back to the skin. This is one of the longest-used products in my practice (over 20 years).
    - 2 oz. tube $10.00 4 oz. jar $18.00
    - *Sombra*: An alcohol-free natural pain relieving gel. This gel comes highly recommended by our clients who participate in lots of sports. They find it to be a great help in treating aches, pains, swelling, inflammation, and soreness of muscles and joints. Arthritic clients find it helps as well. All natural ingredients. It has six botanical extracts to help counteract pain. Cruelty free.
    - 4 oz. jar $10.00
    - *Inflamyar*: By Pekana. A spagyric homeopathic ointment used for sprins, strins, joint problems or inflammation. It is effective for treating bursitis, sciatica, or sports injuries. Supported by a multi-center clinical study conducted by German medical doctors. 3.5 oz. tube $25.00.

TESTS

- Hair Mineral Analysis and Heavy Metal Analysis
- Urine Mineral Analysis and Heavy Metal Analysis
- Parasitology Testing: Yeast, Candida, Bacteria
- Adrenal Hypofunction Testing: Saliva
- Salivary Hormone Testing (Male and Female Hormones)
- Liver Toxicity Profiles
- Oxidative Stress Profiles
- Comprehensive Digestive Stool Analysis
- Yeast and Candida Testing
- Food Allergy Testing (Blood) IGG
- Cardiovascular Risk Profile (10 Biomarkers)
- Nutritional Analysis of Blood Test
- Body Composition Analysis
- Osteoporosis Risk Evaluation (Urine)
- Metabolic Screening Questionnaire
- Health Assessment Questionnaire
- Breast Cancer Risk Assessment (Urine)
- Genomic Tests for osteoporosis, cardiovascular function

NOOTROPIC

Nootropics, also referred to as smart drugs, memory enhancers, and cognitive enhancers, are drugs, supplements, nutraceuticals, and functional foods that are purported to improve mental functions such as cognition, memory, intelligence, motivation, attention, and concentration. The word nootropic was coined in 1964 by the Romanian Dr. Corneliu E. Giurgea, derived from the Greek words noos, or "mind," and tropein meaning "to bend/ turn". Nootropics are thought to work by altering the availability of the brain's supply of neurochemicals (neurotransmitters, enzymes, and hormones) by improving the brain's oxygen supply or by stimulating nerve growth. However the efficacy of nootropic substances in most cases has not been conclusively determined. This is complicated by the difficulty of defining and quantifying cognition and intelligence.

Availability and Prevalence

At present, there are several drugs on the market that improve memory, concentration, planning, and reduce impulsive behaviour. Many more are in different stages of development. The most commonly used class of drug are the stimulants.

These drugs are used primarily to treat people with cognitive difficulties: Alzheimer's disease, Parkinson's disease, ADHD. However, more widespread use is being recommended by some researchers. These drugs have a variety of human enhancement applications as well, and are marketed heavily on the World-Wide Web. Nevertheless, intense marketing may not correlate with efficacy; while scientific studies support some of the claimed benefits, it is worth noting that many of the claims attributed to most nootropics have not been formally tested.

In academia, modafinil has been used to increase productivity, although its long-term effects have not been assessed in healthy individuals. Stimulants such as methylphenidate and atomoxetine are being used on college campuses, and by an increasingly younger group. One survey found that 7 per cent of students had used stimulants for a cognitive edge in the past year, and on some campuses the number is as high as 25 per cent.

Hazards

The main concern with pharmaceutical drugs is adverse effects, and these concerns apply to cognitive-enhancing drugs as well. Cognitive enhancers are often taken for the long-term when little data is available.

Dr. Corneliu E. Giurgea originally coined the word nootropics for brain-enhancing drugs with very few side-effects. Racetams are sometimes cited as an example of a nootropic with few effects and wide therapeutic window; however, any substance ingested could produce harmful effects. An unapproved drug or dietary supplement does not have to have safety or efficacy approval before being sold. (This mainly applies to the USA, but may not apply in the EU or elsewhere.)

Some dangers of nootropics include, but are not limited to:

- Downregulation of neurological activity upon stimulation, resulting in a permanent or temporary hypoactive system and/or addictive properties (applies to dopamine, choline, and many other neurotransmitter systems)
- Serotonin syndrome from serotonergic agents
- Excessive acetylcholine receptor activation
- Heart failure, such as that from stimulants or any substance which alters heart rate
- Organ failure such as liver failure and kidney failure

Examples

The term "drug" here is used as a legal designation. Although some of the effects of these substances may be similar to others, only those substances that have shown cognitive effects are included.

Nootropics and Racetams

The word nootropic was coined upon discovery of the effects of piracetam, developed in the 1960s. Although piracetam is the most commonly taken nootropic, there are many relatives in the family that have different potencies and side-effects. Other common racetams include pramiracetam, oxiracetam, and aniracetam. There is no generally-accepted mechanism for racetams. In general, they show no affinity for the most important receptors, although modulation of most important central neurotransmitters, including acetylcholine and glutamate, have been reported. Although aniracetam and nebracetam show affinity for muscarinic receptors, only nefiracetam shows it at the nanomolar range. Racetams have been called "pharmacologically safe" drugs.

Other substances sometimes classified as nootropics include hydergine, vinpocetine, bifemelane, huperzine A (cholinergic activator below), and dimethylaminoethanol.

Stimulants

Stimulants are often seen as smart drugs, but are actually just productivity enhancers. These typically improve concentration and a few areas of cognitive performance, but only while the drug is still in the blood. Some scientists recommend widespread use of stimulants such as methylphenidate and amphetamines by the general population to increase brain power.

- Amphetamines
  - Amphetamine (Adderall, Dexedrine)—adrenergic, dopaminergic
  - Lisdexamfetamine (Vyvanse)—adrenergic, dopaminergic
  - Methamphetamine (Desoxyn)—adrenergic, dopaminergic
  - Methylphenidate (Ritalin)—adrenergic, dopaminergic
- Cholinergics
  - Arecoline
  - Nicotine
- Eugeroics ("Wakefulness Enhancers")—unproven primary mechanisms but proven efficacy
  - Adrafinil
  - Armodafinil
  - Modafinil
- Xanthines-reduces fatigue perception
  - Caffeine
  - Paraxanthine
  - Theobromine
  - Theophylline

Dopaminergics

Dopaminergics are substances that affect the neurotransmitter dopamine or the components of the nervous system that use dopamine. Attributable effects of dopamine are enhancement of attention, alertness, and antioxidant activity. Dopamine is the primary activity of stimulants like methylphenidate (Ritalin) or amphetamine. Dopaminergic nootropics include dopamine synthesis precursors, dopamine reuptake inhibitors, monoamine oxidase inhibitors, and other compounds:

- Metabolic precursors-raise levels
  - L-Phenylalanine-purported cognitive improvement

    - L-Tyrosine-purported cognitive improvement
- Reuptake inhibitors-stabilize/improve levels
    - Amineptine-mild stimulant
- MAO-B inhibitors-prevent breakdown
    - Selegiline-mild stimulant

Others

- cocaine and the relatives-multiple mechanisms that amplify dopamine release
- amphetamine and relatives
- Yohimbe-purported dopaminergic activity

Memory Enhancement

Memory can come from many different processes, but is dependent on the ability to store and recall information.

Cholinergics

Cholinergics are substances that affect the neurotransmitter acetylcholine or the components of the nervous system that use acetylcholine. Acetylcholine is a facilitator of memory formation. Increasing the availability of this neurotransmitter in the brain may improve these functions. Cholinergic nootropics include acetylcholine precursors and cofactors, and acetylcholinesterase inhibitors:

- Precursors
    - Choline-precursor of acetylcholine
    - Meclofenoxate-probable precursor of acetylcholine, approved for Dementia and Alzheimer's
- Cofactors
    - Acetylcarnitine—amino acid that functions in acetylcholine production by donating the acetyl portion to the acetylcholine molecule
    - Vitamin B5—cofactor in the conversion of choline into acetylcholine
- Acetylcholinesterase inhibitors
    - Galantamine
    - Huperzine A
    - Donepezil

    - Rosemary
    - Sage
- Reuptake inhibitors and enchancers
- Coluracetam—choline uptake enhancer
- Agonists
    - Ispronicline
    - Nicotine
    - Arecoline

GABA Blockers

The $GABA_A$ á5 receptor site has recently displayed memory improvements when inverse agonized.

- á5IA—á5 inverse agonist
- Suritozole—á5 partial inverse agonist

Glutamate Activators

The AMPA transmitter and the AMPA receptors are currently being researched with significant memory improvements and possible alertness enhancement when agonized. The drug class for AMPA system modulation is called Ampakines. Although there are many in-research ones, the main ones mentioned will be the ones possibly coming to market or are significantly notable.

Some racetams have shown this activity

- CX-717—Going through FDA approval for memory-impairing illnesses
- IDRA-21—believed to improve memory by significantly enhancing long-term potentiation but used only in animals—incredibly potent
- LY-503,430—Being developed for Parkinson's but showing increase in BDNF, specifically in areas of memory and higher cognitive skills

cAMP

Cyclic adenosine monophosphate is a secondary messenger that, if increased, has shown memory improvements. One common method is by decreasing the activity of phosphodiesterase-4, an enzyme that breaks down cAMP. Typical effects include wakefulness and memory enhancement.

- Propentofylline—nonselective phosphodiesterase inhibitor with some neuroenhancement
- Rolipram—Drug. shows alertness enhancement, long term memory improvement and neuroprotection
- Mesembrine—PDE4-inhibitor with possible serotonergic activity

Serotonergics

Serotonin is a neurotransmitter with various effects on mood and possible effects on neurogenesis. Serotonergics are substances that affect the neurotransmitter serotonin or the components of the nervous system that use serotonin. Serotonergic nootropics include serotonin precursors and cofactors, and serotonin reuptake inhibitors:

- 5-HTP—precursor
- Tryptophan—Essential amino acid
- SSRIs—Class of antidepressants that increase active serotonin levels by inhibiting its reuptake. Have also been shown to promote Neurogenesis in the hippocampus.
- Tianeptine—paradoxical antidepressant, improves mood and reduces anxiety
- Methamphetamine—some serotonin activity

Anti-depression, Adaptogenic (Antistress), and Mood Stabilization

Stress, depression, and depressed mood negatively affect cognitive performance. It is reasoned that counteracting and preventing depression and stress may be an effective nootropic strategy. The term adaptogen applies to most herbal anti-stress claims.

The substances below may not have been mentioned earlier on the page:

- Beta blockers—anxiolytic
- Kava kava—mild euphoric depressant used in relaxation
- Lemon Balm—Displays adaptogen properties

- Passion Flower—possible MAOI and neurotransmitter reuptake activity
- Rhodiola Rosea—possible MAOI activity
- St John's Wort—herbal MAOI that has been approved (in Europe) to treat mild depression
- Ginseng (including Siberian ginseng)—adaptogenic effects shown
- Sutherlandia frutescens—possible anti-inflammatory reducing pain from those illnesses
- Tea—contains many different adaptogens
- Theanine—GABAergic activity producing relaxation, also increases brain serotonin and dopamine levels
- Grape seed extract—has shown some efficacy in reducing bodily stress
- Adafenoxate—possible anti-anxiety effect
- Valerian—possible anti-anxiety effect
- Butea frondosa—possible anti-anxiety effect
- Gotu Kola—adaptogen and anxiolytic

Blood Flow and Metabolic Function

Brain function is dependent on many basic processes such as the usage of ATP, removal of waste, and intake of new materials. Improving blood flow or altering these processes can benefit brain function. Vasodilators mentioned are only those which have shown, at minimum, probable mental enhancement.

- Blessed Thistle—increases blood circulation, improving memory
- Coenzyme q-10—increases oxygen usage by mitochondria
- Creatine—protects ATP during transport
- Lipoic acid—improves oxygen usage and antioxidant recycling, possibly improving memory
- Pyritinol—Drug. Similar to B vitamin Pyridoxine
- Vinpocetine—increases blood circulation (vasodilator) and metabolism in the brain
- Picamilon—GABA activity and blood flow improver
- Ginkgo biloba—vasodilator

Nerve Growth Stimulation and Brain Cell Protection

Nerves are necessary to the foundation of brain communication and their degeneracy, underperformance, or lacking can have disastrous results on brain functions. Antioxidants are frequently used to prevent oxidative stress, but do not improve brain function if that is their only activity.

- Idebenone—antioxidant
- Melatonin—antioxidant
- Inositol—implicated in memory function, deficit linked to some psychiatric illnesses
- dopamine enhancers—dopamine is an antioxidant and can enhance dendrite extension
- Anticonvulsants inhibit seizure related brain malfunction if a person has seizures
- Phosphatidylserine—possible membrane stabilizer

Recreational Drugs

Many recreational substances that are currently illegal or heavily controlled have effects on the brain or long-term functions that are typically considered secondary to their effects on perception. Note that this list is not intended to be exhaustive. This list include substances which are illegal, or not completely illegal, but are controlled or exempt under a Drug schedule.

- Tetrahydrocannabinol—Anxiolytic and analgesic found in cannabis. Neuroprotectant, possible Alzheimer's prevention and possible neurogenesis inducer
- Amphetamine—type stimulants are described above
- 4-methylaminorex—similar to Modafinil but significantly more abuse potential
- Most Entheogens, including hallucinogens-drugs or substances which have shown value in psychotherapy, like mescaline, MDMA, and LSD.
- MDPV—designer drug, 4x as potent as methylphenidate, greater abuse potential
- Tobacco—Contains nicotine and also has significant MAOI activity

Dietary Nootropics

Diet can have the greatest effect on cognition and the brain, as there are many necessary things that must be consumed. However, other substances have been linked to certain benefits, and may be predominant in certain foods.

Some regular food items contain substances with alleged nootropic benefits:

- Hemp or Flax—seeds as source of omega-3 fatty acids
- Fish—sources of omega-3 fatty acids
- Berries—may contain high levels of antioxidants

Direct Hormones

These are hormones that have activity not necessarily attributable to another specific chemical interaction, but have shown effectiveness. Only specific nootropic effects are stated.

- Vasopressin—memory hormone that improves both memory encoding and recall
- Pregnenolone—increases neurogenesis
- Orexin—Significant wakefulness promoter

Secondary Enhancers

These are substances which by themselves may not improve brain function, but may have benefits for those lacking them (in the case of hormones) or may alter the balance of neurotransmitters.

- DHEA—Precursor to Estrogen and Testosterone

Unknown Enhancement

Other agents purported to have nootropic effects but which do not (yet) have attributable mechanisms or clinically significant effects (but may upon refinement of administration) are mentioned here.

Nootropics with proven or purported benefits:

- *Bacopa monniera*—enhances memory and concentration. Folk use in Ayurvedic medicine purports "enhancement of curiosity".

- *Brahmi rasayana*—improved learning and memory in mice.
- *Ergoloid mesylates*—Drug. Similar to LSD. Used against Dementia and Alzheimers
- *Fipexide*—drug for Dementia
- *Gerovital H3*—famous anti-aging mixture, most effects disproven, but some mind enhancement shown
- *Sulbutiamine*—fat soluble vitamin B1 derivative. Some shown memory improvement
- *Royal Jelly*—Increases brain cell growth and diversity, only proven in-vitro, improbable in-vivo
- *Curcumin*—Significant in-vitro activity, but in-vivo activity is limited by low bioavailability

Other Nootropics

These substances have been linked to better cognitive function, but may not be the cause.

- Moderate use of alcohol—Moderate drinkers tend to have better cognitive function than both abstainers and heavy drinkers.

Brain and Neurology

- Action potential
- Aging and memory
- Central nervous system (CNS)
- Dendrite
- Human brain
- Long-term potentiation
- Nervous system
- Neurite
- Neuron
- Neuroplasticity
- Neuroscience
- Neurotransmitter
- Sensory neuroscience
- Synaptic plasticity

Thought and Thinking (What Nootropics are Used for)

- Abstract thinking
- Attention
- Attitude
- Brainstorming
- Cognition
- Cognitive science
- Creative thinking
- Critical thinking
- Curiosity
- Decision making
- Eidetic memory
- Emotions and feelings
- Emotional intelligence
- Goals and goal setting
- Imagination
- Intelligence
- Introspection
- Lateral thinking
- Learning
- Memory
- Memory-prediction framework
- Mental calculation
- Motivation
- Perception
- Personality
- Recollection (recall)

Health

- Anxiety
- Cognitive psychology
- Clinical depression
- Confusion
- Cosmetic pharmacology
- Drug

- Human enhancement
  - Ergogenic aid
- Life extension
- Neurodegenerative disease
- Sleep disorders
- Stress
- Stress management

6

Food Safety: Microbiology and Related Water Activity

MICROBIOLOGICAL ASPECTS OF FOOD SAFETY

In the filed of food satety, Food microbiology is the study of the microorganisms which inhabit, create or contaminate food. Of major importance is the study of microorganisms causing food spoilage. However "good" bacteria such as probiotics are becoming increasingly important in food science. In addition, microorganisms are essential for the production of foods such as cheese, yoghurt, other fermented foods, bread, beer and wine.

Food safety is a major focus of food microbiology. Pathogenic bacteria, viruses and toxins produced by microorganisms are all possible contaminants of food. However, microorganisms and their products can also be used to combat these pathogenic microbes. Probiotic bacteria, including those which produce bacteriocins, can kill and inhibit pathogens. Alternatively, purified bacteriocins such as nisin can be added directly to food products. Finally, bacteriophage, viruses which only infect bacteria, can be used to kill bacterial pathogens. Thorough preparation of food, including proper cooking will eliminate most bacteria and viruses. However, toxins produced by contaminants may not be heat-labile, and some will not be eliminated by cooking.

Fermentation is one way microorganisms can change a food. Yeast, especially S. cerevisiae, is used to leaven bread, brew beer and make wine. Certain bacteria, including lactic acid bacteria, are used to make yogurt, cheese, hot sauce, pickles and dishes such as kimchi.

A common effect of these fermentations is that the food product is less hospitable to other microorganisms, including pathogens and spoilage-causing microorganisms, thus extending the food's shelf-life. Some cheese varieties also require mold microorganisms to ripen and develop their characteristic flavors.

A variety of biopolymers, such as polysaccharides, polyesters and polyamides, are naturally produced by microorganisms. Several microbially-produced polymers are used in the food industry.

Plant-pathogenic bacteria of the genus Xanthomonas are able to produce the acidic exopolysaccharide xanthan gum. Because of its physical properties, it is widely used as a viscosifer, thickener, emulsifier or stabilizer in the food industry. Xanthan consists of pentasaccharide repeat units composed of D-glucosyl, D-mannosyl, and D-glucuronyl acid residues in a molar ratio of 2:2:1 and variable proportions of O-acetyl and pyruvyl residues.

Alginate is the main representative of a family of polysaccharides that neither show branching nor repeating blocks or unit patterns and this property distinguishes it from to other polymers like xanthan or dextran. Alginates can be used as thickening agents.

Cellulose is a simple polysaccharide, in that it consists only of one type of sugar (glucose), and the units are linearly arranged and linked together by β-1,4 linkages only. The mechanism of biosynthesis is however rather complex, partly because in native celluloses the chains are organized as highly ordered water-insoluble fibers. Currently the key genes involved in cellulose biosynthesis and regulation are known in a number of bacteria, but many details of the biochemistry of its biosynthesis are still not clear. In spite of the enormous abundance of cellulose in plants bacterial celluloses are being investigated for industrial exploitations.

Poly-γ-glutamic acid (γ-PGA) produced by various strains of Bacillus has potential applications as a thickener in the food industry.

Levan, a homopolysaccharide which is composed of D-fructofuranosyl residues joined by 2,6 with multiple branches by 2,1 linkages has great potential as a functional biopolymer in foods, feeds, cosmetics, and the pharmaceutical and chemical industries. Levan can be used as food or a feed additive with prebiotic and hypocholesterolemic effects.

Microorganisms synthesize a wide spectrum of multifunctional polysaccharides including intracellular polysaccharides, structural polysaccharides and extracellular polysaccharides or exopolysaccharides (EPS). Exopolysaccharides generally constitute of monosaccharides and some non-carbohydrate substituents (such as acetate, pyruvate, succinate, and phosphate). Owing to the wide diversity in composition, exopolysaccharides have found multifarious applications in various food and pharmaceutical industries.

Foodborne pathogens are the leading causes of illness and death in less developed countries killing approximately 1.8 million people annually. In developed countries foodborne pathogens are responsible for millions of cases of infectious gastrointestinal diseases each year, costing billions of dollars in medical care and lost productivity. New foodborne pathogens and foodborne diseases are likely to emerge driven by factors such as pathogen evolution, changes in agricultural and food manufacturing practices, and changes to the human host status. There are growing concerns that terrorists could use pathogens to contaminate food and water supplies in attempts to incapacitate thousands of people and disrupt economic growth.

Food and waterborne viruses contribute to a substantial number of illnesses throughout the world. Among those most commonly known are hepatitis A virus, rotavirus, astrovirus, enteric adenovirus, hepatitis E virus, and the human caliciviruses consisting of the noroviruses and the Sapporo viruses. This diverse group are transmitted by the fecal-oral route, often by ingestion of contaminated food and water.

Protozoan parasites associated with food and water can cause illness in humans. Although parasites are more commonly found in developing countries, developed countries have also experienced several foodborne outbreaks. Contaminants may be inadvertently introduced to the foods by inadequate handling practices, either on the farm or during processing of foods. Protozoan parasites can be found worldwide, either infecting wild animals or in water and contaminating crops grown for human consumption. The disease can be much more severe and prolonged in immunocompromissed individuals.

Molds produce mycotoxins, which are secondary metabolites

that can cause acute or chronic diseases in humans when ingested from contaminated foods. Potential diseases include cancers and tumors in different organs (heart, liver, kidney, nerves), gastrointestinal disturbances, alteration of the immune system, and reproductive problems. Species of Aspergillus, Fusarium, Penicillium, and Claviceps grow in agricultural commodities or foods and produce the mycotoxins such as aflatoxins, deoxynivalenol, ochratoxin A, fumonisins, ergot alkaloids, T-2 toxin, and zearalenone and other minor mycotoxins such as cyclopiazonic acid and patulin. Mycotoxins occur mainly in cereal grains (barley, maize, rye, wheat), coffee, dairy products, fruits, nuts and spices. Control of mycotoxins in foods has focused on minimizing mycotoxin production in the field, during storage or destruction once produced. Monitoring foods for mycotoxins is important to manage strategies such as regulations and guidelines, which are used by 77 countries, and for developing exposure assessments essential for accurate risk characterization.

Yersinia enterocolitica includes pathogens and environmental strains that are ubiquitous in terrestrial and fresh water ecosystems. Evidence from large outbreaks of yersiniosis and from epidemiological studies of sporadic cases has shown that Y. enterocolitica is a foodborne pathogen. Pork is often implicated as the source of infection. The pig is the only animal consumed by man that regularly harbours pathogenic Y. enterocolitica. An important property of the bacterium is its ability to multiply at temperatures near to 0°C, and therefore in many chilled foods. The pathogenic serovars (mainly O:3, O:5, 27, O:8 and O:9) show different geographical distribution. However, the appearance of strains of serovars O:3 and O:9 in Europe, Japan in the 1970s, and in North America by the end of the 1980s, is an example of a global pandemic. There is a possible risk of reactive arthritis following infection with Y. enterocolitica.

Vibrio species are prevalent in estuarine and marine environments and seven species can cause foodborne infections associated with seafood. Vibrio cholerae O1 and O139 serovtypes produce cholera toxin and are agents of cholera. However, fecal-oral route infections in the terrestrial environment are responsible for epidemic cholera. V. cholerae non-O1/O139 strains may cause gastroenteritis through production of known toxins or unknown mechanism. Vibrio parahaemolytitucs strains capable of producing thermostable direct hemolysin (TDH) and/or TDH-related hemolysin are most important cause of gastroenteritis associated with seafood consumption. Vibrio vulnificus is responsible for seafoodborne primary septicemia and its infectivity depends primarily on the risk factors of the host. V. vulnificus infection has the highest case fatality rate (50%) of any foodborne pathogen. Four other species (Vibrio mimicus, Vibrio hollisae, Vibrio fluvialis, and Vibrio furnissii) can cause gastroenteritis. Some strains of these species produce known toxins but the pathogenic mechanism is largely not understood. The ecology of and detection and control methods for all seafoodborne Vibrio pathogens are essentially similar.

Staphylococcus aureus is a common cause of bacterial foodborne disease worldwide. Symptoms include vomiting and diarrhea that occur shortly after ingestion of S. aureus-contaminated food. The symptoms arise from ingestion of preformed enterotoxin, which accounts for the short incubation time. Staphylococcal enterotoxins are superantigens and, as such, have adverse effects on the immune system. The enterotoxin genes are accessory genetic elements in S. aureus, meaning that not all strains of this organism are enterotoxin-producing. The enterotoxin genes are found on prophage, plasmids, and pathogenicity islands in different strains of S. aureus. Expression of the enterotoxin genes is often under the control of global virulence gene regulatory systems.

Campylobacter spp., primarily C. jejuni subsp. jejuni is one of the major causes of bacterial gastroenteritis in the U.S. and worldwide. Campylobacter infection is primarily a foodborne illness, usually without complications; however, serious sequelae such as Guillain-Barre Syndrome occur in a small subset of infected patients. Detection of C. jejuni in clinical samples is readily accomplished by culture and non-culture methods.

Listeria monocytogenes is Gram-positive foodborne bacterial pathogen and the causative agent of human listeriosis. Listeriae are acquired primarily through the consumption of contaminated foods including soft cheese, raw milk, deli salads, and ready-to-eat foods such as luncheon meats and frankfurters. Although L.

monocytogenes infection is usually limited to individuals that are immunocompromised, the high mortality rate associated with human listeriosis makes L. monocytogenes the leading cause of death amongst foodborne bacterial pathogens. As a result, tremendous effort has been made at developing methods for the isolation, detection and control of L. monocytogenes in foods.

Salmonella serotypes continue to be a prominent threat to food safety worldwide. Infections are commonly acquired by animal to human transmission though consumption of undercooked food products derived from livestock or domestic fowl. The second half of the 20th century saw the emergence of Salmonella serotypes that became associated with new food sources (i.e. chicken eggs) and the emergence of Salmonella serotypes with resistance against multiple antibiotics.

Shigella species are members of the family Enterobacteriaceae and are Gram negative, non-motile rods. Four subgroups exist based on O-antigen structure and biochemical properties; S. dysenteriae (subgroup A), S. flexneri (subgroup B), S. boydii (subgroup C) and S. sonnei (subgroup D). Symptoms include mild to severe diarrhea with or without blood, fever, tenesmus, and abdominal pain. Further complications of the disease may be seizures, toxic megacolon, reactive arthritis and hemolytic uremic syndrome. Transmission of the pathogen is by the fecal-oral route, commonly through food and water. The infectious dose ranges from 10-100 organisms. Shigella spp. have a sophisticated pathogenic mechanism to invade colonic epithelial cells of the host, man and higher primates, and the ability to multiply intracellularly and spread from cell to adjacent cell via actin polymerization. Shigellae are one of the leading causes of bacterial foodborne illnesses and can spread quickly within a population.

More information is available concerning Escherichia coli than any other organism, thus making E. coli the most thoroughly studied species in the microbial world. For many years, E. coli was considered a commensal of human and animal intestinal tracts with low virulence potential. It is now known that many strains of E. coli act as pathogens inducing serious gastrointestinal diseases and even death in humans. There are six major categories of E. coli strains that cause enteric diseases in humans including the (1) enterohemorrhagic E. coli, which cause hemorrhagic colitis and hemolytic uremic syndrome, (2) enterotoxigenic E. coli, which induce traveler's diarrhea, (3) enteropathogenic E. coli, which cause a persistent diarrhea in children living in developing countries, (4) enteroaggregative E. coli, which provoke diarrhea in children, (5) enteroinvasive E. coli that are biochemically and genetically related to Shigella species and can induce diarrhea, and (6) diffusely adherent E. coli, which cause diarrhea and are distinguished by a characteristic type of adherence to mammalian cells.

Clostridium botulinum produces extremely potent neurotoxins that result in the severe neuroparalytic disease, botulism. The enterotoxin produced by C. perfringens during sporulation of vegetative cells in the host intestine results in debilitating acute diarrhea and abdominal pain. Sales of refrigerated, processed foods of extended durability including sous-vide foods, chilled ready-to-eat meals, and cook-chill foods have increased over recent years. Anaerobic spore-formers have been identified as the primary microbiological concerns in these foods. Heightened awareness over intentional food source tampering with botulinum neurotoxin has arisen with respect to genes encoding the toxins that are capable of transfer to nontoxigenic clostridia.

The Bacillus cereus group comprises six members: B. anthracis, B. cereus, B. mycoides, B. pseudomycoides, B. thuringiensis and B. weihenstephanensis. These species are closely related and should be placed within one species, except for B. anthracis that possesses specific large virulence plasmids. B. cereus is a normal soil inhabitant and is frequently isolated from a variety of foods, including vegetables, dairy products and meat. It causes a vomiting or diarrhoea illness that is becoming increasingly important in the industrialized world. Some patients may experience both types of illness simultaneously. The diarrhoeal type of illness is most prevalent in the western hemisphere, whereas the emetic type is most prevalent in Japan. Desserts, meat dishes, and dairy products are the foods most frequently associated with diarrhoeal illness, whereas rice and pasta are the most common vehicles of emetic illness. The emetic toxin (cereulide) has been isolated and characterized; it is a small ring peptide synthesised non-ribosomally by a peptide synthetase. Three types of B. cereus enterotoxins involved in foodborne outbreaks have been identified. Two of these enterotoxins are three-component proteins and are related, while the last is a one-component protein (CytK). Deaths have been recorded both by strains that produce the emetic toxin and by a strain producing only CytK. Some strains of the B. cereus group are able to grow at refrigeration temperatures. These variants raise concern about the safety of cooked, refrigerated foods with an extended shelf life. B. cereus spores adhere to many surfaces and survive normal washing and disinfection (except for hypochlorite and UVC) procedures. B. cereus foodborne illness is likely underreported because of its relatively mild symptoms, which are of short duration.

It is important to be able to detect microorganisms in food, in particular pathogenic microorganisms or genetically modified microorganisms. Real-time PCR is an accepted analytical tool within the food industry. Its principal role has been one of assisting the legislative authorities, major manufacturers and retailers to confirm the authenticity of foods. The most obvious role is the detection of genetically modified organisms, but real-time PCR makes a significant contribution to other areas of the food industry, including food safety.

CLOSTRIDIUM BOTULINUM

Clostridium botulinum is a Gram-positive, rod shaped bacterium that produces the neurotoxin botulin, which causes the flaccid muscular paralysis seen in botulism. It is also the main paralytic agent in botox. It is an anaerobic spore-former, which produces oval, subterminal endospores and is commonly found in soil.

Microbiology

C. botulinum is a rod-shaped microorganism. It is an obligate anaerobe, meaning that oxygen is poisonous to the cells. However, they tolerate very small traces of oxygen due to an enzyme called superoxide dismutase (SOD) which is an important antioxidant defense in nearly all cells exposed to oxygen. Under unfavourable circumstances they are able to form endospores that allow them to survive in a dormant state until exposed to conditions that can support their growth.

In laboratory the microorganism is usually isolated in Tryptose Sulfite Cycloserine (TSC) growth media, always in an anaerobic environment with less than 2 per cent of Oxygen. This can be achieved by several commercial kits that use a chemical reaction to replace O_2 with CO_2 (E.J. GasPak System). C. botulinum is lipase negative microorganism, it grows between pH values of 4.8 and 7 and it can't use lactose as a primary carbon source, characteristics important during a biochemical identification.

Taxonomy History

C. botulinum was first recognized and isolated in 1896 by Emile van Ermengem from home cured ham implicated in a botulism outbreak. The isolate was originally named Bacillus botulinus. However, isolates from subsequent outbreaks were always found to be anaerobic spore formers, so Bengston proposed that the organism be placed into the genus Clostridium as the Bacillus genus was restricted to aerobic spore-forming rods.

Since 1953 all species producing the botulinum neurotoxins (types A-G) has been designated C. botulinum. Substantial phenotypic and genotypic evidence exist to demonstrate heterogeneity within the species. This has led to the reclassification of C. botulinum type-G strains to a new species Clostridium argentinense.

C. botulinum *strains that do not produce a botulin toxin are referred to as* Clostridium sporogenes.

The complete genome of C. botulinum has now been sequenced Sanger.

Phenotypic Types

The current nomenclature for C. botulinum recognises four physiological groups (I-IV). This is mostly based on the ability of the organism to digest complex proteins. Studies at the DNA and rRNA level support the subdivision of the species into groups I-IV. Most outbreaks of human botulism are caused by group I (proteolytic) or II (non-proteolytic) C. botulinum. Group III organisms mainly cause diseases in animals. There has been no record of Group IV C. botulinum causing human or animal disease.

Neurotoxin Types

Neurotoxin production is the unifying feature of the species C. botulinum. Seven types of toxins have been identified and allocated a letter (A-G). Most strains produce one type of neurotoxin but strains producing multiple toxins has been described. C. botulinum producing B and F toxin types have been isolated from human botulism cases in New Mexico and California. The toxin type has been designated Bf as the type B toxin was found in excess to the type F. Similarly, strains producing Ab and Af toxins have been reported.

Organisms genetically identified as other Clostridium species have caused human botulism; Clostridium butyricum producing type E toxin and Clostridium baratii producing type F toxin. The ability of C. botulinum to naturally transfer neurotoxin genes to other clostridia is concerning, especially in the food industry where preservation systems are designed to destroy or inhibit only C. botulinum but not other Clostridium species.

***Phenotypic Groups of* Clostridium botulinum**

Properties	*Group I*	*Group II*	*Group III*	*Group IV*
Toxin Types	A, B, F	B, E, F	C, D	G
Proteolysis	+	–	weak	–
Saccharolysis	–	+	–	–
Disease host	human	human	animal	–
Toxin gene	chromosome	chromosome	bacteriophage	plasmid
Close relatives	C. sporoge-nes, C. putrifi-cum	C. butyricum, C. beijerinickii	C. haemolyti-cum, C. novyi type A	C. subtermi-nale, C. haemo-lyticum

Clostridium Botulinum *in Different Geographical Locations*

A number of quantitative surveys for C. botulinum spores in the environment have suggested a prevalence of specific toxin types in given geographic areas, which remain unexplained.

North America

Type A C. botulinum predominates the soil samples from the western regions while type B is the major type found in eastern areas. The type B organisms were of the proteolytic type I. Sediments from the Great Lake regions were surveyed after outbreaks of botulism among commercially reared fish and only type E spores were detected. It has been noted in a survey that type A strains were isolated from soils that were neutral to alkaline (average pH 7.5) while type B strains were isolated from slightly acidic soils (average pH 6.25).

Europe

C. botulinum type E is prevalent in aquatic sediments in Norway and Sweden, Denmark, the Netherlands, the Baltic coast of Poland and Russia. It was then suggested that the type E C. botulinum is a true aquatic organism and this was shown by the correlation between the level of type E contamination and flooding of the land with seawater. As the land dried, the level of type E decreased and type B became dominant.

In soil and sediment from the United Kingdom, C. botulinum type B predominates. In general, the incidence is usually lower in soil than in sediment. In Italy, a survey was conducted in the vicinity of Rome, a low level of contamination was found and all strains were proteolytic C. botulinum type A or B.

Australia

C. botulinum type A was found to be present in soil samples from mountain areas of Victoria. Type B organisms were detected in marine mud from Tasmania. Type A C. botulinum have been found in Sydney suburbs and types A and B were isolated from urban areas. In a well defined area of the Darling-Downs region of Queensland a study showed the prevalence and persistence of C. botulinum type B after many cases of botulism in horses.

Other

A "mouse protection" test determines the type of C. botulinum present using monoclonal antibodies.

Clostridium botulinum is also used to prepare Botox, used to selectively paralyze muscles to temporarily relieve wrinkles. It has other "off-label" medical purposes, such as treating severe facial pain, such as that caused by trigeminal neuralgia.

Botulin toxin produced by Clostridium botulinum is often believed to be a potential bioweapon as it is so potent that it takes about 75 nanograms to kill a person (LD50 of 1ng/kg, assuming an average person weighs ~75kg); 500 grams of it would be enough to kill half of the entire human population.

Clostridium botulinum is a soil bacterium. The spores can survive in most environments and are very hard to kill. They can survive the temperature of boiling water at sea level, thus many foods are canned with a pressurized boil that achieves an even higher temperature, sufficient to kill the spores.

Growth of the bacterium can be prevented by high acidity, high ratio of dissolved sugar, high levels of oxygen, very low levels of moisture or storage at temperatures below 38°F (type A). For example in a low acid, canned vegetable such as green beans that are not heated hot enough to kill the spores (i.e., a pressurized environment) may provide an oxygen free medium for the spores to grow and produce the toxin. On the other hand, pickles are sufficiently acidic to prevent growth; even if the spores are present, they pose no danger to the consumer. Honey, corn syrup, and other sweeteners may contain spores but the spores cannot grow in a highly concentrated sugar solution; however, when a sweetener is diluted in the low oxygen, low acid digestive system of an infant, the spores can grow and produce toxin. As soon as infants begin eating solid food, the digestive juices become too acidic for the bacterium to grow.

ESCHERICHIA COLI

Escherichia coli (commonly *E. coli*), is a bacterium that is commonly found in the lower intestine of warm-blooded animals. Most E. coli strains are harmless, but some, such as serotype O157:H7, can cause serious food poisoning in humans, and are occasionally responsible for costly product recalls. The harmless strains are part of the normal flora of the gut, and can benefit their hosts by producing vitamin K_2, or by preventing the establishment of pathogenic bacteria within the intestine.

E. coli are not always confined to the intestine, and their ability to survive for brief periods outside the body makes them an ideal indicator organism to test environmental samples for fecal contamination. The bacteria can also be grown easily and its genetics are comparatively simple and easily-manipulated, making it one of the best-studied prokaryotic model organisms, and an important species in biotechnology. E. coli was discovered by German pediatrician and bacteriologist Theodor Escherich in 1885, and is now classified as part of the Enterobacteriaceae family of gamma-proteobacteria.

Strains

A strain of E. coli is a sub-group within the species that has unique characteristics that distinguish it from other E. coli strains. These differences are often detectable only on the molecular level; however, they may result in changes to the physiology or lifecycle of the bacterium. For example, a strain may gain pathogenic capacity, the ability to use a unique carbon source, the ability to inhabit a particular ecological niche or the ability to resist antimicrobial agents. Different strains of E. coli are often host-specific, making it possible to determine the source of fecal contamination in environmental samples. Depending on which E. coli strains are present in a water sample, for example, assumptions can be made about whether the contamination originated from a human, other mammal or bird source.

New strains of E. coli evolve through the natural biological process of mutation, and some strains develop traits that can be harmful to a host animal. Although virulent strains typically cause no more than a bout of diarrhea in healthy adult humans, particularly virulent strains, such as O157:H7 or O111:B4, can cause serious illness or death in the elderly, the very young or the immunocompromised.

Biology and Biochemistry

E. coli is Gram-negative, facultative anaerobic and non-sporulating.

The cells are about 2 micrometres (ìm) long and 0.5 ìm in diameter, with a cell volume of 0.6—0.7 ìm. It can live on a wide variety of substrates. E. coli uses mixed-acid fermentation in anaerobic conditions, producing lactate, succinate, ethanol, acetate and carbon dioxide. Since many pathways in mixed-acid fermentation produce hydrogen gas, these pathways require the levels of hydrogen to be low, as is the case when E. coli lives together with hydrogen-consuming organisms such as methanogens or sulfate-reducing bacteria.

Optimal growth of E. coli occurs at 37°C, but some laboratory strains can multiply at temperatures of up to 49°C. Growth can be driven by aerobic or anaerobic respiration, using a large variety of redox pairs, including the oxidation of pyruvic acid, formic acid, hydrogen and amino acids, and the reduction of substrates such as oxygen, nitrate, dimethyl sulfoxide and trimethylamine N-oxide.

Strains that possess flagella can swim and are motile, but other strains lack flagellum. The flagella of E. coli have a peritrichous arrangement.

E. coli and related bacteria possess the ability to transfer DNA via bacterial conjugation, transduction or transformation, which allows genetic material to spread horizontally through an existing population. This process led to the spread of the gene encoding shiga toxin from Shigella to E. coli O157:H7, carried by a bacteriophage.

Normal Role

E. coli normally colonizes an infant's gastrointestinal tract within 40 hours of birth, arriving with food or water or with the individuals handling the child. In the bowel, it adheres to the mucus of the large intestine. It is the primary facultative organism of the human gastrointestinal tract. As long as these bacteria do not acquire genetic elements encoding for virulence factors, they remain benign commensals.

Role in Disease

Virulent strains of E. coli can cause gastroenteritis, urinary tract infections, and neonatal meningitis. In rarer cases, virulent strains are also responsible for hæmolytic-uremic syndrome (HUS), peritonitis, mastitis, septicemia and Gram-negative pneumonia.. Recently it is thought that E. coli and certain other foodborne illnesses can sometimes trigger serious health problems months or years after patients survived that initial bout.

Gastrointestinal Infection

Low-temperature electron micrograph of a cluster of E. coli bacteria, magnified 10,000 times. Each individual bacterium is oblong shaped.

Certain strains of E. coli, such as O157:H7, O121 and O104:H21, produce toxins. Food poisoning caused by E. coli are usually associated with eating unwashed vegetables and meat contaminated post-slaughter. O157:H7 is further notorious for causing serious and even life-threatening complications like hemolytic-uremic syndrome (HUS). This particular strain is linked to the 2006 United States E. coli outbreak of fresh spinach. Severity of the illness varies considerably; it can be fatal, particularly to young children, the elderly or the immunocompromised, but is more often mild. E. coli can harbor both heat-stable and heat-labile enterotoxins. The latter, termed LT, contains one 'A' subunit and five 'B' subunits arranged into one holotoxin, and is highly similar in structure and function to Cholera toxins. The B subunits assist in adherence and entry of the toxin into host intestinal cells, while the A subunit is cleaved and prevents cells from absorbing water, causing diarrhea. LT is secreted by the Type 2 secretion pathway.

If E. coli bacteria escape the intestinal tract through a perforation (for example from an ulcer, a ruptured appendix, or a surgical error) and enter the abdomen, they usually cause peritonitis that can be fatal without prompt treatment. However, E. coli are extremely sensitive to such antibiotics as streptomycin or gentamicin. This could change since, as noted below, E. coli quickly acquires drug resistance. Recent research suggests that treatment with antibiotics does not improve the outcome of the disease, and may in fact significantly increase the chance of developing haemolytic uraemic syndrome.

Intestinal mucosa-associated E. coli are observed in increased numbers in the inflammatory bowel diseases, Crohn's disease and ulcerative colitis. Invasive strains of E. coli exist in high numbers in the inflamed tissue, and the number of bacteria in the inflamed regions correlates to the severity of the bowel inflammation.

Virulence Properties

Enteric E. coli (EC) are classified on the basis of serological characteristics and virulence properties. Virotypes include:

- *Enterotoxigenic E. coli (ETEC)*: causative agent of diarrhea (without fever) in humans, pigs, sheep, goats, cattle, dogs, and horses. ETEC uses fimbrial adhesins (projections from the bacterial cell surface) to bind enterocyte cells in the small intestine. ETEC can produce two proteinaceous enterotoxins: the larger of the two proteins, LT enterotoxin, is similar to cholera toxin in structure and function, while the smaller protein, ST enterotoxin causes cGMP accumulation in the target cells and a subsequent secretion of fluid and electrolytes into the intestinal lumen. ETEC strains are non-invasive, and they do not leave the intestinal lumen. ETEC is the leading bacterial cause of diarrhea in children in the developing world, as well as the most common cause of traveler's diarrhea. Each year, ETEC causes more than 200 million cases of diarrhea and 380,000 deaths, mostly in children in developing countries.
- *Enteropathogenic E. coli (EPEC)*: causative agent of diarrhea in humans, rabbits, dogs, cats and horses. Like ETEC, EPEC also causes diarrhea, but the molecular mechanisms of colonization and etiology are different. EPEC lack fimbriae, ST and LT toxins, but they utilize an adhesin known as intimin to bind host intestinal cells. This virotype has an array of virulence factors that are similar to those found in Shigella, and may possess a shiga toxin. Adherence to the intestinal mucosa causes a rearrangement of actin in the host cell, causing significant deformation. EPEC cells are moderately-invasive (i.e. they enter host cells) and elicit an inflammatory response. Changes in intestinal cell ultrastructure due to "attachment and

effacement" is likely the prime cause of diarrhea in those afflicted with EPEC.

- *Enteroinvasive E. coli (EIEC)*: found only in humans. EIEC infection causes a syndrome that is identical to Shigellosis, with profuse diarrhea and high fever. EIEC are highly invasive, and they utilize adhesin proteins to bind to and enter intestinal cells. They produce no toxins, but severely damage the intestinal wall through mechanical cell destruction.
- *Enterohemorrhagic E. coli (EHEC)*: found in humans, cattle, and goats. The sole member of this virotype is strain O157:H7, which causes bloody diarrhea and no fever. EHEC can cause hemolytic-uremic syndrome and sudden kidney failure. It uses bacterial fimbriae for attachment, is moderately-invasive and possesses a phage-encoded Shiga toxin that can elicit an intense inflammatory response.
- *Enteroaggregative E. coli (EAggEC)*: found only in humans. So named because they have fimbriae which aggregate tissue culture cells, EAggEC bind to the intestinal mucosa to cause watery diarrhea without fever. EAggEC are non-invasive. They produce a hemolysin and an ST enterotoxin similar to that of ETEC.

Epidemiology of Gastrointestinal Infection

Transmission of pathogenic E. coli often occurs via fecal-oral transmission. Common routes of transmission include: unhygienic food preparation, farm contamination due to manure fertilization, irrigation of crops with contaminated greywater or raw sewage, feral pigs on cropland, or direct consumption of sewage-contaminated water. Dairy and beef cattle are primary reservoirs of E. coli O157:H7, and they can carry it asymptomatically and shed it in their feces. Food products associated with E. coli outbreaks include raw ground beef, raw seed sprouts or spinach, raw milk, unpasteurized juice, and foods contaminated by infected food workers via fecal-oral route.

According to the U.S. Food and Drug Administration, the fecal-oral cycle of transmission can be disrupted by cooking food properly, preventing cross-contamination, instituting barriers such as gloves for food workers, instituting health care policies so food industry employees seek treatment when they are ill, pasteurization of juice or dairy products and proper hand washing requirements.

Shiga toxin-producing E. coli (STEC), specifically serotype O157:H7, have also been transmitted by flies, as well as direct contact with farm animals, petting zoo animals, and airborne particles found in animal-rearing environments.

Urinary Tract Infection

Uropathogenic E. coli (UPEC) is responsible for approximately 90 per cent of urinary tract infections (UTI) seen in individuals with ordinary anatomy. In ascending infections, fecal bacteria colonize the urethra and spread up the urinary tract to the bladder. Because women have a shorter urethra than men, they are 14-times more likely to suffer from an ascending UTI.

Uropathogenic E. coli utilize P fimbriae (pyelonephritis-associated pili) to bind urinary tract endothelial cells and colonize the bladder. These adhesins specifically bind D-galactose-D-galactose moieties on the P blood group antigen of erythrocytes and uroepithelial cells. Approximately 1 per cent of the human population lacks this receptor, and its presence or absence dictates an individual's susceptibility to E. coli urinary tract infections. Uropathogenic E. coli produce alpha-and beta-hemolysins, which cause lysis of urinary tract cells.

UPEC can evade the body's innate immune defenses (e.g. the complement system) by invading superficial umbrella cells to form intracellular bacterial communities (IBCs). They also have the ability to form K antigen, capsular polysaccharides that contribute to biofilm formation. Biofilm-producing E. coli are recalcitrant to immune factors and antibiotic therapy and are often responsible for chronic urinary tract infections. K antigen-producing E. coli infections are commonly found in the upper urinary tract.

Descending infections, though relatively rare, occur when E. coli cells enter the upper urinary tract organs (kidneys, bladder or ureters) from the blood stream.

Laboratory Diagnosis

In stool samples microscopy will show Gram negative rods, with no particular cell arrangement. Then, either MacConkey agar or EMB agar (or both) are inoculated with the stool. On MacConkey agar, deep red colonies are produced as the organism is lactose positive, and fermentation of this sugar will cause the medium's pH to drop, leading to darkening of the medium. Growth on Levine EMB agar produces black colonies with greenish-black metallic sheen. This is diagnosic of E. coli. The organism is also lysine positive, and grows on TSI slant with a (A/A/g+/H_2S-) profile. Also, IMViC is + +—for E. coli; as it's indol positive (red ring) and methyl red positive (bright red), but VP negative (no change-colourless) and citrate negative (no change-green colour). Tests for toxin production can use mammalian cells in tissue culture, which are rapidly killed by shiga toxin. Although sensitive and very specific, this method is slow and expensive.

Typically diagnosis has been done by culturing on sorbitol-MacConkey medium and then using typing antiserum. However, current latex assays and some typing antiserum have shown cross reactions with non-E. coli O157 colonies. Furthermore, not all E. coli O157 strains associated with HUS are nonsorbitol fermentors.

The Council of State and Territorial Epidemiologists recommend that clinical laboratories screen at least all bloody stools for this pathogen. The American Gastroenterological Association Foundation (AGAF) recommended in July 1994 that all stool specimens should be routinely tested for E. coli O157:H7.15 It is recommended that the clinician check with their state health department or the Centers for Disease Control and Prevention to determine which specimens should be tested and whether the results are reportable.

Other methods for detecting E. coli O157 in stool include ELISA tests, colony immunoblots, direct immunofluorescence microscopy of filters, as well as immunocapture techniques using magnetic beads. These assays are designed as screening tool to allow rapid testing for the presence of E. coli O157 without prior culturing of the stool specimen.

Antibiotic Therapy and Resistance

Bacterial infections are usually treated with antibiotics. However, the antibiotic sensitivities of different strains of E. coli vary widely. As Gram-negative organisms, E. coli are resistant to many antibiotics that are effective against Gram-positive organisms. Antibiotics which may be used to treat E. coli infection include amoxicillin as well as other semi-synthetic penicillins, many cephalosporins, carbapenems, aztreonam, trimethoprim-sulfamethoxazole, ciprofloxacin, nitrofurantoin and the aminoglycosides.

Antibiotic resistance is a growing problem. Some of this is due to overuse of antibiotics in humans, but some of it is probably due to the use of antibiotics as growth promoters in food of animals. A study published in the journal Science in August 2007 found that the rate of adaptative mutations in E. coli is "on the order of 10 per genome per generation, which is 1,000 times as high as previous estimates," a finding which may have significance for the study and management of bacterial antibiotic resistance.

Antibiotic-resistant E. coli may also pass on the genes responsible for antibiotic resistance to other species of bacteria, such as Staphylococcus aureus. E. coli often carry multidrug resistant plasmids and under stress readily transfer those plasmids to other species. Indeed, E. coli is a frequent member of biofilms, where many species of bacteria exist in close proximity to each other. This mixing of species allows E. coli strains that are piliated to accept and transfer plasmids from and to other bacteria. Thus E. coli and the other enterobacteria are important reservoirs of transferable antibiotic resistance.

Beta-lactamase Strains

Resistance to beta-lactam antibiotics has become a particular problem in recent decades, as strains of bacteria that produce extended-spectrum beta-lactamases have become more common. These beta-lactamase enzymes make many, if not all, of the penicillins and cephalosporins ineffective as therapy. Extended-spectrum beta-lactamase-producing E. coli are highly resistant to an array of antibiotics and infections by these strains is difficult to treat. In many instances, only two oral antibiotics and a very limited group of intravenous antibiotics remain effective.

Increased concern about the prevalence of this form of "superbug" in the United Kingdom has led to calls for further monitoring and a UK-wide strategy to deal with infections and the deaths. Susceptibility testing should guide treatment in all infections in which the organism can be isolated for culture.

Phage Therapy

Phage therapy—viruses that specifically target pathogenic bacteria—has been developed over the last 80 years, primarily in the former Soviet Union, where it was used to prevent diarrhea caused by E. coli. Presently, phage therapy for humans is available only at the Phage Therapy Center in the Republic of Georgia and in Poland. However, on January 2 2007, the United States FDA gave Omnilytics approval to apply its E. coli O157:H7 killing phage in a mist, spray or wash on live animals that will be slaughtered for human consumption.

Vaccination

Researchers have actively been working to develop safe, effective vaccines to lower the worldwide incidence of E. coli infection. In March 2006, a vaccine eliciting an immune response against the E. coli O157:H7 O-specific polysaccharide conjugated to recombinant exotoxin A of Pseudomonas aeruginosa (O157-rEPA) was reported to be safe in children two to five years old. Previous work had already indicated that it was safe for adults. A phase III clinical trial to verify the large-scale efficacy of the treatment is planned.

In 2006 Fort Dodge Animal Health (Wyeth) introduced an effective live attenuated vaccine to control airsacculitis and peritonitis in chickens. The vaccine is a genetically modified avirulent vaccine that has demonstrated protection against O78 and untypeable strains.

In January 2007 the Canadian bio-pharmaceutical company Bioniche announced it has developed a cattle vaccine which reduces the number of O157:H7 shed in manure by a factor of 1000, to about 1000 pathogenic bacteria per gram of manure.

Role in Biotechnology

Because of its long history of laboratory culture and ease of manipulation, E. coli also plays an important role in modern biological engineering and industrial microbiology. The work of Stanley Norman Cohen and Herbert Boyer in E. coli, using plasmids and restriction enzymes to create recombinant DNA, became a foundation of biotechnology.

Considered a very versatile host for the production of heterologous proteins, researchers can introduce genes into the microbes using plasmids, allowing for the mass production of proteins in industrial fermentation processes. Genetic systems have also been developed which allow the production of recombinant proteins using E. coli. One of the first useful applications of recombinant DNA technology was the manipulation of E. coli to produce human insulin. Modified E. coli have been used in vaccine development, bioremediation, and production of immobilised enzymes. E. coli cannot, however, be used to produce some of the more large, complex proteins which contain multiple disulfide bonds and, in particular, unpaired thiols, or proteins that also require post-translational modification for activity.

Model Organism

E. coli is frequently used as a model organism in microbiology studies. Cultivated strains (e.g. E. coli K12) are well-adapted to the laboratory environment, and, unlike wild type strains, have lost their ability to thrive in the intestine. Many lab strains lose their ability to form biofilms. These features protect wild type strains from antibodies and other chemical attacks, but require a large expenditure of energy and material resources.

In 1946, Joshua Lederberg and Edward Tatum first described the phenomenon known as bacterial conjugation using E. coli as a model bacterium, and it remains the primary model to study conjugation. E. coli was an integral part of the first experiments to understand phage genetics, and early researchers, such as Seymour Benzer, used E. coli and phage T4 to understand the topography of gene structure. Prior to Benzer's research, it was not known whether the gene was a linear structure, or if it had a branching pattern.

Long-term evolution experiments using E. coli have allowed direct observation of major evolutionary shifts in the laboratory.

HEPATITIS A

Hepatitis A, (formerly known as infectious hepatitis), is an acute infectious disease of the liver caused by Hepatitis A virus, which is most commonly transmitted by the fecal-oral route via contaminated food or drinking water. Every year, approximately 10 million people worldwide are infected with the virus. The time between infection and the appearance of the symptoms, (the incubation period), is between two and six weeks and the average incubation period is 28 days.

In developing countries, and in regions with poor hygiene standards, the incidence of infection with this virus approaches 100 per cent and the illness is usually contracted in early childhood. Hepatitis A infection causes no clinical signs and symptoms in over 90 per cent of these children and since the infection confers lifelong immunity, the disease is of no special significance to the indigenous population. In Europe, the United States and other industrialized countries, on the other hand, the infection is contracted primarily by susceptible young adults, most of whom are infected with the virus during trips to countries with a high incidence of the disease.

Hepatitis A does not have a chronic stage and does not cause permanent liver damage. Following infection, the immune system makes antibodies against the hepatitis A virus that confer immunity against future infection. The disease can be prevented by vaccination and hepatitis A vaccine has been proved effective in controlling outbreaks worldwide.

Virus

The Hepatitis virus (HAV) is a Picornavirus; it is non-enveloped and contains a single-stranded RNA packaged in a protein shell. There is only one type of the virus.

Pathogenesis

Following ingestion, HAV enters the bloodstream through the epithelium of the oropharynx or intestine. The blood carries the virus to its target, the liver, where it lives and multiplies within hepatocytes and Kupffer cells (i.e., liver macrophages). There is no apparent virus-mediated cytotoxicity, and liver pathology is likely immune-mediated. Virions are secreted into the bile and released in stool. HAV is excreted in large quantities approimately 11 days prior to appearance of symptoms or anti-HAV IgM antibodies in the blood. The incubation period is 15-50 days, and mortality is less than 0.5 per cent.

Transmission

The virus spreads by the fecal-oral route and infections often occur in conditions of poor sanitation and overcrowding. Hepatitis A can be transmitted by the parenteral route but very rarely by blood and blood products. Food-borne outbreaks are not uncommon, and ingestion of shellfish cultivated in polluted water is associated with a high risk of infection. Approximately 40 per cent of all acute viral hepatitis is caused by HAV. Infected individuals are infectious prior to onset of symptoms, roughly 10 days following infection. The virus is resistant to detergent, acid (pH 1), solvents (e.g., ether, chloroform), drying, and temperatures up to 60C. It can survive for months in fresh and salt water. Common-source (e.g., water, restaurant) outbreaks are typical. Infection is common in children in developing countries, reaching 100 per cent incidence, but following infection there is life-long immunity. HAV can be inactivated by: chlorine treatment (drinking water), formalin (0.35%, 37C, 72 hours), peracetic acid (2%, 4 hours), beta-propiolactone (0.25%, 1 hour), and UV radiation (2 iW/cm/min).

Symptoms

Early symptoms of hepatitis A infection can be mistaken for influenza, but some sufferers, especially children, exhibit no symptoms at all. Symptoms typically appear 2 to 6 weeks, (the incubation period), after the initial infection.

Symptoms can return over the following 6-9 months which include:

- Fatigue
- Fever

- Abdominal pain
- Nausea
- Diarrhea
- Appetite loss
- Depression
- Jaundice, a yellowing of the skin or whites of the eyes
- Sharp pains in the right-upper quadrant of the abdomen
- Weight loss
- Itching

Diagnosis

Although the virus is excreted in the feces towards the end of the incubation period, specific diagnosis is made by the detection of Hepatitis A virus specific IgM antibodies in the blood. IgM antibody is only present in the blood following an acute hepatitis A infection. It is detectable from one to two weeks after the initial infection and persists for up to 14 weeks. The presence of IgG antibody in the blood means that the acute stage of the illness is past and the person is immune to further infection. IgG antibody to HAV is also found in the blood following vaccination and tests for immunity to the virus are based on the detection of this antibody.

During the acute stage of the infection, the liver enzyme alanine transferase (ALT) is present in the blood at levels much higher than is normal. The enzyme comes from the liver cells that have been damaged by the virus.

Hepatitis A virus is present in the blood, (viremia), and feces of infected people up to two weeks before clinical illness develops.

Treatment

There is no specific treatment for hepatitis A. Sufferers are advised to rest, avoid fatty foods and alcohol (these may be poorly tolerated for some additional months during the recovery phase and cause minor relapses), eat a well-balanced diet, and stay hydrated. Approximately 15 per cent of people diagnosed with hepatitis A may experience one or more symptomatic relapse(s) for up to 24 months after contracting this disease.

Prognosis

The United States Centers for Disease Control and Prevention (CDC) in 1991 reported a low mortality rate for hepatitis A of 4 deaths per 1000 cases for the general population but a higher rate of 17.5 per 1000, in those aged 50 and over. Death usually occurs when the patient contracts Hepatitis A while already suffering from another form of Hepatitis, such as Hepatitis B or Hepatitis C or AIDS.

Young children who are infected with hepatitis A typically have a milder form of the disease, usually lasting from 1-3 weeks, whereas adults tend to experience a much more severe form of the disease.

Prevention

Hepatitis A can be prevented by vaccination, good hygiene and sanitation.

Vaccine

Hepatitis A vaccines protect against the virus. Vaccines contain inactivated Hepatitis A virus providing active immunity against a future infection.

Epidemiology

HAV is found in the feces of infected persons and those who are at higher risk include travelers to developing countries where there is a higher incidence rate, and those having sexual contact or drug use with infected persons. There were 30,000 cases of Hepatitis A reported to the CDC in the U.S. in 1997. The agency estimates that there were as many as 270,000 cases each year from 1980 through 2000.

HAV outbreaks still occur in and caused by poor hand hygiene among infected, sometimes symptomatic restaurant employees failing to wash their hands after toilet breaks.

Epidemics

The most widespread hepatitis A outbreak in the United States afflicted at least 640 people (killing four) in north-eastern Ohio and south-western Pennsylvania in late 2003. The outbreak was blamed on tainted green onions at a restaurant in Monaca, Pennsylvania. In 1988, 300,000 people in Shanghai, China were infected with HAV after eating clams from a contaminated river.

WATER ACTIVITY

Water activity or a_w is a measurement of the energy status of the water in a system. It is defined as the vapor pressure of water above a sample divided by that of pure water at the same temperature; therefore, pure distilled water has a water activity of exactly one.

There are several factors that control water activity in a system. Colligative effects of dissolved species (e.g. salt or sugar) interact with water through dipole-dipole, ionic, and hydrogen bonds. Capillary effect where the vapor pressure of water above a curved liquid meniscus is less than that of pure water because of changes in the hydrogen bonding between water molecules. Surface interactions in which water interacts directly with chemical groups on undissolved ingredients (e.g. starches and proteins) through dipole-dipole forces, ionic bonds (H_3O+ or OH-), van der Waals forces (hydrophobic bonds), and hydrogen bonds. It is a combination of these three factors in a food product that reduces the energy of the water and thus reduces the relative humidity as compared to pure water. These factors can be grouped under two broad categories osmotic and matric effects.

Due to varying degrees of osmotic and matric interactions, water activity describes the continuum of energy states of the water in a system. The water appears "bound" by forces to varying degrees. This is a continuum of energy states rather than a static "boundness". Water activity is sometimes defined as "free", "bound", or "available water" in a system. Although these terms are easier to conceptualize, they fail to adequately define all aspects of the concept of water activity.

Water activity is temperature dependent. Temperature changes water activity due to changes in water binding, dissociation of water, solubility of solutes in water, or the state of the matrix. Although solubility of solutes can be a controlling factor, control is usually from the state of the matrix. Since the state of the matrix (glassy vs.

rubbery state) is dependent on temperature, one should not be surprised that temperature affects the water activity of the food. The effect of temperature on the water activity of a food is product specific. Some products increase water activity with increasing temperature, others decrease aw with increasing temperature, while most high moisture foods have negligible change with temperature. One can therefore not predict even the direction of the change of water activity with temperature, since it depends on how temperature affects the factors that control water activity in the food.

As a potential energy measurement it is a driving force for water movement from regions of high water activity to regions of low water activity. For example, if honey (a_w = 0.6) is exposed to humid air (a_w = 0.7) the honey will absorb water from the air. Other examples of this dynamic property of water activity are; moisture migration in multidomain foods (e.g. cracker-cheese sandwich), the movement of water from soil to the leaves of plants, and cell turgor pressure. Since microbial cells are high concentrations of solute surrounded by semi-permeable membranes, the osmotic effect on the free energy of the water is important for determining microbial water relations and therefore their growth rates.

Higher a_w substances tend to support more microorganisms. Bacteria usually require at least 0.91, and fungi at least 0.7.

Uses for Water Activity

Water activity is an important consideration for food product design and food safety.

Food Product Design

Food designers use water activity to formulate products that are shelf stable. If a product is kept below a certain water activity, then mold growth is inhibited. This results in a longer shelf-life.

Water activity values can also help limit moisture migration within a food product made with different ingredients. If raisins of a higher water activity are packaged with bran flakes of a lower water activity, the water from the raisins will migrate to the bran flakes over time, resulting in hard raisins and soggy bran flakes. Food formulators use water activity to predict how much moisture migration will affect their product.

In addition, water activity helps limit or slow certain undesirable reactions, such as non-enzymatic browning, fat oxidation, vitamin degradation, enzymatic reactions, protein denaturation, starch gelatinization and starch retrogradation. This too maintains product quality and extends shelf life.

Food Safety

Water activity is used in many cases as a Critical Control Point for Hazard Analysis and Critical Control Points (HACCP) programmes. Samples of the food product are periodically taken from the production area and tested to ensure that water activity values are within a specified range for food quality and safety. Measurements can be made in as little as five minutes, and are made regularly in most major food production facilities.

For many years researchers tried to equate bacterial growth potential with moisture content. They found that the values were not universal, but specific to each food product. WJ Scott in 1953 first established that it was water activity, not water content that correlated with bacterial growth. It is firmly established that growth of bacteria is inhibited at specific water activity values. FDA regulations for Intermediate Moisture Foods are based on these values.

Lowering the water activity of a food product should not be seen as a kill step. Studies in powdered milk show that viable cells can exist at much lower water activity values but that they will never grow. Over time bacterial levels will decline.

Water Activity Measurement

Water activity values are obtained by either a capacitance or a dew point hygrometer.

Capacitance Hygrometers

Capacitance hygrometers consist of two charged plates separated by a polymer membrane dielectric. As the membrane adsorbs water, its ability to hold a charge increases and the capacitance is measured.

This value is roughly proportional to the water activity as determined by a sensor-specific calibration.

Capacitance hygrometers are not affected by most volatile chemicals and can be much smaller than other alternative sensors. They do not require cleaning, but are less accurate than dew point hygrometers (+/-.015 a_w). They require regular calibration and can be affected by residual water in the polymer membrane.

Dew Point Hygrometers

The temperature at which dew forms on a clean surface is directly related to the vapor pressure of the air. Dew point hygrometers work by placing a mirror over a closed sample chamber. The mirror is cooled until the dew point temperature is measured by means of an optical sensor. This temperature is then used to find the relative humidity of the chamber using psychrometric charts.

This method is the most accurate (+/- .003 a_w) and often the fastest. The sensor requires cleaning if debris accumulates on the mirror.

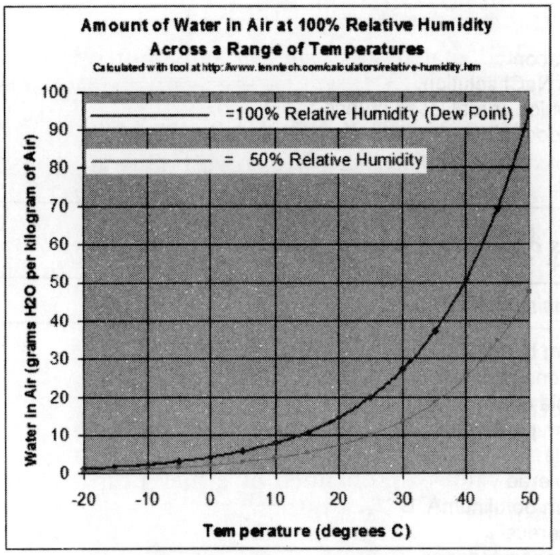

Fig. 6.1: Dark Line Shows Saturation (Caption to be Changed)

Equilibration

With either method, vapor equilibrium must occur in the sample chamber. This will take place over time or can be aided by the addition of a fan in the chamber. Thermal equilibrium must also take place unless the sample temperature is measured.

Water Activity and Moisture Content

Water activity is related to moisture content in a non-linear relationship known as a moisture sorption isotherm curve. These isotherms are substance and temperature specific. Isotherms can be used to help predict product stability over time in different storage conditions.

Selected a_w values

Example Foods

Substance	a_w
Distilled Water	1
Tap water	0.99
Raw meats	0.97-0.99
Milk	0.97
Juice	0.97
Cooked bacon	< 0.85
Saturated NaCl solution	0.75
Point at which cereal loses crunch	0.65
Typical indoor air	0.5-0.7
Honey	0.5-0.7
Dried fruit	0.5-0.6

a_w Values of Microorganism Inhibition

Microorganism Inhibited	a_w
Clostridium botulinum E	.97
Pseudomonas fluorescens	.97
Escherichia coli	.95
Clostridium perfringens	.95
Salmonella	.95
Vibrio cholerae	.95
Clostridium botulinumA, B	.97
Bacillus cereus	.93
Listeria monocytogenes	.92
bacillus subtilis	.91
Staphylococcus aureus	.87
Most Fungi	.70
No microbial proliferation	.50

7

Select Systems of Medicine and Related Dietary Laws

UNANI

'Unani' means medicines which are a symbol of life. The name is derived from the word 'Ionian' which originated in Greece. Unani medicine, like any other form of medical science strives to find the best possible ways by which a person can lead a healthy life with the least or zero sickness. Unani and its allied branches have rational and scientific basic principles. It is distinct from other branches of medicine, as the drugs it uses are natural in their sources and forms. It emphasizes on retaining natural compounds which belong to the human body, and hence prescribes only natural remedies. It involves the use of plants and herbs, these remedies are known to provide cures for diseases such as sinusitis, Leukoderma, rheumatism, jaundice and elephantiasis.

The Origins of Healing

Unani Medicine as a healing system was founded by Hakim Ibn Sina. Yet, because it is a comprehensive system encompassing virtual all of the known healing systems of the world, the threads which comprise Unani Healing can be traced all the way back to Hippocrates. This system has a long and impressive record in India. It was introduced in India around 10th century A.D with the spread of Islamic civilization. Now Unanipathy has become a part of Indian system of Medicine and India is one of the leading countries so far as its practice is concerned. It is very much similar to Ayurveda.

Unani medicine believes that diseases can be kept at bay by the use of clean and fresh water, breathing clean air and consuming fresh food. Likewise, a balance should be maintained between the mind and the body so that the metabolic process can take place easily and the body waste evacuated. Unani medicine also believes that all life forms have originated from the sea.

There are eight specialized branches of Unani medicine—

- Internal medicine (Moalijat)
- Gynecology including Obstetrics and Pediatrics
- Diseases of the head and neck
- Toxicology
- Psychiatry
- Rejuvenation Therapy including Geriatrics
- Sexology
- Regimental Therapy
- Dietotherapy
- Hydrotherapy

According to the Unani discipline as it stands today, the human body is composed of 7 natural and basic components called 'Umoor-e-Tabaiyah' which are responsible for maintenance of health. These are:

- Arkan (Elements)
- Mizaj (Temperament)
- Akhlaat (Humours)
- Aaza (Organs)
- Arwah (Vital forces or Neuro)
- Quwa (Faculties)
- Afaal (Functions)

The loss of any one of these basic components or alteration in their physical state could lead to disease, or even death. It is highly essential to consider all these factors so as to reach the correct diagnosis and consequently the correct line of treatment.

Treatment

The following treatments are done through Unani:

- *Regimental Therapy*—It includes venesection, cupping, diaphoresis, diuresis, turkish bath, massage, cauterisation, purging, emesis, exercise and leeching.
- *Dietotherapy*—It deals with certain ailments by administration of specific diets or by regulating the quantity and quality of food.
- *Pharmacotherapy*—It deals with the use of naturally occurring drugs mostly herbal drugs of animal and mineral origin. Single drugs or their combination in raw form are preferred over compound formulations.

Unanipathy has shown remarkable results in curing diseases like Arthritis, Leucoderma, Jaundice, Bronchial Asthma, Filariasis and several other acute and chronic diseases where other systems do not give the desired level of positive response. The Unani system is a secular system in character and is popular among the masses.

In short, Unani Medicine aims at maintaining proper health by conserving symmetry in the different spheres of a man's life. Unani practitioners not only cure bodily diseases but also act as an ethical instructor.

HOMEOPATHY

Homoeopathy is a complete system of alternative medicine that is safe, simple and effective. It treats the whole person with non toxic remedies to help build up their health such that they are able to heal naturally from whatever disease process they are suffering.

In a world with the bodies of people poisoned by chemicals, radiation, drugs, heavy metals and vaccinations, with modern life styles and poor nutrition, it is far from being a natural world with only simple health problems. In a world with the bodies of people poisoned by chemicals, radiation, drugs, heavy metals and vaccinations, with modern life styles and poor nutrition, it is far from being a natural world with only simple health problems. Many different methods of applying homoeopathic principles, focused on the value of what works rather than adherence to any particular theory of how Homoeopathy should be done, have been developed in the last 20 years in order to simplify and make effective the treatment of 21st century diseases.

Origin

The Homoeopathy way of healing was devised by the Great German physician Dr. Christian Frederick Samuel Hahnemann in the late 18th Century. He came across an old idea of the efficacy of 'Cinchona bark' in treating intermittent fever due to its toxic effect on the stomach and conducted experiments upon himself in order to get the truth. He deduced from the experiment that Cinchona was used as a remedy for intermittent fever and it could produce symptoms similar to those of intermittent fever in healthy people, if taken for a specific period of time. The law of 'Similia Similibus Curentur' or 'let likes be treated by the likes' thus forms the basis of treatment under the Homoeopathic method of drug therapy employed to cure the natural sufferings of person by the administration of drugs which have been experimentally proved to possess the power of producing similar artificial sufferings or symptoms of diseases in healthy human being.

Principals of Homoeopathy

Homeopathic remedies (also called homoeopathic) are a system of medicine based on three principles:

1. Like cures like
2. For example, if the symptoms of your cold are similar to poisoning by mercury, then mercury would be your homeopathic remedy.
3. Minimal Dose
4. The remedy is taken in an extremely dilute form; normally one part of the remedy to around 1,000,000,000,000 parts of water.
5. The Single Remedy

6. No matter how many symptoms are experienced, only one remedy is taken, and that remedy will be aimed at all those symptoms.

How does Homeopathy Differ from Conventional Medicine?

In conventional medical thought, health is seen simply as the absence of disease. You assume that you are healthy if there is nothing wrong with you.

An important basic difference exists between conventional medical therapy and homeopathy. In conventional therapy, the aim often is to control the illness through regular use of medical substances, even if the medication is nothing more than vitamins. If the medication is withdrawn, however, the person returns to illness. There has been no cure. A person who takes a pill for high blood pressure every day is not undergoing a cure but is only controlling the symptoms. Homeopathy's aim is the cure: "The complete restoration of perfect health,"

AYURVEDA

Ayurveda is a traditional system of medicine which originated from India, and is more than 5,000 years old. "Ayur" means life and "Ved" means knowledge. This holistic science is the knowledge of complete balance of the Body, Mind and spirit, including the emotions and psychology, on all levels. It includes in its consideration, longevity, rejuvenation and self-realization therapies through herbs, diet, exercise, yoga, massage, aromas, tantras, mantras, and meditation. It includes diet and herbal remedies and emphasizes the use of body, mind, and spirit in disease prevention and treatment.

Ayurveda and the 3 Gunas

According to the ayurveda, medicines and foods are sattvic, rajasic or tamasic or a combination of these gunas. The gunas are three fundamental attributes that represent the natural evolutionary process through which the subtle becomes gross. In turn, gross objects, by action and interaction among themselves, may again become subtle. Thus the three gunas are defined as:

Sattva : Essence (subtle)
Rajas : Activity
Tamas : Inertia (gross)

Sattvic Foods: Are fresh, juicy, light, unctuous, nourishing, sweet and tasty. Give the necessary energy to the body without taxing it. The foundation of higher states of consciousness etc

Examples: juicy fruits, fresh vegetables that are easily digestible, fresh milk and butter, whole soaked or also sprouted beans, grains and nuts, many herbs and spices in the right combinations with other foods,...

Rajasic Foods: Are bitter, sour, salty, pungent, hot and dry. Increase the speed and excitement of the human organism. The foundation of motion, activity and pain etc

Examples: sattvic foods that have been fried in oil or cooked too much or eaten in excess, specific foods and spices that are strongly exciting etc.

Tamasic Foods: Are dry, old, decaying, distasteful and/or unpalatable. Consume a large amount of energy while being digested. The foundation of ignorance, doubt, pessimism etc

Examples: foods that have been strongly processed, canned or frozen and/or are old, stale or incompatible with each other—meat, fish, eggs and liquor are especially tamasic.

Ayurveda and the 3 Doshas

In Ayurveda, different people with the same disease sometimes receive different diets and herbal plans. Each person's constitution and the imbalance found in each individual are taken into account.

With Ayurveda, we acknowledge that beneficial daily habits are different for each person, because each person is a unique combination of the 3 fundamental biological principles, which are called "Doshas": Vata, Pitta and Kapha. Everybody has all 3 energies—although people experience each of them to a lesser or greater degree.

NATUROPATHY

Naturopathy is the technique of treatment of human disease which emphasizes assisting nature. It can embrace minor surgery and the use of nature's agencies, forces, processes, and products, introducing them to the human body by any means that will produce health-yielding results. Naturopathy is based upon the tendency of the body to maintain a balance and to heal itself. The purpose of naturopathic medicine is to further this process by using natural remedies. It is a holistic approach to health care based on a belief in the healing power of nature. It is a system of therapy and treatment which relies exclusively on natural remedies, such as sunlight, air, water, supplemented with diet and therapies such as massage. Naturopaths work closely with you to improve your health by making lifestyle such as improving your diet and reducing stress. They also employ alternative therapies, including herbal remedies, homeopathy, and hands-on techniques such as massage to stimulate your body's ability to heal itself. Naturopathy is organized around three fundamental principles:

1. The physician should strive to aid the body's natural healing abilities;
2. The root cause of an illness should be addressed rather than its symptoms;
3. And above all, only therapies that cause no harm should be used (which means that toxic drugs and surgery are avoided whenever possible).

Naturopathy is based on the belief that the body is self-healing. The body will repair itself and recover from illness spontaneously if it is in a healthy environment. Naturopaths have many remedies and recommendations for creating a healthy environment so the body can spontaneously heal itself. In treating patients, the naturopathic practitioner may use a number of alternative therapies, including homeopathy, herbal remedies, traditional Chinese medicine, spinal manipulation, nutrition, hydrotherapy, massage and exercise.

With the discovery of penicillin and synthetic drugs, suddenly we found that there could be a faster way to cure illness. Hence, naturopathy went into a decline—not because it is ineffective, but rather because synthetic drugs give a much faster relief. But today, naturopathy is revived, and many people are turning back to it.

HINDU DIETARY LAW

Food in Hindu law is traditionally governed by the rules laid out in the Dharmaśāstras, a genre of Sanskrit texts pertaining to Hindu religious and legal duty. The Dharmaśāstras has put much emphasis on Bhojana ("that which is enjoyed"). Others have attached additional Hindu Law instructions and taboos to food. Together, these address areas such as how many times food was to be taken, the kinds of foods and drinks allowed or forbidden, what causes food defilement, whose food was to be eaten, and etiquette and ceremonies before taking food both at the time of taking it as well as after taking it.

'Food in the Dharmaśāstras'

Food is the essence of life, from which things unfold. "Everything is centered in food, the evil deeds of man resort to their food. Whoever eats the food of another partakes of that man's sin." It is because of this that elaborate restrictions are laid out for Indian society about everything relating to food. Some obscure commands do exist in the Dharmaśāstras about food. For example, Manu says that one should face east when partaking in food and the Visnu KH. S. 68 goes on to say that a man is allowed to do so facing south, except when the diner's mother is alive. Food does, however, play a useful role in the concept of life for Hindu society. Manu II. 5 goes on to tell which direction, when eating, promotes which asset in life. Someone facing the south would eat food that would lead to fame, as one who faces west eats food to produce wealth, and so on.

It is also instructed that one who is about to eat food should greet the food when it is served to him. In performing this act, he should pay honour to it, and never find fault in it.

The injuctions found in the Dharmaśāstras are summarized more clearly by Patrick Olivelle in his article "From Feast to Fast:

Food and the Indian Ascetic." In his work, Olivelle breaks down more clearly what the Dharmaúâstra prescribes for individual parts of Hindu society. All the topics that Kane touched on, mentioned above, are explained here in a way which relates food to both everyday life for Hindus as well as life in the cosmic realm.

The production, preparation, exchange and consumption of food have very particular processes of execution. These aspects of food are all commanded in order to protect kinship, purity, ritual, ethical values, and social stratification, each of which play a huge part in Hindu society. Food plays a central role in explaining the Hindu conception of the cosmos and creation itself. Ancient creation stories portray the creator god of the Brahmins as the creator as well as the actual food for his creatures. The production of food is the immediate concern after the creation of the very first beings. Other creation myths exist, each of which, however, connect creation, food, and sacrifice. Food was held in high respects, according to the Dharmaúâstra, from the very beginning. Manu "From the sun comes rain, and from rain food, and therefrom the living creatures derive their subsistence"

Kane and Olivelle both reference the command that "One should not speak ill of food. That is the rule" to further the point that food is established upon food. Food being established upon food in this text is the ancient way of describing the correlation between food and eater, that one cannot exist without the other. "The whole of creation, therefore, is a vast food chain."

As well as being the source of creation, food is also seen as a danger in Hindu society. As food is the source of creation at the cosmic level, so is it the source of immorality at a social level. Food is central to sacrificial offerings to the gods. Even of the five daily sacrifices, four of them involve transaction of food. In this way, since the cosmos represents a giant food cycle, the interdependence of all beings is expressed in the transaction of food.

Although in most Dharmaśāstras texts the behaviour towards food is described more for Brahmins, the elite caste, recent studies of these texts show that similar behavioural patterns existed at all levels of Hindu society. This culture has formulated many prohibitions and classifications with regard to food as a critical mechanism for the formation of social groups and the expression of leadership. Other such social classes in society that are to obey injunctions of food are the mendicant world renouncers and the sedentary forest hermits.

Food and Asceticism

The world renouncer is not allowed to produce, store, or prepare food. He obtains his daily food solely by begging. Because there is a proper time for this begging, which is after the householders of the upper classes have finished their food, his meals consist of their left-overs. Distinct types of begging exist, with each different method pertaining to a different subclass of these mendicants. The lowest class eats at the house of his son or his relative, the next class does not go to the house of his relative, but rather begs his food from seven other houses. The highest, archetypal renouncer begs randomly, but obtains just a morsel from each of the houses from which he begs. As these classes of people cannot produce or store food, their relationship to this entity is one-way. The renoucer does not engage in any form of food transaction, only reception.

The forest hermits, on the other hand, are not mediated in their food habits by culture. Their food is wild and uncultivated. Their diet would consist mainly of fruits, roots, leaves, and anything that grows naturally in the forest. Forbidden to them is anything that is cultivated. Gaut. III 32 and Baudh II.6.11 state that 'He shall not step on plowed land; he shall not enter a village'.'. Like the renouncers, the forest hermits are further subdivided into those who cook their food and those who do not cook their food. Each of these subcategories are even further divided into five classes based upon whether they only grains, or only roots, and so on for those that cook. For those who do not cook their food, their five classes are based more on how they eat their food: with hands only, with mouth only and so on.

Observing ascetical food codes and habits allows scholars to make generalizations regarding food according to these patterns. For instance, Olivelle claims that four distinct areas of Hindu relationships to food exist in ascetical food practices. These would be procurement, storage, preparation, and consumption. In these areas, humans put forth much effort and energy to follow them correctly. This then, becomes a social as well as cultural endeavor for which to practice. The rules of the ascetics show that they take and eat only that which is enough for their sustenance. The creation myths at the cosmic levels show that the ideal world with provide everything humans need, so long as humans take only what is necessary to them. Taking more than one needs or what is commanded of one's caste results in greed and the overall deterioration of the world. Food then, is a dangerous substance, as well as the source of all things in being. The relationship between a man and his food, then, is his relationship to the cosmos.

ISLAMIC DIETARY LAWS

Islamic dietary laws provide a set of rules as to what Muslims eat in their diet and other areas.

Overview

Islamic jurisprudence specifies which foods are halâl (lawful) and which are harâm (unlawful). This is based on rules found in the Qur'an, the holy book of Islam. Other rules are added to these in fatwas by Mujtahids with various degrees of strictness, but they are not always held to be authoritative by all. According to the Quran, the only foods explicitly forbidden are meat from animals that die of themselves, blood, the meat of pigs, and animals dedicated to other than God.(Quran 5:3) Stated in the Qur'an is an exception in case of hardship or lack of alternatives.

Healthy Diet

A healthy diet is considered important in Islam, although what constitutes such might not be necessarily in consideration of Western standards. Some Muslim scholars consider an excess of eating is a sin due to an interpretation of the following verse in the Qur'an:

It is He Who produceth gardens, with trellises and without, and dates, and tilth with produce of all kinds, and olives and pomegranates, similar (in kind) and different (in variety): eat of their fruit in their season, but render the dues that are proper on the day that the harvest is gathered. But waste not by excess: for Allah loveth not the wasters. (Qur'an 6:141)

The following authentic hadith (saying of the Prophet) also states:

> Man fills no vessel worse than his stomach. It is sufficient for the son of Adam to have a few mouthfuls to give him the strength he needs. If he has to fill his stomach, then let him ? leave to one-third for food, one-third for drink and one-third for air. (Reported by al-Tirmidhi and Ibn Maajah. Saheeh al-Jaami', 5674).

Food and Cooking Hygiene

Food and cooking hygiene is an important part of Islamic dietary laws.

Slaughter

Dhabî?ah is the prescribed method of ritual slaughter of all animals excluding fish and most sea-life per Islamic law. For such a method the animal must be slaughtered by a Muslim or by the People of the Book (Christian and Jew), while mentioning the name of God (Allah in Arabic). According to some fatwas, the animal must be slaughtered only by a Muslim. However, some different fatwas dispute this, and rule from the Qur'anic position, according to verse 5:5 of the Qur'an, that an animal properly slaughtered by People of the Book (Jews, Christians or Sabians) is dhabiha. Thus, many observant Muslims will accept kosher meat if dhabiha options are not available. Other main references in Qur'an include 2:173, 5:3, 5:5, 5:90, 6:118, 6:145, 16:115.

If there is doubt to anything being regarded as halâl or haram, Muslims are generally advised to refrain from consumption until clarification or permissiveness is given by another Muslim learned in Fiqh.

Animals for food may not be killed by being boiled or electrocuted, and the carcass should be hung upside down for long enough to be blood-free. Different rules apply to fish; for instance, fish with scales are always halâl, while it has been debated whether shellfish and scaleless fishes, such as catfish, are halâl, haram or makruh (prohibitively disliked).

There are no restrictions on vegetarianism or veganism, with muslims affiliated with the Hardline straight edge doctrine having promoted veganism from an Islamic perspective.

Food Certification

Due to the recent rise in Muslim populations in the United States and Europe, certain organizations have emerged that can certify dhabiha food products and ingredients for Muslim consumers. The Muslim Consumer Group is an example of an organization that places certification labels such as the H-MCG symbol to identify the dhabiha status of different edible and non-edible consumer products.

Prohibited Food

Some animals and manners of death or preparation can make certain things haram to eat, that is, taboo food and drink. These include what are regarded as unclean animals.

Alcohol

In Islam, alcoholic beverages—or any intoxicant—is generally forbidden. Intoxicants were forbidden in the Qur'an through several separate verses revealed at different times over a period of years. At first, it was forbidden for Muslims to attend to prayers while intoxicated (4:43). Then a later verse was revealed which said that alcohol contains some good and some evil, but the evil is greater than the good (In Surah Al-Baqarah: 219, it states "They ask Thee concerning Wine and Gambling, Say: In them is great sin, and some profit, for men; but the sin is greater than the profit."). This was the next step in turning people away from consumption of it. Finally, "intoxicants and games of chance" were called "abominations of Satan's handiwork," intended to turn people away from God and forget about prayer, and Muslims were ordered to abstain (5:90-91). In addition to this, observant Muslims refrain from consuming food products that contain pure vanilla extract or soy sauce if these food products contain alcohol.

However, there are no prohibitions on using alcohol for

scientific, industrial or automotive use (either as a biofuel, solvent or a coolant, for instance).

In Turkey, which has an official Muslim population of 99 per cent, alcohol is not seen as taboo as it is in other Muslim countries. The sale of alcohol is legal and it is not uncommon to see Turkish Muslims drinking. However Turks who usually enjoy alcoholic beverages will refrain from them during the holy month of Ramadan.

Blood

Drinking blood and its by-products is forbidden. This includes meats that have not been drained of blood. However, this does not apply to blood transfusions or organ transplants because they are not eaten and digested.

Pork

Consumption of pork and products made from pork is strictly forbidden in Islam.

The origin of this belief is derived from the chapter of the Cow (Al Baqara) speaks of this: Quran 2.173 which states: He hath only forbidden you dead meat, and blood, and the flesh of swine, and that on which any other name hath been invoked besides that of Allah. But if one is forced by necessity, without wilful disobedience, nor transgressing due limits, then is he guiltless. For Allah is Oft-forgiving Most Merciful.

Gelatin: Gelatin made from porcine skin or bones, which makes up roughly 50 per cent of the supply of gelatin on the market, is forbidden.

Gelatin made from other animals, for example, fish is acceptable. Kosher gelatin comes from certain fish to avoid the Kashrut (Jewish) prohibition against mixing meat (fish is not considered meat) and dairy in the same meal. (Muslims can mix meat and dairy.) Therefore, gelatin in food items certified as Kosher is halâl, as it is from fish. However, it is typical to use algal sources of thickeners, in the home or in commercial products, to ensure they are hal-l.

8

Food Scarcity, Famine, Foodgrains' Management, Food Security and Food Policy

FAMINE

A famine is a widespread shortage of food that may apply to any faunal species, which phenomenon is usually accompanied by regional malnutrition, starvation, epidemic, and increased mortality.

Although most famines coincide with regional shortages of food, famine in some human populations has occurred amid plenty or on account of acts of economic or military policy that have deprived certain populations of sufficient food to ensure survival. Historically, famines have occurred because of drought, crop failure, pestilence, and man-made causes such as war or misguided economic policies. Bad harvests, overpopulation, and epidemic diseases like the Black Death helped cause hundreds of famines in Europe during the Middle Ages, including 95 in the British Isles and 75 in France.

During the 20th century, an estimated 70 million people died from famines across the world, of whom an estimated 30 million died during the famine of 1958-61 in China. The other most notable famines of the century included the 1942-1945 disaster in Bengal, famines in China in 1928 and 1942, and a sequence of famines in the Soviet Union, including the Holodomor, Stalin's famine inflicted on Ukraine in 1932-33. A few of the great famines of the late 20th century were: the Biafran famine in the 1960s, the disaster in Cambodia in the 1970s, the Ethiopian famine of 1983-85 and the North Korean famine of the 1990s.

Famine is typically induced by a human population exceeding the regional carrying capacity to provide food resources. An alternate view of famine is a failure of the poor to command sufficient resources to acquire essential food (the "entitlement theory" of Amartya Sen), analyses of famine that focused on the political-economic processes, an understanding of the reasons for mortality in famines, an appreciation of the extent to which famine-vulnerable communities have strategies for coping with the threat of famine, and the role of warfare and terrorism in creating famine. Modern relief agencies categorize various gradations of famine according to a famine scale.

Many areas that suffered famines in the past have protected themselves through technological and social development. The first area in Europe to eliminate famine was the Netherlands, which saw its last peacetime famines in the early 17th century as it became a major economic power and established a complex economic organization. Noting that many famines occur under dictatorship, colonial rule, or during war, Amartya Sen has posited that no functioning democracy has suffered a famine in modern times.

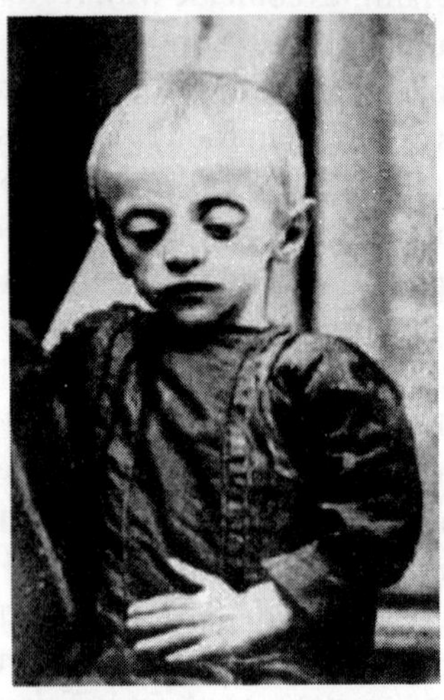

Fig. 8.1: Child Victim of the Holodomor Famine

Characteristics of Famine

Today, famine strikes Sub-Saharan African countries the hardest, but with exhaustion of food resources, overdrafting of groundwater, wars, internal struggles, and economic failure, famine continues to be a worldwide problem with millions of individuals suffering. These famines cause widespread malnutrition and impoverishment; The famine in Ethiopia in the 1980s had an immense death toll, although Asian famines of the 20th century have also produced extensive death tolls. Modern African famines are characterized by widespread destitution and malnutrition, with heightened mortality confined to young children. Relief technologies including immunization, improved public health infrastructure, general food rations and supplementary feeding for vulnerable children, has blunted the mortality impacts of famines, while leaving their economic consequences unchanged. Humanitarian crises also arise from civil wars, refugee flows and episodes of extreme violence and state collapse, creating famine conditions among the affected populations.

Despite repeated stated intentions by the world's leaders to end hunger and famine, famine remains a chronic threat in much of Africa and Asia. In July 2005, the Famine Early Warning Systems Network labelled Niger with emergency status, as well as Chad, Ethiopia, South Sudan, Somalia and Zimbabwe. In January 2006, the United Nations Food and Agriculture Organization warned that 11 million people in Somalia, Kenya, Djibouti and Ethiopia were in danger of starvation due to the combination of severe drought and military conflicts. In 2006, the most serious humanitarian crisis in Africa is in Sudan's region Darfur.

Some believe that the Green Revolution was an answer to famine in the 1970s and 1980s. The Green Revolution began in the 20th century with hybrid strains of high-yielding crops. Between 1950 and 1984, as the Green Revolution transformed agriculture around the globe, world grain production increased by 250 per cent. Some criticize the process, stating that these new high-yielding crops require more chemical fertilizers and pesticides, which can harm the environment. However, it was an option for developing nations suffering from famine. These high-yielding crops make it technically possible to feed much of the world population. They can be developed to provide enhanced nutrition, and a well-nourished, well-developed population would emerge. Some say that the problems of famine and ill-nourishment are the results of ethical dilemmas over using the technologies we have, as well as cultural and class differences. Furthermore, there are indications that regional food production has peaked in many world sectors, due to certain strategies associated with intensive agriculture such as groundwater overdrafting and overuse of pesticides and other agricultural chemicals.

Frances Moore Lappé, later co-founder of the Institute for Food and Development Policy (Food First) argued in Diet for a Small Planet (1971) that vegetarian diets can provide food for larger populations, with the same resources, compared to omnivorous diets.

Noting that modern famines are sometimes the outcome of misguided economic policies, political design to impoverish or marginalize certain populations, or acts of war, political economists have investigated the political conditions under which famine is prevented. Amartya Sen states that the liberal institutions that exist in India, including competitive elections and a free press, have played a major role in preventing famine in that country since independence. Alex de Waal has developed this theory to focus on the "political contract" between rulers and people that ensures famine prevention, noting the rarity of such political contracts in Africa, and the danger that international relief agencies will undermine such contracts through removing the locus of accountability for famines from national governments.

Causes of Famine

In biological terms, a population beyond its regional carrying capacity causes famine. While the operative cause of famine is an imbalance of population with respect to food supply, some famines are caused by a combination of political, economic, and biological factors. Famines can be exacerbated by poor governance or inadequate logistics for food distribution. In some modern cases, it is political strife, poverty, and violence that disrupts the agricultural and food distribution processes. Modern famines have often occurred in nations that, as a whole, were not initially suffering a shortage of food. One of the largest historical famines (proportional to the affected population) was the Great Irish Famine, 1845-1849, which began in 1845 and occurred as food was being shipped from Ireland to England because the English could afford to pay higher prices. The largest famine ever (in absolute terms) was the Chinese famine of 1958-61 that occurred as a result of the Great Leap Forward. In a similar manner, the 1973 famine in Ethiopia was concentrated in the Wollo region, although food was being shipped out of Wollo to the capital city of Addis Ababa where it could command higher prices. In contrast, at the same time that the citizens of the dictatorships of Ethiopia and Sudan had massive famines in the late-1970s and early-1980s, the democracies of Botswana and Zimbabwe avoided them, despite having worse drops in national food production. This was possible through the simple step of creating short-term employment for the worst-affected groups, thus ensuring a minimal amount of income to buy food, for the duration of the localized food disruption and was taken under criticism from opposition political parties and intense media coverage.

The failure of a harvest or the change in conditions, such as drought, can create a situation whereby large numbers of people live where the carrying capacity of the land has dropped radically. Famine is often associated with subsistence agriculture, that is, where most farming is aimed at producing enough food energy to survive. The total absence of agriculture in an economically strong area does not cause famine; Arizona and other wealthy regions import the vast majority of their food, since such regions produce sufficient economic goods for trade.

Disasters, whether natural or man-made, have been associated with conditions of famine ever since humankind has been keeping written records. The Torah describes how "seven lean years" consumed the seven fat years, and "plagues of locusts" could eat all of the available food stuffs. War, in particular, was associated with famine, particularly in those times and places where warfare included attacks on land, by burning or salting fields, or on those who tilled the soil.

As observed by the economist Amartya Sen, famine is sometimes a problem of food distribution and poverty. In certain cases, such as the Great Leap Forward, North Korea in the mid-1990s, or Zimbabwe in the early-2000s, famine can be caused as an unintentional result of government policy. Famine is sometimes used as a tool of repressive governments as a means to eliminate opponents, as in the Ukrainian famine of the 1930s. In other cases, such as Somalia, famine is a consequence of civil disorder as food distribution systems break down. Most cases are not simply the result of the excedence of the Earth's carrying capacity.

Approximately 40 per cent of the world's agricultural land is seriously degraded. In Africa, if current trends of soil degradation continue, the continent might be able to feed just 25 per cent of its population by 2025, according to UNU's Ghana-based Institute for Natural Resources in Africa. As of late 2007, increased farming for use in biofuels, along with world oil prices at nearly $100 a barrel, has pushed up the price of grain used to feed poultry and dairy cows and other cattle, causing higher prices of wheat (up 58%), soybean (up 32%), and maize (up 11%) over the year. Food riots have recently taken place in many countries across the world. An epidemic of stem rust on wheat caused by race Ug99 is currently spreading across Africa and into Asia and is causing major concern.

There are a number of ongoing famines caused by overpopulation, loss of arable land, war or political intervention. Beginning in the 20th century, nitrogen fertilizers, new pesticides, desert farming, and other agricultural technologies began to be used as weapons against famine. Between 1950 and 1984, as the Green Revolution transformed agriculture around the globe, world grain production increased by 250 per cent. These agricultural technologies temporarily increased crop yields, but there are signs as early as 1995 that not only are these technologies reaching their peak of assistance, but they may now be contributing to the decline of arable land (e.g. persistence of pesticides leading to soil contamination and decline of area available for farming. Developed nations have shared these technologies with developing nations with a famine problem, but there are ethical limits to pushing such technologies on lesser developed countries. This is often attributed to an association of inorganic fertilizers and pesticides with a lack of sustainability. In any case, these technological advances might not be influential in those famines which are the result of war. Similarly so, increased yield may not be helpful with certain distribution problems, especially those arising from political intervention.

David Pimentel, professor of ecology and agriculture at Cornell University, and Mario Giampietro, senior researcher at the National Research Institute on Food and Nutrition (INRAN), place in their study Food, Land, Population and the U.S. Economy the maximum U.S. population for a sustainable economy at 200 million. To achieve a sustainable economy and avert disaster, the United States must reduce its population by at least one-third, and world population will have to be reduced by two-thirds, says study.

The authors of this study believe that the mentioned agricultural crisis will only begin to impact us after 2020, and will not become critical until 2050. The oncoming peaking of global oil production (and subsequent decline of production), along with the peak of North American natural gas production will very likely precipitate this agricultural crisis much sooner than expected. Geologist Dale Allen Pfeiffer claims that coming decades could see spiraling food prices without relief and massive starvation on a global level such as never experienced before.

Water deficits, which are already spurring heavy grain imports in numerous smaller countries, may soon do the same in larger countries, such as China or India. The water tables are falling in scores of countries (including Northern China, the US, and India) due to widespread overpumping using powerful diesel and electric pumps. Other countries affected include Pakistan, Iran, and Mexico. This will eventually lead to water scarcity and cutbacks in grain harvest. Even with the overpumping of its aquifers, China has developed a grain deficit, contributing to the upward pressure on grain prices. Most of the three billion people projected to be added worldwide by mid-century will be born in countries already experiencing water shortages. After China and India, there is a second tier of smaller countries with large water deficits — Algeria, Egypt, Iran, Mexico, and Pakistan. Four of these already import a large share of their grain. Only Pakistan remains marginally self-sufficient. But with a population expanding by 4 million a year, it will also soon turn to the world market for grain.

According to a UN climate report, the Himalayan glaciers that are the principal dry-season water sources of Asia's biggest rivers—Ganges, Indus, Brahmaputra, Yangtze, Mekong, Salween and Yellow—could disappear by 2035 as temperatures rise and human demand rises. Approximately 2.4 billion people live in the drainage basin of the Himalayan rivers. India, China, Pakistan, Afghanistan, Bangladesh, Nepal and Myanmar could experience floods followed by severe droughts in coming decades. In India alone, the Ganges provides water for drinking and farming for more than 500 million people.

Effects of Famine

The demographic impacts of famine are sharp. Mortality is concentrated among children and the elderly. A consistent demographic fact is that in all recorded famines, male mortality exceeds female, even in those populations (such as northern India and Pakistan) where there is a normal times male longevity advantage. Reasons for this may include greater female resilience under the pressure of malnutrition, and the fact that women are more skilled at gathering and processing wild foods and other fall-back famine foods. Famine is also accompanied by lower fertility. Famines therefore leave the reproductive core of a population—adult women—lesser affected compared to other population categories, and post-famine periods are often characterized a "rebound" with increased births. Even though the theories of Thomas Malthus would predict that famines reduce the size of the population commensurate with available food resources, in fact even the most severe famines have rarely dented population growth for more than a few years. The mortality in China in 1958-61, Bengal in 1943, and Ethiopia in 1983-85 was all made up by a growing population over just a few years. Of greater long-term demographic impact is emigration: Ireland was chiefly depopulated after the 1840s famines by waves of emigration.

Levels of Food Insecurity

In modern times, governments and non-governmental organizations that deliver famine relief have limited resources with which to address the multiple situations of food insecurity that are occurring simultaneously. Various methods of categorizing the gradations of food security have thus been used in order to most efficiently allocate food relief. One of the earliest were the Indian Famine Codes devised by the British in the 1880s. The Codes listed three stages of food insecurity: near-scarcity, scarcity and famine, and were highly influential in the creation of subsequent famine warning or measurement systems. The early warning system developed to monitor the region inhabited by the Turkana people in northern Kenya also has three levels, but links each stage to a pre-planned response to mitigate the crisis and prevent its deterioration.

The experiences of famine relief organizations throughout the world over the 1980s and 1990s resulted in at least two major developments: the "livelihoods approach" and the increased use of nutrition indicators to determine the severity of a crisis. Individuals and groups in food stressful situations will attempt to cope by rationing consumption, finding alternative means to supplement income, etc. before taking desperate measures, such as selling off plots of agricultural land. When all means of self-support are exhausted, the affected population begins to migrate in search of food or fall victim to outright mass starvation. Famine may thus be viewed partially as a social phenomenon, involving markets, the price of food, and social support structures. A second lesson drawn was the increased use of rapid nutrition assessments, in particular of children, to give a quantitative measure of the famine's severity.

Since 2004, many of the most important organizations in famine relief, such as the World Food Programme, Thom Bauermann and the U.S. Agency for International Development chris Scott, have adopted a five-level scale measuring intensity and magnitude. The intensity scale uses both livelihoods' measures and measurements of mortality and child malnutrition to categorize a situation as food secure, food insecure, food crisis, famine, severe famine, and extreme famine. The number of deaths determines the magnitude designation, with under 1000 fatalities defining a "minor famine" and a "catastrophic famine" resulting in over 1,000,000 deaths.

Historical Famine, by Region

Famine in Africa

In the mid-22nd century BC, a sudden and short-lived climatic change that caused reduced rainfall resulted in several decades of drought in Upper Egypt. The resulting famine and civil strife is believed to have been a major cause of the collapse of the Old

Kingdom. An account from the First Intermediate Period states, "All of Upper Egypt was dying of hunger and people were eating their children." In 1680s, famine extended across the entire Sahel, and in 1738 half the population of Timbuktu died of famine.

Historians of African famine have documented repeated famines in Ethiopia. Possibly the worst episode occurred in 1888 and succeeding years, as the epizootic rinderpest, introduced into Eritrea by infected cattle, spread southwards reaching ultimately as far as South Africa. In Ethiopia it was estimated that as much as 90 per cent of the national herd died, rendering rich farmers and herders destitute overnight. This coincided with drought associated with an el Nino oscillation, human epidemics of smallpox, and in several countries, intense war. The great famine that afflicted Ethiopia from 1888 to 1892 cost it roughly one-third of its population. In Sudan the year 1888 is remembered as the worst famine in history, on account of these factors and also the exactions imposed by the Mahdist state. Colonial "pacification" efforts often caused severe famine, as for example with the repression of the Maji Maji revolt in Tanganyika in 1906. The introduction of cash crops such as cotton, and forcible measures to impel farmers to grow these crops, also impoverished the peasantry in many areas, such as northern Nigeria, contributing to greater vulnerability to famine when severe drought struck in 1913.

However, for the middle part of the 20th century, agriculturalists, economists and geographers did not consider Africa to be famine prone (they were much more concerned about Asia). There were notable counter-examples, such as the famine in Rwanda during World War II and the Malawi famine of 1949, but most famines were localized and brief food shortages. The specter of famine recurred only in the early 1970s, when Ethiopia and the west African Sahel suffered drought and famine. The Ethiopian famine of that time was closely linked to the crisis of feudalism in that country, and in due course helped to bring about the downfall of the Emperor Haile Selassie. The Sahelian famine was associated with the slowly growing crisis of pastoralism in Africa, which has seen livestock herding decline as a viable way of life over the last two generations.

Since then, African famines have become more frequent, more

widespread and more severe. Many African countries are not self-sufficient in food production, relying on income from cash crops to import food. Agriculture in Africa is susceptible to climatic fluctuations, especially droughts which can reduce the amount of food produced locally. Other agricultural problems include soil infertility, land degradation and erosion, and swarms of desert locusts which can destroy whole crops and livestock diseases. The most serious famines have been caused by a combination of drought, misguided economic policies, and conflict. The 1983-85 famine in Ethiopia, for example, was the outcome of all these three factors, made worse by the Communist government's censorship of the emerging crisis. In Sudan at the same date, drought and economic crisis combined with denials of any food shortage by the then-government of President Gaafar Nimeiry, to create a crisis that killed perhaps 250,000 people—and helped bring about a popular uprising that overthrew Nimeiry.

Numerous factors make the food security situation in Africa tenuous, including political instability, armed conflict and civil war, corruption and mismanagement in handling food supplies, and trade policies that harm African agriculture. An example of a famine created by human rights abuses is the 1998 Sudan famine. AIDS is also having long-term economic effects on agriculture by reducing the available workforce, and is creating new vulnerabilities to famine by overburdening poor households. On the other hand, in the modern history of Africa on quite a few occasions famines acted as a major source of acute political instability. In Africa, if current trends of population growth and soil degradation continue, the continent might be able to feed just 25 per cent of its population by 2025, according to UNU's Ghana-based Institute for Natural Resources in Africa.

Recent examples include Ethiopia in 1973 and mid-1980s, Sudan in the late-1970s and again in 1990 and 1998. The 1980 famine in Karamoja, Uganda was, in terms of mortality rates, one of the worst in history. 21 per cent of the population died, including 60 per cent of the infants.

In October 1984, television reports around the world carried footage of starving Ethiopians whose plight was centered around a feeding station near the town of Korem. BBC newsreader Michael

Buerk gave moving commentary of the tragedy on 23 October 1984, which he described as a "biblical famine". This prompted the Band Aid single, which was organised by Bob Geldof and featured more than 20 other pop stars. The Live Aid concerts in London and Philadelphia raised further funds for the cause. An estimated 900,000 people die within one year as a result of the famine, but the tens of millions of pounds raised by Band Aid and Live Aid are widely believed to have saved the lives of around 6,000,000 more Ethiopians who were in danger of death.

More than 20 years on, famine and other forms of poverty are still affecting Ethiopia, but all concerned have insisted that the problems would have been far worse had it not been for Geldof and his fundraising causes.

Famine in Asia

China

Chinese scholars had kept count of 1,828 rampages by the famine since 108 B.C. to 1911 in one province or another — an average of close to one famine per year. From 1333 to 1337 a terrible famine killed 6,000,000 Chinese. The four famines of 1810, 1811, 1846, and 1849 are said to have killed not less than 45,000,000 people. The period from 1850 to 1873 saw, as a result of Taiping Rebellion, drought, and famine, the population of China drop by over 60 million people. China's Qing Dynasty bureaucracy, which devoted extensive attention to minimizing famines, is credited with averting a series of famines following El Niño-Southern Oscillation-linked droughts and floods. These events are comparable, though somewhat smaller in scale, to the ecological trigger events of China's vast 19th century famines. (Pierre-Etienne Will, Bureaucracy and Famine) Qing China carried out its relief efforts, which included vast shipments of food, a requirement that the rich open their storehouses to the poor, and price regulation, as part of a state guarantee of subsistence to the peasantry (known as ming-sheng).

When a stressed monarchy shifted from state management and direct shipments of grain to monetary charity in the mid-nineteenth century, the system broke down. Thus the 1867-68 famine under the Tongzhi Restoration was successfully relieved but the Great North China Famine of 1877-78, caused by drought across northern

China, was a vast catastrophe. The province of Shanxi was substantially depopulated as grains ran out, and desperately starving people stripped forests, fields, and their very houses for food. Estimated mortality is 9.5 to 13 million people.(Mike Davis, Late Victorian Holocausts)

The largest famine of the 20th century, and almost certainly of all time, was the 1958-61 Great Leap Forward famine in China. The immediate causes of this famine lay in Chairman Mao Zedong‘s ill-fated attempt to transform China from an agricultural nation, Communist Party cadres across China insisted that peasants abandon their farms for collective farms, and begin to produce steel in small foundries, often melting down their farm instruments in the process. Collectivization undermined incentives for the investment of labour and resources in agriculture; unrealistic plans for decentralized metal production sapped needed labour; unfavourable weather conditions; and communal dining halls encouraged overconsumption of available food, "Communal dining and the Chinese Famine 1958-1961“). Such was the centralized control of information and the intense pressure on party cadres to report only good news—such as production quotas met or exceeded—that information about the escalating disaster was effectively suppressed. When the leadership did become aware of the scale of the famine, it did little to respond, and continued to ban any discussion of the cataclysm. This blanket suppression of news was so effective that very few Chinese citizens were aware of the scale of the famine, and the greatest peacetime demographic disaster of the 20th century only became widely known twenty years later, when the veil of censorship began to lift.

The 1958-61 famine is estimated to have caused excess mortality of about 30 million, with a further 30 million cancelled or delayed births. It was only when the famine had wrought its worst that Mao reversed the agricultural collectivization policies, which were effectively dismantled in 1978. China has not experienced a major famine since 1961 (Woo-Cummings, 2002).

India

Owing to its almost entire dependence upon the monsoon rains, India is more liable than any other country in the world to crop failures, which upon occasion deepen into famine. There were 14 famines in India between 11th and 17th century (Bhatia, 1985). For example, during the 1022-1033 Great famines in India entire provinces were depopulated. Famine in Deccan killed at least 2 million people in 1702-1704. B.M. Bhatia believes that the earlier famines were localised, and it was only after 1860, during the British rule, that famine came to signify general shortage of foodgrains in the country. There were approximately 25 major famines spread through states such as Tamil Nadu in the south, and Bihar and Bengal in the east during the latter half of the 19th century.

Romesh Dutt argued as early as 1900, and present-day scholars such as Amartya Sen agree, that the famines were a product of both uneven rainfall and British economic and administrative policies, which since 1857 had led to the seizure and conversion of local farmland to foreign-owned plantations, restrictions on internal trade, heavy taxation of Indian citizens to support unsuccessful British expeditions in Afghanistan, inflationary measures that increased the price of food, and substantial exports of staple crops from India to Britain. (Dutt, 1900 and 1902; Srivastava, 1968; Sen, 1982; Bhatia, 1985.) Some British citizens, such as William Digby, agitated for policy reforms and famine relief, but Lord Lytton, the governing British viceroy in India, opposed such changes in the belief that they would stimulate shirking by Indian workers. The first, the Bengal famine of 1770, is estimated to have taken around 10 million lives—one-third of Bengal's population at the time. The famines continued until independence in 1947, with the Bengal Famine of 1943-44—even though there were no crop failures—killing 1.5 million to 3 million Bengalis during World War II.

The observations of the Famine Commission of 1880 support the notion that food distribution is more to blame for famines than food scarcity. They observed that each province in British India, including Burma, had a surplus of foodgrains, and the annual surplus was 5.16 million tons (Bhatia, 1970). At that time, annual export of rice and other grains from India was approximately one million tons.

In 1966, there was a close call in Bihar, when the United States allocated 900,000 tons of grain to fight the famine.

North Korea

Famine struck North Korea in the mid-1990s, set off by

unprecedented floods. This autarkic urban, industrial society had achieved food self-sufficiency in prior decades through a massive industrialization of agriculture. However, the economic system relied on massive concessionary inputs of fossil fuels, primarily from the Soviet Union and the People's Republic of China. When the Soviet collapse and China's marketization switched trade to a hard currency, full price basis, North Korea's economy collapsed. The vulnerable agricultural sector experienced a massive failure in 1995-96, expanding to full-fledged famine by 1996-99. An estimated 600,000 died of starvation (other estimates range from 200,000 to 3.5 million). North Korea has not yet resumed its food self-sufficiency and relies on external food aid from China, Japan, South Korea and the United States. Recently, North Korea requested that food supplies no longer be delivered. (Woo-Cummings, 2002)

Vietnam

Various famines have occurred in Vietnam. Japanese occupation during World War II caused the Vietnamese Famine of 1945, which caused 2 million deaths. Following the unification of the country after the Vietnam War, Vietnam briefly experienced a food shortage in the 1980s, which prompted many people to flee the country.

Famine in Europe

Western Europe

The Great Famine of 1315-1317 (or to 1322) was the first crisis that would strike Europe in the 14th century, millions in northern Europe would die over an extended number of years, marking a clear end to the earlier period of growth and prosperity during the 11th and 12th centuries. Starting with bad weather in the spring of 1315, universal crop failures lasted until the summer of 1317, from which Europe did not fully recover until 1322. It was a period marked by extreme levels of criminal activity, disease and mass death, infanticide, and cannibalism. It had consequences for Church, State, European society and future calamities to follow in the 14th century.

The 17th century was a period of change for the food producers of Europe. For centuries they had lived primarily as subsistence farmers in a feudal system. They had obligations to their lords, who had suzerainty over the land tilled by their peasants. The lord of a fief would take a portion of the crops and livestock produced during the year. Peasants generally tried to minimize the amount of work they had to put into agricultural food production. Their lords rarely pressured them to increase their food output, except when the population started to increase, at which time the peasants were likely to increase the production themselves. More land would be added to cultivation until there was no more available and the peasants were forced to take up more labour-intensive methods of production. Nonetheless, they generally tried to work as little as possible, valuing their time to do other things, such as hunting, fishing or relaxing, as long as they had enough food to feed their families. It was not in their interest to produce more than they could eat or store themselves.

During the 17th century, continuing the trend of previous centuries, there was an increase in market-driven agriculture. Farmers, people who rented land in order to make a profit off of the product of the land, employing wage labour, became increasingly common, particularly in western Europe. It was in their interest to produce as much as possible on their land in order to sell it to areas that demanded that product. They produced guaranteed surpluses of their crop every year if they could. Farmers paid their labourers in money, increasing the commercialization of rural society. This commercialization had a profound impact on the behaviour of peasants. Farmers were interested in increasing labour input into their lands, not decreasing it as subsistence peasants were.

Subsistence peasants were also increasingly forced to commercialize their activities because of increasing taxes. Taxes that had to be paid to central governments in money forced the peasants to produce crops to sell. Sometimes they produced industrial crops, but they would find ways to increase their production in order to meet both their subsistence requirements as well as their tax obligations. Peasants also used the new money to purchase manufactured goods. The agricultural and social developments encouraging increased food production were gradually taking place throughout the sixteenth century, but were spurred on more directly by the adverse conditions for food production that Europe found itself in the early seventeenth century — there was a general cooling trend in the Earth's temperature starting at the beginning end of the sixteenth century.

The 1590s saw the worst famines in centuries across all of Europe, except in certain areas, notably the Netherlands. Famine had been relatively rare during the 16th century. The economy and population had grown steadily as subsistence populations tend to when there is an extended period of relative peace (most of the time). Subsistence peasant populations will almost always increase when possible since the peasants will try to spread the work to as many hands as possible. Although peasants in areas of high population density, such as northern Italy, had learned to increase the yields of their lands through techniques such as promiscuous culture, they were still quite vulnerable to famines, forcing them to work their land even more intensively.

Famine is a very destabilizing and devastating occurrence. The prospect of starvation led people to take desperate measures. When scarcity of food became apparent to peasants, they would sacrifice long-term prosperity for short-term survival. They would kill their draught animals, leading to lowered production in subsequent years. They would eat their seed corn, sacrificing next year's crop in the hope that more seed could be found. Once those means had been exhausted, they would take to the road in search of food. They migrated to the cities where merchants from other areas would be more likely to sell their food, as cities had a stronger purchasing power than did rural areas. Cities also administered relief programmes and bought grain for their populations so that they could keep order. With the confusion and desperation of the migrants, crime would often follow them. Many peasants resorted to banditry in order to acquire enough to eat.

One famine would often lead to difficulties in following years because of lack of seed stock or disruption of routine, or perhaps because of less-available labour. Famines were often interpreted as signs of God's displeasure. They were seen as the removal, by God, of His gifts to the people of the Earth. Elaborate religious processions and rituals were made to prevent God's wrath in the form of famine.

The great famine of the 1590s began the period of famine and decline in the 17th century. The price of grain, all over Europe was high, as was the population. Various types of people were vulnerable to the succession of bad harvests that occurred throughout the 1590s in different regions. The increasing number of wage labourers in the countryside were vulnerable because they had no food of their own, and their meager living was not enough to purchase the expensive grain of a bad-crop year. Town labourers were also at risk because their wages would be insufficient to cover the cost of grain, and, to make matters worse, they often received less money in bad-crop years since the disposable income of the wealthy was spent on grain. Often, unemployment would be the result of the increase in grain prices, leading to ever-increasing numbers of urban poor.

All areas of Europe were badly affected by the famine in these periods, especially rural areas. The Netherlands was able to escape most of the damaging effects of the famine, though the 1590s were still difficult years there. Actual famine did not occur, for the Amsterdam grain trade [with the Baltic] guaranteed that there would always be something to eat in the Netherlands although hunger was prevalent.

The Netherlands had the most commercialized agriculture in all of Europe at this time, growing many industrial crops, such as flax, hemp, and hops. Agriculture became increasingly specialized and efficient. As a result, productivity and wealth increased, allowing the Netherlands to maintain a steady food supply. By the 1620s, the economy was even more developed, so the country was able to avoid the hardships of that period of famine with even greater impunity.

The years around 1620 saw another period of famines sweep across Europe. These famines were generally less severe than the famines of twenty-five years earlier, but they were nonetheless quite serious in many areas. Perhaps the worst famine since 1600, the great famine in Finland in 1696, killed a third of the population.

The period of 1740-43 saw frigid winters and summer droughts which led to famine across Europe leading to a major spike in mortality.(cited in Davis, Late Victorian Holocausts, 281)

Other areas of Europe have known famines much more recently. France saw famines as recently as the nineteenth century. Famine still occurred in eastern Europe during the 20th century.

The frequency of famine can vary with climate changes. For example, during the little ice age of the 15th century to the 18th century, European famines grew more frequent than they had been during previous centuries.

Because of the frequency of famine in many societies, it has long been a chief concern of governments and other authorities. In pre-industrial Europe, preventing famine, and ensuring timely food supplies, was one of the chief concerns of many governments, which employed various tools to alleviate famines, including price controls, purchasing stockpiles of food from other areas, rationing, and regulation of production. Most governments were concerned by famine because it could lead to revolt and other forms of social disruption.

In contrast, the Great Irish Famine, 1845-1849, was in no small part the result of policies of the Whig government of the United Kingdom under Lord Russell. Unlike in Britain, the land in Ireland was owned mostly by Anglican people of English descent, who did not identify culturally or ethnically with the Irish population. The landlords were known as the Anglo-Irish. As the landowners felt no compunction to use their political clout to aid their tenants, the British government‘s expedient response to the food crisis in Ireland was to leave the matter solely to market forces to decide. A strict free-market approach, aided by the British army guarding ports and food depots from the starving crowds, ensured food exports continued as before, and even increased during the famine period. The immediate effect was 1,000,000 dead and another 1,000,000 refugees fleeing to Britain and the United States. After the famine passed, infertility caused by famine, diseases and immigration spurred by the landlord-run economy being so thoroughly undermined, caused the population to enter into a 100-year decline. It was not until the 1970's that the population of Ireland, then at half of what it had been before the famine, began to rise again. This period of Irish population decline after the famine was at a time when the European population doubled and the English population increased fourfold. This left the country severely underpopulated. The population decline continued in parts of the country worst affected by the famine until the 1990s-150 years after the famine and the British government‘s laissez-faire economic policy. Before the Hunger, Ireland's population was over half of England‘s. Today it is an eighth. The population of Ireland is 6 million but there are over 80 million more people of Irish descent outside of Ireland. That is 20 more times the population of Ireland.

Others state it was not the free market that caused the Irish famine, because at the time, Ireland did not have a free market. Irish Catholic citizens were prohibited by law from owning land, from leasing land, from voting, from holding political office, from living in a corporate town or within five miles of a corporate town, from obtaining education, from entering a profession, and from doing many other things that are necessary in order to succeed and prosper in life.

Famine returned to the Netherlands during World War II in what was known as the Hongerwinter. It was the last famine of Europe, in which approximately 30,000 people died of starvation. Some other areas of Europe also experienced famine at the same time.

Italy

The harvest failures were devastating for the northern Italian economy. The economy of the area had recovered well from the previous famines, but the famines from 1618 to 1621 coincided because of a period of war in the area. The economy did not recover fully for centuries. There were serious famines in the late-1640s and less severe ones in the 1670s throughout northern Italy.

England

From 1536 England began legislating Poor Laws which put a legal responsibility on the rich, at a parish level, to maintain the poor of that parish. English agriculture lagged behind the Netherlands, but by 1650 their agricultural industry was commercialized on a wide scale. The last peace-time famine in England was in 1623-24. There were still periods of hunger, as in the Netherlands, but there were no more famines as such. Rising population levels continued to put a strain on food security, despite potatoes becoming increasingly important in the diet of the poor. On balance, potatoes increased food security in England where they never replaced bread as the staple of the poor. Climate conditions were never likely to simultaneously be catastrophic for both the wheat and potato crops.

Iceland

In 1783 the volcano Laki in south-central Iceland erupted. The lava caused little direct damage, but ash and sulfur dioxide spewed out over most of the country, causing three-quarters of the island's livestock to perish. In the following famine, around ten thousand people died, one-fifth of the population of Iceland. [Asimov, 1984, 152-153]

Russia and the USSR

Droughts and famines in Imperial Russia are known to have happened every 10 to 13 years, with average droughts happening every 5 to 7 years. Famines continued in the Soviet era, the most notorious being the Holodomor in Ukraine (1932-1933). The last major famine in the USSR happened in 1947 due to the severe drought.

LIST OF FAMINES

5th Century BC

- 440 BC famine in Ancient Rome.

2nd Century BC

- Between 108 BC and 1911 AD there were no fewer than 1828 major famines in China, or one nearly every year in one or another province, which however varied greatly in severity.

5th Century AD

- Famine in Western Europe associated with the Fall of Rome and its sack by Alaric I. Between 400 and 800 AD, the population of the city of Rome fell by over 90 per cent, mainly because of famine and plague.

7th Century AD

- 639 AD—Famine in Arabia during the Caliphate of 'Umar ibn Al-Khattab
- 650 Famine throughout India

8th Century

- 750's famine in Spain

9th Century

- 800-1000 AD, severe drought killed millions of Maya people with famine and thirst and initiated a cascade of internal collapses that destroyed their civilization
- 809 famine in Frankish Empire
- 875-884 peasant rebellion in China inspired by famine; Huang Chao captured capital

10th Century

- 927 famine in Byzantine Empire

11th Century

- 1005 Famine in England There were 95 famines in the Middle Ages.
- 1016 Famine throughout Europe
- 1022,1033 Great famines in India, in which entire provinces were depopulated
- 1064-1072 Seven years' famine in Egypt
- 1051 famine forced the Toltecs to migrate from a stricken region in what is now central Mexico
- 1066 famine in England

13th Century

- 1199-1202 famine in Egypt
- 1230 famine in Novgorod
- 1231-1232 famine in Japan
- 1235 famine in England. 20,000 die in London, alone
- 1255 famine in Portugal
- 1258 famine in Germany and Italy
- 1294 famine in England

14th Century

- 1315-1317 Great Famine in Europe.
- 1333 famine in Portugal
- 1333-1334 famine in Spain
- 1333-1337 famine in China
- 1344-1345 Great famine in India
- 1387 after Timur the Lame left Asia Minor, severe famine ensued
- 1390 famine in England
- 1396-1407 The Durga Devi famine in India, lasting twelve years

15th Century

- 1403-1404 famine in Egypt
- 1441 famine in Mayapan, Mexico
- 1445 famine in Korea
- 1450-1454 famine in Aztec Empire
- 1460-1461 Kanshô famine in Japan

16th Century

- 1504 famine in Spain
- 1518 famine in Venice
- 1528 famine in Languedoc, France
- 1540 famine in Spain
- 1555 famine in England
- 1567-1570 famine in Harar in Ethiopia, combined with plague. Emir of Harar, died.
- 1574-1576 famine in Istanbul and Anatolia
- 1586 famine in England which gave rise to the Poor Law system
- 1590s famines in Europe

17th Century

- 1599-1600 famine in Spain
- 1601-1603 one of the worst famines in all of Russian

history; famine killed as many as 100,000 in Moscow and up to one-third of Tsar Godunov's subjects. Same famine killed about half Estonian population.

- 1611 famine in Anatolia
- 1618-1648 famines in Europe caused by Thirty Years' War
- 1619 famine in Japan. During the Tokugawa period, there were 154 famines, of which 21 were widespread and serious.
- 1623-1624 famine in England
- 1630-1631 Deccan famine in India kills 2,000,000 (Note: There was a corresponding famine in northwestern China, eventually causing the Ming dynasty to collapse in 1644.)
- 1636 famine in Spain
- 1648-1660 Poland lost an estimated 1/3 of its population due to the wars, famine, and plague
- 1649 famine in northern England
- 1650-1652 famine in the east of France
- 1651-1653 famine throughout much of Ireland during the Cromwellian conquest of Ireland
- 1661 famine in India, when not a drop of rain fell for two years
- 1661-1662 famine in Morocco
- 1661-1662 famine in France
- 1669 famine in Bengal
- 1680 famine in Sardinia
- 1680 famine in Japan
- 1680s famine in Sahel
- 1690s famine in Scotland which may have killed 15 per cent of the population
- 1693-1694 famine in France which killed 2 million people
- 1695-1697 famine killed about a fifth of Estonian population (70 000-75 000 people). Famine also hit Sweden (80 000-100 000 dead)
- 1696-1697 famine in Finland wiped out almost a third of the population

18th Century

- 1702-1704 famine in Deccan, India, killed 2 million people

- 1706-1707 famine in France
- 1708-1711 famine in East Prussia killed 250,000 people or 41 per cent of its population
- 1709-1710 famine in France
- 1740-1741 famine in Ireland
- 1722 famine in Arabia
- 1727-1728 famine in England
- 1732 famine in Japan
- 1738-1739 famine in France
- 1738-1756 famine in West Africa, half the population of Timbuktu died of starvation
- 1741 famine in Norway
- 1750 famine in Spain
- 1764 famine in Naples
- 1769-1773 Bengal famine of 1770
- 1770-1771 famine in Czech lands killed hundreds of thousands people
- 1771-1772 famine in Saxony and southern Germany
- 1773 famine in Sweden
- 1779 famine in Rabat, Morocco
- *1780s Great* Tenmei *Famine in Japan*
- 1783 famine in Iceland caused by Laki (volcano) eruption killed one-fifth of Iceland's population
- 1784 widespread famine throughout Egypt
- 1784-1785 famine in Tunisia killed up to one-fifth of all Tunisians
- 1788 famine in France. The two years previous to the French Revolution saw bad harvests and harsh winters, possibly because of a strong El Niño cycle caused by the 1783 Laki eruption at Iceland.

19th Century

- 1800-1801 famine in Ireland
- Four famines—in 1810, 1811, 1846, and 1849—in China claimed nearly 45 million lives.
- 1811-1812 famine devastated Madrid, taking nearly 20,000 lives

- 1815 eruption Tambora, Indonesia. Tens of thousands died of subsequent famine
- 1816-1817 famine in Europe (Year Without a Summer)
- 1830 famine killed almost half the population of Cape Verde
- 1830s Tenpo famine (Japan)
- 1835 famine in Egypt killed 200,000
- 1845-1849 Great Irish Famine killed more than 1 million people
- 1846 famine led to the peasant revolt known as"Maria da Fonte" in the north of Portugal
- 1846-1857 Highland Potato Famine in Scotland
- 1850-1873 as a result of Taiping Rebellion, drought, and famine, the population of China drop by over 60 million people
- 1866 Orissa famine of 1866 in India; one million perished
- 1866-1868 Famine in Finland. About 15 per cent of the entire population died
- 1869 famine in Rajputana; one million and a half perished
- 1870-1871 famine in Persia is believed to have caused the death of 2 million persons
- 1873-1874 famine in Anatolia
- 1879 Famine in Ireland
- 1876-1879 Famine in India, China, Brazil, Northern Africa (and other countries). Famine in northern China killed 13 million people, 12-29 million died in India
- 1888 famine in Sudan
- 1888-1892 Ethiopian Great famine. About one-third of the population died. Conditions worsen with cholera outbreaks (1889-92), a typhus epidemic, and a major smallpox epidemic (1889-90).
- 1891-1892 famine in Russia caused 375,000 to 500,000 deaths
- 1896-1897 famine in northern China
- 1896-1902 famine in India

20th Century

- 1907 famine in east-central China

- 1914-1918 Mount Lebanon famine during World War I which killed about a third of the population
- 1914-1918 famine in Belgium
- 1916-1917 famine caused by the British blockade of Germany in WWI; up to 750,000 Germans starved to death
- 1916-1917 winter famine in Russia
- 1917-1919 famine in Persia. As much as 1/4 of the population living in the north of Iran died in the famine
- 1917-1921 a series of famines in Turkestan at the time of the Bolshevik revolution killed about a sixth of the population
- 1921 famine in Russia killed 5 million
- 1921-1922 Famine in Tatarstan
- 1921-1922 famine in Volga German colonies in Russia. One-third of the entire population perished
- 1928-1929 famine in northern China. The drought resulted in 3 million deaths
- 1928-1929 famine in Ruanda-Burundi, causing large migrations to the Congo
- 1932-1933 famine in Ukraine (Holodomor), some parts of Russia and North Caucasus area. As many as 10 million people may have died
- 1932-1933 famine in Kazakhstan killed 1.2-1.5 million
- 1936 famine in China, with an estimated 5 million fatalities
- 1940-1943 famine in Warsaw Ghetto
- 1941-44 Leningrad famine caused by a 900-day blockade by Nazi and Finnish troops. About one million Leningrad residents starved, froze, or were bombed to death in the winter of 1941-42, when supply routes to the city were cut off and temperatures dropped to –40 degrees.
- 1941-1942 famine in Greece caused by Nazi occupation. An estimated 300,000 people perished
- 1942-1943 famine killed one million in China
- 1943 famine in Bengal
- 1943 famine in Ruanda-Urundi, causing migrations to the Congo
- 1944 famine in the Netherlands during World War II, more than 20,000 deaths
- 1945 famine in Vietnam

- 1946-1947 famine in Soviet Union
- 1959-1961 Great Leap Forward/The Great Chinese Famine (China). The official statistic is 20 million deaths, as given by Hu Yaobang
- 1967-1970 Biafran famine caused by Nigerian blockade
- 1968-1972 Sahel drought
- 1973 famine in Ethiopia; failure of the government to handle this crisis led to fall of Haile Selassie and to Derg rule
- 1974 famine in Bangladesh
- 1975-1979 Khmer Rouge. An estimated 2 million Cambodians lost their lives to murder, forced labour and famine
- 1980 famine in Karamoja, Uganda
- 1984 famine in Ethiopia
- 1991-1993 Somalian famine
- 1996 North Korean famine
- 1998 famine in Sudan caused by war and drought
- 1998-2000 famine in Ethiopia. The situation worsened by Eritrean-Ethiopian War
- 1998-2004 Second Congo War. 3.8 million people died, mostly from starvation and disease
- 2000-2007 Zimbabwe's food crisis caused by Mugabe's land reform policies

21st Century

- 2003-famine in Sudan/Darfur (Darfur conflict)
- 2005 Malawi food crisis
- 2005-06 Niger food crisis
- 2006 Horn of Africa food crisis

ASSESSMENT AND RESPONSE OF FOOD SCARCITY AND FAMINE

Description

Over the years Oxfam has been involved in a wide variety of health-related projects. The Practical Health Guides draw on this experience to put forward ideas on best practice in the provision of health care and services in developing countries.

Where people are suffering from food scarcity or famine, the obvious response seems to be food aid. This may indeed be necessary, but handing out food may not be the best solution, and other actions could be equally urgent, such as public health or income support measures. This book provides a new approach to assessing and responding to situations of food scarcity and gives a comprehensive explanation of how to assess these situations in order to judge which interventions will be most effective.

This book offers advice on carrying out initial assessments and nutrition surveys, and emphasises the importance of finding out the underlying causes of food scarcity by seeking out the views of those affected. Food distribution, and how to target the people who need it most, supplementary and therapeutic feeding programmes, are also covered.

EUROPE: Subsidies Feeding Food Scarcity

> "Farmers in countries of the South cannot compete with subsidised agricultural products from Europe," said Thilo Bode, director of the German non-government organisation Foodwatch. "The subsidies the EU pays to farmers in France, Germany, Britain, Spain and elsewhere cheapen European food production in such a way that small farmers in say, Senegal, can no longer exist."

Bode said the EU, the U.S. and other industrialised countries pay their farmers a billion dollars a day in subsidies. "These very same countries have forced developing countries through international organisations to eliminate their customs duties and their trade barriers, constraining them to import subsidised food."

The economic consequences of such policies are increasing unemployment and poverty among farmers in Africa, Asia and Latin America, Bode said. This leads on to food scarcity because farmers lose the means to grow more, he told IPS.

The EU channels more than 50 billion dollars a year to its farmers in subsidies under the Common Agricultural Policy (CAP).

These subsidies represent about 45 per cent of the European Commission's budget.

The CAP guarantees a minimum price to European farmers, imposes import tariffs and quotas on certain foods, and provides direct subsidy payment for cultivated land. Following an agreement in 2005, the CAP is due to be phased out by 2013.

Other industrialised countries, especially the U.S., also pay substantial subsidies to their farmers, and protect their local markets with import tariffs and quotas.

These subsidies have been at the core of debates in international forums such as the World Trade Organisation, the Organisation for Economic Cooperation and Development, and the United Nations. But now with prices of basic foods like rice, wheat and corn rising sharply, industrialised countries' subsidies for agriculture are increasingly under the spotlight.

Wheat prices have risen on average 130 per cent since March 2007, according to the United Nations Educational, Scientific, Cultural Organisation (UNESCO), while soy prices have jumped 87 per cent. Food prices have risen 83 per cent over the past three years, the World Bank reported this month.

This increase in food prices has fuelled protests in several countries, including Haiti, Egypt, Cameroon, Cote d'Ivoire, Mauritania, Ethiopia, Uzbekistan, Yemen, the Philippines, Thailand, Indonesia and Italy.

Voices are rising within Europe against such subsidies. Renate Kuenast, leader of the German Green party, said during a debate in the Bundestag, the lower chamber of the German parliament, that EU subsidies are substantially responsible for the global food scarcity.

Kuenast called for a new agricultural revolution. "The European Commission must stop as soon as possible all subsidies, including export credits to agriculture," she said.

Kuenast said before German parliamentarians that "if the EU would not cut artificially the prices of its own agricultural products, there would be no hunger and food scarcity in the world, because the small farmers in developing countries would still be producing their own food."

Bode and Kuenast backed several reports that have called for radical reform of agriculture in Europe and North America in order to tackle food scarcity.

In a UNESCO report released Apr. 15, a body of 400 experts called for a revolution in agriculture to avoid social explosions around the world from rising food prices.

The report, officially known as the International Assessment of Agricultural Science and Technology for Development (IAASTD), explores ways of finding an equilibrium between the economic efficiency of agriculture, its social and welfare benefits, and the environmental consequences of economic activities.

A typical example of the difficulties in finding such balance is the search for carbon-free fuel for automobiles. Biofuels, once a hope for reducing greenhouse gas emissions through transport, and thus helping to cut global warming, are now under heavy criticism because their environmental footprint is seen as negative by many studies.

But production of biofuels has boomed, driven by rising world fuel prices and the growing demand for energy. And this boom has contributed to creating conditions for the present food scarcity in many regions by crowding out production of grains such as maize and wheat.

The IAASTD recognises this, saying that the diversion of crops to fuel "can raise food prices and reduce our ability to alleviate hunger throughout the world."

The IAASTD authors affirm in the report that "we are now in a good position to reflect on (all these) consequences and to outline various policy options to meet the challenges ahead, perhaps best characterised as the need for food and livelihood security under increasingly constrained environmental conditions from within and outside the realm of agriculture and globalised economic systems."

Salvatore Arico, a UNESCO biodiversity expert and co-author of the report, put it more bluntly. "Modern agriculture will have to change radically if the international community wants to cope with growing populations and climate change, while avoiding social fragmentation and irreversible deterioration of the environment," he told IPS.

The IAASTD assessment, while admitting that modern agriculture has brought significant increases in food production, also says these benefits have been spread unevenly, at "an increasingly intolerable price, paid by small-scale farmers, workers, rural communities and the environment." (END/2008)

CASE STUDY: NIGERIAN FOOD SCARCITY

THE Federal Ministry of Agriculture and Water Resources said yesterday the Federal Government had entered into an agreement with the Republic of Thailand to import tones of rice to stave off an impending food crisis in the country.

The Ministry of Agriculture would also release 11,000 metric tones of grains to the market at half of the market price, Agriculture Minister, Dr Said Abba Ruma disclosed yesterday.

The minister made the disclosure while briefing members of the House Committee on Agriculture on government's response to the food scarcity in the country. According to the minister, the imported rice from Thailand would arrive Nigeria within the next three months.

"Right now we are now making a survey of the quantum of rice available in this country and we have been made to understand that we have about 800,000 metric tones of paddy which probably when processed might lead us to either 200,000 metric tones taking into consideration the nature of seaving, wastages, the broken ones and all that.

"But government has taken a position to commence immediately the purchase of rice on ground in Nigeria and to express also a request to the Thailand government for the importation of rice in order to immediately within the next two to three months alleviate the sufferings of Nigerians while we intensify efforts at production", he stated.

He said Government was worried about the "food scarcity and has decided to embark on massive importation of Thailand rice to meet the immediate needs of the populace while it embarks on other far-reaching measures to ensure food availability and accessibility."

The government, he said chose Thailand rice, because according to him, other major producers were not ready to export their yields, when they had not yet satisfied their respective local markets, while he noted that some Nigerian crops had comparative advantage.

"It is certainly clear that in the crops which have comparative advantage, which we produce in this country, maize, cassava, sorghum, millet and to some extent soya beans and others.

"We have released assorted grains, I think more than 40,000 metric tones and will continue to do so. Immediately within this week we are also realizing about 11,000 metric tones in addition to the 40,000 metric tones that we have realized to the states for them to effectively supervise public sales at half the price it is currently obtained in the market.

"But Nigerians are also so much dependent on other staple foods that we still import and which by the realities of what we are facing today those countries from where we bring in those items have placed a ban on exports of those products. I think probably with the exception of Thailand that has earmarked about three to four million metric tones of rice, taking into consideration the vulnerability of most African countries, most of the countries have stopped importation of rice.

"And a number of Nigerians especially the middle class and the upper class are of course used to rice and that is the basis of the concern now about rice. And of course in addition to this is the easy nature in processing. In the event of emergency rice certainly is one of the staple food that could be easily prepared with little stress or none at all. We do produce rice to a reasonable quantity in this country but one of the fundamental challenge is rice processing.

"We also working on market development outlets for agricultural produce. Other responsibilities which include promoting private sector participation which government in best practice agriculture must make effort to do and which we believe in is the issue of guaranteed minimum price. We have been contending with this issue for a very long time in this country.

"We do not have a sustainable funding mechanism for guaranteed minimum price. By the grace of God beginning from this year we hope to have a sustainable funding framework for biome sustenance to the tune of N10 billion. And with states coming along to participate it becomes a much bigger fund". he said

CASE STUDY: KENYAN FOOD SECURITY

The Grand Coalition Cabinet meeting on Thursday failed to reach a decision on how to handle Mungiki and other armed groups.

President Kibaki chairs the first session of the Grand Coalition Cabinet meeting at State House, Nairobi on Thursday. Top on the agenda was the need to boost security and ensure there was enough food in the wake of rising prices. Photo/PPS

The meeting, chaired by President Kibaki at State House, Nairobi, also resolved that food security would be the government's top priority.

It was the first formal coming together of the 42-member Cabinet.

Talks centred on the agenda and policies of the Government that brings together PNU, ODM and ODM Kenya.

It is understood that the meeting had on its agenda how to handle the security threat posed by the Sabaot Land Defence Force in Mt Elgon District, Mungiki and other outlawed armed groups and the fate of youths who were arrested during the post-election violence in the Rift Valley. Also on the agenda was the need to promote harmony among the ministers from various political parties.

Corruption

Sources said that other issues on the agenda included resettlement of internally displaced people, corruption and the question of protocol in Government.

The attempts by backbenchers to form a grand opposition coalition also featured as did debate on adoption of a harmonised Government manifesto to provide policy guidelines for the next four-and-a-half years.

Thursday's meeting had been postponed twice; once because Prime minster Odinga was out of the country for treatment and on another occasion to create time to heal differences among the ministers from different political camps.

To promote harmony in the Cabinet, an induction and bonding session was organised in Nairobi was last week held with the aim of getting the Cabinet ministers, assistant ministers and permanent secretaries to work as a team and drive the reform agenda of the Grand Coalition.

President Kibaki convened Thursday's meeting to drive the

agenda of the coalition and find ways to tackle challenges posed by post-election violence, including finding solutions to the challenges posed by Mungiki, the Sabaot Land Defence Force and other armed groups.

Mr Odinga has in the past said he would hold talks with leaders of the sect. But in a ministerial statement earlier this week, Internal Security minister George Saitoti ruled out talks with the sect.

Protect Lives

Although a plan for talks with Mungiki leaders was being put in place, it is understood that Prof Saitoti told the sitting that he was faced with the dilemma of accepting to start talks with outlawed gangs when the Constitution requires him to use the law to protect the lives of Kenyans and their property.

Those pushing for dialogue said the armed gangs had developed into complex outfits and using force to crush them would not succeed as the crackdown on Mungiki had showed. The final decision on the issue was put off until next week.

However, the meeting resolved that making the country food situation secure would be among the top priority of the Government. In this regard it was resolved that the country must urgently increase its food reserves, which will see the strategic maize reserves increased from four million bags to eight million bags in the next two years.

It was further decided that due to an anticipated grain shortage later in the year, the National Cereals and Produce Board should import three million bags of maize in the next few weeks as a precautionary measure.

The Cabinet noted that escalating international food prices were posing a serious threat to Kenya's food security hence the need to take immediate measures to cushion wananchi.

In recent months, consumers have raised concerns over rising prices of food and other basic products. Inflation, post-election violence and rising oil prices globally have been blamed for the high cost of food and other basic consumer goods.

Ministers agreed that the importation of grains would only be a temporary measure as the Government seeks ways of increasing food production.

The Cabinet also reviewed the re-settlement of internally displaced families. Members expressed satisfaction with the four-week old resettlement drive that has taken an estimated 70 per cent of displaced families back to their homes.

CASE STUDY: CHINA AND INDIA

The world is now facing a climate-driven shrinkage of river-based irrigation water supplies. Mountain glaciers in the Himalayas and on the Tibet-Qinghai Plateau are melting and could soon deprive the major rivers of India and China of the ice melt needed to sustain them during the dry season. In the Ganges, the Yellow, and the Yangtze river basins, where irrigated agriculture depends heavily on rivers, this loss of dry-season flow will shrink harvests.

The world has never faced such a predictably massive threat to food production as that posed by the melting mountain glaciers of Asia. China and India are the world's leading producers of both wheat and rice—humanity's food staples. China's wheat harvest is nearly double that of the United States, which ranks third after India. With rice, these two countries are far and away the leading producers, together accounting for over half of the world harvest.

The Intergovernmental Panel on Climate Change reports that Himalayan glaciers are receding rapidly and that many could melt entirely by 2035. If the giant Gangotri Glacier that supplies 70 per cent of the Ganges flow during the dry season disappears, the Ganges could become a seasonal river, flowing during the rainy season but not during the summer dry season when irrigation water needs are greatest.

Yao Tandong, a leading Chinese glaciologist, reports that the glaciers on the Tibet-Qinghai Plateau in western China are now melting at an accelerating rate. He believes that two thirds of these glaciers could be gone by 2060, greatly reducing the dry-season flow of the Yellow and Yangtze rivers. Like the Ganges, the Yellow River, which flows through the arid northern part of China, could become seasonal. If this melting of glaciers continues, Yao says, "[it] will eventually lead to an ecological catastrophe."

Even as India and China face these future disruptions in river flows, overpumping is depleting the underground water resources that both countries also use for irrigation. For example, water tables are falling everywhere under the North China Plain, the country's principal grain-producing region. When an aquifer is depleted, the rate of pumping is necessarily reduced to the rate of recharge. In India, water tables are falling and wells are going dry in almost every state.

On top of this already grim shrinkage of underground water resources, losing the river water used for irrigation could lead to politically unmanageable food shortages. The Ganges River, for example, which is the largest source of surface water irrigation in India, is a leading source of water for the 407 million people living in the Gangetic Basin.

In China, both the Yellow and Yangtze rivers depend heavily on ice melt for their dry-season flow. The Yellow River basin is home to 147 million people whose fate is closely tied to the river because of low rainfall in the basin. The Yangtze is China's leading source of surface irrigation water, helping to produce half or more of China's 130-million-ton rice harvest. It also meets many of the other water needs of the watershed's 368 million people.

The population in either the Yangtze or Gangetic river basin is larger than that of any country other than China or India. And the ongoing shrinkage of underground water supplies and the prospective shrinkage of river water supplies are occurring against a startling demographic backdrop: by 2050 India is projected to add 490 million people and China 80 million.

In a world where grain prices have recently climbed to record highs, with no relief in sight, any disruption of the wheat or rice harvests due to water shortages in these two leading grain producers will greatly affect not only people living there but consumers everywhere. In both of these countries, food prices will likely rise and grain consumption per person can be expected to fall. In India, where just over 40 per cent of all children under five years of age are underweight and undernourished, hunger will intensify and child mortality will likely climb.

For China, a country already struggling to contain food price inflation, there may well be spreading social unrest as food supplies tighten. Food security in China is a highly sensitive issue. Anyone in China who is 50 years of age or older is a survivor of the Great

Famine of 1959-61, when, according to official figures, 30 million Chinese starved to death. This is also why Beijing has worked so hard in recent decades to try and maintain grain self-sufficiency.

As food shortages unfold, China will try to hold down domestic food prices by using its massive dollar holdings to import grain, most of it from the United States, the world's leading grain exporter. Even now, China, which a decade or so ago was essentially self-sufficient in soybeans, is importing 70 per cent of its supply, helping drive world soybean prices to an all-time high. As irrigation water supplies shrink, Chinese consumers will be competing with Americans for the U.S. grain harvest. India, too, may try to import large quantities of grain, although it may lack the economic resources to do so, especially if grain prices keep climbing. Many Indians will be forced to tighten their belts further, including those who have no notches left.

The glaciologists have given us a clear sense of how fast glaciers are shrinking. The challenge now is to translate their findings into national energy policies designed to save the glaciers. At issue is not just the future of mountain glaciers, but the future of world grain harvests.

The alternative to this civilization-threatening scenario is to abandon business-as-usual energy policies and move to cut carbon emissions 80 per cent—not by 2050 as many political leaders suggest, because that will be too late, but by 2020, as outlined in Plan B 3.0: Mobilizing to Save Civilization. The first step is to ban new coal-fired power plants, a move that is fast gaining momentum in the United States.

Ironically, the two countries that are planning to build most of the new coal-fired power plants, China and India, are precisely the ones whose food security is most massively threatened by the carbon emitted from burning coal. It is now in their interest to try and save their mountain glaciers by shifting energy investment from coal-fired power plants into energy efficiency and into wind farms, solar thermal power plants, and geothermal power plants. China, for example, can double its current electrical generating capacity from wind alone.

We know from studying earlier civilizations that declined and collapsed that it was often shrinking harvests that were responsible.

For the Sumerians, it was rising salt concentrations in the soil that lowered wheat and barley yields and brought down this remarkable early civilization. For the Mayans, it was soil erosion following deforestation that undermined their agriculture and set the stage for their demise. For our twenty-first century civilization, it is rising atmospheric carbon dioxide (CO2) concentrations and the associated rise in temperature that threatens future harvests.

At issue is whether we can mobilize to lower atmospheric CO2 concentrations before higher temperatures melt the mountain glaciers that feed the major rivers of Asia and elsewhere, and before shrinking harvests lead to an unraveling of our civilization. The good news is that we have the energy efficiency and renewable energy technologies to dramatically reduce CO2 concentrations if we choose to do so.

FCI'S INTEGRATED INFORMATION SYSTEM FOR FOODGRAINS MANAGEMENT PROJECT

The IISFM Project with total estimated cost of Rs 97.66 Crores is being implemented in three (3) phases commencing from 2003-04 and to be completed by 2005-06 under the 10 Five-Year Plan. A tripartite Agreement has been entered into between Food Corporation of India (FCI), National Informatics Centre (NIC), and National Informatics Centre Services Incorporated (NICSI) on 24/9/2003 for implementation of IISFM Project.

So far, Hardware and Software has been installed in FCI Headquarters, 5 Zonal Offices, 23 Regional Offices, all FCI District Offices and 462 Depots. Besides orders have also been placed with NICSI for hardware/software supplies at 224 FCI hired Depots [CWC/SWC/ARDC/St Govt hired/Private hired] where installation of Hardware is expected shortly. Balance FCI Depots are being linked to the nearby Depots on the basis of recommendation from FCI Zonal Offices/Regional Offices.

Out of 164 FCI District Offices, 154 District offices have fed the data online in the District Stock Accounting Software for July 2005. This data is being fed online by about 1700 trained Data Entry Operators under the supervision of trained 344 FCI Technical Supervisors (FTSs) and 102 Technical Support Persons (TSPs) provided by NIC/NICSI. The data feeding status as well as stock position can be viewed on the IISFM website http://iisfm.nic.in/ which is being maintained and updated by NIC. The stock reports pertaining to the central pool balance sheet for wheat, rice, paddy, sugar and coarse grain are also available on the IISFM website.

Based on suggestions by FCI field functionaries, the IISFM Depot Module Version-I Software has been modified/tested by NIC and released for depots on 10.8.2005.

Virtual Private Network [VPN] connectivity from District office level upwards to FCI Headquarters at 194 locations is also being established through BSNL. This will enable speedy and secure data transfer. Besides Video Conferencing facility is also being established from FCI Headquarters to FCI Zonal/Regional Offices to enable fast and cost effective means for conducting meetings/ reviews etc.

Action is also being taken for widening the scope of IISFM Project in FCI to include data of Central Pool Stocks with State Agencies particularly in States that have adopted de-Centralized procurement and distribution scheme and financial accounting of FCI.

FCI'S VISION 2020

- To aggressively promote Decentralized Procurement by State Governments with special emphasis in non-traditional areas and commodities.
- To initiate procurement of non-MSP governed commodities on commercial principles.
- To ensure adequate buffer for meeting requirements under TPDS and Other Welfare Schemes.
- To dispose off surplus and un-storage worthy godowns and introduce concepts of mechanized handling in the conventional godowns.
- To undertake R&D for conversion of some of the existing capacity to bulk and cost effective utilization of existing bulk capacity.
- To optimize monthly movement programme with existing state of art of computerization within the country at various locations as per corporate policies and priorities.

- Modernization of Quality Control equipments and systems for food preservation in order to increase the shelf life of food grain.
- To venture in the fields of Forward Trading and Exports of both surplus stocks of food grains in Central Pool and no-traditional commodities.
- To introduce state of art of financial management in order to reduce the dependency on the present banking system in the country.
- To initiate systems for settlement of storage loss and transit loss through insurance coverage and revised inventory mechanism.
- To develop efficiency in human resource management both in staff/officers and workers with changed circumstances in the work approach of P.S.U.s.
- To achieve state of art in computerized communication between different offices/depots through out the country.

OPPORTUNITIES AS PERCEIVED BY FCI

- After nearly four decades of varied experience in food management, FCI can now play a wider role in being a food advisor to the Central/State Govts.
- The Corporation can also play a more proactive role in the sphere of commercial ventures.
- To diversify into non traditional commodities/activities.

STRENGTH OF FCI

Facilitator for Food Security

- Provider of price and market assurance to the farmer
- Ensuring steady food grain supplies to 5 Lakhs Fair Price Shops for PDS to cover 141 million APL/67 million card holders.
- Ensuring food for All other Welfare Schemes.

Management Capability and Experience

- Large pool of talent managing world's largest food grain operation on behalf of Govt. of India

Enormity of Scale

- Countrywide network of offices and strategically located Food Storage Depots.
- Operates in mandis/purchase centres located within 10 kms. proximity of farmers.
- Undertakes purchases of 30 to 40 million tonnes annually making it the largest buyer in the world.

Effective Market Intervention to Stabilize Prices

State of the Art Experience on Food Grain preservation/ Warehousing/Transportation Management

- Maintains the health of millions of tonnes of food grain in storage. Quality acknowledge by International buyers.
- Excellent Storage Management.
- Timely movement of food grains from procuring States to consuming States.

CASE STUDY: SAARC'S COMPOSITE FOOD POLICY

Facing the common challenge of feeding the poor in this region of over 1.2 billion people, policymakers from Saarc nations favour a composite policy for ensuring food security in the region.

Facing the common challenge of feeding the poor in this region of over 1.2 billion people, policymakers from Saarc nations favour a composite policy for ensuring food security in the region.

'It is time for us to initiate collective measures to provide food security to our people. The Saarc members must have a comprehensive food policy, and we must work towards that,' Pakistan's former agriculture minister Amir Mohammad told IANS.

'Let's move forward fast. Agriculture is the mainstay of our people. In Pakistan, 65 per cent of people living in villages are engaged in varied agriculture activities. India faces a similar situation. How to augment farmers' income by enhancing productivity is a challenge before us.'

Mohammad was among the 100 delegates from Afghanistan, Sri Lanka, Bhutan, Bangladesh, the Maldives, Nepal, Pakistan and India who took part in a three-day conference on 'Science-based Agricultural Transformation Towards Alleviation of Hunger and Poverty in Saarc countries'.

The South Asian Association for Regional Cooperation is made up of these eight countries. The delegates were unanimous on the need to respond to the foodgrain crunch in the Saarc nations on a priority basis.

'We should supply foodgrains first to the neighbouring countries if there is a need,' said M.K.A. Chowdhury, member director (crops) of the Bangladesh Agricultural Research Council (BARC).

'Sixty per cent people out of Bangladesh's 140 million population is engaged in agriculture, and still nearly 50 per cent of the total population lives below the poverty line. Identical problems dog other Saarc nations too.'

According to India's Planning Commission, over 22 per cent people in the country live below the poverty line.

According to the United Nations Food and Agriculture Organisation (FAO), record world prices for most staple foods have led to an 18 per cent food price inflation in China, 13 per cent in Indonesia and Pakistan, and 10 per cent or more in Latin America, Russia and India.

'We will not be able to ensure food security without a fine-tuned food policy. I hope to have some solution in the near future. Each of us will impress upon our respective governments to do the needful,' Afghanistan's Agriculture Minister Obaidullah Ramin told IANS.

Suresh Prabhu, chairman of the steering committee of the first Saarc meet on agriculture and a former Indian minister, said: 'The Saarc region needs a policy that not only ensures food security but also makes agriculture a profitable enterprise. We must join hands to improve agricultural productivity and respond to one another's needs in enhancing livelihoods for food security.'

Mohammad suggested the member nations 'adopt a policy

which guarantees quality seeds and investments in technological upgradation in agriculture. A common strategy is needed to meet multifarious challenges'.

Scientists also advocated better use of technology to meet the rising demand.

'The global warming and deceleration in agro productivity call for a policy that makes agriculture economically sound. A synergy between agriculture and technology has become the need of the hour,' India's noted agri-scientist M.S. Swaminathan told IANS.

9

Hunger, Global Hunger Crisis and Related Facts: Evaluating Role of Food Aid and Food Security

HUNGER

Definition

Hunger is a feeling experienced when the glycogen level of the liver falls below a threshold, usually followed by a desire to eat. The often unpleasant feeling originates in the hypothalamus and is released through receptors in the liver. Although an average nourished individual can survive weeks without food intake, the sensation of hunger typically begins after a couple of hours without eating and is generally considered quite uncomfortable. The sensation of hunger can often be alleviated and even mitigated entirely with the consumption of food.

Hunger Pangs

When hunger contractions occur in the stomach, these are called hunger pangs. Hunger pangs usually do not begin until 12 to 24 hours after the last ingestion of food, in starvation. A single hunger contraction lasts about 30 seconds, and pangs continue for around 30-45 minutes, then hunger subsides for around 30-150 minutes. Individual contractions are separated at first, but are almost continuous after a certain amount of time. Emotional states (anger, joy etc.) may inhibit hunger contractions. Levels of hunger are increased by lower blood sugar levels, and are higher in diabetics. They reach their greatest intensity in 3 to 4 days and may weaken in the succeeding days, though hunger never disappears. Hunger contractions are most intense in young, healthy people who have high degrees of gastrointestinal tonus. Periods between contractions increase with old age.

Biological Mechanisms

The fluctuation of leptin and ghrelin hormone levels results in the motivation of an organism to consume food. When an organism eats, adipocytes trigger the release of leptin into the body. Increasing levels of leptin results in a reduction of one's motivation to eat. After hours of non-consumption, leptin levels drop significantly. These low levels of leptin cause the release of secondary hormone, ghrelin, which in turn reinitiates the feeling of hunger.

Some studies have suggested that an increased production of grehlin may enhance desire towards perceptive food cues, while an increase in stress may also influence the hormone's production. These findings support why hunger can prevail under stressful situations.

Behavioural Response

Hunger appears to increase activity and movement in many animals—for example, an experiment on spiders showed increased activity and predation in starved spiders, resulting in larger weight gain. This pattern is seen in many animals, including humans while sleeping. It even occurs in rats with their cerebral cortex or stomachs completely removed. Increased activity on hamster wheels occurred when rats were deprived not only of food, but also water or B vitamins such as thiamine This response may increase the animal's chance of finding food, though it has also been speculated the reaction relieves pressure on the home population.

UNDERSTANDING KEY HUNGER TERMS

Hunger: A condition in which people do not get enough food to provide the nutrients for fully productive, active and healthy lives. People living in households where there is hunger are often forced to go without food because they cannot afford to buy it or cannot provide enough for everyone in the household.

Malnutrition: A condition resulting from inadequate consumption (undernutrition) or excessive consumption of one or more nutrients that can impair mental and physical health, and cause or be the consequence of infectious disease.

• *Undernutrition*: A condition resulting from inadequate consumption of calories, protein and/or nutrients to meet the basic physical requirements for an active and healthy life.

Food Insecurity: The limited or uncertain availability or ability to acquire safe, nutritious food in a socially acceptable way. People living in households that are food insecure do not always know how to provide for their next meal and are often forced to cut back on meals or food portions to stretch resources.

Food Security: Assured access to enough nutritious food to sustain an active and healthy life, including: food availability (adequate food supply); food access (people can get to food); and appropriate food use (the body absorption of essential nutrients).

Child Nutrition Programmes: Five federal programmes developed to ensure that children have access to enough nutritious food to grow and learn. The programmes include the Special Supplemental Nutrition Programme for Women, Infants and Children (WIC), the Child and Adult Care Food Programme, the National School Lunch Programme, School Breakfast Programme, and the Summer Food Service Programme.

Elderly Nutrition Programmes: Federal programmes that provide health services and nutritious food to low-income senior citizens including meals delivered to homes or served at church.

Emergency Food: Services provided to people who have no other source of food. Often community-based organizations provide food boxes or hot meals on a periodic basis. Many services use donated food and surplus commodities purchased and distributed by the federal government.

GLOBAL HUNGER CRISIS

Global Crisis

WFP warns that the immediate hunger crisis may ignite more civil unrest as already seen in many developing countries. Here are examples of how the global hunger crisis is affecting many of these nations.

Africa

- High prices of basic commodities in West Africa are impacting people's purchasing power, especially in countries such as Mauritania that depend on imports to feed themselves. If the prices continue to rise, the 2008 'lean' season— the months before the harvest when stocks are low—could start early for many households.
- WFP's food and operations costs are now 30 per cent higher than at the same time last year because of increases in basic food commodities. An additional $183 million are therefore needed for the region.
- Food traders at the Baidoa market in Somalia say the price of the local staple food sorghum and imported rice almost doubled from February to March because of rising global food and fuel prices, widespread insecurity, the record weakness of the Somali shilling against the dollar and a series of poor harvests. Shop keepers say they now have to change their prices twice a day—usually upwards.
- Mauritania's president announced a $112 million emergency plan to fight the impact of high food prices on April 5th. The plan aims to increase food assistance to the poor, increase availability of basic food commodities in the domestic market and boost local agricultural production.
- Mauritania depends on imports for 70 per cent of its food needs. High cereal prices on the international market are leading to an access crisis. Traders are having serious problems importing, mainly due to cash flow constraints. Wheat and sorghum prices have increased by 40 per cent since May 2007 and vegetable oil prices by 25 per cent during the same period.
- In Sierra Leone the price of rice rose by almost 40 per cent during 2007. In the same period the price of palm oil increased by about 50 per cent, and that of bread (wheat

flour) by 25 per cent. In January 2008, the Bread Manufacturers Association called its members out on strike against the rising price of wheat flour, which is manufactured locally with imported wheat.

- In Guinea Bissau the price of imported rice remains 25 per cent above the October 2007 level. The high prices for the national staple may cause hardship when household cereal stocks from the 2007 harvest run out. The most recent food security monitoring survey indicated that some 14 per cent of rural households are either moderately or severely food insecure, with that proportion expected to rise as the lean season (June to October) approaches.

Mideast

- The high price phenomenon comes against a background of worrying food production forecasts. A report issued in March by the Food and Agriculture Organization states that agriculture in the Middle East is likely to suffer losses because of high temperatures, droughts, floods and soil degradation.
- Price rises have an impact on WFP's operations in the region. At present we are providing food to nearly four million people in the Mideast — in Iraq, Syria, Yemen, Egypt and the occupied Palestinian territory.
- Food price rises are having a catastrophic effect on the Syrian economy and the ability of the Government to introduce economic reform measures. Price rises are coinciding with a reduction in oil production (the Government's main source of income). The result is an increase in the number of people needing support and mounting pressure on the social welfare system.
- Newspapers in Egypt are reporting that people have started to go for inferior commodities lacking in nutritional value; they are buying less and less meat/poultry/cheese and they are also cutting down on expenses for education and health expenses, etc. March and April saw several price-related protests.

- To address the concerns about rising food prices, the Government of Egypt has had to boost its spending on subsidies to the poor from 20 billion Egyptian pounds ($4 billion) to 30 billion Egyptian pounds ($6 billion). This includes increased spending on bread subsidies from 9 billion Egyptian pounds to 15 billion Egyptian pounds.
- On 13 February, the Iraq Parliament approved the 2008 Budget and allocated $3.6 billion to the Public Distribution System (PDS) to ensure that food distribution would continue to people in Iraq. Due to commodity price rises worldwide it is difficult to say whether this allocation will be enough to cover the entire year.
- WFP has requested $87.5 million to help feed its caseload of more than 750,000 displaced people in Iraq. It has recently estimated it needs an additional $9 million to cope with rising food and fuel prices.
- Yemen, which imports around 75 per cent of its food requirements, is feeling the impact of rising food prices as so many households spend a large proportion of their income on food. The price of wheat has doubled since February. Other consumer goods have also seen sharp price rises.
- The Government of Yemen is trying to stabilize the market by encouraging more local wheat production and the creation of more silos to store the wheat. It's also encouraging the production and/or importation of mixed (red) wheat which is more nutritious than white (soft) wheat.

Latin America and Caribbean

- Protests in Haiti, which started in early April when rioters attacked UN peacekeepers in Les Cayes, were marked by several deaths. In the wake of the protests the government announced a $10 million package aimed at cutting the cost of living.
- WFP has reiterated its appeal to the international community for urgent funds to support its operations in Haiti, the western hemisphere's poorest country, following the rioting over rising food prices. Riots in Haiti underline

the additional need for lifesaving food assistance. WFP has received so far only 13 per cent ($12.4 million) of the $96 million necessary to assist 1.7 million people in Haiti—barely enough to support operations throughout April. Due to rising costs, WFP recently revised its funding requirements upwards by 22 per cent.

- Due to escalating market prices, in rural El Salvador, with the same amount of money today people can purchase 50 per cent less food than they did 18 months ago. This means that in principle their nutritional intake, on an already poor diet, is being cut by half.
- In Nicaragua the price of tortilla went up 54 per cent between January 2007 and January 2008. In Guatemala the price rose 17 per cent over the same period.
- Price rises have been particularly harsh in Central America where in the past year the price of maize, the key staple food crop, has nearly doubled. The price of beans, another staple commodity, also reached unprecedented levels, partly because of unfavourable weather conditions.
- In response to this situation, WFP is trying to determine the impact of rising food prices on the region's poor in order to anticipate future trends and support national Governments in the region in the adoption of effective intervention and mitigation strategies.
- According to a USDA study, Latin America could bear the brunt of a food price shock. The food gap (the amount of food needed to raise consumption of all income groups to the recognized minimum) could rise 24 per cent by 2016, compared to 8.7 per cent in Asia and 6 per cent in Sub-Saharan Africa.

Asia

- WFP's purchase cost for rice in Bangkok was $ 460 per metric ton on March 3. Five weeks later, it is now $ 780.
- At the end of January, Afghanistan President Hamid Karzai appealed for $77 million to help feed an additional 2.5 million people, now hungry because of rising food prices.

. WFP Food distributions to urban Afghans unable to afford staples began in March.

- Average wheat prices in Afghanistan have increased by 67 per cent since the start of 2007; on average, Afghans who are not engaged in agriculture now spend 75 per cent of their income on food.
- Wheat prices in Tajikistan have increased by 128 per cent over the last year, whilst wheat flour prices increased on average by 76 per cent. The prices of vegetable oil have increased by 126 per cent during this period.
- The Tajikistan government has appealed to the international community for help with fuel and food, reporting to WFP that up to two million people might be in need of food assistance in the coming weeks.
- The price of rice has risen between 25 and 30 per cent throughout Bangladesh over the last three months. In 2007, the price of rice rose around 70 per cent.
- Cambodia has been producing a rice surplus since 1996. However, in 2007, so much rice was exported to neighboring countries to cash in on the higher prices paid by foreign traders that normally self-sufficient Cambodians now face a rice gap.
- WFP in Cambodia risks having to cutting school feeding activities mainly due to price increases. Existing donations had been expected to last until August 2008 but price rises could make the school breakfast programme for 450,000 children unfeasible.
- Partly as a result of increased commodity prices and connected unrest, the Indonesian Government has recently expanded its rice subsidy programme by 50 per cent. The Government plans to provide subsidized rice to an estimated 80 million people.

INTERNATIONAL HUNGER FACTS

World Hunger and Poverty: How They Fit Together

- 854 million people across the world are hungry, up from 852 million a year ago.

- Every day, almost 16,000 children die from hunger-related causes—one child every five seconds.
- In essence, hunger is the most extreme form of poverty, where individuals or families cannot afford to meet their most basic need for food.
- Hunger manifests itself in many ways other than starvation and famine. Most poor people who battle hunger deal with chronic undernourishment and vitamin or mineral deficiencies, which result in stunted growth, weakness and heightened susceptibility to illness.
- Countries in which a large portion of the population battles hunger daily are usually poor and often lack the social safety nets we enjoy, such as soup kitchens, food stamps, and job training programmes. When a family that lives in a poor country cannot grow enough food or earn enough money to buy food, there is nowhere to turn for help.

Facts and Figures on Population

- Today our world houses 6.55 billion people.
- The United States is a part of the developed or industrialized world, which consists of about 57 countries with a combined population of about 1 billion, less than one sixth of the worldâ™s population.
- In contrast, approximately 5.1 billion people live in the developing world. This world is made up of about 125 low and middle-income countries in which people generally have a lower standard of living with access to fewer goods and services than people in high-income countries.
- The remaining 0.4 billion live in countries in transition, which include the Baltic states, eastern Europe and the Commonwealth of Independent States.

Facts and Figures on Hunger and Poverty

- In 2004, almost 1 billion people lived below the international poverty line, earning less than $1 per day.
- Among this group of poor people, many have problems

obtaining adequate, nutritious food for themselves and their families. As a result, 820 million people in the developing world are undernourished. They consume less than the minimum amount of calories essential for sound health and growth.

- Undernourishment negatively affects peopleâ™s health, productivity, sense of hope and overall well-being. A lack of food can stunt growth, slow thinking, sap energy, hinder fetal development and contribute to mental retardation.
- Economically, the constant securing of food consumes valuable time and energy of poor people, allowing less time for work and earning income.
- Socially, the lack of food erodes relationships and feeds shame so that those most in need of support are often least able to call on it.
- Go to the World Food Programme website and click on either "Counting the Hungry" or "Interactive Hunger Map" for presentations on hunger and poverty around the world.

Facts and Figures on Health

- Poor nutrition and calorie deficiencies cause nearly one in three people to die prematurely or have disabilities, according to the World Health Organization.
- Pregnant women, new mothers who breastfeed infants, and children are among the most at risk of undernourishment.
- In 2005, about 10.1 million children died before they reached their fifth birthday. Almost all of these deaths occured in developing countries, 3/4 of them in sub-Saharan Africa and South Asia, the two regions that also suffer from the highest rates of hunger and malnutrition.
- Most of these deaths are attributed, not to outright starvation, but to diseases that move in on vulnerable children whose bodies have been weakened by hunger.
- Every year, more than 20 million low-birth weight babies are born in developing countries. These babies risk dying in infancy, while those who survive often suffer lifelong physical and cognitive disabilities.

- The four most common childhood illnesses are diarrhea, acute respiratory illness, malaria and measles. Each of these illnesses is both preventable and treatable. Yet, again, poverty interferes in parents ability to access immunizations and medicines. Chronic undernourishment on top of insufficient treatment greatly increases a child risk of death.
- In the developing world, 27 per cent of children under 5 are moderately to severely underweight. 10 per cent are severely underweight. 10 per cent of children under 5 are moderately to severely wasted, or seriously below weight for one height, and an overwhelming 31 per cent are moderately to severely stunted, or seriously below normal height for one age.

Facts and Figures on HIV/AIDS

- The spreading HIV/AIDS epidemic has quickly become a major obstacle in the fight against hunger and poverty in developing countries.
- Because the majority of those falling sick with AIDS are young adults who normally harvest crops, food production has dropped dramatically in countries with high HIV/AIDS prevalence rates.
- In half of the countries in sub-Saharan Africa, per capita economic growth is estimated to be falling by between 0.5 and 1.2 per cent each year as a direct result of AIDS.
- Infected adults also leave behind children and elderly relatives, who have little means to provide for themselves. In 2003, 12 million children were newly orphaned in southern Africa, a number expected to rise to 18 million in 2010.
- Since the epidemic began, 25 million people have died from AIDS, which has caused more than 15 million children to lose at least one parent. For its analysis, UNICEF uses a term that illustrates the gravity of the situation; child-headed households, or minors orphaned by HIV/AIDS who are raising their siblings.,
- 1 per cent (ages 15-49) of the world is HIV prevalent (2005 data).

- 1.1 per cent (ages 15-49) of developing countries are HIV prevalent (2005 data).
- Approximately 39.5 million people are living with HIV/ AIDS in the world. Of this figure, 63 per cent live in Sub-Saharan Africa.
- In 2006, 4.3 million people become infected with HIV and 2.9 million people died of AIDS.

VISION FOR FOOD AID IN THE 21ST CENTURY

At the World Food Summit (WFS) in 1996, 186 nations came together and pledged to provide the moral and political leadership needed to alleviate extreme hunger and malnutrition. WFS participant countries pledged to reduce by half the number of undernourished people in the world. Nearly 10 years on, there has been minimal progress toward this historic goal. Globally, undernourishment has declined by 3 per cent.

That means that there are presently more than 850 million people who do not have enough food to eat and 2.7 billion people living on less than $2 a day. And in sub-Saharan Africa the situation has actually worsened since the WFS. There, the combination of political unrest, conflict, drought and disease â□" principally AIDS â□" and continued high population growth adds up to a grim scenario for the coming years.

As countries rich and poor take stock of these tasks, debate continues about the kinds of resources and efforts that will best achieve these goals and the levels required. Part of this debate has focused on food aid. Over the past 50 years, food aid has been one of the principal resources deployed in the effort to end hunger, and a number of donor countries, the United States prominent among them, have channeled billions of dollars' worth of food to developing countries.

This report focuses on the benefits and costs of food aid and set forth recommendations for making food aid more efficient and effective. It is an opportune moment to reflect on how food aid programmes, those of the United States in particular, may be strengthened to achieve hunger and poverty reduction more effectively. U.S. food aid programmes, authorized through the federal farm bill, are on track to be renegotiated in 2007. The United States is also actively engaged in World Trade Organization (WTO) trade negotiations, which will very likely affect food aid practices. Through the dual avenues of the U.S. farm bill and WTO negotiations, it should be possible to improve developing countries' prospects for food security and sustainable development while strengthening donor support for effective food aid programmes.

CASE STUDY: U.S. FOOD AID' ROLE IN REDUCING WORLD HUNGER

In 1996, the World Food Summit set its sights on reducing by half the number of hungry people in the world by 2015. But 8 years after the signing of this declaration, the international community is coming to grips with the fact that it will fall far short of its goal. All indicators developed by ERS lead to the inescapable conclusion that the aggregate food security situation—measured by food availability of many low-income countries—has hardly improved at all in the last decade. Reports from the Food and Agriculture Organization (FAO) of the United Nations tell the same story.

Among the reasons for chronic undernutrition in the poorest countries are slow growth in domestic food production, high population growth, inadequate purchasing power, and frequent setbacks associated with natural and manmade shocks, such as drought, hurricanes, and civil strife. To counter the trend, the ultimate goal is to reduce the impacts of shocks, which reduce food production and consume too many resources in countries with too few to spare. Until that long-term goal can be met, it is critical to strengthen the food safety net in the most vulnerable countries. Because most poor countries do not have national food safety net programmes, they depend on international food aid. But food aid increasingly falls short of needs: quantities change annually, and overall levels have grown only minimally during the life of the programmes. The uncertain availability of food aid, though worrisome, is just one reason why food aid has not played a larger role in reducing world hunger. Differing objectives in food aid programmes, lack of consistency among donors' approaches to food aid, and types of food donated are just a few factors that limit the effectiveness (the degree to which it reduces a country's food gaps) of food aid.

Future of Food Aid Programmes is Uncertain

The global quantity of food aid has fluctuated during the last two decades, and its share has declined relative to both total agricultural exports from food aid suppliers and total food imports of low-income countries. The virtual stagnation in the level of food aid over time is not likely to change, and it may even decline if budgets remain tight. As major donor nations reduce market support to agriculture due to budget constraints as well as to comply with their commitments to the World Trade Organization, decreases in surplus food production will likely follow. The costs of food aid may increase as a result.

As the trend in supplies of food aid has remained relatively flat, the gap between food production and food consumption in low-income countries, and thus the demand for food aid, has widened. According to ERS, the gap between recommended nutritional requirements and purchasing power of the populations in the world's poorest countries was more than 32 million tons in 2003, about four times larger than the supply of food aid in 2002. While this gap is projected to narrow to less than 28 million tons during the next decade, it will likely remain far above the level of available food aid, which may decline.

According to the World Bank, about 1 billion people in developing countries live in poverty with annual per capita incomes of less than $370. In some regions, particularly Sub-Saharan Africa, per capita food consumption has declined in the last two decades, but food aid supplies have not changed since the late 1980s. For these countries, further declines in food consumption from already low levels can lead to severe food shortages, malnutrition, and political instability.

These estimates, however, do not necessarily mean that significant increases in food aid would be able to close these gaps. Given the poor distribution systems in these countries, absorption of large quantities of food imports would be difficult, if not impossible. Nevertheless, targeting efforts in the distribution of food aid need to be improved in order to increase its effectiveness and reduce hunger. There are growing and unresolved questions related to the impacts and the role of food aid. Despite 50 years of food donations, food aid's role in reducing world hunger remains unclear.

How Effective is Food Aid in Improving Food Consumption?

There are three types of food aid, each with a differing objective. Programme food aid is a government-to-government donation that aims to reduce food import costs for the recipient country. Project food aid is used by a government or nongovernment organization to provide support for development projects. Emergency food aid is used to augment food supplies or assist in rebuilding productive assets for countries affected by political or natural disasters.

The different uses of food aid have generated debates on the positive (additional food supplies) and negative (production disincentive due to the decline in local prices) effects of the programmes. Still, food aid is regarded as a valuable resource for increasing food consumption by providing temporary relief from food shortages. But has food aid reduced consumption instability over time? Since the quantities of food aid fall short of the aggregate needs of the study countries, the next question is whether food aid is provided to those who need it the most.

What does food aid contribute to consumption? The overall contribution of food aid to total food consumption in the 70 countries included in ERS's annual Food Security Assessment is small, but the importance of food aid is more pronounced when it is measured at the country level at particular points in time. The 70 countries covered in this exercise include 4 in North Africa, 37 in Sub-Saharan Africa, 10 in Asia, 11 in Latin America and the Caribbean, and 8 in the Commonwealth of Independent States (CIS). Food aid, on average, provided less than 4 per cent of food consumption (grain equivalent) for the 70 countries in the last decade, but the share varied greatly by country and tended to be more significant during emergencies.

- During Somalia's 1992-93 civil war, food aid contributed to about 70 per cent of its consumption.

- When Mozambique was faced with prolonged economic and political difficulties (early 1980s through early 1990s), it often relied on food aid to supplement more than a third of its food consumption.
- In Rwanda during 1997-99, food aid contributed to more than a third of food consumption.
- Since 2000, Eritrea has relied on food aid for about half of its consumption.
- During 2000-02, the largest recipients of food aid were North Korea (4.2 million tons total for the 3 years), Ethiopia (4.0 million tons), Bangladesh (1.4 million tons), and Afghanistan (1.1 million tons). In North Korea, food aid contributed to about 20 per cent of food consumption. In Ethiopia and Bangladesh, food aid's contribution to consumption was less than 10 per cent.

Has food aid stabilized consumption? Food aid clearly had a significant role in reducing the loss of life during food emergencies in such countries as Ethiopia, Sudan, Somalia, Afghanistan, Rwanda, and Haiti. However, over time and at the aggregate level, the impact was less apparent. Based on food consumption data (grain only) in 62 low-income countries, the annual consumption shortfalls from trend in each country (excluding food aid) during 1981-99 exceeded the cumulative quantity of food aid received over the same period by 8 per cent. Ideally, the volume of food aid would have matched the consumption shortfalls. In practice, however, food aid followed a declining trend while consumption shortfalls varied annually: in 5 of the 19 years, aggregate food aid exceeded the consumption shortfalls; in 12 of the years, it was less than the shortfalls; and in only 2 years (1986 and 1992) did the quantities match. The comparisons are much more uneven at the country level.

The Evolution of the 50-Year U.S Initiative

The U.S. food aid programme began in the early 1950s with the enactment of the Agricultural Trade Development and Assistance Act of 1954 (P.L. 480). The programme's objectives include the provision of humanitarian assistance and the support of economic development (project aid) in recipient countries. These objectives are carried out under three broad programmes:

- Title I consists of government-to-government commodity sales and sales to private entities in developing countries under long-term, low-interest credit arrangements.
- Title II provides food as a grant for emergency relief and economic development projects.
- Title III provides for government-to-government grants to support economic development in the least developed countries (1977 amendment); this programme has not received funding since 2001.

The goals of food aid have changed through time, and the importance of food aid as an export outlet has diminished substantially. For example, during the early 1970s, as commercial demand for grains increased dramatically, fewer commodities were available for food aid, and donations fell to their lowest level since the enactment of P.L. 480. During the mid-1980s, increased U.S. grain stocks did not translate into increased food aid because the U.S. Government adopted a targeted export subsidy programme that boosted agricultural exports. With the decline in food aid as a share of exports, the U.S. food aid programme has become more focused toward humanitarian goals. In 1991, for the first time since the start of U.S. food aid programmes, the largest share of the P.L. 480 budget was allocated to Title II to support humanitarian concerns. Between 2001 and 2003, Title II received 85 per cent, on average, of the P.L. 480 budget.

Other food aid programmes include:

- Food for Progress, which provides for the donation or credit sale of U.S. commodities to developing countries and emerging democracies,
- Section 416(b) of the Agricultural Act of 1949, which provides for overseas donations of surplus commodities acquired by the Commodity Credit Corporation, and
- McGovern-Dole International Food for Education and Child Nutrition, which helps support education, child

development, and food security for some of the world's poorest children.

Does food aid respond to needs? The effectiveness of food aid depends on whether it is provided to those who need it most. Distribution food gaps, as estimated by ERS, reflect the amount of food needed to raise consumption of all income groups within a country to the nutritional requirement. This measure captures the differences in purchasing power within a country. Food aid effectiveness is measured on a scale of 0 to 100 per cent, with 0 per cent reflecting food aid given to a country with no needs and 100 per cent reflecting food aid that reduces a country's food gap by its full amount. This method measures actual consumption as related to purchasing power within the countries at the national level and may not capture micro-level specific programmes, such as food for work, which could be location specific.

During 1991-2000, the average effectiveness of food aid was 66 per cent, meaning two-thirds of food aid went toward reducing and/or eliminating the recipient countries' food gaps. The remaining 34 per cent went to countries that either did not have food needs or that had needs less than the amount of food actually received. Regionally, food aid deliveries in Sub-Saharan Africa and Latin America were highly effective in reducing food gaps, averaging about 80 per cent, compared with 40-46 per cent in Asia and the CIS.

The effectiveness of food aid in meeting nutritional needs depends highly on how food aid is allocated and what criteria are used to make allocation decisions. The largest nutritional gain is realized when food aid is targeted to the lowest income group—thus indirectly increasing this group's purchasing power—either in emergency situations or in support of supplementary feeding programmes, such as food stamps. In these cases, food aid changes a country's income distribution indirectly because it allows the lower income group to consume more than expected given its income level. In 2000, about half of food aid was used for emergencies, which can be categorized as targeted. It is not clear how much of the other half was targeted—the effectiveness of other uses of food aid in reducing hunger is difficult to estimate. All food aid reduces food costs in the market, making food more affordable; but without targeting to the most vulnerable group, the benefits of food aid tend to be distributed across the entire population of a country.

What Prevents the Programme From Achieving Its Full Potential?

There are many unresolved issues relating to food aid. After 50 years, there are neither uniform approaches nor transparent criteria among donors regarding decisions to allocate food aid. Programme eligibility criteria are loosely defined, and it is not always clear when an activity stops, and why. Many countries receive food aid for reasons that are not clear. For example, China received wheat in 2000-02 as food aid to finance development projects, but, in turn, donated food (wheat, rice, corn, oils) to North Korea and several African countries during the same period. In addition, it is not clear what governs donor decisions to shift from the use of food aid for development purposes to emergency relief (or vice versa) both within a country and across countries. Such changes have implications (positive or negative) on the coordination and management of food aid between donors and recipients. In each case, it is difficult to measure which potential goals are met (cost effectiveness, meeting recipient needs) and to what extent. Compounding the problem are the changes in annual availability of food aid stemming from donors' political and budgetary considerations. It is an open question whether a programme with this type of characteristic can provide a reliable food safety net, let alone a reliable source of development.

Another issue of concern is the producer disincentive impact of food aid when it is sold for development activities. In such cases, food aid results in lower producer prices, which reduces incentives to produce, thereby creating a growing dependency on food aid. The selection of commodities used for food aid is also raising questions. The growing share of noncereal food aid products, such as vegetable oil, pasta, dried potatoes, dried fish, pulses, sugar, and fresh vegetables, is potentially worrisome. As recently as the early 1990s, these products accounted for only 9 per cent of total food aid donations; 10 years later, the share had jumped to more than 14 per cent. This is problematic because these commodities are higher priced than cereals and, therefore, are not likely to reach the poorest segment of the population. In some cases, these commodities now account for a larger share of the food aid package than cereals. For example, in 2000, noncereals accounted for two-thirds of Georgia's food aid receipts (67,739 tons in grain equivalent).

Toward Improving Effectiveness of Food Aid

The goal of the World Food Summit was to halve global hunger in a little over a decade. Each and every signatory country bears the responsibility of meeting this goal, but short-term economic and political shocks around the world remain serious obstacles. The United States plays a pivotal role within the international food aid system, and its actions have a profound effect on the actions of other donors and the system as a whole. The 50th anniversary of the U.S. food aid programme in 2004 is a timely point to appraise the programme and reexamine plans for the future. The U.S. Action Plan on Food Security, released in March 1999, outlines policies and actions aimed at alleviating hunger at home and abroad. To improve the effectiveness of the international food assistance programme, the action plan made aid to the most food-insecure countries a priority. It is too early to evaluate the impacts of this policy change, but steps are being taken by the U.S. Government to develop transparent methods to monitor the effectiveness of food aid in reducing hunger in recipient countries.

Lessons from the past could be useful toward improving the effectiveness of food aid. For example, emergency food aid has saved lives (response to drought in Ethiopia, 1984-85, 1991, 1999-2000, and Zambia, 1992; response to civil strife in Somalia, 1991-92, and Rwanda, mid-late 1990s; response to Hurricane Mitch in Honduras in 1998-99; response to financial crisis in Indonesia in 1998). Food aid has also proved effective in post-emergency situations.

Who Are the Major Food Aid Donors and Where Does the Aid Go?

The major food aid donors are the United States, European Union (EU), Japan, Canada, and Australia. In the late 1980s, the U.S. provided roughly 7 million tons of food aid per year, or nearly 60 per cent of global food aid donations during the period. The EU share at that time was about 25 per cent. U.S. donations fell considerably from the late 1980s through the mid-1990s, and the U.S. share of world food aid slipped below 50 per cent in 1994-96. This decline was offset by the EU, whose share rose to 35 per cent, and Japan, whose share jumped from less than 4 to nearly 6 per cent. U.S. donations have rebounded considerably, however, and since 2000, the U.S. share of world food aid has surpassed levels of the late 1980s. Conversely, EU donations have slipped, with the EU share averaging less than 20 per cent in recent years.

Countries in Sub-Saharan Africa (SSA) and Asia have been by far the largest recipients of food aid, receiving more than 60 per cent of the volume of food aid during the last 15 years. The food aid share of the two regions has changed over time, depending on the economic and political developments in their respective countries. Severe droughts in the early 1990s resulted in higher food aid shipments to SSA, while political, financial, and natural disasters in the late 1990s triggered a shift in donations to Asia. On a per capita basis, however, food aid receipts are much higher in SSA than in Asia because of differences in population: SSA countries have less than half of the population of lower income Asian countries.

Donors' Shares of Global Food Aid

	U.S.	*EU*	*Japan*	*Canada*
	Percent			
1988	58.1	22.5	3.6	8.6
1989	56.6	27.2	3.9	6.7
1990	59.7	24.6	3.6	7.2
1991	58.1	25.4	3.3	7.3
1992	49.7	35.2	3.0	6.9
1993	63.5	24.4	2.4	3.6
1994	56.1	29.0	2.4	7.1
1995	41.7	39.5	8.7	4.9
1996	44.3	35.5	6.4	5.2
1997	43.3	30.6	4.5	7.3
1998	48.2	22.8	13.7	4.8
1999	63.9	24.3	2.9	2.7
2000	61.5	18.9	4.8	2.7
2001	59.0	18.8	8.8	2.6
2002	64.9	13.8	3.2	1.7
1988-89	57.4	24.8	3.8	7.6
1994-96	47.3	34.7	5.8	5.8
2000-02	61.8	17.2	5.6	2.4

Other uses of food aid, however, have had mixed results, particularly programme food aid, that is, government-to-government donations that are commonly sold in recipient country markets. Programme food aid is a resource transfer and is often used to reduce financial constraints of recipient countries. Therefore, it is not targeted to any specific nutritional or development objectives. Another drawback of programme food aid is the potential for interfering with market functions. The most prevalent food aid commodities are cereals and vegetable oils, commodities most often imported commercially by the recipient. The injection of food aid in this circumstance can disrupt markets and depress producer prices.

There is also evidence that programme food aid, in some instances, has created structural import dependency. For example, programme food aid has encouraged the development of industries, such as poultry farming or wheat milling, that require imports to continue operations even after the termination of the food aid programme.

Overall, the impact of food aid in reducing hunger has fallen short of its potential and, in some cases, has negatively affected the economies of the recipient countries. A more important problem lies in the fact that there is no coordination among donors to establish guidelines for distribution and need-based targeting of food aid. It is an annual budgetary programme, which hinders its flexibility to expand or contract in response to the needs of recipients. However, steps toward transparent goals and criteria for food aid eligibility, length of the programme, and type of programme could enhance its effectiveness and pave the road to improved coordination among donors.

CASE STUDY: FOOD SECURITY IN THE UNITED STATES: HUNGER AND FOOD SECURITY

New Labels Describe Ranges of Food Security

In 2006, USDA introduced new language to describe ranges of severity of food insecurity. USDA made these changes in response to recommendations by an expert panel convened at USDA request by the Committee on National Statistics (CNSTAT) of the National Academies. Even though new labels have been introduced, the methods used to assess households food security have remained unchanged, so statistics for 2005 and later years are directly comparable with those for earlier years for the corresponding categories.

USDA's Revised Labels Describe Ranges of Food Security

General Categories (Old and New Labels are the Same)	*Detailed categories*		
	Old Label	*New Label*	*Description of Conditions in the Household*
Food security	Food security	High food security	No reported indications of food-access problems or limitations
		Marginal food security	One or two reported indications typically of anxiety over food sufficiency or shortage of food in the house. Little or no indication of changes in diets or food intake
Food insecurity	Food insecurity without hunger	Low food security	Reports of reduced quality, variety, or desirability of diet. Little or no indication of reduced food intake
	Food insecurity with hunger	Very low food security	Reports of multiple indications of disrupted eating patterns and reduced food intake

CNSTAT Review and Recommendations

USDA requested the review by CNSTAT to ensure that the measurement methods USDA uses to assess households access or lack of access to adequate food and the language used to describe those conditions are conceptually and operationally sound and that they convey useful and relevant information to policy officials and the public. The panel convened by CNSTAT to conduct this study included economists, sociologists, nutritionists, statisticians, and other researchers. One of the central issues the CNSTAT panel addressed was whether the concepts and definitions underlying the measurement methods especially the concept and definition of hunger and the relationship between hunger and food insecurity were appropriate for the policy context in which food security statistics are used.

The CNSTAT Panel:

- Recommended that USDA continue to measure and monitor food insecurity regularly in a household survey
- Affirmed the appropriateness of the general methodology currently used to measure food insecurity
- Suggested several ways in which the methodology might be refined (contingent on confirmatory research). Research on these issues is currently underway at ERS.

The CNSTAT panel also recommended that USDA make a clear and explicit distinction between food insecurity and hunger. "Food insecurity" the condition assessed in the food security survey and represented in USDA food security reports is a household-level economic and social condition of limited or uncertain access to adequate food. Hunger is an individual-level physiological condition that may result from food insecurity. The word "hunger," the panel stated in its final report, "...should refer to a potential consequence of food insecurity that, because of prolonged, involuntary lack of food, results in discomfort, illness, weakness, or pain that goes beyond the usual uneasy sensation." To measure hunger in this sense would require collection of more detailed and extensive information on physiological experiences of individual household members than could be accomplished effectively in the context of the CPS. The panel recommended, therefore, that new methods be developed to measure hunger and that a national assessment of hunger be conducted using an appropriate survey of individuals rather than a survey of households.

The CNSTAT panel also recommended that USDA consider alternative labels to convey the severity of food insecurity without using the word "hunger," since hunger is not adequately assessed in the food security survey. USDA concurs with this recommendation and, accordingly, has introduced the new labels "low food security" and "very low food security."

Characteristics of Households with Very Low Food Security

Conditions reported by households with very low food security are compared with those reported by food-secure households and by households with low (but not very low) food security.

The defining characteristic of very low food security is that, at times during the year, the food intake of household members is reduced and their normal eating patterns are disrupted because the household lacks money and other resources for food. Very low food security can be characterized in terms of the conditions that households in this category typically report in the annual food security survey. In the 2006 survey, households classified as having very low food security reported the following specific conditions:

- 98 per cent reported having worried that their food would run out before they got money to buy more.
- 96 per cent reported that the food they bought just did not last and they did not have money to get more.
- 94 per cent reported that they could not afford to eat balanced meals.
- 95 per cent reported that an adult had cut the size of meals or skipped meals because there was not enough money for food.
- 85 per cent reported that this had occurred in 3 or more months.
- 95 per cent of respondents reported that they had eaten less than they felt they should because there was not enough money for food.
- 69 per cent of respondents reported that they had been hungry but did not eat because they could not afford enough food.
- 46 per cent of respondents reported having lost weight because they did not have enough money for food.

- 33 per cent reported that an adult did not eat for a whole day because there was not enough money for food.
- 24 per cent reported that this had occurred in 3 or more months.

All households without children that were classified as having very low food security reported at least six of these conditions, and 71 per cent reported seven or more. Conditions in households with children were similar, but the reported food-insecure conditions of both adults and children were taken into account.

10

Food/Livelihood Security and Food Shortage Challenges: Role of Agricultural Production, Demand and Trade

FOOD SECURITY AS A GLOBAL CONCERN

In recent decades, demographic and economic growth have challenged the limits of economic, social, and ecological sustainability, giving rise to questions about food security at the global level. Despite technological advances that have modernized the conditions of production and distribution of food, hunger and malnutrition still threaten the health and well-being of millions of people around the world.

Access to food is still perceived by many as a privilege, rather than a basic human right, and it is estimated that about 35,000 people around the world die each day from hunger. An even larger number of people (mainly women, children, and the elderly) suffer from malnutrition. Far from disappearing, hunger and malnutrition are on the increase, even in advanced industrialized countries like Canada, where each year an estimated 2.5 million people depend on food banks. About 30 million people in the United States are reported to be unable to buy enough food to maintain good health. The continuing reality of hunger and the unsustainability of current practices, both locally and globally, make food security an essential concern.

According to the United Nations Food and Agriculture Organization's (FAO's) widely accepted definition,

"Food security" means that food is available at all times; that all persons have means of access to it; that it is nutritionally adequate in terms of quantity, quality and variety; and that it is acceptable within the given culture. Only when all these conditions are in place can a population be considered "food secure."

To achieve lasting self-reliance at the national and household levels, initiatives must be founded on the principles of economic feasibility, equity, broad participation, and the sustainable use of natural resources.

In recent years, most of the research initiatives for food security have focused on four key components of the FAO's definition:

- *Availability*: Providing a sufficient supply of food for all people at all times has historically been a major challenge. Although technical and scientific innovations have made important contributions focused on quantity and economies of scale, little attention has been paid to the sustainability of such practices.
- *Accessibility*: The equality of access to food is a dimension of food security. Within and between societies, inequities have resulted in serious entitlement problems, reflecting class, gender, ethnic, racial, and age differentials, as well as national and regional gaps in development. Most measures to provide emergency food aid have attempted to help the disadvantaged but have had limited success in overcoming the structural conditions that perpetuate such inequities.
- *Acceptability*: As essential ingredients in human health and well-being, food and food practices reflect the social and cultural diversity of humanity. Efforts to provide food without paying attention to the symbolic role of food in people's lives have failed to solve food-security problems. This dimension of food security is also important in determining whether information and food-system innovations will be accepted in a country, given the social and ecological concerns of its citizens.
- *Adequacy*: Food security also requires that adequate measures are in place at all levels of the food system to guarantee the sustainability of production, distribution, consumption, and waste management. A sustainable food

> system should help to satisfy basic human needs, without compromising the ability of future generations to meet their needs. It must therefore maintain ecological integrity and integrate conservation and development.

Unfortunately, a number of global economic and ecological problems continue to limit the prospect of global food security. World per capita cereal production (62% of least-developed countries' [LDCs'] food consumption), for example, has been increasing only marginally in recent years. In fact, it has even been on the decline in sub-Saharan Africa and in Latin America and the Caribbean, particularly in low-income countries struck by economic reforms, natural and other disasters, and other factors. The LDCs' dependence on net food imports has been growing and is set to continue to grow; currently, 104 of 132 LDCs are net importers, although imports have brought little relief overall (Singer 1997). In sub-Saharan Africa, the number of chronically undernourished people more than doubled in 1970-91, notwithstanding that this region depended on food aid for half its total food imports. The population of this region is expected to more than double by 2020 (de Haen and Lindland 1997).

Regional and global economic crises and chronic problems of underdevelopment make the situation particularly bad in the developing world. The overall mean per capita income of so-called Black Africa, for example, is, at its best, no higher than it was in 1960, and the region has less weight in the global economy today than it did in the 1960s (Brandt 1997). Economic informalization clearly accompanies an economy's disintegration. Real prices in domestic food markets have increased over the last few years and are set to increase further. To improve food security and global food supplies, policy scenarios of the 2020 Vision Initiative require increased exports of staple foods from industrialized countries to the LDCs (von Braun 1997). But insufficient purchasing power among the world's poorest 800 million people remains a primary obstacle to such strategies.

Multilateral agreements in trade and investment further threaten the availability and accessibility of food for large segments of the world's population. Many experts agree that the reduction in world surpluses and the increase in international prices encouraged by the Uruguay Round of the General Agreement on Tariffs and Trade pose an immediate threat to regions already suffering severe food insecurity. The duration of this threat is unknown.

Global prospects for improving food security are further threatened by environmental limitations on production increases, even in Green Revolution countries, and by growing poverty. In Asia, a large share of the population will soon be without access to adequate food supplies (Zarges 1997). So, despite the technical modernization of food production and distribution, hunger and malnutrition still undermine the health and well-being of millions of people and actually seem to be worsening, particularly among low-income urban residents. This led Dr Uwe Werblow (1997) of the European Commission in Brussels to recommend favouring production of more traditional food crops in rural areas and developing non-land-using production in peri-urban and urban areas.

Food Security and Urban Populations

Although the consequences can be visible, the causes and the scope of food-security problems for urban populations may not be apparent. From production to consumption, the food system comprises complex interrelated and interdependent parts: social and economic elements, agencies, processes, and structures. Their interdependent relationship requires a structural and systemic analysis focusing on global as well as local linkages. The rural-urban and local-global interrelationships make it impossible to study urban food-security issues in isolation. Yet, it is also clear that the extraordinary urban growth in the 20th century and increasing threats to food security for millions of urban dwellers merits particular attention. The scope and urgency of the problems require analyses of food-security questions for urban areas and new policies and practices to encourage the adoption of sustainable urban food systems.

Food security has become an increasing concern of urban populations. We identify four major challenges to focus our analysis. First, urban centres have expanded enormously, in population and in size. In the 20th century, urban growth has reached unprecedented levels in most parts of the world. In three recent decades alone, the urban population in developed countries doubled, from 448 million in 1950 to 875 million in 1990. In the same period the urban population in developing countries more than quintupled, from 280 million to 1.6 billion. In 1990, 33 per cent of the world's urban population was living in cities with 1 million or more inhabitants. By the end of this century, six of the largest cities will be found in the developing world. Having urban settlements approaching 30 million people will likely strain already overburdened services in countries with limited resources and extreme income inequalities. Urban expansion has converted a significant portion of green space and good-quality, often scarce, agricultural land. It has already increased water and air pollution and created serious waste-disposal problems. Also, zoning bylaws, speculative land markets, and soil and water contamination have created obstacles to effective local food systems and urban agriculture.

A second challenge has been the unevenness of access to food. Historically, poverty has been predominantly a rural phenomenon. Yet, as the majority of the world's population moves to urban areas, we are seeing a reversal in the regional distribution of poverty. World Bank (1990) figures indicated that in 1988 about 25 per cent of the poorest segments of the developing world were living in urban areas. The World Bank also estimated that by 2000 this will reach 50 per cent (World Bank 1990). In developing countries, the ranks of the urban poor have swelled as a result of such factors as the continuous migration of the rural poor into the cities, the limited ability of the urban informal sector to absorb the unemployed, the limited employment opportunities in formal labour markets, negative impacts of the global economic crisis, and the austerity measures adopted to deal with foreign debt. In Eastern Europe and the industrialized West the situation is not much better. A decline in full-time, secure, well-paid employment (the result of economic downsizing), the dismantling of the welfare state and social programmes, and the feminization of poverty have turned urban poverty into a truly global phenomenon. Most observers agree that the increase in poverty has been the biggest threat to food security. Unfortunately, most of the solutions have been limited to patchwork remedies, such as food banks, food aid, and similar emergency responses.

The third challenge is overcoming the inability of the existing market and service agencies to respond to the highly diverse social and cultural mosaic of the urban population. The complexity of cities — the diversity of their class, gender, ethnic, and demographic characteristics and their corresponding needs and access problems— creates new challenges in the attempt to ensure urban food security. Although the markets and traditional service agencies target certain "consumers," thousands of others are marginalized. Food retail chains often ignore poor neighbourhoods in the North and South alike, and the location of bulk-produce stores in suburbs limits the access of smaller families, elderly people, people with disabilities, and those who depend on public transit. The diversity of food practices arising from most cities' complex ethnic composition also creates distinct access problems. Unfortunately, most retailers, food banks, and public-service agencies fail to respond to the unique traditions of cultural minorities and thereby pressure people into making significant dietary changes to conform to what the dominant food system provides.

The fourth challenge is the growing commodification and globalization of the agrifood system. The majority of people in urban populations have very little understanding of how their food is produced, transported, processed, or distributed. The dominant structures of production, distribution, and marketing of food often ignore local solutions for efficient and accessible production and distribution. Although the global food system claims to offer more choice at an affordable cost for the individual consumer, it has actually created obstacles for more sustainable local food systems. In many places, even in-season, locally grown foods tend to be more expensive or more difficult to find than those shipped in from thousands of miles away (Bonanno et al. 1994; McMichael 1994; Goodman and Watts 1997). Often food grown locally is exported while thousands of local residents may be suffering hunger and malnutrition. Questions can be raised about the long-term economic, ecological, and political sustainability of the so-called success of the current food system, with its global division of labour, commodified food economy, increasing regional specialization, industrialized agriculture, and transcontinental networks of distribution.

Most of the papers in this section were presented at the International Conference on Sustainable Urban Food Systems, organized by the Centre for Studies in Food Security, at Ryerson Polytechnic University, Toronto, with the cooperation of the International Development Research Centre, FoodShare Toronto, Oxfam Canada, and the Toronto Food Policy Council. The conference was hosted by the university in May 1997, and the aim was to include research papers, opinion pieces, and visionary papers to create a forum to stimulate further discussion and generate new ideas in this field. This volume reflects the original intention of the conference by bringing together the contributions of a group of academics, community organizers, policymakers, practitioners, and youth representatives. The authors are concerned about food-security issues and have been involved in research and applied projects in the field. These projects, grounded in the practices of everyday life, involve the work of street vendors, antihunger advocates, environmentally conscious chefs, and urban gardeners. However trivial they may be, they have generated a sense of hope in others involved in similar small-scale projects all over the world.

This section aims to develop a conceptual and practical framework for sustainable urban food systems. Several papers propose ways to improve the availability and accessibility of food for urban residents and the feasibility of various forms of more self-reliant local food systems. For instance, the book contains insights on how existing structures for marketing and distribution can improve accessibility, why and how different forms of urban food production and distribution are emerging, and how these structures can become part of local food systems that better respond to food-security needs, especially those of urban dwellers.

To reflect the global nature of the dominant food system, the conference participants were drawn from both the North and the South to share their concerns about food security and their experiences of local and global initiatives for sustainable food systems worldwide. The book covers a range of issues, such as urban food systems, local food systems, urban and community agriculture, gender roles in food-security strategies, hunger and income insecurities, and health and ecological concerns, and points out the linkages among these. The reader can learn from the rich sample of case studies.

This volume, like the conference, is more of an open invitation to scholars, practitioners, and policymakers to focus their attention on urban food-security concerns. Food is an essential part of life. Therefore, food-security concerns require public awareness. Changes in the food system require public regulation and cannot be left to the vagaries of the marketplace. Although the achievements of the dominant food system are worth acknowledging, its fairness, sustainability, and feasibility are highly questionable. Given the rising populations of megacities, the food-security needs of urban populations will require governments to develop comprehensive and participatory interventions to avoid future catastrophes. The surest ways to avoid disaster are to be prepared and to understand the nature of the problems, as well as the available opportunities. Most of the papers included in this volume identify a number of common concerns and solutions:

- Local food systems offer long-term sustainable solutions, both for the environment and for local and regional economic development. By linking the productive activities in the surrounding bioregion to the consumers in metropolitan centres, local food systems can reduce greenhouse gases and other pollutants caused by long-distance transportation and storage. They can reduce the vulnerability of food-supply systems to the impacts of weather and market-related supply problems of distant producers, offer greater choice through regional variations in biodiversity, provide fresher and more nutritious products in season, allow for more effective regional control of quality and chemical inputs, and create the potential for local development and employment opportunities. A regional or national network of local food systems does not necessarily diminish the possible advantages of the global food system for food security; rather, it would enhance these advantages.

- Cities need to encourage urban and peri-urban agriculture, aquaculture, food forestry, and animal husbandry, as well as safe waste recycling, as elements of more self-reliant local food-system initiatives. Food and nonfood production can tap idle resources and, through income and savings, improve food security, local employment, and urban resource management. From a food-democracy viewpoint, one's right to be fed needs to embrace one's right to feed oneself. Future plans for the flexible, creative, and combined use of urban space and form need to include permanent and temporary food production within metropolitan regions and to create land reserves for productive green space.
- Cities and metropolitan regions need to give priority to the availability and accessibility of food and develop their own food-security plans as part of their social and economic planning. Food-policy councils should be formed to advise local governments and planners.
- Food banks and other community assistance programmes should only be relied on as emergency measures, rather than being institutionalized as permanent mechanisms for food access. Food banks often serve two goals: to assist low-income consumers and to distribute surplus food. To reduce poverty and inequities in access, structural measures need to be undertaken to provide long-term food security. At the same time, mechanisms for distribution of surplus food can be developed to respond to specific community needs, without stigmatizing the poor.
- No single solution will solve the problem of food insecurity. What is needed is a list of choices and a commitment to the principles of food security (listed above). The best recipe we can offer is to establish globally interlinked local food systems that use diverse technical, social, and economic resources to improve the availability and accessibility of sustainably produced and distributed, culturally acceptable food. Reaching this goal requires unique local solutions, as well as global cooperation to solve common problems.

- Finally, the concept of food democracy was the central theme of the conference's keynote speaker, Tim Lang. Moving beyond the notion that consumers act as rational beings who focus on their individual interests, the concept of food democracy (or food citizenship) recognizes that consumers can identify the interests of others (food workers, other consumers, future generations, and other species). As citizens, we can participate in shaping the food system and the ways consumption of food in our communities expresses the values of family and culture.

Given the complexity of the food chain and the limitations of a conference setting, it is practically impossible to include or even claim to do justice to all dimensions of urban food-security questions. Our goal was to create a forum by inviting people who share similar concerns and a similar desire to achieve a sustainable food system. We accept and respect the diversity of opinions on this issue, and we do not claim to offer all the answers. While focusing on urban food systems we recognize that cities have evolved as hubs of economic and cultural life — their success in terms of dense populations is also the source of their vulnerability — and that their survival depends on the ways they relate to their local, regional, national, and global contexts.

NEW CHALLENGE ON FOOD FRONT

A fast-unfolding food shortage is engulfing the entire world, driving food prices to record highs. Over the past half-century grain prices have spiked from time to time because of weather-related events, such as the 1972 Soviet crop failure that led to a doubling of world wheat, rice, and corn prices. The situation today is entirely different, however. The current doubling of grain prices is trend-driven, the cumulative effect of some trends that are accelerating growth in demand and other trends that are slowing the growth in supply.

The world has not experienced anything quite like this before. In the face of rising food prices and spreading hunger, the social order is beginning to break down in some countries. In several provinces in Thailand, for instance, rustlers steal rice by harvesting fields during the night. In response, Thai villagers with distant fields have taken to guarding ripe rice fields at night with loaded shotguns.

In Sudan, the U.N. World Food Programme (WFP), which is responsible for supplying grain to 2 million people in Darfur refugee camps, is facing a difficult mission to say the least. During the first three months of this year, 56 grain-laden trucks were hijacked. Thus far, only 20 of the trucks have been recovered and some 24 drivers are still unaccounted for. This threat to U.N.-supplied food to the Darfur camps has reduced the flow of food into the region by half, raising the specter of starvation if supply lines cannot be secured.

In Pakistan, where flour prices have doubled, food insecurity is a national concern. Thousands of armed Pakistani troops have been assigned to guard grain elevators and to accompany the trucks that transport grain.

Food riots are now becoming commonplace. In Egypt, the bread lines at bakeries that distribute state-subsidized bread are often the scene of fights. In Morocco, 34 food rioters were jailed. In Yemen, food riots turned deadly, taking at least a dozen lives. In Cameroon, dozens of people have died in food riots and hundreds have been arrested. Other countries with food riots include Ethiopia, Haiti, Indonesia, Mexico, the Philippines, and Senegal.

The doubling of world wheat, rice, and corn prices has sharply reduced the availability of food aid, putting the 37 countries that depend on the WFP's emergency food assistance at risk. In March, the WFP issued an urgent appeal for $500 million of additional funds.

Around the world, a politics of food scarcity is emerging. Most fundamentally, it involves the restriction of grain exports by countries that want to check the rise in their domestic food prices. Russia, the Ukraine, and Argentina are among the governments that are currently restricting wheat exports. Countries restricting rice exports include Viet Nam, Cambodia, and Egypt. These export restrictions simply drive prices higher in the world market.

The chronically tight food supply the world is now facing is driven by the cumulative effect of several well established trends that are affecting both global demand and supply. On the demand side, the trends include the continuing addition of 70 million people per year to the earth's population, the desire of some 4 billion people to move up the food chain and consume more grain-intensive livestock products, and the recent sharp acceleration in the U.S. use of grain to produce ethanol for cars. Since 2005, this last source of demand has raised the annual growth in world grain consumption from roughly 20 million tons to 50 million tons.

Meanwhile, on the supply side, there is little new land to be brought under the plow unless it comes from clearing tropical rainforests in the Amazon and Congo basins and in Indonesia, or from clearing land in the Brazilian cerrado, a savannah-like region south of the Amazon rainforest. Unfortunately, this has heavy environmental costs: the release of sequestered carbon, the loss of plant and animal species, and increased rainfall runoff and soil erosion. And in scores of countries prime cropland is being lost to both industrial and residential construction and to the paving of land for roads, highways, and parking lots for fast-growing automobile fleets.

New sources of irrigation water are even more scarce than new land to plow. During the last half of the twentieth century, world irrigated area nearly tripled, expanding from 94 million hectares in 1950 to 276 million hectares in 2000. In the years since then there has been little, if any, growth. As a result, irrigated area per person is shrinking by 1 per cent a year.

Meanwhile, the backlog of agricultural technology that can be used to raise cropland productivity is dwindling. Between 1950 and 1990 the world's farmers raised grainland productivity by 2.1 per cent a year, but from 1990 until 2007 this growth rate slowed to 1.2 per cent a year. And the rising price of oil is boosting the costs of both food production and transport while at the same time making it more profitable to convert grain into fuel for cars.

Beyond this, climate change presents new risks. Crop-withering heat waves, more-destructive storms, and the melting of the Asian mountain glaciers that sustain the dry-season flow of that region's major rivers, are combining to make harvest expansion more difficult. In the past the negative effect of unusual weather events was always temporary; within a year or two things would return to normal. But with climate in flux, there is no norm to return to.

The collective effect of these trends makes it more and more difficult for farmers to keep pace with the growth in demand. During seven of the last eight years, grain consumption exceeded production. After seven years of drawing down stocks, world grain carryover stocks in 2008 have fallen to 55 days of world consumption, the lowest on record. The result is a new era of tightening food supplies, rising food prices, and political instability. With grain stocks at an all-time low, the world is only one poor harvest away from total chaos in world grain markets.

Business-as-usual is no longer a viable option. Food security will deteriorate further unless leading countries can collectively mobilize to stabilize population, restrict the use of grain to produce automotive fuel, stabilize climate, stabilize water tables and aquifers, protect cropland, and conserve soils. Stabilizing population is not simply a matter of providing reproductive health care and family planning services. It requires a worldwide effort to eradicate poverty. Eliminating water shortages depends on a global attempt to raise water productivity similar to the effort launched a half-century ago to raise land productivity, an initiative that has nearly tripled the world grain yield per hectare. None of these goals can be achieved quickly, but progress toward all is essential to restoring a semblance of food security.

This troubling situation is unlike any the world has faced before. The challenge is not simply to deal with a temporary rise in grain prices, as in the past, but rather to quickly alter those trends whose cumulative effects collectively threaten the food security that is a hallmark of civilization. If food security cannot be restored quickly, social unrest and political instability will spread and the number of failing states will likely increase dramatically, threatening the very stability of civilization itself.

GLOBAL FOOD SHORTAGE

Food prices have risen steeply over the past two years and farmers last week warned the cost of basic items such as bread, milk and meat would jump again this year, mainly due to soaring commodity prices. "Year on year, humanity now eats more than it produces," he said.

And the need for protein, especially from China and India, was growing faster still with demand expected to more than double by 2050.

"Cities are now taking much of the water that was used to grow food, while ground water levels are falling in every country where it is used for food," he said.

"We are losing land. We are building on it, eroding and degrading it or locking it in conservation reserves.

"By 2050 we will have to feed the equivalent of 13 billion people at today's level of nutrition," he said.

Also in National

- Bingle eulogy: 'I love my Dad'-Lara's tribute
- Sydney: More terror raids tipped
- Pay talks: Qantas staff call off strike
- Extradition: Mokbel begins journey home
- Animal attack: Man gored by 100kg stag
- Ooops: Arsonist torches himself
- Embryo agony: Girl's twin found inside her
- Sad goodbye: Saddle Club star farewelled
- Topless protest: Pensioners strip off
- Police shooting: 'Sorry you had to kill my son'
- Taxes targeted but: Nelson 'won't block budget'
- Drug charges: McKenney's court no-show
- Binge drinking: 'Lift beer tax too'—Coke
- Logged off: Hacker shuts down government
- Final viewing: Woman buried in wrong grave
- Font size: Decrease Increase
- Email article: Email
- Print article: Print

WORLD AGRICULTURAL PRODUCTION, DEMAND AND TRADE

Global Trends in Production and Demand

World agricultural production has been increasing steadily, outstripping world population growth by a widening margin since the 1960s. However, world agricultural growth (for all products) has actually been slowing down, from 3 per cent per annum (p.a.) in the 1960s to 2 per cent p.a. in the mid-1990s. But the deceleration in world population growth over the same period was even greater, falling from the peak of 2.07 per cent p.a. to its current level of 1.34 per cent in 1995-2000. There have been significant inter-regional disparities in production growth and demographic profiles which underlie the geographical distribution of global demand.

World production of and demand for agricultural products have shown a declining growth trend since the 1970s. While production grew on average at 2.28 per cent p.a. during the 1970s and consumption by 2.3 per cent, their rates of expansion slowed during the 1980s to stand, in the eight years up to 1997, at 1.97 per cent and 1.91 per cent, respectively. The picture varies among products. Production growth rates increased significantly for vegetables, fats and oils, tropical fruit, roots crops and eggs, and since the 1980s for millet and sorghum also; they fell notably for most basic foodstuffs (i.e. cereals, meats and dairy products) and declined sharply for other agricultural products during the 1980s; but they have since rebounded (not always to pre-1980s rates) in 1990-1997.

In the developing countries (taken as a group), production and consumption have been growing at much higher (and increasing) rates than in either the developed countries or the economies in transition. In fact, in the economies in transition there were sharp absolute declines in both production and consumption in 1990-1997, reflecting the economic dislocations associated with systemic changes in these countries. Demand in developing countries as a whole accelerated from an annual rise of around 3 per cent in 1970-1979 to about 4.1 per cent in 1990-1997. Production growth lagged somewhat behind, but rose nevertheless from 2.8 per cent to about 3.9 per cent over the same period. By contrast, the developed countries' production growth rate decelerated to 0.68 per cent from 1.8 per cent in the 1970s and recovered somewhat in the 1990s. Their growth of consumption of agricultural products also decelerated, falling from 1.5 per cent to around 0.5 per cent.

The developing countries accounted for much of the growth in overall commodity demand since the 1970s because of their higher population growth, their comparatively buoyant per caput GDP expansion and the greater responsiveness of their demand to income growth. By contrast, a slower growth in demand occurred in the developed countries, because already high current per caput consumption and slow growth of population had a dampening effect on demand for many commodities. As a result of these relative growth rates, developing countries have steadily increased their share in world production and consumption of nearly all the main agricultural commodities. Nevertheless, in per caput terms, their production and particularly consumption (in kilograms per person) remain far below those of both the developed countries and the economies in transition.

Among the developing countries, East and South Asia have made the most impressive gains in production since 1970, more than doubling their cereals production and increasing their share of global cereals output from 31 per cent to 38 per cent. They increased output of vegetable oils more than five-fold and raised their share of global production from 25 per cent to 44 per cent. Their production of livestock products more than trebled, raising their share of global production from 25 per cent to 45 per cent. However, their production still lags behind consumption, so that East and South Asia have not increased their presence in world export markets, with the exception of vegetable oils. They have tended rather to increase imports as well as production to supply rapidly growing domestic markets. In contrast with the other commodities, vegetable oil exports from East and South Asia have increased from 19 per cent to 44 per cent of the world market.

The developing countries of Latin America and the Caribbean also increased production faster than the world average, raising their shares of global production, consumption and trade for a number of commodities. Their share of global vegetable oils production increased from 9 per cent to 13 per cent and exports from 11 per cent to 15 per cent. Although their share in global production of fruit and vegetables was unchanged during the period, their exports of these products increased from 20 per cent of world exports to 32 per cent. However, Latin American and Caribbean countries raised their domestic consumption faster than the world average, increasing their share of global consumption for all commodity categories except fruit and vegetables.

The countries of North Africa and the Near East have made

few gains in production (or exports) of agricultural products, relative to world totals. However, some expansion of production and much higher imports brought about a substantial increase in domestic consumption from 1970 to 1997 in cereals, vegetable oils, livestock products and fruit and vegetables.

The countries of sub-Saharan Africa have had little success in increasing their share in world agricultural production, consumption, imports or exports. In some cases their small share of world consumption has declined further. Between 1970 and 1997, their production of cereals and livestock products grew slightly faster than the global average, increasing their share of global production by less than one percentage point. Their share of global cereals and livestock product consumption also grew by less than one percentage point. Production of vegetable oils and fruit and vegetables grew considerably slower, shrinking the region's share of global production from 9 per cent to 5 per cent for vegetable oils and from 7 per cent to 5 per cent for fruit and vegetables. The region's consumption of these products grew at a slower pace than the world average and thus shrank as a share of global consumption.

CASE STUDY: DEVELOPMENTS IN GLOBAL AGRICULTURAL MARKETS

Introduction

Developments in agricultural markets for the period 1995-1998 and considers whether any changes of note may be attributable to the implementation of the Uruguay Round (UR) Agreement on Agriculture (AoA). The analysis covers products that have generally been subject to high levels of protection and support (e.g. cereals, meat and dairy products and sugar) as well as some commodities that have faced relatively lower barriers, such as primary tropical products (coffee, cocoa, tea). This is followed by an analysis of changes in price variability for particular products.

For several commodities, the period 1995-1998 was a reasonably buoyant one for trade and prices and, in a number of cases, the resilient market was due partly to the implementation of commitments made in the Uruguay Round. This is mainly the case for cereals and meat, where export subsidy reductions, the opening of minimum access commitments and income-induced demand effects have had some impact. Prices of many products rose during the period because stocks had been drawn down, in part because of the gradual reduction of government intervention in agricultural commodity markets. However, in the case of most of the other major agricultural commodities, developments in 1995-1998 had more to do with special factors, such as weather, the phase of the commodity cycle or developments in other markets, e.g. synthetics or competing products.

The subsequent weakness of many agricultural prices in 1998 underlines the important role of other factors, including the financial crises and resulting economic slowdown that have affected many countries. Still, the trend towards liberalisation and the reduced government intervention in commodity markets—whether or not due to the UR—have also played a role.

Analysis by Commodity

Wheat

In 1995-1998, world wheat production was about 10 per cent above the average for 1984-1994, while both world trade and opening stocks were below the average (Table 1 and Figure 1). World prices rose strongly in 1995-1996 because of successive poor crops in 1994 and 1995 and the low level of stocks in major exporting countries. The latter was due largely to a deliberate policy to cut carryover stocks, which was associated with the adoption of market-oriented policies consistent with the UR in a number countries. In addition, export subsidies fell well below UR commitments (in 1995 only 6 per cent of the total allowed was used). The surge in prices caused a strong expansion in output in 1996 and 1997, which led to stock replenishment and falling prices. Despite falling in 1997 and 1998, prices in 1995-1998 were on average nearly 9 per cent higher than in 1984-1994.

Table 10.1: Agricultural Commodities in 1985-94 and 1995-98: Average World Production, Trade, Stocks and Prices

Commodity	*Period*	*Production*	*Trade*	*Stocks*	*Prices US$/Tonne*
		Million Tonnes			
Wheat	1985-94	538	96	143	140
	1995-98	588	94	118	166
Coarse Grains	1985-94	825	90	167	102
	1995-98	885	91	130	125
Rice (milled)	1985-94	337	13	58	258
	1995-98	378	22	54	330
Sugar	1985-94	107	28	36	205
	1995-98	124	35	43	252
Fats and Oils	1985-94	74.6	26.9		490
	1995-98	96.2	43.6		592
Oilmeals	1985-94	124.1	57.1		206
	1995-98	152.7	72.8		228
Bovine meat	1985-94	54.0	5.81		2575
	1995-98	42.1	6.7		1831
Pigmeat	1985-94	68.6	4.1		3077
	1995-98	80.8	5.7		2532
Poultry	1985-94	40.3	2.8		1009
	1995-98	57.8	6.7		881
Ovine meat	1985-94	6.8	0.87		2708
	1995-98	7.3	0.88		3151
Milk	1985-94	529	53.1		1386
	1995-98	543	63.6		1867
Coffee	1985-94	5.9	4.5		2221
	1995-98	6.0	4.6		2662
Cocoa	1985-94	2.4	1.8		1524
	1995-98	3.0	2.0		1546
Tea	1985-94	2.5	1.1		1901
	1995-98	2.8	1.2		1882
Bananas	1985-94	47.2	8.4		561
	1995-98	57.9	11.7		590
Jute	1985-94	3.6	0.4		334
	1995-98	3.2	0.4		344
Cotton	1985-94	19.2	5.8		1498
	1995-98	19.2	5.8		1785
Rubber	1985-94	5.3	3.5		918
	1995-98	6.6	4.8		1226

Source: FAO

For wheat and coarse grains (maize) prices are for crop years ending in June. Wheat, HRW No. 2. Maize, US yellow No. 2. Milled rice, Thai 100 per cent. Sugar, raw ISA. Soybean oil./Soybeanmeal. SMP.

Coarse Grains

During 1995-1998, global production of coarse grains was 7 per cent higher and trade was 2 per cent higher than in 1985-1994. On the other hand, opening carryover stocks were as much as 28 per cent below the average for the previous decade. During 1995-1998, export prices for maize of United States and Argentine origin were above the pre-UR average.

World prices of coarse grains increased steeply in 1995-1996. This rise can be explained by a 10 per cent decrease in production—due to a combination of bad weather and policy measures—precisely at a moment when stocks had been drawn down and demand was firm. Furthermore, during 1995, imports by Japan, the Republic of Korea and Thailand exceeded their tariff quota levels, and WTO members used only 27 per cent of their export subsidy ceilings, putting additional upward pressure on prices. Following the sharp price rise, production of coarse grains recovered during 1996-1997 and demand weakened, causing prices to fall. Some of the recent price declines can be ascribed to relatively weak demand for livestock products, in part due to the Asian financial crisis.

Rice

Compared with the 1985-1994 average, production of rice (in its milled equivalent) in 1995-1998 was 12 per cent (41 million tonnes) higher, trade as much as 70 per cent higher, and stocks 7 per cent lower. Prices of Thai long grain rice were well above the previous period levels and remained so in 1998. The same was true of US long grain and Thai broken rice.

It would be inappropriate to ascribe the tightness of global rice markets during 1995-1998 entirely to the UR, because other factors have also played a role. For example, the sharp price increase observed in 1994 and part of 1995 was mainly related to the drought in Japan. Some slackening of prices during 1996 and 1997 reflected a general improvement in production in all major importing countries. Conversely, the price increases in 1998 reflected the poor harvests in major rice-importing countries in Southeast Asia and in South America, due to El Niño-related weather anomalies, which offset the price-depressing effects of the Asian financial crisis.

Sugar

Broadly speaking, the UR was not expected to have a significant effect on the world sugar economy because concessions on market access by the major consuming developed countries were limited. The reduction in subsidized exports was not expected to have much effect as these exports accounted for only 5 per cent of world trade. The main stimulus to sugar trade was expected to come from tariff reductions in the developing countries. Production, trade and prices were all expected to be slightly higher, but for reasons not necessarily linked to the AoA. During 1995-1998 world sugar production, trade, stocks and prices were all higher than in 1985-1994. Nevertheless, with record crops again in 1998, prices decreased significantly in that year.

The rise in production and stocks was due to relatively favourable producer prices, while economic growth and, sometimes, subsidized consumer prices stimulated demand and trade. Weaker import demand in 1998 in the Russian Federation, China and some other countries in Asia affected by the financial crisis, along with expectations of large crops in 1998-1999, led to a significant fall in prices in 1998. Greater availability from Brazil, due to the devaluation of its currency, further exacerbated the over-supply situation, driving world prices to their lowest levels in 20 years. During the decade 1985-1994 there was some tendency for price stability to improve, with the exception of the late 1980s, when the full impact of the termination of the economic provisions of the International Sugar Agreement (ISA) was felt.

Fats and Oils

In 1995-1998, world production of and trade in fats and oils exceeded significantly the levels reached in 1985-1994. Although prices declined from their 1994 peak, they were higher in 1995-1998 than in the previous ten years.

Expectations were that the UR would give a slight boost to production and trade partly because of the reduction in export subsidies and partly because of the effects of higher incomes on demand. The main expectation was for a boost to production and exports of palm and palm kernel oils in South-East Asia and, to a lesser extent, soybean oil in South America.

Oilmeals

In 1995-1998 world production of and trade in oilmeals were well above the levels attained in 1985-1994. The UR was not expected to have a significant direct effect on volumes or prices because oilmeals were already traded with few major distortions, although some relatively small indirect effects were expected due to changes foreseen in livestock products and other feedstuffs. The increases in production, prices and trade in 1995-1998 were largely due to continuing expansion of demand from the livestock sector and to the boost provided to demand by the surge in feed grain prices in 1995-1996. The short-term outlook is for a decline in prices to pre-1995 levels because of the higher production of 1998. Indeed, some significant price falls took place in 1998. For the medium term, continuing fairly strong demand is foreseen, tempered, nonetheless, by the effects of the slowdown in economic growth on the livestock sector in South and East Asia.

Meat

Bovine meat production, trade and prices were generally below trend during the 1995-1998, and production and prices were below the averages of the previous ten years. Most of the decline in prices was due to factors such as the Bovine Spongiform Encephalitis (BSE) crisis and other health-scares that depressed demand for beef. Before the UR, export subsidies and non-tariff barriers were more prevalent in the global beef market and the commitments under the AoA on export subsidies and market access were stronger than for other types of meat.

The European Community (EC), the world's second largest meat exporter, used export subsidies for nearly all of its beef shipments before the UR. Its beef exports are presently limited by ceilings on both the subsidized volume and value, which suggests that in the absence of such limitations subsidized exports would have been higher and world prices lower than they actually were. The recent rebuilding of EC beef stocks, after they had been almost eliminated before the implementation of the UR, confirms the important role the UR has played in constraining the volume of subsidized supplies on global markets.

Tariff quota access opportunities for beef exceed, by far, those for the competing types of meat taken together. Consequently, improved market access commitments, mainly in the United States and the Republic of Korea, were expected to boost beef both trade and beef prices. Nevertheless, trade and prices weakened in 1996 and early 1997, due to health-related reductions in demand. This situation was subsequently further aggravated by the financial crises in Asia, the Russian Federation and elsewhere. The general slowdown in beef production was the consequence of downsizing of the meat sectors in many countries in transition.

In the case of pigmeat, prices in 1995-1998 were significantly below the 1985-1994 average, while world trade and production were above average. The AoA was expected to boost trade and prices on the basis of improved market access commitments and disciplines on the use of export subsidies.

In 1995, and even more in 1996, trade was boosted by a reduction in minimum import prices ("gate prices") and tariffs in Japan and by substantial purchases by the Russian Federation. Subsequently, however, the surge in Japanese import volumes triggered the UR special safeguard clause, resulting in much higher gate prices that cut imports. The strong gains in global pork trade receded in 1997 and 1998 due to a number of health scares and to the economic slowdown that depressed import demand in Asia. Record supplies of pork in the major exporting countries exerted further downward pressure on prices in 1998.

The AoA provided some flexibility in terms of export subsidy utilisation. The EC used this flexibility to roll over the unused portion of previous years' commitments for pork, thereby exporting more in 1998/99 than their ceiling for the year would have permitted, perhaps putting additional downward pressure on global pork prices.

In the poultry sector, world production and trade in 1995-1998 were significantly above the averages for the previous ten years, although prices were below average. The main effect of the UR was expected to be some firming of prices, reflecting higher incomes, higher feed prices and reduced export subsidies. Among the meat sectors, the fewest market access commitments were created for poultry. Overall, the strong performance of the poultry sector cannot be attributed to the UR. Rather, growing demand from the Russian

Federation and China—neither of which are WTO members—accounted for nearly 80 per cent of the gains in trade in 1995-1998.

For sheepmeat, world production trade and prices were all above the 1984-1994 levels. The UR was not expected to have much effect on production and trade, although prices were expected to be firmer. Tariff quota access opportunities in this sector reflect almost entirely the conversion of the EC's previous access agreements. Some boost to trade appears to have occurred in the United States following the abolition of the Meat Import Law, but this was offset by negative market developments in other countries unrelated to the UR.

Milk

For milk and milk products, little change was foreseen as a result of the AoA for the volume of world production and trade, but prices were expected to be slightly higher because of minimum access commitments and reduced export subsidies. The period 1995-1998 saw production and trade above the 1985-1994 levels. Developments in production largely reflected, on the one hand, the continued decline of output in the Commonwealth of Independent States (CIS) and, on the other, the rising output in Australia and New Zealand and in several developing countries in Asia and Latin America.

Prices during 1995-1998 were, to varying degrees, above the levels of previous years, including those of skim milk powder, butter, and cheese. The prices for cheese on world markets were helped to some extent by the reduction in export subsidies. However, the prices for most other products were affected by factors unrelated to the UR, as commitments to reduce export subsidies were in general easily met within patterns of trade prevailing over the period. In particular, the prices of butter have been influenced by the much lower levels of surplus stocks in recent years—compared with the levels in the early 1990s—as well as by the strong import demand from the Russian Federation. Since 1998, international dairy prices have fallen as a result of a decline in demand, due to the economic slowdown in Southeast Asia, the Russian Federation and Brazil, all of which are important net importers of dairy products.

Dairy products have been the subject of two WTO panel cases: one concerning the Canadian pricing system for milk (which complainants argue cross-subsidises exports via high returns from the domestic market) and the other concerning imports of spreadable butter from New Zealand into the EC.

Bananas

The volume of banana exports in 1995-1998 was above the 1985-1994 levels. The trend in global trade over that ten-year period had been strongly upwards, particularly as shipments to the EC were unusually high in the period preceding the mid-1993 entry into force of the common market regime for bananas, with countries seeking to establish quota positions prior to the coming into force of the tariff quotas. Since then, global trade has continued to grow on trend. Slower growth in imports into the EC coincided with faster growth in exports to some other regions and countries, notably Eastern Europe, the CIS and China.

Three markets (the United States, the EC and Japan) account for more than two thirds of world banana imports. The United States, the world largest banana import market, applies no duties or quantitative restrictions to banana imports. Japan has no quantitative restrictions on banana imports, but does apply a seasonal import tariff. As a result of its UR commitments, its MFN tariff rates are being gradually lowered; however, practically all banana imports into Japan enter at preferential tariff rates lower than the MFN rates. Expectations of the impact of the UR on the banana market were largely based on the likely effect of the EC Framework Agreement, including its tariff quotas.

Through the Dispute Settlement mechanism, the UR has had an important indirect effect on the world banana economy. Based on cases brought by the United States and Ecuador against the EC, the Dispute Settlement Panel (DSP) of WTO found that the EC banana import regime violated several sections of the General Agreement on Tariffs and Trade (GATT), particularly Article XIII, and also elements of the General Agreement on Trade in Services (GATS). The Panel ruled that, due to the EC banana import regime, the United States had suffered losses equal to US$191.4 million. This ruling enabled the United States to impose tariffs totalling an equivalent amount on a series of EC products.

The EC is currently working towards adopting a banana import regime compatible with WTO provisions. Although it has not yet decided on an alternative import policy for bananas, a revised regime may open up the possibility for some developing countries to sell more fruit in the EC market, and thus increase their export earnings. At the same time, it may lift some of the protection that the current system provides to other developing countries, which in turn may lose some market share and corresponding export earnings.

Citrus

The UR has not had a significant short-term effect on world fresh citrus trade. While exports had grown at the annual average rate of 7 per cent in 1991-1994 period, they grew at only 1 per cent annually in 1994-1997.

In the EC, the world's largest fresh citrus importer, the AoA resulted in a change in the import regime for fruits and vegetables. The new regime has substituted entry prices and maximum tariff equivalents for the former reference prices and countervailing duties. However, the new system works in a similar (though not identical) fashion to the former one, and the entry prices for citrus fruit were fixed at similar levels to those of the former reference prices (except for oranges, where they set higher). As a result, there has been no major change in the EC's total imports of citrus since 1995.

Under the AoA, the United States is to reduce its MFN import tariff for frozen concentrated orange juice (FCOJ) by 15 per cent by the year 2000. This concession however, has had no major impact on the FCOJ market so far. "New" groves planted in Florida to replace those lost by freezes in the mid-1980s have reached full maturity and as a result record crops were harvested in recent seasons. As domestic output of orange juice has grown in the United States, the demand for imports has declined.

In the longer run, the main effects of the UR on global citrus trade may well be through the Sanitary and Phytosanitary (SPS) Agreement. The current process of harmonising testing procedures may lead to freer trade and should benefit citrus exports. Several major importing countries have recently agreed to lift bans on citrus imports that were based on phytosanitary grounds when it could be demonstrated that risks were kept very low. For example, Japan has agreed on import protocols for Australian mandarins while the

United States Department of Agriculture (USDA) has proposed to allow imports of Argentine citrus into the United States. In the EC, SPS negotiations continue with Argentina and Uruguay, with a view to further opening the EC market for citrus fruit from those countries.

Tropical Beverages

The volumes of coffee production and trade in 1995-1998 were slightly above those of 1985-1994. Coffee prices had been on a pronounced downward trend from the mid-1980s to 1993 when weather damage to crops led to severe shortages. The UR was not expected to have much effect as trade in coffee was almost free of non-tariff barriers and tariffs were generally low. Price developments of 1995-1998 thus mainly reflected the cyclical nature of the crop, the incidence of frosts in Brazil, as well as to some extent, the operation of the export retention scheme.

The situation in cocoa closely mirrors that of coffee, with world production and trade slightly above the 1985-1994 values. Again, prices had been on a strongly declining path during the decade prior to the signing of the International Cocoa Agreement (ICA) in 1993. The UR was expected to have only a small positive effect on trade and prices via the effect of higher incomes. Hence, the rather high prices in 1995-1998 were mainly the result of a cyclical upturn following the new cocoa agreement and concerns about production constraints in some of the main supplying countries.

For tea, world production and trade were above the 1985-1994 levels; but prices were below them. It was expected that the UR would have little impact on the global tea economy because import tariffs are already low or zero in major import markets. Nevertheless, there is scope for some expansion in potential growth markets in developing countries. The current global economic crisis has stifled growth somewhat.

Agricultural Raw Materials

Agricultural raw materials are generally traded with few tariff restrictions, and have not been directly affected by the UR Agreements. Cotton, rubber, hides and skins, as well as natural fibres such as jute, have not been subject directly to any significant changes.

Many of these materials are suffering from low prices caused in some cases, such as rubber and hides and skins, by the economic difficulties faced by some importers in the past year or two, and in others, such as cotton and jute, by cyclical factors associated with high levels of production and an accumulation of stocks in recent years.

However, products manufactured from these materials will be affected, sometimes quite significantly, by the UR Agreements. The Agreement on Textiles and Clothing (ATC), in particular, is likely to result in a considerably increased trade in textiles and consequently in changes to the geographical pattern of trade in cotton. Some increase in overall demand for cotton is expected to result, but any impact is unlikely to be felt until the Agreement is fully implemented in 2005. In addition, tariffs on imports of some leather products, particularly footwear, have been reduced. This also is likely to affect mainly the pattern of trade, as processing is further concentrated away from the consuming countries, but may result in some increase in demand for these products and hence for raw hides and skins.

The period 1995-1998 saw global cotton production, trade and prices rise above the 1985-1994 levels. The recent weakness of cotton prices from 1997 to 1998 has had more to do with competition from man-made fibres in China and India, increased cotton supplies and the Asian financial crisis, than with the phasing out of the Multi-Fibre Arrangement (MFA).

While jute trade volumes were at levels similar to those reached in 1985-1994, production was below them. Jute was not included in the AoA and any changes occurring to the jute industry because of the UR were expected to be mostly those associated with improved access for synthetic fibres as a result of the implementation of the ATC. The increase in prices in 1995-1996 has been followed by extremely low prices from 1997 through and into 1998-1999.

Rubber production, trade and prices in 1995-1998 were above the 1985-1994 levels. This was not due to the UR, as rubber was already traded fairly freely and the price-boosting effects of higher incomes flowing from the UR on demand for motor vehicles, and hence of rubber, were estimated to be limited. The relative firmness of prices in 1995 and 1996 was attributed to the strengthening of the import demand for rubber in the major motor vehicle exporting countries, although prices fell in 1998 and have remained weak due to increased supplies and the effects of the Asian financial crisis.

Analysis of Changes in Agricultural Price Instability

This section analyzes the variability of international agricultural prices in the period 1995-1998 in comparison with the period 1990-1994, immediately prior to the coming into effect of the AoA. The focus is on within-year price instability, based on the 48 months of data for 1995-1998 compared with corresponding data for 1990-1994. The results are reported in Table 10.2.

Table 10.2: Coefficients of Variation of Monthly Nominal Prices of Different Commodities (%)

Commodity	*Average 1990-94*	*Average 1995-98*
Wheat (HRW2)	6.8	7.9
Maize (USYellow2)	5.3	12
Rice (Thai 100%)	10.3	8.6
Rice (Thai A1)	7.6	9.7
White sugar	7.9	7.0
Raw sugar (ISA)	11.0	8.4
Soybean oil	5.5	5.3
Palm oil	9.2	4.6
Sunflower oil	6.1	8.3
Rapeseed oil	5.2	5.9
Skim milk powder	11.7	5.4
Whole milk powder	9.8	5.1
Butter	9.1	9.5
Cheese	10.6	2.4
Bovine	4.8	5.8
Lamb/mutton	4.7	8.8
Pork	10.9	11.0
Poultry	4.4	5.0
Coffee	14.4	12.0
Cocoa	9.9	5.0
Tea	10.8	11.2
Cotton	7.2	6.4
Rubber	7.6	10.7
Jute	14.5	14.4
Hides and skins	8.9	9.4

The variability of monthly international prices as measured by within-year coefficients of variations is fairly evenly distributed across agricultural products; some (13 commodities) were higher in 1995-1998 than in 1990-1994, while others (12) were lower. There was no overall trend and, although some of the changes would seem to be significant statistically, they cannot be fully explained by the entry into force of the UR. In the case of cereals, there were significant increases in the coefficients of variation of wheat, maize and one variety of rice, as there were true for meat and some vegetable oils Although these increases might not be directly attributable to the entry into force of the UR, they can be partly explained by the adoption in the main grain-exporting countries of market-oriented UR-compatible agricultural policies, which have led to declining stocks and increasing price volatility. For most of the other commodities, price instability actually declined.

Conclusions

From the foregoing analyses, two major conclusions stand out:

- First, for a number of agricultural commodities, the reasonably buoyant market conditions in the second half of the 1990s can be partly attributed to the UR. This is true mainly for the cereals and meat sectors, where the boost was due to export subsidy reductions, the opening of minimum access, reduced intervention in the market and hence lower stocks, and the effect of higher incomes. For most other agricultural commodities, however, the impact of the UR on the volume of trade and level of prices was probably negligible. Developments in 1998 illustrate the degree to which agricultural markets are affected by sudden changes in weather or in economic conditions, which can offset the more gradual effects associated with structural changes, such as those due to the UR.
- Second, there is little evidence that there has been a significant across-the-board change in within-year world

price instability since 1995. However, the view of experts is that during the next few years, while policies adjust to the new trading environment, prices are likely to be unstable. Compared to the past, the outlook is for the new international trading environment to be characterised by lower levels of overall stocks; however, markets are likely to be more resilient due to faster response to production/demand shocks. Hence, it is not clear whether price instability will be higher or lower in the future or whether the probability of price spikes will be greater or smaller. The variability of prices in the new market environment will depend on several factors, including the effect of the implementation of the commitments agreed under the UR, as well as other factors affecting market developments.

ISSUES AT STAKE RELATING TO AGRICULTURAL DEVELOPMENT, TRADE AND FOOD SECURITY

The Current Agricultural Situation of the Developing Countries

For a large number of developing countries, especially the 82 low-income food-deficit countries (LIFDCs) currently identified by FAO, the agricultural sector remains largely underdeveloped, in respect of production both for the domestic market and for export. At the same time, in most of these countries, the agricultural sector lies at the centre of their economies. It accounts for a large share of GDP, employs a large proportion of the labour force, represents a major source of foreign exchange earnings, supplies the bulk of basic food required by the population and provides subsistence and other income for large rural populations (see Table 10.3). Thus, significant progress in promoting economic growth, reducing poverty and enhancing food security cannot be achieved in most of these countries without realising more fully the productive potential of the agricultural sector and its contribution to overall economic development.

Table 10.3: Relative Importance of Agriculture in Developing Countries

Country	*Share of Agriculture in GDP, 1997 (%)*	*Country*	*Agricultural Population as % of Total Population (1995-97)*	*Country*	*Share of Agricultural In Total Merchandise Exports, 1995-97 (%)*
(1)	(2)	(3)	(4)	(5)	(6)
LIFDCs		LIFDCs		LIFDCs	
Congo, Dem Rep. of	64.0	Bhutan	93.3	Burundi	95.3
Burundi	58.0	Nepal	93.3	Sudan	94.2
Ethiopia	56.0	Burkina Faso	92.3	Ethiopia	93.1
Albania	55.0	Rwanda	90.9	Malawi	74.6
Central African Rep.	54.0	Burundi	90.8	Chad	67.8
Guinea-Bissau	54.0	Niger	88.7	Guinea-Bissau	64.9
Kyrgyzstan	52.0	Guinea	85.3	Guatemala	62.4
Lao PDR	52.0	Ethiopia	84.0	Afghanistan	62.3
Cambodia	50.0	Guinea-Bissau	83.8	Tanzania, Uni. Rep. of	61.6
Mali	49.0	Mali	83.1	Mali	59.2
Tanzania, Uni. Rep of.	48.0	Gambia	80.2	Togo	56.7
Ghana	47.0	Tanzania, Uni. Rep of	79.9	Cuba	55.7
Nigeria	45.0	Malawi	79.4	Côte d'Ivoire	54.8
Armenia	44.0	Papua New Guinea	78.9	Kenya	54.5
Sierra Leone	44.0	Chad	78.7	Comoros	52.0
Nepal	43.0	Eritrea	78.7	Somalia	50.9
Haiti	42.0	Kenya	77.1	Nicaragua	49.1
Cameroon	41.0	Lao PDR	77.1	Benin	47.4

(Contd.)

(1)	(2)	(3)	(4)	(5)	(6)
Togo	40.0	Mozambique	77.1	Madagascar	45.4
Chad	39.0	Central African Rep	75.9	Burkina Faso	40.6
Mozambique	39.0	Madagascar	75.9	Gambia	40.0
Rwanda	39.0	Comoros	75.2	Honduras	38.5
Benin	38.0	Senegal	75.0	Rwanda	37.1
Niger	38.0	Solomon Islands	74.6	Ghana	36.9
Malawi	36.0	Angola	72.9	Kyrgyzstan	36.0
Burkina Faso	35.0	Somalia	72.9	Ecuador	34.5
Georgia	35.0	Equatorial Guinea	72.3	Swaziland	33.0
Nicaragua	34.0	Cambodia	71.6	Cameroon	32.4
Madagascar	32.0	Zambia	71.6	Bolivia	29.6
Mongolia	31.0	China	70.0	Mozambique	28.7
Bangladesh	30.0	Liberia	69.5	Macedonia, FYR of	27.5
Kenya	29.0	Afghanistan	68.3	Congo, Dem. Rep. of	24.4
Côte d'Ivoire	27.0	Congo, Dem Rep. of	65.1	Central African Rep.	24.2
India	27.0	Haiti	64.8	Syrian Arab Rep.	22.2
Guinea	26.0	Sudan	64.6	Haiti	21.5
Pakistan	26.0	Sierra Leone	64.3	Sri Lanka	20.8
Papua New Guinea	26.0	Togo	62.1	Lao PDR	18.5
Mauritania	25.0	Bangladesh	59.6	Morocco	17.9
Guatemala	24.0	Benin	57.9	Papua New Guinea	17.4
Azerbaijan	22.0	Ghana	57.1	Nepal	17.3
Sri Lanka	22.0	Cameroon	56.8	Solomon Islands	17.1
China	20.0	India	56.8	Georgia	16.7
Honduras	20.0	Yemen	54.6	Niger	16.5
Morocco	20.0	Mauritania	53.8	Mongolia	16.5
Philippines	20.0	Côte d'Ivoire	53.6	India	16.5

(Contd.)

(1)	(2)	(3)	(4)	(5)	(6)
Senegal	18.0	Pakistan	52.6	Bhutan	16.0
Yemen	18.0	Sri Lanka	47.5	Egypt	13.8
Egypt	16.0	Indonesia	46.7	Pakistan	13.4
Indonesia	16.0	Congo, Dem. Rep. of	44.0	Cambodia	13.2
Zambia	16.0	Bolivia	43.6	Sierra Leone	13.1
Lesotho	14.0	Philippines	41.8	Albania	12.2
Bolivia	13.0	Morocco	40.3	Indonesia	11.7
Ecuador	12.0	Egypt	39.3	Azerbaijan	11.5
Macedonia, FYR of	11.0	Honduras	39.1	Senegal	10.3
Congo, Dem. Rep. of	10.0	Lesotho	38.8	Korea, Dem. People's Rep. of	9.0
Angola	7.0	Nigeria	37.1	Philippines	8.9
Korea, Dem. People's Rep. of	6.0	Swaziland	36.2	Mauritania	8.6
Eritrea	na	Korea, Dem. People's Rep of	33.2	Guinea	7.1
Afghanistan	na	Ecuador	30.3	Equatorial Guinea	6.8
Bhutan	na	Syrian Arab Rep	29.8	Lesotho	5.9
Comoros	na	Mongolia	27.2	Liberia	5.8
Cuba	na	Nicaragua	25.4	Armenia	5.5
Equatorial Guinea	na	Cuba	18.0	China	5.1
Gambia	na	Albania	na	Zambia	3.6
Liberia	na	Armenia	na	Bangladesh	3.4
Solomon Islands	na	Azerbaijan	na	Nigeria	3.2
Somalia	na	Georgia	na	Yemen	2.9
Sudan	na	Guatemala	na	Eritrea	2.7
Swaziland	na	Kyrgyzstan	na	Congo, Dem. Rep. of	0.7

(Contd.)

(1)	(2)	(3)	(4)	(5)	(6)
Syrian Arab Rep	na	Macedonia, FYR of	na	Angola	0.1
Other Developing Countries	13.2	Other Developing Countries	29.1	Other Developing Countries	22.9
Uganda	44.0	Uganda	80.8	Uganda	76.3
Zimbabwe	28.0	Myanmar	71.5	Paraguay	72.1
Viet Nam	27.0	Viet Nam	69.0	Costa Rica	61.9
Paraguay	23.0	Zimbabwe	64.9	Cyprus	56.7
Turkey	17.0	Namibia	52.0	Uruguay	56.2
Colombia	16.0	Thailand	52.0	Panama	53.0
Costa Rica	15.0	Botswana	45.3	Dominican Rep.	47.7
Brazil	14.0	Gabon	43.1	Zimbabwe	46.1
Namibia	14.0	Paraguay	42.7	Argentina	45.2
Tunisia	14.0	Fiji	42.0	Myanmar	41.1
Dominican Rep	13.0	Oman	39.4	Colombia	32.9
El Salvador	13.0	El Salvador	36.1	El Salvador	30.1
Malaysia	13.0	Turkey	33.2	Brazil	29.9
Algeria	12.0	Peru	32.0	Mauritius	25.1
Lebanon	12.0	Iran, Islamic Rep. of	29.3	Viet Nam	23.2
Thailand	11.0	Tunisia	26.1	Jamaica	21.0
Mauritius	10.0	Mexico	26.0	Turkey	20.0
Uruguay	9.0	Panama	25.3	Chile	15.2
Jamaica	8.0	Algeria	24.7	Lebanon	15.0
Panama	8.0	Costa Rica	23.2	Namibia	14.6
Peru	7.0	Colombia	23.1	Thailand	14.1
Argentina	6.0	Jamaica	22.2	Mexico	10.2
Korea, Rep. of	6.0	Dominican Rep	20.7	Jordan	10.1
Jordan	5.0	Malaysia	20.6	Malaysia	10.1

(Contd.)

(1)	(2)	(3)	(4)	(5)	(6)
Mexico	5.0	Brazil	18.7	Peru	9.4
Venezuela	4.0	Chile	16.5	Tunisia	8.0
Gabon	2.0	Mauritius	13.3	Botswana	5.0
Botswana	na	Saudi Arabia	13.1	Iran, Islamic Rep. of	4.8
Chile	na	Jordan	12.8	Iraq	3.7
Cyprus	na	Iraq	12.2	Oman	3.5
Fiji	na	Uruguay	11.5	Venezuela	2.2
Iran, Islamic Rep. of	na	Argentina	11.4	Un. Arab Emirates	2.2
Iraq	na	Korea, Rep. of	11.2	Fiji	1.6
Libyan Arab Jam.	na	Venezuela	11.2	Korea, Rep. of	1.3
Myanmar	na	Cyprus	10.4	Saudi Arabia	0.8
Oman	na	Libyan Arab Jam.	7.6	Algeria	0.8
Saudi Arabia	na	Un. Arab Emirates	5.9	Libyan Arab. Jam.	0.5
Un. Arab Emirates	na	Lebanon	4.9	Gabon	0.4
Developing Countries	26.3	Developing Countries	50.4	Developing Countries	27.3
-LIFDCs:	32.5	-LIFDCs:	63.2	-LIFDCs:	29.7
Developed Countries:	3.0	Developed Countries	8.7	Developed Countries	8.3

Source: GDP: Oxford University Press for the World Bank (1999), *World Development Report 1998/89;* Population and exports: FAOSTAT (1999).

The agricultural population is defined as all persons depending for their livelihood on agriculture, hunting, fishing or forestry. It comprises all persons actively engaged in agriculture and their non-working dependants.

Simple average of the countries listed.

Several factors have contributed, in varying degrees in different countries, to this underdevelopment of the agricultural sector. However, two key factors stand out: the past policy bias against agriculture in these countries and the major distortions on world agricultural markets due to the protection and subsidization of this sector in many developed countries. While progress has been made in both areas in recent years, much remains to be done. Developing countries have a crucial stake in the next round of WTO negotiations on agriculture, as these will largely determine whether meaningful reforms that address these issues are achieved.

The traditional policy bias in most developing countries against agriculture, reflected in direct and indirect taxation of agricultural production and exports, was due to a variety of reasons. Revenue considerations were one major factor, as agriculture was the only economic activity that could be relatively easily taxed in many countries in immediate post-independence years. A second important factor was the socio-political imperative of maintaining low food prices, most often through state-controlled marketing boards. Indirect taxation of agricultural exports occurred principally through overvalued exchange rates. These factors, taken together, had the unintended consequence of depressing farm prices and profitability, thus reducing incentives for investment.

Since the late 1980s and early 1990s, many developing countries have implemented domestic policy reforms which have reduced the policy bias against agriculture. Further agricultural reform remains high on the agenda of many developing countries. The common objectives of these reforms are to: (i) enhance productivity; (ii) increase domestic production of basic foods; iii) improve the quality and standards of products; and (iv) diversify production and exports by promoting the development of new crops and the processing of primary products. Achieving these objectives requires building farming capacity, attracting new investment, promoting innovation and ensuring the provision of infrastructure, farm inputs and credit. While many challenges remain for these countries in achieving the full productive potential of their agricultural sectors, the main domestic policy impediments are being greatly reduced.

The second key factor constraining agriculture in developing countries, namely the high levels of subsidies and protection provided to agriculture in the developed world, continue to pose serious problems in several respects. Domestic support to agriculture in developed countries encourages over-production, which in turn increases supplies on world markets (by reducing import demand or increasing export supply) and depresses world prices. Low prices make it harder for producers in developing countries to compete in their home markets, as well as in international markets, thus reducing incentives for production and retarding the development of the agricultural sector.

Export subsidies further distort global markets and often destabilise world prices, as developed countries tend to use subsidies more when world prices are low, thus further depressing prices. On the other hand, subsidised exports tend to fall when world prices are high, just at the time when developing countries might be said to "benefit" from subsidised supplies. Developing countries thus have an interest in the reduction of both domestic support and export subsidies in the developed countries. They have a concomitant interest, however, in ensuring that disciplines intended to restrain the excesses of some developed countries do not interfere with their own ability to adopt appropriate development policies for the agricultural sector.

High levels of border protection in many developed countries are an additional impediment to exports from developing countries. However, because some developing country exporters benefit from preferential access to these markets in some heavily protected products, it is difficult to achieve consensus among developing countries on reducing the barriers in those cases. Trade preferences other than those under the Generalized System of Preferences (GSP) are being challenged within the WTO, and there is growing pressure to convert these non-reciprocal programmes—e.g. the Lomé Convention—into free trade agreements. Furthermore, as multilateral trade reform proceeds, the value of trade preferences will continue to diminish. Thus, an export strategy based solely on preferential access is unlikely to be successful in the long run. Nevertheless, at present, several developing countries depend on trade preferences for a substantial share of their export earnings and their interests need to be taken into account. The reduction of border protection in the developed countries consequently needs to ensure that the current beneficiaries of preferential arrangements are compensated and assisted in adjusting to a more competitive environment.

The Agreement on Agriculture began a process of bringing the trade-distorting agricultural policies of developed countries under multilateral rules and disciplines. However, much remains to be done before developing countries can benefit significantly. For this reason, the next round of negotiations will have a direct bearing on agricultural development, trade and food security in the developing countries. Issues arising from the implementation of the UR agreements, as well as those emerging for the forthcoming negotiations on agriculture, are outlined below from the perspective of the ability of developing countries to enhance their domestic food security and to take advantage of new trading opportunities.

Issues Relating to Developing Domestic Capacities in Agriculture

In view of the overriding role of agriculture in the developing economies, enhancing the domestic capacities of the sector is crucial for their socio-economic development. While the Agreement on Agriculture acknowledges the need for special and differential treatment (SDT) for developing countries and has a number of provisions on the subject, these provisions have been seen by many developing countries as falling short of what is necessary and as failing to provide the requisite policy flexibility. In this context, developing countries have drawn a distinction between the protection and support measures used in developed countries that distort world markets and those used by developing countries to ensure food security, to promote broader economic development, or to diversify their agricultural exports. In developing countries where market institutions are not fully developed, or function only imperfectly, a degree of support and protection is considered necessary. However, their need for policy flexibility should not be used as an argument for the continuation of trade-distorting policies in the developed countries. This section addresses some of the issues at stake regarding domestic policy flexibility to develop the agricultural potential of developing countries.

Domestic Support

The policy flexibility of developing countries under the Agreement on Agriculture involves four elements: reduction commitments on domestic support, exemptions under the de minimis threshold, special and differential treatment provisions, and "green box" policies. Most developing countries do not have reduction commitments on domestic support because, as noted above, they typically did not provide support to agriculture. Under the de minimis provisions, they may exclude from their calculation, and hence from their reduction commitments, support that would otherwise be subject to disciplines if such support constitutes less than 10 per cent of the value of production. For product-specific programmes, the de minimis limit is based on production of the specified product, whereas for non-product-specific programmes, the limit refers to the value of total agricultural production.

Some of the particular needs of developing countries in the area of domestic support are taken into account in the provisions for special and differential treatment. Article 6 of the Agreement excludes from the reduction commitment some support measures that are considered developmental, namely measures taken in the context of programmes designed to encourage agricultural and rural development and constituting an integral part of national development programmes. Such measures include: investment subsidies which are generally available to agriculture in developing countries; agricultural input subsidies generally available to low-income or resource-poor producers in developing countries; and domestic support to producers in developing countries to encourage diversification from growing illicit narcotic crops.

Also exempt from reduction commitments, for all WTO members, are the "green box" measures outlined in Annex 2 of the Agreement. These are measures that are considered to have no, or at most minimal, trade-distorting effects or effects on production.

The "green box" includes, inter alia, general services to agriculture such as research and extension, and pest and disease control; public stockholding for food security purposes; structural adjustment programmes; environmental programmes; crop and income insurance schemes; and certain direct payments and income supports that are not linked to agricultural production. Support must be provided through publicly-funded government programmes (including government revenue forgone), and must neither involve transfers from consumers nor have the effect of providing price support to producers.

The domestic support reduction commitments of developed countries were an important first step toward addressing the high levels of support and protection prevailing in many of them. Nevertheless, the global level of this "amber box" support remains quite high and the distribution is skewed against developing countries. The trade-distorting agricultural policies of developed countries impose significant costs on developing countries, as has been well documented, and further reforms are needed before the latter can benefit significantly.

In contrast, the overwhelming majority of developing countries, as shown in Table 10.4, have reported zero or less than de minimis total base AMS levels. Most of these countries, constituting about two thirds of the current WTO membership, have no reduction commitments on domestic support but neither do they have WTO "rights" to use "amber box" support in excess of the de minimis level in the future. Although many of these countries are not currently constrained by the domestic support provisions of the Agreement, they may find their policy options limited in the future. Only 20 developing countries (out of more than 100) have reported positive total base AMS and, of these, only 12 reported that it was in excess of the 10 per cent de minimis allowance. Furthermore, depending on the interpretation of Article 13 (b) of the Agreement, their rights to product-specific de minimis support could be further constrained if the support given in the 1992 marketing year was less than the de minimis level.

Table 10.4: Base Total AMS as Reported by Selected Developing Countries (by Region)

Region	*Reported Base Total AMS*		
	Above de Minimis	*Positive but Less than de Minimis*	*Zero or Negative*
Africa	Morocco, Tunisia	Mauritius	Angola, Benin, Botswana, Burkina Faso, Burundi, Cameroon, Central African Rep., Chad, Côte d'Ivoire, Democratic Republic of the Congo, Djibouti, Egypt, Gabon, Gambia, Ghana, Guinea, Guinea-Bissau, Kenya, Lesotho, Madagascar, Malawi, Mali, Mauritania, Mozambique, Namibia, Niger, Nigeria, Rwanda, Senegal, Sierra Leone, Swaziland, Tanzania, Togo, Uganda, Zambia, Zimbabwe
America	Brazil, Colombia, Costa Rica, Mexico, Venezuela	Argentina, Panama, Uruguay	Antigua and Barbuda, Barbados, Belize, Bolivia, Chile, Cuba, Dominica, Dominican Republic, Ecuador, El Salvador, Grenada, Guatemala, Guyana, Haiti, Honduras, Jamaica, Nicaragua, Paraguay, Peru, Saint Kitts and Nevis, Saint Lucia, Saint Vincent and the Grenadines, Suriname, Trinidad and Tobago
Asia	Republic of Korea, Thailand	India, Pakistan, Philippines	Bahrain, Bangladesh, Brunei Darussalam, Hong Kong, China, Indonesia, Kuwait, Macao, Malaysia, Maldives, Mongolia, Myanmar, Qatar, Singapore, Sri Lanka, United Arab Emirates
Europe	Bulgaria, Cyprus	Turkey	Malta, Romania
Oceania	Papua New Guinea		Solomon Islands, Fiji
Number of Countries	12	8	80

Source: Compilations based on background documentation of the WTO Secretariat.

A second issue of concern for developing countries is related to the fact that product-specific support is generally devoted mainly to production of basic foodstuffs. On average, more than 70 per cent of the Current Total AMS notified by developing countries during 1995 and 1996 was allocated to the production of cereals. For several countries, such support is near the allowed product-specific de minimis level. Thus, while the de minimis exemption is unused for many products in these countries, it may constrain their support of basic food production. Furthermore, the extent of flexibility in non-product specific support for developing countries may be inadequate. Sector-wide support in areas such as agricultural credit, transport, irrigation and fuel are important aspects of the development strategies of many countries, and additional flexibility in their use may be needed.

A third issue is that, because the base year AMS is expressed in fixed nominal prices, several developing countries have difficulties remaining within their currently allowed AMS levels on account of high inflation and currency depreciation, despite the fact that the real level of support to agriculture has not increased. Although the Agreement (Article 18, paragraph 4) recognises the need to "give due consideration to the influence of excessive rates of inflation" on the ability to abide by domestic support commitments, how that should be done and precisely what is meant by "excessive rates of inflation" are not spelled out. Some of these countries have therefore raised the issue of being allowed to maintain support levels in real terms.

The interpretation of certain other terms associated with domestic support may be an important issue for developing countries. In general, countries have not been consistent in their interpretation of the term 'eligible production': some used total production, others used marketed amounts and still others used the amount procured by a parastatal. As a result, the AMS and its respective de minimis levels may change considerably if a different interpretation is made on what production level to include in the calculation. Other problems have arisen regarding lack of clarity in the definition of "low-income" or "resource-poor" producers. Most of the developing countries have referred to the exemption of input subsidies for poor farmers and excluded almost all of their input subsidies, a practice that has been intensively questioned at the WTO. For many developing countries, input subsidies are an essential component of their broader agricultural development strategies and are used to facilitate the adoption of improved farming technology. Therefore, how this issue is clarified is important for them.

A critical issue of concern to developing countries is the need for a more precise definition of measures that qualify for inclusion in the "green box". Although such measures are described as having, at most, only minimal distorting effects on production or trade, that is probably not the case, at least in the long run, for many policies currently justified under the green box. In view of the limited financial ability of many developing countries to provide such support, their expenditures remain insignificant compared with those of the developed countries (see Table 10.5). Since there is currently no WTO limit on the total amount of expenditure on green box measures, developing countries have an interest in clarifying, and perhaps tightening, the definition of such policies.

Table 10.5: Total Expenditure on Green Box Measures by WTO Members in 1995 and 1996

WTO Member	*1995*		*1996*	
	Amount (US$ Million)	*Percentage Share in Total Reported Expenditure of WTO Members*	*Amount (US$ Million)*	*Percentage Share in Total Reported Expenditure of WTO Members*
(1)	(2)	(3)	(4)	(5)
Total reported expenditure of WTO members:	129 440	100.00	126 735	100.00
Developed countries	110 173	85.10	110 958	87.60
Developing countries	19 266	14.91	15 776	12.50
Developing countries				
Argentina		0.00	137	0.11
Bahrain		0.00	0	0.00
Botswana	11	0.01		0.00
Brazil	4 883	3.77	2 600	2.05

(Contd.)

(1)	(2)	(3)	(4)	(5)
Chile	176	0.14	170	0.13
Colombia	318	0.25	578	0.46
Cuba	908	0.70	1 090	0.86
Cyprus	130	0.10	128	0.10
Fiji	-	0.00	16	0.01
Gambia	n.a.			0.00
Guyana		0.00		0.00
India	2 196	1.70		0.00
Jamaica		0.00	7	0.01
Kenya	53	0.04	66	0.05
Korea, Rep. of	5 174	4.00	6 443	5.08
Malaysia	244	0.19	300	0.24
Malta	1	0.00		0.00
Mexico	1 626	1.26		0.00
Mongolia	n.a.		n.a.	
Morocco	157	0.12	378	0.30
Namibia	50	0.04		0.00
Pakistan	440	0.34	392	0.31
Paraguay	23	0.02	9	0.01
Philippines	136	0.11	282	0.22
Romania	730	0.56	756	0.60
Thailand	1 353	1.05	1624	1.28
Trinidad and Tobago	61	0.05	98	0.08
Tunisia	30	0.02	39	0.03
Uruguay	18	0.01	33	0.03
Venezuela	539	0.42	618	0.49
Zimbabwe	14	0.01	12	0.01
Developed countries				
Australia	707	0.55	740	0.58
Canada	1539	1.19		0.00
Czech Republic	132	0.10	197	0.16
EC	24 110	18.63	28 378	22.39
Hungary	105	0.08	-	0.00
Iceland	30	0.02	50	0.04
Israel	292	0.23	414	0.33
Japan	32 859	25.39	25 020	19.74
New Zealand	128	0.10	136	0.11
Norway	647	0.50	638	0.50
Poland	436	0.34	549	0.43
Slovak Republic	1	0.00	1	0.00
Slovenia	85	0.07	91	0.07
South Africa	763	0.59	525	0.41
Switzerland-Liechtenstein	2 299	1.78	2 404	1.90
United States	46 041	35.57	51 815	40.88

Source: See Table 10.2. Including the transition economies of Central and Eastern Europe (other than Romania).

Note: Countries are listed in the alphabetical order and categorization used by WTO.

Border Protection

It is sometimes necessary to maintain a degree of border protection in order to implement a domestic support policy, particularly when there is an administered price support system. Even when there is no such system, producer prices may still be supported through tariffs. In general, the bound tariffs of developing countries are sufficiently high to allow for a considerable degree of protection at the border. However, there are issues in this area that need to be noted.

First, most developing countries chose to offer a uniform, single rate of binding for all agricultural products. With the tariffs now bound and facing further reductions in the next round, some of these countries might need to approach tariff reductions carefully. In particular, an across-the-board reduction could leave little room to provide a degree of protection for sensitive sectors, an aspect which needs to be taken into account in the choice of a reduction formula. Second, some countries have bound their tariffs at very low levels and consequently now have little room for manoeuvre in the use of the tariff as a contingency measure against price fluctuations on world markets. Third, there are some anomalies in the schedule of bound tariffs of some developing countries. For example, for some products the bound rates are very low (even zero) while for others—e.g. substitute commodities—they are very high, implying that the high bound rates have no practical significance. Some rationalization of tariff bindings seems necessary.

Export Subsidies

There are two main concerns regarding the export subsidy provisions of the Agreement on Agriculture. One is that they legitimise the use of export subsidies in agriculture (such subsidies are prohibited in other sectors), and the other is that they effectively favour exporters that used subsidies in the past (predominantly developed countries), although the level of subsidy must be reduced, while prohibiting others from using them. Developing countries are, however, entitled to use subsidies (without a reduction commitment) for marketing costs and internal transport and freight costs. For developing countries, a primary rationale for the use of trade policies is the need to support infant industries. Thus, in view of their severe supply bottlenecks and technological constraints, agricultural export subsidy schemes could have relevance in some cases, as they would allow the targeting of incentives to specific, selected agro-industries. Few developing countries have the financial resources necessary to use export subsidies as a market-development tool, and what is generally more important for them is the need to discipline the use of export subsidies by developed countries.

Trade-related Aspects of Intellectual Property Rights (TRIPS)

The acquisition and adaptation of technology, particularly for production, is an issue of vital concern for developing countries, notably in respect of the requirement under the TRIPS Agreement to provide for the protection of property rights to plant and animal varieties, either by patents or by effective sui generis legislation. The issue of the patentability of plant and animal varieties, as well as of genetically modified organisms (GMOs), raises questions beyond the mere protection of intellectual property rights, such as the rights of local communities and indigenous peoples, sovereign rights over natural genetic resources, biosafety and food security. Developing countries face two sets of difficulties in this area. On the one hand, most of them, particularly the LDCs, lack the scientific capability to innovate and patent new materials—and are not even in a position to fully catalogue the natural resources of bio-materials that they currently possess. They also do not have appropriate legislation in this area. On the other hand, there is a growing concentration of transnational corporations in bio-tech industries, notably in the seed sector. This concentration or lack of competition (reinforced by global patentability) enables these industries to exact monopoly rents from farmers worldwide. In addition, aside from the issue of costs, many countries feel it is unsafe to rely entirely on external sources for an input as important as seeds.

The Agreement recognised these problems and addressed them through special and differential treatment provisions for developing countries. However, in the view of many developing countries, these provisions have not resulted in any concrete benefits to them, particularly regarding financial and technical assistance and access on favourable terms to new technologies.

Imbalances in Support Levels

As noted above, if developing countries are to develop fully their agricultural potential, they need to rectify their past policy bias against agriculture as well as seek a reform of policies in developed countries that distort world agricultural markets. While both sets of reforms are essential, their sequencing could be crucial in determining whether the situation of the developing countries progressively improves or worsens. As was also noted, there is a substantial imbalance in the remaining levels of domestic support and export subsidies allowed to developed countries, on the one hand, and developing countries, on the other, under the Agreement on Agriculture. The "standstill and roll back" principle underlying that Agreement consequently implies that developed countries have WTO "rights" to use their remaining high levels of support and protection, while developing countries' "rights" to similar support and protection are subject to their considerably lower levels. The issue of concern is that, unless the levels of support and protection of the developed countries can be brought down quickly, the imbalance in support levels, together with the constraints on developing countries' policies, could make adjustment in the latter much slower and more difficult.

Issues Relating to Market Access

The major markets for the agricultural exports of developing countries are in the developed world (primarily, Europe, Japan and North America). However, improved access is important for them not only in those markets but also in the markets of the higher-income developing countries.

Continuing High Agricultural Tariffs

In principle, tariffication was intended to result in bound tariffs no more protective than the non-trade barriers that existed in the base period. And since all tariffs are being reduced, market access terms should have improved. However, a recent OECD study found that actual border protection to agriculture was higher in 1996 than in 1993 in eight of the (then) 10 member countries (EC being treated as a single country) and that tariff protection was substantially higher on food and beverages than on agricultural products as a whole. It should be noted that the study used production-weighted averages of applied MFN tariffs; since bound rates cannot be below the applied rates, border protection based on bound rates would be even higher.

The post-UR tariff profile of many developed countries is typically characterised by relatively high rates on temperate-zone food products and lower rates on tropical products. Tariff reductions were generally lower for temperate-zone products (cuts on tropical products averaged 43 per cent; cuts were lower for other product groups, the lowest being 26 per cent for dairy products). Developing countries as a whole have a high stake in the export of temperate-zone products as these are also the products where the market is still expanding. Tariff peaks in agriculture are most common in three product groups: major food staples; fruit and vegetables; and processed foods. For all agricultural and fisheries products taken together (HS chapters 1-24) the tariff lines for which duties exceed 20 per cent constitute about one quarter of all tariff lines for both the EC and Japan and about one tenth for the United States (see Table 10.6).

Tariff Escalation

Tariff escalation (i.e. progressive increases in tariffs as the processing chain advances) can result in significant effective protection to processed products, depending on the share of value added in the final output. Tariff escalation as a barrier to trade will matter more in the coming years as trade is rapidly shifting to processed products. The developing countries have a strong interest in this matter as they are trying to escape from the circle of producing and exporting primary products. As noted above, the post-UR bound tariffs are relatively very high on processed foods. Several studies have shown that although tariff escalation was reduced post-UR, it still prevails in several important product chains, notably coffee, cocoa, oilseeds, vegetables, fruit and nuts and hides and skins.

Complexity of Tariffs

The post-UR agricultural tariff structure of several major developed countries remains complex, contrary to the promise of a simple

Table 10.6: Distribution of Tariff Peaks by Agricultural Product Group in the European Community, Japan and the United States

Product Group	*Number of Tariff Items*				*Tariff Peaks*	
	Total	*20-29 %*	*30-99 %*	*>100 %*	*No. of peaks*	*Share in total (%)*
European Community (EC)						
Meat, live animals (1-2)	351	68	79	14	161	46
Fish and crustaceans (3)	373	45	0	0	45	12
Dairy products (4)	197	21	77	9	107	54
Fruit and vegetables (7-8)	407	10	5	1	16	4
Cereals, flours etc. (10-11)	174	29	75	0	104	60
Veg. oils, fats, oilseeds (12,15)	211	0	8	2	10	5
Canned and prep.meat, fish (16)	105	17	8	0	25	24
Sugar, cocoa and prep. (17,18)	75	34	6	0	40	53
Prepared fruit, vegetables (20)	310	70	39	1	110	35
Other food industry prod. (19,21)	90	27	8	0	35	39
Beverages and tobacco (22,24)	202	9	15	2	26	13
Other agri.prod (5-6, 9, 13-14, 23)	231	4	14	4	22	10
All agri., fishery products (1-24)	2726	343	334	33	701	26
Japan						
Meat, live animals (1-2)	136	3	19	7	29	21
Fish and crustaceans (3)	189	0	0	0	0	0
Dairy products (4)	146	45	57	22	122	84
Fruit and vegetables (7-8)	209	1	2	7	10	5
Cereals, flour etc. (10-11)	132	37	24	10	71	54
Veg. oils, fats, oilseeds (12,15)	161	1	1	3	5	3
Canned and prep.meat, fish (16)	101	21	3	3	27	27
Sugar, cocoa and prep. (17,18)	80	26	19	6	51	64

(Contd.)

Product Group	Number of Tariff Items				Tariff Peaks	
	Total	20-29 %	30-99 %	>100 %	No. of peaks	Share in total (%)
Prepared fruit, vegetables (20)	231	52	5	2	59	26
Other food industry prod. (19,21)	232	113	2	15	130	56
Beverages and tobacco (22,24)	65	8	0	0	8	12
Other agri. prod (5-6, 9, 13-14, 23)	208	0	0	0	0	0
All agri., fishery products (1-24)	1890	307	132	75	514	27
United States						
Meat, live animals (1-2)	116	6	0	0	6	5
Fish and crustaceans (3)	114	0	0	0	0	0
Dairy products (4)	251	29	58	9	96	38
Fruit and vegetables (7-8)	269	13	0	0	13	5
Cereals, flour etc. (10-11)	59	0	0	0	0	0
Veg. oils, fats, oilseeds (12,15)	124	0	2	2	4	3
Canned and prep.meat, fish (16)	90	1	1	0	2	2
Sugar, cocoa and prep. (17,18)	144	6	13	2	21	15
Prepared fruit, vegetables (20)	169	3	2	3	8	5
Other food industry prod. (19,21)	156	11	18	2	31	20
Beverages and tobacco (22,24)	126	1	3	8	12	10
Other agri. prod. (5-6, 9, 13-14, 23)	161	0	2	0	2	1
All agri., fishery products (1-24)	1779	70	99	26	195	11

Tariff peaks are defined as MFN tariff rates that are 20 per cent or more.
HS chapters are shown in parentheses.

Source: Calculations by the FAO Secretariat based on data in UNCTAD/WTO (1997), "The post-Uruguay Round tariff environment for developing countries" (TD/B/COM.1/14), tables 1-3.

"tariff-only" regime. Apart from in-quota and above-quota duties, tariffs that are not ad valorem are used quite frequently. Often, they also vary for one or more technical reasons such as sugar content or alcohol content, making them even less transparent. Such tariffs are obviously more complex than ad valorem only and complicate the comparison of trade restrictiveness across products and countries which is essential for trade negotiations. Specific tariffs also weigh more heavily against lower-priced imports—their degree of restrictiveness varies inversely with the unit price of the imported product, while it remains constant in the case of an ad valorem tariff.

Some cases of more complex import arrangements continue. One notable example is the "entry price" system applied by the EC on fruit and vegetables. This regime also uses seasonal tariffs, complicating it further. The developing countries are increasingly becoming competitive in these products and so the regime is seen by many as a source of disguised protection. A second example is the cereal import regime of the Communities, which is operated in a way similar to the previous variable levy system. Several developing countries are important exporters of grains and rice.

Tariff Rate Quotas

Tariff rate quotas (TRQs) were intended to ease the process of tariffication. Thirty-six WTO members have tariff quota commitments in their Schedules, with a total of 1 370 individual quotas for agricultural products. The total volume of their TRQs in 1995 as a percentage of world trade in the products concerned typically ranged from 3 per cent to 7 per cent. For some product groups, e.g. dairy, meat and sugar, it exceeded 10 per cent and so how the TRQs are used is a matter of great importance.

While TRQs have potentially created some new trading opportunities, a number of conceptual and implementation issues have arisen, including: the lack of transparency in their administration (e.g. not all the many ways of administering TRQs provide effective market access); allocation to traditional (historical) suppliers and not on an MFN basis, and counting existing preferential access schemes as part of minimum access commitments; counting allocations to non-members of WTO;

allocation to state-trading enterprises and producer organizations, etc. All of these have presented difficulties for new entrants. Also, the broad product classification of TRQs that is permitted has prevented opening up minimum access in some sub-products of a product category. Finally, the setting of within-quota tariffs under the UR has been very uneven and, although many of the quotas have been opened at low or zero tariffs, some within-quota tariffs are so high that imports may not take place. All these problems have been responsible for an under-utilization of TRQs (some 60-65 per cent overall), although market conditions have also sometimes been identified as the main reason.

> The developing countries have a stake in reforming the TRQ system, but perhaps what is most important for them is ensuring that they have effective access. Data on quota utilization for 1995-98 have yet to be analysed to examine the extent to which the developing countries were able to access the new quotas. Such an analysis remains a priority.

Special Safeguard Provisions

The special safeguard (SSG) provisions allow an importer to increase tariffs above bound levels in response to a surge in imports or a decline in import prices. Because the agricultural SSG measures were reserved for countries undertaking tariffication, most developing countries do not have access to such measures (Table 10.7). Close to 80 per cent of the tariffied items of the OECD countries are subject to SSGs. The right to have recourse to SSGs is more common in meat, cereals, fruit and vegetables, oilseeds and oil products and dairy products (Table 10.8).

Maintaining the SSG under present conditions (existing country and product eligibility) will perpetuate discrimination against WTO Members that do not have the right to safeguard measures, largely developing countries. Thus, some suggestions have been made for the elimination of the SSG altogether, also on grounds that resort is possible to the other WTO safeguards. However, the general WTO safeguards are not automatic. They require proof of "injury test", are costly and involve delays. Hence, in general,

Table 10.7: Special Safeguard Measures for Agriculture (SSG): Potential Application and Action by WTO Members

Member	*Potential Application of SSG*		*Grounds for Action Taken and Number of Tariff Items Involved, 1995-98*	
	Number of Tariff Items	*Number of Product Groups (HS 4-Digit Headings)*	*Price*	*Volume*
(1)	(2)	(3)	(4)	(5)
Developed Countries*				
Australia	10	2		
Bulgaria	21	9		
Canada	150	37		
Czech Republic	236	29		
EC	539	72	26	47
Hungary	117	117		
Iceland	462	121		
Israel	41	14		
Japan	121	27	4	73
New Zealand	4	2		
Norway	581	141		
Poland	144	133	10	1
Slovak Republic	114	28		1
South Africa	166	75		
Switzerland-Liechtenstein	961	134		
United States	189	26	24	6
Sub-total	**3856**	**967**	**64**	**128**
Developing Countries				
Barbados	37	24		
Botswana	161	71		
Colombia	56	55		
Costa Rica	87	24		
Ecuador	7	1		
El Salvador	84	23		
Guatemala	107	35		
Indonesia	13	4		
Korea, Rep. of	111	34	8	
Malaysia	72	12		
Mexico	293	83		
Morocco	374	46		
Namibia	166	75		
Nicaragua	21	14		
Panama	6	2		

(Contd.)

(1)	(2)	(3)	(4)	(5)
Philippines	118	36		
Romania	175	14		
Swaziland	166	75		
Thailand	52	23		
Tunisia	32	13		
Developing Countries				
Uruguay	2	1		
Venezuela	76	63		
Sub-total	**2216**	**728**	**8**	**0**
All WTO members	**6072**	**1695**	**74**	**128**

Source: see Table 2.

Note: Countries are listed in the alphabetical order and categorization used by WTO.

HS 8-digit, HS 9-digit, HS 6-digit

*Including the transition economies of Central and Eastern Europe (other than Romania).

Table 10.8: Special Safeguard Measures (SSG) for Agriculture: Potential Application and Action by WTO Members by Product Category

Product Category	*Potential Application of SSG*		*Grounds for Action Taken and Number of Tariff Items Involved, 1996-98*	
	Number of Tariff Items	*Percentage of Total Number of Tariff Items*	*Price*	*Volume*
Cereals	1087	17.9	7	2
Oilseeds, fats and oils and products	706	11.6	5	
Sugar and confectionery	291	4.8	23	
Dairy products	715	11.8	15	20
Animal and products thereof	1327	21.9	5	47
Eggs	74	1.2	1	
Beverages and spirits	329	5.4	1	
Fruit and vegetables	809	13.3	1	48
Tobacco	73	1.2		
Agricultural fibres	13	0.2		5
Coffee, tea, mate, cocoa and preparations; spices and other food preparations	277	4.6	6	1
Other agricultural products	371	6.1	8	
All product categories	6072	100.0	72	123

Source: See Table 10.2.

available WTO safeguards (set out in the Agreement on Safeguards) are not a viable option for many developing countries and for them the SSG option in the Agreement on Agriculture would be highly desirable. Thus, from the point of view of many developing countries it would be desirable for the SSG to become a permanent instrument in the multilateral trading system, but preferably limited to a specified number of basic foodstuffs, i.e. those that are considered sensitive on the grounds of domestic food security, as discussed above. At the same time, some tightening of "triggers" may be desirable so that the safeguards are not used too often.

SPS and TBT

The SPS and TBT Agreements define rules for setting national standards and regulations relating to sanitary and phytosanitary measures as well as technical requirements for food safety and quality so that such regulations do not unduly restrict trade.

A major challenge faced by the developing countries is raising the SPS/TBT standards of their exports to at least internationally recognized levels. For example, the import detention list for the United States for the period 1996-97 shows that the majority of detentions and rejections of products related to microbiological contamination and filth (Table 10.9) rather than to strictly technical considerations. Although the gap in the ability of those countries to meet such standards is wide, the lack of compliance with standards in the developed countries has not been the only reason for the detention and rejection of food imports from the developing countries. The latter face an additional challenge where the developed countries, on risk assessment grounds, adopt higher standards than those currently recognized by international standard-setting bodies. In addition, rising consumer concerns in the affluent countries over food safety and quality compound the difficulty of the developing countries in meeting ever higher standards.

It would no doubt be counter-productive for the developing countries to press for exemption from, or a weakening of, WTO rules relating to SPS/TBT or for that matter for lower international standards. That would merely have an adverse effect on consumer confidence in importing countries. Hence, a positive approach appears essential. However, many developing countries require

Table 10.9: United Stated Imports: Number of Contraventions Cited for Import Detention by the Food and Drug Administration and Their Relative Importance, July 1996-June 1997

Reason for Contravention	*Africa*		*Latin America and Caribbean*		*Europe*		*Asia*		*Total*	
	No.	%	No.	%	No.	%	No.	%	No.	%
Food additives	2	0.7	57	1.5	69	5.8	426	7.4	554	5.0
Pesticide residues	0	0.0	821	21.1	20	1.7	23	0.4	864	7.7
Heavy metals	1	0.3	426	10.9	26	2.2	84	1.5	537	4.8
Mould	19	6.3	475	12.2	27	2.3	49	0.8	570	5.1
Microbiological contamination	125	41.3	246	6.3	159	13.4	895	15.5	1 425	12.8
Decomposition	9	3.0	206	5.3	7	0.6	668	11.5	890	8.0
Filth	54	17.8	1 253	32.2	175	14.8	2037	35.2	3 519	31.5
Low-acid canned food	4	1.3	142	3.6	425	35.9	829	14.3	1400	12.5
Labelling	38	12.5	201	5.2	237	20.0	622	10.8	1098	9.8
Other	51	16.8	68	1.7	39	3.3	151	2.6	309	2.8
Totals	303	100	3895	100	1184	100	5784	100	11166	100

Source: FAO (1999), "The importance of food quality and safety for developing countries", Committee on World Food Security (CFS: 99/3).

assistance to meet these standards. Thus the support of the developing countries for the strengthening of the SPS/TBT Agreements could be predicated on effective mechanisms being put into place to assist them in upgrading their SPS standards. The SPS and TBT agreements contain promises of financial and technical assistance for the developing countries; translating these promises into concrete action would be one issue to pursue. In addition, some mechanism (e.g. an international ombudsman/arbitrator) may be required to minimize "trade harassment". Finally, the limited participation of these countries, in both number and effectiveness, in international standard-setting bodies remains an issue at stake.

Domestic Market Stability

Although price instability on world markets affects all countries, the consequences can be much greater for developing countries for two reasons: i) much of the rural population still earns a living from food production; and ii) food accounts for a relatively large share of household expenditure (see Table 10.10). While the Agreement on Agriculture may contribute to stability,in world prices because of the disciplines imposed on trade-distorting policies and the greater integration of markets, it may also lead to increased fluctuations in world prices because of reduced world stocks and a shift in the location of production from countries with high levels of support to those with low or no support. However, its net impact on world prices remains uncertain.

In any case, world agricultural market instability remains a major problem for LIFDCs because of their high dependence on imports and the weakness of their agricultural sectors. Thus, access of these countries to WTO-compatible safeguard measures remains an issue of great concern to them. Three possibilities are worthy of consideration in this respect. First, for basic foods, many developing countries favour having access to the SSG, which is simpler to use, rather than the general WTO safeguard mechanism, which is not easy to apply in practice. Second, price bands provide an appropriate and tested instrument for these countries. It is, however important to ensure that domestic markets are not thereby fully insulated from movements in world prices. Also, the legality of a price band policy is not entirely clear: applying a duty within the bound rate is permitted, but the Agreement in Agriculture prohibits "variable import duties". This is an issue on which developing countries could seek clarification in the next round. Third, risk management instruments are yet another option to hedge against market instability. Market-based instruments such as forward and futures price contracts and options are fully compatible with the WTO régime.

Reliability of World Food Markets

Another issue relating to world market stability concerns possible disruptions in world supplies for a variety of possible reasons: food exporters may restrict exports, trade embargoes may be imposed, large changes in exchange rates can make imports extremely expensive and wars, civil conflict or natural disasters can disrupt supplies. Thus, strengthening the provisions on export prohibition (Article 12 of the Agreement on Agriculture) would be highly desirable.

Table 10.10: Food Expenditure as a Percentage of Household Consumption Expenditure in Low-Income Food-Deficit Countries and Other Developing and Transition Economies

Country	Share of Expenditure on Food in Total Household Expenditure	Year/period	Country	Share of Expenditure on Food in Total Household Expenditure	Year/Period
	(%)			(%)	
Low-income Food-deficit Countries (LIFDCs):			*Other Developing Countries:*		
Rwanda	80.6	1982/83	Uganda	68.0	1989/90
Zambia	80.2	1974/75	Peru	54.5	1985/86
Albania	75.0	1997	Algeria	52.6	1988
Togo	69.2	1988/89	Mexico	50.6	1984
Ghana	66.4	1987/88	Morocco	50.6	1984/85
India	65.4	1986/87	Jamaica	50.5	1984
Bangladesh	63.4	1988/89	Seychelles	49.4	1983/84
Tanzania, U.R. of	62.5	1969	Latvia	49.0	1997
Sri Lanka	61.4	1985/86	Fiji	45.9	1977
Egypt	60.1	1981/82	Mauritius	45.8	1986/87
Nepal	59.4	1984/85	Iran, Islam Rep. of	45.2	1989
Indonesia	56.8	1987	Colombia	44.5	1972
China	56.2	1990	Tunisia	44.0	1985
Samoa	55.2	1971/72	Macao	42.7	1981/82
Guatemala	54.8	1979/81	Thailand	41.7	1988
Philippines	53.9	1988	Jordan	40.4	1986/87
Haiti	53.6	1986/87	Uruguay	39.2	1982/83

(Contd.)

Nigeria	50.6	1980/81	Hong Kong, China	39.0	1989/90
Côte d'Ivoire	49.1	1979	Costa Rica	38.7	1987/88
Pakistan	44.5	1987/88	Malaysia	38.6	1980/82
Lesotho	37.8	1986/87	Singapore	37.3	1987/88
Swaziland	31.6	1985	New Caledonia	36.3	1980/81
Bahamas	30.5	1973	Botswana	36.2	1985/86
Sierra Leone	30.3	1969/70	French Guiana	33.3	1984/85
			Panama	33.3	1983/84
Transition economies:			Other developing countries:		
			Martinique	33.2	1984/85
Romania	58.6	1997	Turkey	33.0	1987
Bulgaria	54.3	1997	Rep. of Korea	32.0	1990
Lithuania	52.2	1997	Guadeloupe	30.9	1984/85
Croatia	40.1	1991	Kuwait	29.7	1986/87
Estonia	39.9	1997	Cyprus	29.4	1984/85
Slovakia	37.3	1997	Brazil	28.7	1987/88
Czech Republic	30.5	1996	Trinidad and Tobago	28.3	1981/82
Poland	28.0	1995	Netherlands Antilles	27.9	1981
Slovenia	22.5	1997	Reunion	23.3	1986/87
Hungary	17.7	1995	Cayman Islands	22.1	1983/84
			Bermuda	18.8	1982

Source: Data on LIFDCs and other developing countries are from FAO (1994) "Compendium of food consumption statistics from household surveys in developing countries", volumes 1 and 2, (*FAO Economic and Social Development Paper 116*); data for the transition economies are from OECD (1998).

Note: The FAO data are based on national household surveys which differ significantly in terms of survey coverage, concepts, definitions and year and mode of data collection. Hence, this table should be taken to reflect the broad range across the selected countries.

The Marrakesh Decision

The implementation of the Marrakesh Decision in favour of LDCs and NFIDCs is a matter of concern, particularly for potential beneficiaries. To date, the Decision has not been implemented, despite the fact that food aid has dropped to very low levels and food import bills of these countries have risen. Implementation has so far been hampered by several factors which include, the requirement of undisputed proof of the need for assistance (and whether the need resulted from the reform process under the UR) and the variety of instruments called under the Decision to respond to such needs, without precise specification of the respective responsibilities of all concerned. More basically, however the Decision addresses a transitional problem whereas the food security problem in the countries concerned is long-term and complex and encompasses broader development issues that go beyond just trade.

Accession to WTO

The overwhelming concern of developing countries not yet members of WTO has been the terms of accession to the Organization. Treating countries on the basis of the most recent three years for which data are available and imposing hard terms in the negotiation of tariff ceiling bindings and access to special and differential treatment appear to be tighter conditions than those of previous negotiations, and may impose undue restraint on their flexibility to design domestic food and agricultural policies.

New Issues

Finally, new issues such as state trading, competition policy, environmental considerations and labour standards present a multitude of challenges to developing countries. What is important is that legitimate concerns should be divorced from the increasing invocation of these issues by some countries for protectionist purposes.

In conclusion, there are many issues at stake for the developing countries in the forthcoming WTO negotiations. In many cases, improvements could be straightforward, while in others they may entail some hard negotiations and bargaining.

FOOD SECURITY AND THE WTO TRADE NEGOTIATIONS

In the context of the forthcoming trade negotiations, the key issues arising from the outcome of the World Food Summit, without taking a position on any of these issues. In its Article 20 the Agreement on Agriculture states that the reform process will take into account also non-trade concerns. Such concerns, addressed in the preamble to the Agreement, include food security and the need to protect the environment, and taking into account the possible negative effects of the implementation of the reform process on the least-developed and net food-importing developing countries. Food security was the focus of the WFS, particularly in respect of the developing and least-developed countries. The Summit also gave due attention to environmental protection in the context of underpinning the longer-term sustainability of food production systems.

The following section of this paper recalls the outcome of the WFS and discusses briefly the complex, multifaceted issue of food security, inevitably involving a consideration of questions such as market access and food quality and safety as well as sanitary requirements which, strictly speaking, are trade rather than non-trade concerns. The intention is to separate out the food security—trade concerns in a broad sense from the Summit's outcome. The WFS also defined agriculture broadly to include fisheries and forestry. However, without discussing classification issues, this paper focuses mainly on land-based food production systems.

The Outcome of the World Food Summit

The main achievement of the 186 Heads of State and Government or their representatives attending the Summit was their approval on 13 November 1996, by consensus, of the Rome Declaration on World Food Security and the World Food Summit Plan of Action. Fifteen delegations made reservations and/or interpretative statements on these texts, which are recorded in the Summit's report. However, these do not substantively change the thrust of the Summit's outcome. The Declaration, which notes the agreement of participating governments that trade is a key element in achieving food security, contains seven commitments covering the key components of a food security strategy: an enabling political, social and economic environment; improved access to food; sustainable food production; food, agricultural trade and overall trade policies; preparedness for natural disasters and man-made emergencies; investment; and implementation, monitoring and follow-up. Each of these commitments is elaborated on by a 'basis for action' and a series of 'objectives and actions'.

Of the seven commitments, those concerning access, sustainable food production and trade are of greatest relevance to the issue of food security. They will be reviewed in the next section in more detail, but some further points should first be noted:

(a) The adopted texts build on a prior internationally agreed definition of food security. Thus the Summit stated that: "Food security exists when all people, at all times, have physical and economic access to sufficient, safe and nutritious food to meet their dietary needs and food preferences for an active and healthy life." To achieve food security, concerted action is required at all levels—the individual, household, national, regional and global. It is the totality of this 'concerted action' which the Summit addressed.

(b) While the Rome Declaration reaffirmed the "right of everyone to have access to safe and nutritious food, consistent with the right to adequate food and the fundamental right of everyone to be free from hunger", neither it nor the Plan of Action is an elaboration of the right to food. However, Objective 7.4 of the Plan of Action sets out to clarify the content of the right to adequate food and the fundamental right of everyone to be free from hunger. It emphasises the full and progressive realisation of this right as a means to achieving food security for all.

(c) The outcome of the Summit reflects the evolution in thinking—in both the industrialised and the developing countries—about the process of development. The environment—development—food security nexus had been explored in the annual sessions of the Commission for Sustainable Development (CSD) established by the United Nations Conference on the Environment and Development (UNCED), held in Rio di Janeiro in June 1992. The Rome Summit, however, focused on the food and agricultural and rural development perspective.

Review of Selected Commitments

(i) Commitment Four: Food, Agricultural Trade and Overall Trade Policies

This commitment is taken first because it is the one which has the most relevance to this paper. The 'basis for action' under this commitment begins with the statement that "Trade is a key element in achieving world food security." The term 'trade' is used without any qualification and thus refers to trade in general and not only in agricultural and food products. The text continues by saying that trade contributes to food security by stimulating "... economic growth, which is critical to improving food security", and that it has a major bearing on access to food through its positive effect on economic growth, income and employment. Yet it also recognises that such benefits might not reach the poorest. Therefore it calls for "appropriate domestic economic and social policies" to better ensure that all, including the poor, benefit from economic growth" stimulated by a more liberal trade regime.

Commitment Four, while stating that trade "allows food consumption to exceed food production," implicitly recognises that trade also allows food (and agricultural non-food) production to exceed consumption, leading to the well-known 'vent for surplus' argument explaining the role of agricultural trade in economic development. Hence, food trade not only improves the physical and economic access to food, on the side of supply, by increasing food availability, which also contributes to lower food prices for domestic consumers, but also promotes, on the side of demand, the international exchange of surplus food and agricultural products. In other words, it improves entitlements through exchange and, in so doing, widens the range of food available for consumption, improving diets and satisfying food preferences. But food and agricultural trade may also have, through the effects of competition, harmful effects on traditional food production systems and those engaged in them. In this context, the Commitment (Objective 4.1) specifically refers, inter alia, to seeking to avoid the adverse trade-induced impacts "on women's new and traditional economic activities towards food security."

Objective 4.1 also expresses a concern about the possible conflict between trade and environmental policies and states that the international community will endeavour to ensure the "mutual supportiveness of trade and environment policies in support of sustainable food security." The Marrakesh Ministerial Decision on Trade and Environment of 14 April 1994 represents a shift in perspective, towards ensuring that environmental measures do not unfairly affect market access for developing countries' food and agricultural exports, including fish and fishery products. These two concerns are separate, the first relating to the longer-term sustainability of food security with the needed conservation of the integrity of the underpinning natural resources, together with the human resources—knowledge and experience—required to manage them. This important issue is discussed below, in the context of Commitment Three. The second concern relates to market access needed to exploit the income-earning potential to be derived on the basis of the 'vent for surplus' argument. Improved food security may indeed result from unimpeded market access.

Two further concerns addressed by Commitment Four, and linked also to Commitment Three, relate to food safety and sanitary requirements, where the international community pledged to continue to assist countries to "adjust their institutions and standards" to such requirements. The issue of food safety has taken on particular significance in recent years with the outbreak of Bovine Spongiform Encephalitis (BSE) in cattle (mad cow disease), with its believed transmittal to human beings. Even more recently dioxin has been allegedly found in some traded animal products in Europe and traced to contaminated feeds. The food safety issue was even addressed at the G7 meeting in Cologne in June 1999. Food safety including, from the consumer point of view, the issue of genetically modified organisms (GMOs) constitutes a major challenge to the proponents of a more liberalized food and agricultural trading regime. The Agreement on the Application of Sanitary and

Phytosanitary Measures (SPS) aimed at furthering the use of harmonised measures on the basis of international standards, guidelines and recommendations, appears to fail to prevent faulty domestic control of standards from affecting the quality of exported food products, particularly those with a longer production-processing chain typical for animal food products. In this regard, FAO has developed a draft Code of Practice for Good Animal Feeding, through the Codex Alimentarius Commission, but all such codes need the appropriate national monitoring and control measures to be effective. If the recent, most publicised, international food safety scares are a correct indication of the actual situation, assistance to countries to "adjust their institutions and standards...to food safety and sanitary requirements" needs to be strongly underlined.

International trade not only permits food consumption in a country to exceed production (it need not have self-sufficiency in food) but also offers a means (which is likely to be less costly than holding strategic reserves of food) to even out fluctuations in domestic supplies even when self-sufficiency is broadly achieved. Such generalizations have been supported during the past half century or more by the secular decline in world prices of traded food products relative to those of manufactures and by lower transport and port handling costs. All of this is largely self-evident, but the key issue remains the reliability of supply of key food commodities and the level and variability of world market prices. Memories of the World Food Crisis of 1973-74 linger on as well as the spectre of food embargoes.

In this regard Commitment Four sets the objective (Objective 4.2) of meeting "essential food import needs in all countries, considering world price and supply fluctuations and taking especially into account food consumption of vulnerable groups in developing countries." The admonition that food exporting countries should act as reliable sources of supplies to their trading partners and administer all export-related trade policies and programmes responsibly is consistent with the decision that governments and the international community should examine "WTO-compatible options and take any appropriate steps to safeguard the ability of importing developing countries...to purchase adequate supplies of basic foodstuffs from external sources on reasonable terms and conditions." Facilities already exist to assist the least-developed and net food-importing developing countries in financing essential food imports, through international financial institutions (mainly the International Monetary Fund), but they are not automatically accessible. It is possible, and it would perhaps be desirable, that such issues will receive attention under Article 20 of the Agreement on Agriculture, with the continuing negotiations taking into account the experience to date in implementing the reduction commitments and the effect of such commitments on world trade in agriculture. It is to be hoped that what will be included in such 'experience' is not defined on such a narrow basis as to cover only the application of the reduction commitments. It should also include other factors that may have adversely effected the reliability of trade as a support to improved food security and which may be susceptible to changes in trade policy in exporting countries.

Commitment Four recalls Article 12 of the Agreement on Agriculture, which refers to export prohibitions and restrictions in the context of domestic supply shortfalls in the exporting country rather than the application of trade embargoes for political or military motives. There is, moreover, the affirmation of the Rome Declaration that "Food should not be used as an instrument for political or economic pressure" and of "the necessity of refraining from unilateral measures not in accordance with the international law and the Charter of the United Nations and that endanger food security".

Commitment Three: Sustainable Food, Agriculture, Fisheries, Forestry and Rural Development, Policies and Practices

Commitment Three is of key importance because it is concerned with the expansion of food production (and hence with the issue of a certain degree of self-sufficiency in food), and with the sustainability of policies (and hence with the natural resource-use aspects of food production); it also refers specifically to the multifunctional character of agriculture, but without explicitly stating what that involves. These issues, along with those arising from Commitment Two relating to access to food, lie at the core of the debate on non-trade concerns (NTCs) which the Summit itself, probably deliberately, did not enter into. It is not possible to avoid the NTC issue in this paper. Moreover, it is useful to consider what is meant by the multifunctional character of agriculture.

Commitment Three relates more to the typical food-deficit, developing country situation where expanding food production is one of the primary means to increase the availability of food and income for those living in poverty. The issue of food self-sufficiency is not directly addressed, and rightly so. The approach is linked to improving access to food through raising effective demand and is linked to rural development: stimulating production and promoting economic diversification. It is also particularly concerned with protecting fragile environments and with the sustainable management of natural resources. In this respect, the links between the concept of sustainable agricultural and rural development (SARD) and food security-focused development of the Rome Plan of Action are clear. Key phrases used in 'Objectives and Actions' of Commitment Three are:

- "To pursue, through participatory means, sustainable, intensified and diversified food production,...taking fully into account the need to sustain natural resources."
- "To combat environmental threats to food security, in particular ... erosion of biological diversity ... to achieve greater production."
- "To promote sound policies and programmes on transfer and use of technologies.compatible with sustainable development..."
- Action to "strengthen and broaden research and scientific cooperation...to increase productive potential and maintain the natural resource base...to eradicate poverty and promote food security."
- "... formulate and implement integrated rural development strategies....that promote rural employment, skill formation,...that reinforce the local productive capacity of farmers, fishers and foresters ... including members of vulnerable and disadvantaged groups, women and indigenous people ...and that ensure their effective participation."

This is a complex agenda because it is a statement on human-centred, gender-sensitive, participatory, resource-conserving, small-scale, local knowledge-using, bottom-up agricultural and rural development into which food security is woven as an integral part. It may be contrasted with an efficiency-seeking, large-scale, technology and profit-driven, top-down development where food security may well improve, but not necessarily equitably so, either spatially (i.e. between rural and urban areas or between richly endowed regions and marginal ones) or within the society (essentially the poor and less well-off compared to the affluent). Perhaps unjustly, liberalized food and agricultural trade has come to be associated with the second rather than the first development paradigm. Of course, it can be argued that even if this latter link holds, then less optimal or desirable situations that emerge can and should be corrected by domestic food and agricultural and rural development policies rather than by international trade policies.

Within Commitment Three, unlike the NTC approach, food security and environmental concerns and objectives are interwoven and considered in a holistic way. Promoting the conservation and sustainable use of biological diversity in general, and plant genetic resources in particular, receives particular attention mainly because the vision of agricultural development is one where farmer-developed land and traditional varieties of major crops continue to provide the core food production systems, with modern varieties broadening but not replacing indigenous cultivated plant germplasm. Nevertheless, a utilitarian approach is fostered through integrating conservation and sustainable utilisation of plant genetic resources for food and agriculture, by appropriate in situ and ex situ approaches. Conservation through in situ approaches is particularly important because the aim is to conserve the diversity of cultivated plants while using them, along with their wild relatives, within productive landscapes to maintain evolutionary processes. Ex situ conservation cannot replicate these processes. Much of this thinking derives from the Fourth International Technical Conference on Plant Genetic Resources, held in Leipzig in June 1996. There are similar concerns relating to animal genetic resources, although the problems naturally differ and formal intergovernmental discussion of them has only recently got under way.

These issues have direct bearing on the Agreement on Trade-

Related Aspects of Intellectual Property Rights (TRIPS), to which the Rome Plan of Action, again probably deliberately, does not directly refer. The TRIPS Agreement is distinct from the Agreement on Agriculture and lays down its own review process. The key issue here is how to confer adequate plant variety protection (PVP) so as not to inhibit the transfer of needed plant germplasm while protecting local and possibly vulnerable farming systems. While the review process is under way, States can continue to avail themselves of Article 27, paragraph 3(b), of the TRIPS Agreement, which allows for the exclusion from patentability of plants and animals other than micro-organisms. However, PVP itself has to be provided for either by patents or by an effective sui generis system or by any combination of them. It has been observed that the terms used in the Article are not defined and are open to varying interpretations.

Commitment Two: Improving Physical and Economic Access by All, at All Times, to Food

This commitment is mentioned because it emphasises the human-centred, gender-sensitive approach of the Plan of Action. The issue of physical access to food and the role of trade in this connection was discussed above under Commitment Four. This Commitment broadens the scope, to focus additionally on economic access to food and hence the need for "secure and gainful employment" as well as "equitable and equal access to productive resources such as land, water and credit." Underlying this concern is the need to focus attention on "vulnerable and disadvantaged individuals, households and groups", among which women predominate. Such focused attention raises at least two issues relating to trade. Firstly, imported food products are accessible to different groups of people compared to food domestically produced, especially through self-provisioning. Secondly, the gender issue in this context underlines that proceeds from traded food products, and particularly from higher value products aimed at export markets, may not accrue to the women in poor households and thereby may not contribute to improved food security. Indeed women's scarce time may be diverted from self-provisioning activities to producing such traded products. Such issues were alluded to under Commitment Three and are only flagged again here.

The safety of food and its 'appropriateness' also come to the fore in Commitment Two: "...ensure that food supplies are safe, ... appropriate and adequate to meet the needs...of the population" and again "Encourage...the production and use of culturally appropriate, traditional and under-utilized food crops... and the sustainable utilization of unused or under-utilized fish resources". Specific reference is made to the Agreement on the Application of Sanitary and Phytosanitary Measures and "other relevant international agreements that ensure the quality and safety of food..."

The issue of food quality, particularly in the context of international food trade, is a challenge that has to be met. That of the interaction between such trade and the use of culturally "appropriate, traditional and under-utilized food crops" and fish products does not appear to have been given due attention in the Agreement on Agriculture.

Some Preliminary Conclusions

From the above discussion, the following key issues emerge relating to food security in the context of the forthcoming trade negotiations. They may be divided into what may be termed 'general' and 'specific' issues. The general ones are the following:

- What is the net impact of the further liberalization of food and agricultural trade—set within the broader context of globalization and considering the wide range of situations found in developing countries—on global goals such as the Rome Summit's target of halving the number of undernourished people in the world by 2015?
- To what extent can domestic economic and social policies—specifically, food, agricultural and rural development policies—offset the diverse (and possibly negative) impacts of international policies such as those relating to international trade?

These are indeed wide-ranging issues; the more specific issues are:

- How to ensure that the overall economic gains from trade benefit the poorest people—those who are most likely to be suffering from food insecurity. Can we rely on trickle down of these gains to enhance economic access to food by the poor?
- How to ensure that trade improves physical access to food by all. Imported food may ensure food supplies for urban people, but it may not be distributed adequately to undernourished rural people, whose greater need may be to produce more food for themselves through improved access to resources.
- How to ensure that food and agricultural production and trade do not contribute to the over exploitation of natural resources which may jeopardise domestic food security in the long term.
- How to ensure that food trade flows are not subject to supply disruptions such as embargoes or similar restrictions; i.e. that they are reliable.
- How to ensure that imported food products are of acceptable quality and are safe to eat.

Finally, it should be noted that the trade-food security interface, as revealed by the above analysis and in the context of international law, is not limited to the Agreement on Agriculture alone but also involves other UR Agreements, such as that on TRIPS.

Box 1: The Seven Commitments of the World Food Summit (Rome, 13-17 November 1996)

One....ensure an enabling political, social and economic environment designed to create the best conditions for the eradication of poverty and for durable peace, based on full and equal participation of women and men, which is most conducive to achieving sustainable food security for all;

Two.... implement policies aimed at eradicating poverty and inequality and improving physical and economic access by all, at all times, to sufficient, nutritionally adequate and safe food and its effective utilization;

Three .... pursue participatory and sustainable food, agriculture, fisheries, forestry and rural development policies and practices in high and low potential areas, which are essential to adequate and reliable

(*Contd.*)

food supplies at the household, national, regional and global levels, and combat pests, drought and desertification, considering the multifunctional character of agriculture;

Four.... strive to ensure that food, agricultural trade and overall trade policies are conducive to fostering food security for all through a fair and market-oriented world trade system;

Five .... endeavour to prevent and be prepared for natural disasters and man-made emergencies and to meet transitory and emergency food requirements in ways that encourage recovery, rehabilitation, development and a capacity to satisfy future needs;

Six .... promote optimal allocation and use of public and private investments to foster human resources, sustainable food, agriculture, fisheries and forestry systems, and rural development, in high and low potential areas;

Seven .... implement, monitor and follow-up this Plan of Action at all levels in cooperation with the international community.

Box 2: Defining Food Security

The Rome Summit built on the definition of food security endorsed by the FAO/WHO International Conference on Nutrition held in Rome in December 1992, namely: "access for all people at all times to enough food for an active, healthy life." The Summit elaborated on this definition by adding the ideas of having both physical and economic access rather than just 'access'; having both safe and nutritious as well as sufficient food; and stating that the food should meet people's dietary needs as well as their food preferences for an active and healthy life. The Summit thus fleshed out the earlier definition, linking food security to trade through the notions of 'access' and 'sufficiency'.

An alternative approach to defining food security is that of 'entitlements' to food, and has been put forward by A.K. Sen. Each person has an entitlement to food derived from his or her own *production*, from *exchange* through barter, markets or working in non-food production activities, or from *transfer* (of food) either from the family, the community, civil society or the State. The direct link between trade and this approach is through the entitlement of *exchange*.

Box 3: The Multifunctional Character of Agriculture

Agricultural activities, apart from producing food and fibre etc for which there is a market and which therefore have a monetary value, also involve externalities for which there are no identified markets—i.e. they are subject to market failure. Such externalities may be positive or negative. Of course, all economic activities to some degree share this characteristic, although it seems that agriculture is unique in the range of externalities ascribed to it. Such externalities also may be termed public goods (or public bads, if negative) as opposed to private goods.

(*Contd.*)

The distintinction is important in as much as public goods (or bads) and their associated market failures may justify government intervention to ensure or control their supply through subsidies or regulation or taxation. In practice agriculture is often held to produce a public good, in order to justify continued intervention by the State, although strictly speaking there are no grounds for such a claim.

Until relatively recently, it was agriculture's negative environmental externalities—pollution of surface and ground water and air, loss of habitats and biodiversity, soil erosion, etc—which received most attention from policymakers, involving taxes or regulations to correct for market failures. Now it is being increasingly argued that agriculture also produces positive externalities, alternatively known as multiple functions, the related market failures of which merit policy interventions such as subsidies or other means of agricultural support to ensure their continued 'production'.

There is a broad consensus on what these multiple functions are, although there is a variety of taxonomies by which they are organized. The main point is that they should be genuine externalities and not simply extensions of agriculture's economic primary function of producing food, fibre etc, although they may be in joint supply with them. If this strict definition is applied, the following is a shortlist of functions:

- Food security, including nutritional and food safety aspects, sometimes termed 'strategic' functions.
- Environmental: protection of natural resources, including natural habitats and biodiversity and so contributing to the sustainability of food production systems; disaster prevention (floods and landslides); protecting rural landscapes.
- Social and cultural: linked to employment and income generation in rural areas and hence sustaining the viability of rural communities and maintaining rural society.

Some of these functions are interrelated or synergistic. For example, protecting rural landscapes may promote tourism and hence generate employment and so maintain rural communities. Some observers contend that agriculture's multiple functions cannot be separated and therefore must be performed "on the same spot", but that would rule out the use of tradable permits between agricultural regions. These positive externalities or multiple functions have also been described in general international usage as non-trade concerns—(NTCs) for example, in Article 20 of the Agreement on Agriculture. However, as has been seen, when the multifaceted issue of food security is opened up, as it was at the Rome Summit, there are several clear links between trade and food security. Setting such semantic considerations aside, the next step is to examine what are NTCs commonly cited under the three headings above—food security, environment and social—and relate them to the Rome Plan of Action and particularly its Commitment Three which, as noted above, sets out to pursue, *inter alia,* sustainable

(*Contd.*)

food and agricultural policies and practices, considering the multifunctional character of agriculture. A pertinent observation at this point is that some of the main proponents of NTCs are industrialised countries, in particular those with what may be termed 'difficult' agricultural production environments (harsh climate, mountainous terrain, etc) and with an enduring rural tradition and concern for the conservation of rural landscapes. They also possess the financial means to subsidise their agricultural sectors and their populations generally spend a small share of their disposable income on food.

Food security. This objective or peacetime function receives high priority in several industrialised countries, mainly for strategic reasons because their food security as such, in normal conditions, is hardly in question. For example, Norway recognises that because of high food production costs, it would be much more cost-efficient for several countries, including Norway, *under ordinary circumstances*, to rely entirely on world markets for their food supplies. However, based on historical experience and due to the uncertainty associated with future international supplies, national production policies have been *and will always be* (author's highlighting) a central element in Norway's food security policy. National stocking of food can only partly compensate for the risk that a tight international food supply situation may be of long duration. This risk applies not only to a situation of war but also to peacetime crises such as plant and animal diseases, extensive radioactive fallout, or major shifts in global demand and supply. Food security policies based on a minimum level of self-sufficiency, by preserving the capacity to produce, can be regarded as a risk insurance, with the public costs involved related to the population's risk aversion and its willingness to pay for that insurance.

There are four components to Norway's food security policy: firstly, the need to protect arable land from degradation and alternative use; secondly, to maintain food self-sufficiency from domestic production, measured in terms of calories, at the minimum current level of 50 per cent (57 per cent including fish products); thirdly, to maintain a "fairly sizeable", well trained and experienced farming population; and fourthly, to maintain a decentralised food production structure as being less vulnerable in times of crises.

Does food security in fact increase with the level of self-sufficiency? It can indeed be argued that a policy of self-sufficiency is likely to make domestic food prices more rather than less unstable. Also, by promoting food self-sufficiency, the agricultural sector is likely to become more dependent on inputs with a high import content, particularly with regard to energy. In turn, energy, i.e. fuel, is more likely than food commodities to be subject to effective trade embargoes or sudden price hikes. Yet political support for a food self-sufficiency policy still remains strong in some countries. However, the government response could be a more rational food security policy based on a range of options. Such a policy would be based on an assessment of the main sources of food supply uncertainty: firstly, unforeseen variations in supply caused by natural

(*Contd.*)

events—adverse weather or outbreaks of pests and diseases of important food crops in major producing countries; secondly, man-made events such as hostilities or disasters (such as another Chernobyl) of a sufficient magnitude to affect trade flows; and thirdly, political interventions short of war such as trade embargoes. In the face of such uncertainties, there is a range of possible policy interventions, other than only promoting self-sufficiency; they relate to consumption (e.g. promoting the substitution between foods), production (e.g. making it more responsive to a sudden need to increase supply), storage and marketing (strengthening supplier-importer links). Such policies need not be discussed further here.

The environmental function. The potential for agriculture to yield environmental services is now widely recognized among the OECD countries. Thus a recent OECD paper states: "The provision of environmental benefits and amenities is increasingly seen as an element of the 'multifunctionality' of the [agricultural] sector." The word 'amenities' is significant because it differentiates the industrialised and developing country concerns, with those of the former focusing primarily on protecting agricultural landscapes and those of the latter focusing on the resource-protecting services—prevention of soil erosion and watershed protection, for example—without which food security may be threatened. Indeed, Commitment Three refers to the need "To combat environmental threats to food security....erosion of biological diversity, and degradation of land and aquatic-based natural resources...to achieve greater production." The Commitment does not, however, explicitly ascribe these needs to the multifunctionality of agriculture.

The socio-cultural function. Again, the respective industrialised—developing country interpretations of this function are nuanced differently. The former are primarily concerned with avoiding the depopulation of the countryside which uncontrolled social and economic forces would probably bring about. They are also concerned with maintaining populated rural landscapes and viable rural communities for tourism purposes while also noting that an agrarian structure based on many relatively small, owner-occupied family farms is more conducive to social stability and cultural preservation than one dominated by relatively few large holdings. Food security also is thought to be promoted by a decentralised, evenly distributed, production structure. The developing countries, and many developed countries also, tend to refer to agriculture as being a traditional 'way of life' which has cultural and societal connotations. Rapid rural-urban migration is also cited as a potential disruptive force in a developing country society, contributing to urban unemployment, crime, etc.

Increasingly, discussions on the multifunctionality of agriculture have come to take on a 'normative' stance. They do so by implying that there is some desirable typology of agriculture or agricultural and rural development paradigm that would maximise these functions or positive externalities. This typology has become known as 'multifunctional agriculture'.

(*Contd.*)

These issues cannot be examined too closely here. The Rome Summit only 'considered' the multifunctional character of agriculture in passing, probably not wishing to get involved in a debate on the subject. However, it is pertinent to ask, while not denying the validity of certain of the arguments for a multifunctional agriculture, what is the appropriate area of policy to achieve the benefits or services sought: food, agricultural, rural, social, regional? In all of these areas of policy, international trade has a bearing, of course. Another issue is: Are all of the functions listed above in joint supply with agriculture's primary function of producing food, fibre, etc.? In other words, is it necessary to produce these products to achieve the externalities sought? The answer must be: not always. Furthermore, there is the "necessity test": should a policy measure designed to promote the positive externality be challenged as being inconsistent under the GATT? Article XX of the GATT requires that the measure in question must not only be allowable under the exceptions relating to the protection of the environment and human health, but also be necessary to fulfil the policy objective. Thus far, no dispute panel has accepted the necessity of a measure inconsistent with other provisions of the GATT even if the objective of the policy complied with the allowable exceptions. Hence, the potential importance of the NTC arguments for those industrialised countries seeking to protect their agricultural sectors. Of course, developing countries, and particularly the LDCs, are allowed varying latitude in their policy support measures to agriculture, as provided for in Article 15 of the Agreement on Agriculture.

CASE STUDY: ENHANCING AGRICULTURAL DEVELOPMENT, TRADE AND FOOD SECURITY

Introduction

The rules and disciplines of the Agreement on Agriculture are intended to restrict the use by countries of policy measures that distort world agricultural markets. Nevertheless, there is still flexibility to use a wide range of policy options to pursue national agricultural policy objectives. For each country, the precise extent of this flexibility is determined by its specific commitments on market access, domestic support and export subsidies. With the next round of negotiations about to begin, concern has been expressed by many developing countries that their policy options for the future may be limited by the general provisions of the Agreement as well as by their specific commitments. These concerns, which are related to the issues at stake in the forthcoming negotiations, were reviewed in Paper No. 4. This paper continues that debate and identifies measures that developing countries may pursue in the forthcoming negotiations in order to preserve sufficient flexibility to achieve their agricultural production, trade and food security goals.

Domestic Agricultural Production

In the context of the Agreement on Agriculture, a country has basically two broad policy options to support domestic production and agricultural development: border measures, i.e. through tariffs, as long as they remain within the tariff bindings; and domestic support measures, i.e. price and non-price support to farmers, again within the limits of WTO rules and commitments.

As regards border measures, in general, bound tariffs of the developing countries on agricultural products are at a level sufficiently high to allow them considerable flexibility in stabilising domestic markets or protecting producers. However, there are some problem areas. For example, very few developing countries rationalised their bound tariffs and as a result a number of anomalies have been noted in their commitments. For many net food-importing developing countries with large numbers of low-income households, raising tariffs has also limitations for socio-political reasons.

As regards domestic support, the Agreement distinguishes several categories of measures: "amber" box measures (both product and non-product-specific), "green" and "blue" box measures, and (for developing countries) a special category of agricultural development measures. Of these, quantitative limits have been set only for amber box measures (through the AMS)—the exact amount depending upon each country's reported base-period (1986-88) AMS. Many developing countries reported a zero level base-period AMS. Regarding other measures, no limits on outlays have been placed; but there is a lack of clarity in the definition of these measures. As with bound tariffs, the extent of flexibility in the support of agriculture therefore depends upon what has been committed in the UR.

Besides the current WTO Members, flexibility for domestic support is needed also by developing countries negotiating their accession to WTO, particularly taking into account their developmental and food security concerns.

On both of these broad policy options, developing countries may need to pursue a two-pronged strategy. The first would be to remove some of the imbalances in existing provisions in the Agreement on Agriculture that have allowed considerable production and trade-distorting support by countries that can afford it. In this respect, the following reforms may be considered:

- Significant reductions in total AMS, as these have not been binding at all;
- Further limitations on switching support between products, preferably making AMS reduction commitments product-specific;
- *Elimination or reduction of* de minimis *allowances for countries with large AMS levels;*
- Tightening of the criteria for inclusion in the green box, including a more concise/measurable notion of what is "minimal effect on production and trade";
- Acknowledging blue box measures as trade-distorting and counting them under Current Total AMS for reduction purposes;
- Limitations on the applicability of Article 13 ("Peace Clause");
- Pushing for a substantial reduction or elimination of export subsidies that displace domestic production, with due consideration of possible negative effects (e.g. strengthening the Marrakesh Decision) in order to help food importers adjust to change.

The second component of the strategy would be to ensure that the developing countries have the necessary degree of flexibility to pursue agricultural development and food security policies. This may require clarifications/interpretations/adjustments to the current provisions of the Agreement on Agriculture, as follows:

- Allowing them the option of recalculating their AMS and revising their Schedules where deemed necessary;

- Higher de minimis allowances for non-product-specific AMS, especially when there is a large negative product-specific AMS;
- Granting some "credit" for negative product-specific AMS by excluding from the AMS calculation specific food security expenditures;
- Extension of the green box, on SDT basis, to include food security measures specifically for developing countries;
- Clarification of definitions and methodological problems, e.g. eligible production, excessive inflation, "low-income" and "resource-poor farmers";
- Allowing them the option of rationalising their tariff commitments on agricultural products and rebalancing tariffs (i.e. raising some tariffs, e.g. on sensitive commodities, and reducing others);
- Extending to all acceding developing countries the current (SDT) flexibility in respect of domestic support;
- Extending more financial and technical assistance (through international financial institutions and specialized agencies) to help them develop human resources, to meet SPS standards and to strengthen their legal and administrative capacity on trade issues.

Access to World Markets

For a country dependent on agricultural exports, increasing agricultural export earnings is essential to economic development and food security, and particularly so for developing countries. Their combined share of agricultural exports is not only low (about 30 per cent of the world total), but has also been stagnant, and many of them depend on the world market for satisfying much of their food needs. While the results of the UR have contributed to improving market access for products of export interest to developing countries, much remains to be done, including further reductions in tariff levels and tariff escalation, improved access to tariff rate quotas (TRQs), and curtailment of the use of safeguards and new non-tariff measures. Some reforms to be considered include the following:

- Reducing tariff peaks and tariff escalation on products of export interest to developing countries, which may require the use of a harmonization formula for tariff cuts;
- Eliminating the use of complex tariffs (including the banning of specific tariffs, as these give more protection to lower-priced imports);
- Expanding the TRQs and agreeing to rules for setting the in-quota tariff rate;
- Ensuring access to new TRQs for developing countries, also taking into account the specific interests of those currently benefiting from preferential access arrangements in developed country markets;
- Considering ways of compensating countries for the erosion of preferential tariff margins during the adjustment phase;
- Making the administration of TRQs more transparent so that developing country exporters are able to take advantage of new trading opportunities;
- Adding product specificity in minimum access commitments by disaggregating further the TRQs.

Domestic Market Stability

The reforms outlined above should provide considerable room for increasing domestic food production. Improved market access and other related reforms should contribute to raising export earnings, which are fundamental for improving the capacity to import food, particularly by LDCs and NFIDCs.

Although these reforms can be expected to contribute somewhat to the stability of global agricultural markets, these markets are by nature volatile. There are general WTO provisions for stabilising domestic markets (e.g. anti-dumping and safeguard measures), but they are not useful for many developing countries, which need more accessible and simpler instruments. Thus, the following reforms may be sought:

- If the time allowed for recourse to special safeguard measures were to be extended, it would be only right that this facility be available to all WTO members, but perhaps only for a limited number of sensitive basic foodstuffs and perhaps only with some tightening of "triggers" so that there is no abuse;

- Support the use of price bands as a means of cushioning the impact of world market variability on the domestic market, i.e. for stabilization and not for protection;
- Seek exemption from AMS disciplines of expenditures related to the acquisition and maintenance of food security stocks;
- Seek to strengthen Article 12 of the Agreement on Agriculture by supporting the prohibition of export taxes in addition to export bans.

Complementary Measures

The Marrakesh Decision

The Decision on Measures Concerning the Possible Negative Effects of the Reform Programme on Least Developed and Net Food-Importing Developing Countries calls for assistance to be given to these countries if they are adversely affected by the reform process. To date, there has not been any concrete benefit stemming from the Decision. Accordingly, LDCs and NFIDCs could aim to include, in a revised Decision, provisions that would make it more effective and responsive to their needs:

- Establish the Decision as a legally binding instrument on an equal footing with other commitments under the Agreement on Agriculture;
- Establish mechanisms, that would allow LDCs and NFIDCs to become automatically eligible for assistance when world market prices rise above a certain level;
- Seek to set up an on-going programme or fund to provide financial and technical assistance to LDCs and NFIDCs in order to improve their agricultural productivity and infrastructure and reduce their dependence on food imports;
- Seek to clarify the role of the WTO in the implementation

and monitoring of compensating measures, through, for instance, the creation of institutional mechanisms and mandatory notification requirements.

Capacity Building

Finally, despite improvements in recent years, the participation of many developing countries in multilateral trade negotiations remains weak and their capacity to implement the various agreements and to take advantage of trade opportunities is limited. Clearly, much needs to be done in this area to level the playing field. Technical and financial assistance on capacity building is essential, some of the priority areas being as follows:

- Strengthening the capacity of developing countries in multilateral negotiations, assisting them to deal with problems they confront in their effort to keep pace with their WTO commitments and to take advantage of trade opportunities;
- Assisting non-members of WTO to achieve accession on terms consistent with their development and food security needs;
- Implementing the Integrated Framework for trade-related technical assistance to LDCs as recognised in the Plan of Action for the Least Developed Countries adopted in Singapore in December 1996 by the first WTO Ministerial Conference.

CASE STUDY: ASIA AND THE PACIFIC

The focus of this chapter is on improving productivity and food availability as the first step towards sustainable food security in Asia and the Pacific. The overall purpose of this study is to determine how to promote agricultural productivity growth to achieve sustainable food security most efficiently in Asia and the Pacific. The specific objectives are:

1. to examine the trends in agricultural production and productivity growth in Asia and the Pacific;

2. to isolate the sources of agricultural productivity growth; and
3. to determine the relative significance of these factors in determining the success in agriculture of member countries.

Special attention is paid to the role of investment, both in physical and human capital, in maintaining and increasing agricultural productivity. The analysis provides policy implications useful for improving food security.

Introduction

Ensuring food for all, today and in generations to come, is one of the greatest challenges facing the world community. Food security is defined as the ability of people to meet their required level of food consumption at all times; it is considered by many to be a basic human right. However, about 1.1 thousand million people in low-income, food-deficit developing countries cannot meet such basic needs (FAO, 1997a). Among them, more than 800 million live in rural areas, depending directly on agriculture for their food supply, employment and income. Therefore, boosting the rural economy, particularly through increased agricultural production, is one of the chief means of alleviating poverty and increasing food security (Pinstrup-Andersen and Pandya-Lorch, 1998).

Food security consists of three major components: availability (associated with production and trade); accessibility (associated with income and wealth); and utilization (associated with health and nutrition) (Asenso-Okyere, Benneh and Tims, 1997). While there seems to be a consensus among analysts that current global food production is adequate to avoid widespread famine and malnutrition (Rosegrant and Ringler, 1997), the overall positive trends disguise the disparities in production and distribution of food between regions. The disparities are described by Rosegrant, Agcaoili-Sombilla and Perez (1995) as a two-tiered system of food security, in which rich and rapidly growing economies enjoy abundant, affordable food supplies, while poor, slow-growing countries suffer from food scarcity and malnutrition. This means that the food security problem is, in the main, not one of shortage but of imbalance and distribution.

Another aspect of food security is sustainability. The concerns are: "can food production continue to keep up with demand in generations to come?" and "is the prosperity of the current generation at the expense of the future?" Some analysts believe that the rapid growth in agricultural production in the last few decades has occurred at great environmental cost (Anderson, 1994). That is, over-exploitation has resulted in natural resources being depleted and the environment being damaged. Indeed, the greater intensity of use of land and water resources and chemicals has created problems such as soil salinization, soil erosion, water pollution, pest resistance, etc. As a result, there are signs of declining rates of growth in yields. For example, it has been shown that the average annual growth rate of paddy rice yield in the world declined from 2.42 per cent in 1974-82 to 1.78 per cent in 1982-90 (Rosegrant, Agcaoili-Sombilla and Perez, 1995). The corresponding figures were 2.62 and 1.66 per cent for Asia and 4 and 1.6 per cent for China (Pinstrup-Andersen, 1994). Similar results were found for other crops, including wheat, maize, sorghum and other coarse grains.

Similarly, externalities from agricultural production, and related environmental or "green" issues such as climate change, preservation of wilderness areas and biodiversity, animal welfare and food safety, have received increasing attention in the discussion of agricultural policy in recent years (Alston, Norton and Pardey, 1995).

These concerns suggest that sustainable food security is not only about meeting the increasing and changing demand for food now, but about protecting the environment for future generations. Whether and how this is to be achieved depends on a number of economic, social and political factors, both at the national and international levels. Socio-economic factors with potentially significant effects on future developments in the world food situation include: population and income growth, demographic changes and urbanization on the demand side, as well as technological change and productivity growth on the supply side (Rosegrant, Agcaoili-Sombilla and Perez, 1995). Therefore, future agricultural production and productivity growth depend on, among others, a combination of agricultural, environmental, trade and macro-economic policies at the global level.

Although food security issues are multi-faceted, the discussion here focuses on food availability and production in Asia and the Pacific as a first step towards resolving such issues. Particular attention is paid to the role of investment and agricultural productivity in meeting the challenge of sustainable food security.

Seven member countries in this region were selected for in-depth examination: Australia, the United States, China, India, Indonesia, Japan and South Korea. These countries are chosen because of their importance in the food balance both in the world and the region. For example, China and India are predicted jointly to account for more than 30 per cent of the estimated global increase in cereal demand (718 million metric tons) between 1993 and 2020 (Rosegrant and Ringler, 1997). The estimated demand increase from China has raised concerns over China's ability to feed itself and the impact of changes in China's trade position on global food balances and prices (Alexandratos, 1996; Brown, 1995; Fan and Agcaoili-Sombilla, 1997). Indonesia is chosen for similar reasons. Together, these three countries account for nearly 70 per cent and 40 per cent of the population in Asia and in the world in 1996, respectively (FAO, 1997b).

In addition, Australia and the United States are chosen because of their role as major food exporters to the region. Japan and South Korea, on the other hand, represent (newly) industrialized countries that are major food importers. These differences among the selected countries in the stage of economic development, resource endowments and government policy are central to identifying factors in affecting agricultural productivity growth and the role of government policy.

Production and Productivity Growth in Agriculture

When evaluating the performance of a production unit or the agricultural sector, it is common to use production (the level of output), productivity (output per unit of input) or efficiency (actual output relative to the potential output or best practices) as indicators. Although these measures are closely related, they can yield different rankings in measuring performance. In general, productivity is the most commonly used measure, be it measured in terms of total factor productivity (TFP) or in partial terms such as labour productivity (output per labour) and yield (output per hectare) for its relative ease in calculation and interpretation.

In the following sections, changes over time in output and productivity growth in different regions are compared and the causes for variations are discussed.

Agricultural Development and Input Use

Agricultural output and productivity vary greatly with the stage of economic development, resource endowments, government policy and agronomic-ecological conditions. However, there is a similar path in agricultural development over time and across countries. Pingali and Heisey (1996) categorized the technological transformation of cereal crop production system into three distinct phases:

(i) the land-augmentation phase;
(ii) the labour-substitution phase; and
(iii) the knowledge-and management-intensity phase.

The basic assumption is that the transition from one phase to another is determined by growing factor scarcity, first for land, then for labour and finally for other factors of production, such as machinery and management skills.

The first phase is characterized by area expansion being the main source of output growth, as was seen during the pre-Green Revolution era of the 1950s and 1960s. However, as opportunities for area expansion decline over time, cropping intensity is increased, along with increasing use of water, fertilizers, pesticides and high yielding varieties. This was indeed the case during the Green-Revolution period in the 1970s and early 1980s. Such intensive production results in an increased demand for labour and mechanization, as the production system moves from single-cropping to double-and triple-cropping with increased application of purchased inputs.

Eventually, production reaches the point of diminishing

marginal returns to further intensification, as was the case in the late 1980s, the post-Green Revolution phase. Here, better technical knowledge and management skills are used to substitute for traditional inputs. Variety selection, fertilizer timing and placement, water management and pesticide application are some areas in which productivity has improved with reduction in unit cost of production.

The model just outlined is used in the following analysis as the basic framework to explain the changes in input use and in productivity between the 1960s and the 1990s. First, it is applied to various regions in the world, then to the developing and developed countries, and finally to the selected countries in Asia and the Pacific.

Comparisons of Agricultural Output and Input Use by Regions

Agricultural output along with usage rates for conventional inputs, including land, labour, tractor and fertilizer, in various regions are presented in Table 11. It can be seen that in 1994, Asia produced 47 per cent of the world's agricultural output and had most of the agricultural (40%) and irrigated land (70%) and highest total fertilizer use (47%). Only in terms of total tractor use does it rank second, following Europe. In terms of input use per hectare, Asia ranks third for both fertilizer and tractors, following Europe and North America.

Notably, output in Asia tripled between 1961 and 1994. This three-fold increase can be attributed to the increase in input use (an 81% increase in irrigated land, a 13-fold increase in fertilizer usage, and a 27-fold increase in tractor usage). However, there was only a slight increase (eight percent) in the amount of land used. In terms of factor productivity in Asia, it appears that fertilizer productivity declined by 80 per cent from 1961 to 1994 while land productivity increased by 184 per cent. Because of the interaction between inputs used, these results should be interpreted with caution. Overall, the information presented in Table below suggests that although fertilizer usage in Asia is approaching the levels used in Europe and North America, land productivity can be improved further by increasing the degree of mechanization.

Table 10.11: Agricultural Output, Input Use and Productivity by Regions, 1961 and 1994

Input Use, 1961 and 1994	*Africa*	*Asia*	*Europe*	*Latin America*	*North America*
1961					
Net ag output (89-91 thousand million US$)	36.68	161.42	123.37	50.79	84.59
Land (million hectares)	155.12	436.21	151.37	102.27	225.71
Irrigated land (million hectares)	7.36	90.17	8.32	8.13	14.35
Percent of land irrigated	4.75	20.67	5.50	7.95	6.36
Tractors (million)	0.26	0.26	5.38	0.46	6.42
Fertilizer (million tonnes)	0.73	3.89	14.29	1.06	14.09
Fertilizer per hectare (kg)	4.68	8.92	94.43	10.33	62.45
Tractor per 1 000 ha (number)	1.65	0.60	35.53	4.53	28.45
1994					
Net ag output (89-91 thousand million US$)	78.81	496.74	186.14	122.42	162.68
Land (million hectares)	190.02	472.56	135.43	156.01	233.28
Irrigated land (million hectares)	12.20	163.17	16.77	17.65	22.11
Percent of land irrigated	6.42	34.53	12.38	11.32	9.48
Tractors (million)	0.59	7.87	12.35	1.67	6.36
Fertilizer (million tonnes)	3.47	61.08	21.98	9.23	32.86
Fertilizer per hectare (kg)	18.26	129.26	162.34	59.17	140.86
Tractor per 1 000 ha (number)	3.12	16.66	91.19	10.73	27.25

(*Contd.*)

Input Use, 1961 and 1994

	Africa	*Asia*	*Europe*	*Latin America*	*North America*

Factor Productivity, 1961 and 1994

	Africa	*Asia*	*Europe*	*Latin America*	*North America*
1961					
Net output/fertilizer(US$1 000/mt)	50.48	41.47	8.63	48.08	6.00
Net output/HA (US$/ha)	236.49	370.06	815.04	496.66	374.79
1994					
Net output/fertilizer(US$1 000/mt)	22.71	8.13	8.47	13.26	4.95
Net output/HA (US$/ha)	414.72	1,051.18	1,374.48	784.70	697.37

Source: FAO (1997b).

Comparisons of Agricultural Output and Input Use, Developing Versus Developed Countries

In this section, comparisons were made for trends in land use, production and yield between developing and developed countries and across four commodities (rice, wheat, maize and other grains) for the period 1967-1994. The data were split into two subperiods, which coincided with the peak-green revolution period (1967-1982) and the post-green revolution period (1982-1994). The results are summarized in Table 10.12.

Several points can be drawn from Table 10.2. First, there are substantial variations in growth rates across all commodities, between developing and developed countries, and over time between the two subperiods. Secondly, the growth rates of cereal production and yield show a significant slowdown nearly across the board in the second subperiod. Thirdly, the crop area has been declining, again with only a few exceptions. Finally, the growth rates in yield

Table 10.12: Annual Growth Rates of Crop Area, Production and Yield 1967-1994 (percent)

	Area		*Production*		*Yield*		
	1967-82	*1982-94*	*1967-82*	*1982-94*	*1967-82*	*1982-94*	*1993-2020*
Wheat							
Developed	–0.12	–1.38	1.73	–0.03	1.87	1.35	1.06
Developing	1.45	0.42	5.39	2.94	3.88	2.52	1.30
World	0.48	–0.59	2.88	1.20	2.40	1.80	1.17
Maize							
Developed	0.64	–0.26	3.05	0.69	2.33	1.01	0.84
Developing	0.65	1.36*	3.46	3.66*	2.80	2.27	1.36
World	0.64	0.77*	3.20	1.93	2.52	1.16	1.03
Paddy Rice							
Developed	–0.23	–0.28	–0.14	0.34*	0.09	0.61*	0.53
Developing	0.81	0.21	3.21	2.03	2.38	1.81	1.08
World	0.78	0.20	2.96	1.94	2.17	1.74	1.05
Other Grains							
Developed	0.52	–1.63	1.32	–0.78	0.79	0.85*	0.78
Developing	–0.87	0.12	1.20	0.03	2.08	–0.09	1.24
World	–0.15	–0.79	1.28	–0.52	1.43	0.26	0.85

Source: Rosegrant and Ringler (1997).
p indicates projected, not observed, figures.
* indicates increases in growth rates between 1967-82 and 1982-94.

between 1993 and 2020 are projected to be lower than what they were previously, with the exception of "other grains." Those exceptional cases are highlighted with asterisks in Table 10.2.

According to Rosegrant and Ringler (1997), the reduction in land area and production of wheat and other grains in developed countries was primarily policy-induced. It reflects the changes in price support programmes in North America and the Common Agricultural Policy in the European Union, as well as economic and political reforms in the formally centrally planned economies of Eastern Europe and the former Soviet Union. On the other hand, the slowdown of cereal productivity growth in developing countries, particularly in Asia, since the 1980s, was attributed to declining world prices and over-intensification of cereal production. Specifically, declining cereal prices had caused a shift of land out of cereals and into more profitable cropping alternatives, such as horticultural products. Furthermore, the intensity of land use in the late 1960s and 1970s, when the Green Revolution was in full swing, led to input usage beyond the optimal levels, reducing yield in the later period.

From these observations, it seems apparent that land area available for cropping is unlikely to increase and may fall even further as more agricultural land is diverted to residential and industrial uses. A decrease in cropping area means that a greater burden will be placed on growth in crop yield to meet future cereal demand. Moreover, it appears that over-intensification may have led to resource degradation and hence a slowdown in yield growth. The implication is that, to maintain or increase yield in the future, more emphasis on sustainable agriculture is essential.

The Asian-Pacific Countries

The data presented here focus on seven Asian-Pacific countries and, where appropriate, use the United States as a benchmark. Moreover, comparisons are made based on agriculture as a whole rather than by commodity. The countries included are Australia, the United States, China, India, Indonesia, Japan, and South Korea.

Trends in input use, in terms of arable land and labour, and final agricultural output are presented in Table 10.13. The growth rates in labour use are variable. While there tended to be negative or little growth in labour input use in the United States, Japan, Australia and South Korea, there was slight to moderate growth in China, India and Indonesia. In terms of arable land use, the overall picture displayed little to negative growth. In addition, the negative growth was quite substantial in Indonesia and South Korea during 1987-94. The latter result could be attributable to fast industrialization in these two countries.

Table 10.13: Annual Average Growth Rates of Labour, Land Use and Agricultural Output (Percent)

	USA	*Japan*	*Australia*	*China*	*Indonesia*	*India*	*South Korea*
Labour							
1961-75	-3.27	-3.66	-0.39	3.39	0.51	2.22	0.79
1975-87	-2.48	-2.53	0.22	0.59	1.60	1.50	-3.40
1987-94	0.86	-7.29	-1.10	0.98	2.08	2.55	-4.54
Arable Land							
1961-75	0.23	-1.55	2.43	-0.39	0.00	0.36	0.10
1975-87	-0.03	-0.53	0.89	-0.38	1.36	0.11	-0.22
1987-94	0.00	-0.64	0.02	-0.23	-2.98	0.00	-1.17
Final Agricultural Output							
1961-75	2.26	2.42	3.61	4.09	2.91	2.42	4.65
1975-87	1.00	0.86	0.93	4.99	4.42	2.58	3.10
1987-94	2.71	-0.42	1.73	5.15	3.38	4.64	2.29

Source: Rao and Lee (1997); FAO (1997b).

Agricultural output growth has remained positive from 1961 to 1994 (Table 10.3), with only one exception (Japan). Comparisons of growth rates are more variable, however. For example, during 1975-87, the developed economies (United States, Japan and Australia) experienced a slowdown in production while production in less developed economies (China, India, South Korea and Indonesia) accelerated (Table 10.3).

The slowdown during the period 1975-1987 coincides with the growth deceleration in OECD countries during 1973-1987 in response to the oil shocks and resulting changes in macroeconomic policies (Maddison, 1989). Maddison claims that Asian countries did not suffer as much from the oil price increases because of generally more flexible commodity and labour markets and less institutional rigidity that magnify external price shocks compared to OECD countries. Another reason for strong growth in Asian countries was because of high levels of investment and rising educational levels during that period.

After the recession, during 1987-1994, Japan continued its slide to register a negative output growth (-0.42 percent), the United States showed a strong recovery and Australia recovered but only to half the rate it was before the slowdown. In comparison, China and India had shown strong output growth throughout the observation period. Also, it can be seen from Table 5.3 that, although during 1987-1994 the output growth rate was negative (-0.42 percent) in Japan, labour productivity grew by an impressive 7.41 per cent, the highest among the countries listed. The increase in productivity stemmed from the fact that the reduction in output was more than offset by the savings in labour use. In China, output grew at a rate of 4.09 per cent per year during 1961-1975 while labour productivity grew only marginally at a rate of 0.68 per cent. The differing rates imply that increases in output may have been due to greater use of labour rather than from productivity increases. In contrast, output growth in Japan comes mainly from productivity growth.

Table 10.14 shows the growth rates for partial factor productivity in terms of land and labour. It should be noted that both China and India showed strong growth in output between 1961 and 1994 (4.09 to 5.15 per cent per annum for China and 2.42 to 4.64 per cent for India, Table 10.3) but the results for productivity growth were somewhat different. In particular, China registered a dramatic

Table 10.14: Annual Average Growth Rates in Labour and Land Productivity (percent) (1987 Geary-Khamis Prices with Shadow Prices)

	USA	*Japan*	*Australia*	*China*	*Indonesia*	*India*	*South Korea*
Labour Productivity							
1961-75	5.72	6.32	4.02	0.68	2.39	0.20	3.83
1975-87	3.57	3.48	0.72	4.37	2.77	1.07	6.74
1987-94	1.84	7.41	2.87	4.13	1.28	2.04	7.16
Land Productivity							
1961-75	2.03	4.03	1.16	4.51	2.91	2.05	4.54
1975-87	1.03	1.40	0.05	5.39	3.02	2.47	3.33
1987-94	2.71	0.22	1.71	5.39	6.56	4.65	3.51

Source: Rao and Lee (1997); FAO (1997b).

increase in labour productivity from 0.68 per cent per annum in 1961-1975 to 4.37 per cent in 1975-1987 and 4.13 per cent in 1987-1994; the comparable figures for India were 0.20, 1.07 and 2.04 per cent. In general, output growth in both countries was due to the increased use of water and purchased inputs such as high yielding varieties and fertilizers (Wong, 1989).

South Korea and Japan both encountered a slowdown in output growth between 1961-1975 and 1987-1994, but labour productivity grew at impressive rates of 7.41 per cent in Japan and 7.16 per cent in South Korea during 1987-1994. Despite their high levels of labour productivity, Australia and the United States both encountered a slowdown during the period 1975-1987 in output and labour productivity growth. Although labour productivity picked up again during the period 1987-1994 for Australia, the United States continued its decline.

Growth rates of land productivity, presented in Table 10.4, show that in general less developed countries experienced higher growth than developed countries. Japan from 1961 to 1975 is an exception. This could be the result of land intensification where input-intensive multiple cropping was a common practice to compensate for the scarcity of cultivated land. The national index of multiple cropping in China was 1.31 in 1952, 1.5 in 1978 and 1.58 in 1996 (Lin, 1998). In comparison, the index in India was 1.18 in 1970 and 1.24 in 1980 (Wong, 1989). These figures may explain some of the growth in land productivity in these two countries. Wong (1989) also claims that land reforms in China from collectivization to private ownership had a larger impact on land productivity than in India where land reform changed the land tenure system but not ownership.

Despite strong growth in output and partial factor productivity of labour and land, total factor productivity growth has been found to be negative for China (Tang, 1984; Wen, 1993; Wong, 1989) and India (Wong, 1989). These results indicate clearly that output growth was generated primarily from the expansion of inputs, rather than productivity increases.

Table 10.15 shows the relative labour productivity and yields in the selected Asian-Pacific countries using the 1961 figures for the United States as a benchmark. First, it can be seen that most countries have become more productive over time. Secondly, there are wide disparities among countries with three possible divisions. The first group includes the United States and Australia; the second, Japan and South Korea; and the third, China, Indonesia and India. For example, in 1961, agricultural labour in the United States was two-thirds as productive as that in Australia, nearly 15 to 25 times as productive as that in Japan and South Korea and more than 30 to 40 to times as productive as that in China, Indonesia and India. In 1994, the agricultural labour force in the United States was equally productive as that of Australia, 10 to 20 times as productive as Japanese and Korean agricultural labour and 60 to 80 times as productive as Chinese, Indonesian and Indian agricultural labour. The differences in mechanization and labour quality may explain the differences in the level of and changes in productivity in these countries.

Table 10.15: Indices of Agricultural Labour and Land Productivity in Selected Countries (USA 1961 = 100)

	USA	*Japan*	*Australia*	*China*	*Indonesia*	*India*	*South Korea*
Labour Productivity							
1961	100.0	6.1	149.2	2.3	2.9	3.4	3.6
1975	217.9	14.3	258.9	2.5	4.0	3.5	6.2
1978	252.3	15.1	334.4	2.8	4.3	4.0	8.1
1987		21.6	282.1	4.2	5.5	3.9	13.5
1994	377.3	35.7	343.8	5.6	6.0	4.5	21.8
Land Productivity							
1961	100.0	415.9	51.9	06.1	106.0	63.6	227.0
1975	132.5	723.5	60.9	196.7	158.3	84.6	422.8
1978	138.1	751.5	74.4	218.4	174.5	93.3	525.6
1987	149.9	855.2	61.3	369.4	226.3	113.3	626.4
1994	180.8	868.4	69.0	533.3	352.8	155.7	797.3

Source: Rao and Lee (1997); FAO (1997b).

The comparative performance in terms of land productivity (or yield) of arable land shows a different picture (Table 10.15). In this case, Japan and South Korea have the highest yields, followed by China, then by Indonesia, the United States, India and Australia. These results indicate that countries with limited land resources tend to farm their lands more intensively and hence have higher output per unit of arable land. They also reflect differences in climate and water availability.

In summary, it appears that there are substantial variations in input use and productivity among countries and over time. The only trend that is common to the countries examined is perhaps the negative growth in arable land use. Secondly, there are substantial variations in the level of productivity and the rate of productivity growth among developing countries (China, India, and Indonesia), newly industrialized countries (Japan and South Korea) and developed countries (Australia and the United States).

This suggests that there is ample room for productivity improvements in the less developed countries. Meanwhile, the gaps in productivity, as presented in Table 15, are closing. Furthermore, the fact that growth in output and various measures of productivity can sometimes move in opposite directions confirms the important distinctions between output growth and productivity growth, and between total and partial factor productivity.

Finally, it is apparent that the slowing or negative growth in global crop area will increasingly place the burden of meeting future cereal demand on productivity improvements. Productivity improvement can come either from using existing inputs more efficiently (moving closer to the production frontier) or from technological change (shifting the production frontier upward), or a combination of both. It has been shown that, with existing technology, efficiency is primarily influenced by human capital, such as farmers' education and experience, access to credit and extension services (Coelli and Battese, 1996). Technological change depends, on the other hand, on investments in agricultural research and extension (Alston, Norton and Pardey, 1995; Antle and Capalbo, 1988; Pray and Evenson, 1991). In the next section, sources of productivity growth are discussed based on a survey of existing literature.

Factors Affecting Productivity Growth

In explaining productivity growth, economists originally limited themselves to the role of conventional inputs such as land, labour, physical capital, water and chemical inputs. However, the failure to explain productivity growth adequately led them to examine the role of human capital and public goods, such as education, agricultural research and extension and publicly provided infrastructure (Griliches, 1963; Mankiw, Romer and Weil, 1992; Nelson, 1964 and 1981; Solow, 1957). Public policies that have a strong link to agricultural productivity such as policy reforms were also examined (Auraujo, Chambas and Foirry, 1997; Lachaal, 1994; Lin, 1992; McMillan, Whalley and Zhu, 1989; Wiens, 1983).

The rationale for considering research is the belief that investments in research result in increases in the stock of knowledge, which, in turn, either facilitate the use of existing knowledge or generate new technology. Technological advances, whether resulting from changes in input quality or how inputs are combined, lead to productivity gains. Education, training and extension also increase productivity by increasing people's knowledge and skill base, which are essential for technology adoption and efficient use of inputs. Public infrastructure, on the other hand, increases productivity by facilitating the exchange of goods and services.

Technological Change

Technological change is recognized by many as one of the most important sources of productivity growth (Antle and Capalbo, 1988). It refers to the changes in the production process that come about from the application of innovation and newly acquired scientific knowledge and technical and management skills. Technological change increases agricultural productivity either by shifting the production frontier upward so that more measured output can be produced with the same amount of inputs or by moving closer to the production frontier so that the same amount of output can be produced with a smaller amount of inputs. Better organizational and management skills not only improve input-output combinations but enable producers to respond more quickly to changing market circumstances (Alston, Norton and Pardey, 1995).

While generation of new technology or knowledge comes from investments in research and development, adoption of technology involves investments by the potential users in both physical and human capital (Antle and Capalbo, 1988). Therefore, adoption of technology depends principally on their applicability and expected returns of the innovation. However, there may be a long lag between development, adoption and productivity gains. Chavas and Cox (1992) found the lag to be up to 15 years between making an investment in research and having an effect on productivity. However, after taking effect, the benefits from an innovation may persist for thirty years or more.

The lag between generation of new technology and its widespread adoption by farmers has important policy implications. First, the adverse effects of reduced public funding to agricultural research and extension on productivity may be under-estimated if the lagged effects are not accounted for. Secondly, the complementarity between research and extension should be taken into account. The former helps the development of new technology, while the latter helps speed up the rate of diffusion and adoption of new technology. Extension can be done more effectively by identifying factors that contribute to technology adoption. As an example, innovators in a farming community can be identified and targeted for extension services.

Since better-educated farmers are found to be more likely to adopt new technology, human capital is a pre-condition for technology adoption and hence productivity growth. Further, if adoption of new technology requires additional investments, lack of access to credit and additional inputs may prevent or slow down technology adoption. Finally, because potential users of new technology often differ in the agronomic-ecological conditions in which they operate, new technology may require adaptive research before it can be transferred successfully to different locations. These impediments to technology adoption mean careful planning and provision of necessary infrastructure are essential to capture the full benefits of new technology.

Agricultural Research and Extension

Many researchers have explored the roles of research and extension in promoting agricultural growth. Rosegrant and Evenson (1992) found that in South Asia, public research accounted for 30 per cent of the output growth, and extension for about 25 per cent, with corresponding rates of return being 63 per cent and 52 per cent, respectively. Pray and Evenson's (1991) survey of Asia found the rates of return to national research investment ranged from 19 to 218 per cent, returns to national extension investment from 15 to 215 per cent, and returns to international research investment from 68 to 108 per cent.

Evenson and McKinsey (1991) found that public investment in research accounted for over half of the output growth in India and extension contributed about one-third. The calculated internal rates of return were 218 per cent for public research and 177 per cent for extension. However, they found that little output growth was attributable to infrastructure. Jamison and Lau (1982) also found that physical capital had little impact on production or profits, as compared to farmer's education and extension services.

Fan (1996) found that public research expenditures accounted for about 20 per cent of total production growth in Chinese agriculture during the period 1965 to 1994. The annual rates of return to agricultural research investment in China ranged from 44 per cent to 83 per cent. Fan (1996) concluded that the rapid growth in agricultural output in China during the 1980s and 1990s was the result of public investments in R&D as well as the institutional and market reforms that began in 1979. He concluded that increases in agricultural research were justifiable; not only did they stimulate additional output growth, but the rate of return to agricultural research was much higher than commercial interest rates.

Despite the high rates of returns from public research investments, agricultural research intensity (ARI), measured as a percentage of Chinese agricultural GDP, was found to have declined from 0.56 per cent for the period 1958-1965 to 0.43, 0.44, 0.39 and 0.40 per cent, respectively, for 1966-1976, 1977-1985, 1986-1990 and 1991-1993 (Fan, 1996). Lin (1998) reported that, as part of the overall market reform, the Chinese Government had reduced its fiscal appropriation for agricultural research, shifting funding from institutional supports to competitive grants and cost recovery. As such, it can be expected that an increasing proportion of research activities will move from the public to the private domain.

Other studies on output growth have also shown a high payoff from agricultural research and extension (Table 10.16). The results indicate that the rate of return on research, in most cases, ranged from 15 to 50 per cent for both developed and developing countries, but some estimates were as high as 218 per cent. The wide disparity among the estimates raises questions regarding the sensitivity of these estimates to the commodity of interest and the use of different time periods and methodologies. Estimates for Asian countries appear to be higher and show a much wider variation than those of studies in the United States. This could be due to the diverse nature of Asian agriculture, which differs from country to country in economic, social and agronomic-ecological conditions. Because of inconsistency in the data and methodology used, it is not possible to make direct comparisons across countries or over time. Nevertheless, the general conclusion that R&D yields relatively high returns seems indisputable.

Table 10.16: Internal Rate of Return to Public and Private Investments to Raise Agricultural Productivity

	Time Period	*Country Studied*	*Public R&D (Percent)*	*Private R&D (Percent)*	*Extension (Percent)*
Makki, Tweeten and Thraen (1996)	1930-90	USA	27	6	—
Huffman and Evenson (1993)	1950-82	USA	41	46	—
Chavas and Cox (1992)	1950-82	USA	28	17	—
Davis (1981)	1964-74	USA	28-52	—	—
Griliches (1963)	1949-59	USA	30-50	—	—
Mullen and Cox (1995)	1953-88	Australia	15-40	—	—
Mullen and Strappa-zzon (1996)	1953-94	Australia	18-39	—	—
Thirtle (1996)	1954-92	UK	15-20	—	—
Maredia and Byerlee (1996)	1965-90	37 LDCs	5-34	—	—
Rosegrant and Evenson (1992)	Various	S. Asia	63	—	52
Pray and Evenson (1991)	Various	Asia	19-218	—	15-215
Fan (1996)	1975-94	China	44-83	—	—
Salmon (1991)	1965-77	Indonesia	151	—	—
Evenson and McKinsey (1991)	1966-86	India	218	95	—

Source: Adapted from Makki, Tweeten and Thraen (1996).

Human Capital

Human capital refers to knowledge, experience and skills possessed by people involved in the production process. It is influenced directly by education, training and extension. Its importance lies in the fact that it has a significant impact on the adoption and the utilization of technology, which in turn, affect the allocation of resources and productivity. A well-trained and well-educated labour force is said to be in a better position to assess changing conditions and make necessary adjustments. This ability is becoming ever more important in an increasingly deregulated and global economy where changes in the commodity markets are frequent and quick responses are required.

The concept of investment in human capital covers not only investments in formal schooling and post-school and on-the-job training, but also investment in the form of improved health and family care. Social capital, on the other hand, refers to one's ability to utilize social networks and institutions. Social status, education and the range of social institutions available can influence one's social capital. Social capital is important in that it affects access to physical capital, land title, credit and cooperatives, all of which have implications for resource allocation and, hence, productivity.

Women appear to suffer most severely from having limited access to human and social capital in some developing countries, although a larger proportion of women than men are engaged in agriculture (Quisumbing et al., 1995). For example, women account for 70 to 80 per cent of household food production in sub-Saharan Africa, 65 per cent in Asia, and 45 per cent in Latin America and the Caribbean. As such, it has been suggested that empowerment of women and gender equality are important factors for raising productivity and promoting food security in developing countries. Jahnke, Kirschke and Lagemann (1987) also found that low adoption of high yield varieties (HYV) in Africa is attributable to lack of appropriate technology development and few extension services directed to women. These findings suggest that acknowledging the critical role of rural women in Asia and providing them with greater access to resources and human capital are crucial in promoting sustainable agriculture and food security.

Policy Reform and Prices

The importance of policy reform is increasingly viewed as fundamental for agricultural productivity gains, especially for countries where government intervention in agriculture has been strong. Removing market distortions and allowing market signals to be transmitted to producers is the main objective of structural adjustment programmes by international organizations for economies in transition and countries in debt. Land reform and most land policies, which assign property rights to users so that efficient and responsible use of resources can take place, are other cases where changes in policy can have a significant impact on productivity.

A good example of policy reform is the implementation of China's responsibility system (RS) in the late 1970s, which linked productivity with material rewards. The policy reform was found to have resulted in increased incentives to produce and hence there were increases in crop yields for every major crop (Wiens, 1983). McMillan, Whalley and Zhu (1989) also reported that in response to the RS and price reforms, output in the Chinese agricultural sector increased by over 61 per cent and productivity by 32 per cent between 1978 and 1984. Moreover, 78 per cent of the output growth was attributed to the RS and 22 per cent to higher prices for crops. Lin (1992) also found that 47 per cent of the growth in agricultural output was attributable to the RS during the same period.

However, Lin (1992) acknowledged that benefits from the RS reform had disappeared by 1984-1987. Similar results were found by Huang, Rosegrant and Rozelle (1996), who indicated that the growth rate of rice production was much higher during the reform period (4.5 per cent) than afterwards, during 1984-1992 (1.3 per cent). Moreover, while the reform was the most significant source of output growth during the reform period, technology was the most significant source of growth later during 1984-1992. Based on these results, Kalirajan, Obwona and Zhao (1996) concluded that despite the substantial impacts of policy reform on output and productivity growth, they provide only a one-shot boost to agricultural productivity. As such, long-term productivity gains depend more on technical change, investments in agricultural research and human capital and, to a lesser extent, on infrastructure.

By contrast, some government policies have been found to have detrimental effects on productivity. Lachaal (1994) found that direct input subsidies to agriculture reduce productivity growth and were a source of technical inefficiency. In this case, the subsidies encouraged using subsidized materials at the expense of other inputs. It was found that with each 10 per cent increase in subsidy, the cost of production increased by 1.8 per cent. Similarly, Makki, Tweeten and Thraen (1996) found that government commodity programmes had had little effect on improving agricultural productivity in the United States. They concluded that the interest of United States' agriculture in international competitiveness and low food costs would be better served by focusing on research, extension and education than by commodity programmes. They also cautioned that the debate to reduce public spending on agricultural research and extension should carefully consider the potential long-term implications of such a policy.

International Trade

Facilitated by improvements in transportation and communication technology, trade has also been important in diffusing new products and new technologies. It is also clear that opening of economies is strongly associated with rapid economic growth. A case in point is the rapid post-war growth of the most dynamic Asian countries, such as Japan, South Korea and Taiwan, and the low growth of inward-looking economies such as China (before the open-door policy) and India. Statistics have shown that during 1950-1973, the annual average compound growth rate in export volume were relatively high in Japan, South Korea and Taiwan as compared to China, Indonesia and India (Table 10.17). During 1973-1986, export growth declined relative to the previous period in Japan, South Korea, Taiwan and Indonesia, was unchanged in India, and climbed dramatically in China.

However, the opening of an economy does not come without risks, particularly where macro-economic, financial and lending policies are not well in place. The recent Asian financial crises underscore how weak financial policies can undermine much of the gains from trade.

Table 10.17: Average Compound Growth Rate in Export Volume (Per cent)

	1950-1973	1973-1986
Japan	15.4	7.6
South Korea	20.3	14.0
Taiwan	16.3	11.6
China	2.7	10.4
Indonesia	6.5	3.3
India	2.5	2.5

Source: Maddison (1989).

Natural Resources

Natural resources are critical determinants of food supply. Degradation of natural resources, such as land and water, undermines production capacity and threatens the sustainability of the natural ecosystem (Pinstrup-Andersen and Pandya-Lorch, 1998). Land degradation has been severe in the past few decades. It was found that since 1945, about two thousand million of the world's 8.7 thousand million hectares of agricultural land, permanent pastures, forest and woodland have been degraded through inappropriate agricultural practices, overgrazing and deforestation (Oldeman, 1992).

One major contributing factor to land degradation is the overuse and misuse of irrigation water (Anderson, 1994). Asia contains the majority of the world's irrigated land. Water for irrigation is essentially free, however. Research into various water allocation mechanisms such as attempts to structure economic incentives for water use must be undertaken. To a large extent, these problems can be alleviated by assigning property rights. Poverty reduction as well as government policies to provide access to markets and credit for land improvements and technology would also reduce misuse of water resources. Therefore, agricultural research is a critical input into sustainable agricultural development, particularly as related to land and water management issues.

Role of Investment

Investments in agricultural research and development (R&D) from both the public and private sectors can lead to technology generation and productivity improvements. The impact of investment on agricultural research can be seen most clearly from Rosegrant, Agcaoili-Sombilla, and Perez (1995). In their global food projections to 2020, they assumed a baseline scenario of US$10 thousand million public investment in national agricultural research and extension services. The low-investment scenario, which assumed an annual cut of US$1.5 billion to the current level of public investment, resulted in a fall of 15 per cent in crop and livestock yield growth rates by 2020. In contrast, if funding of national and international research were to rise by US$750 million per year, crop yield growth would be six per cent higher in 2020 than under the baseline scenario. Although these figures are projections and their accuracy is subject to underlying assumptions, they indicate strongly the negative effects of reduced public investment in research and extension, and the crucial role of investment in increasing agricultural productivity.

Private versus Public Investments

Table 5.6 indicated that the rate of return is, in most cases, greater from public research than private research (Chavas and Cox, 1992; Evenson and McKinsey, 1991; Huffman and Evenson, 1993; Makki, Tweeten, Thraen, 1996). The higher rate of return from public research is, in part, attributed to economies of scale in the production of new agricultural technology and the spill-over and externalities associated with such research (Schultz, 1964). One example of such externalities is the international flow of germplasm. In this case, research benefits from breeding programmes of one country or research institute are appropriated by users who do not incur the full research costs. Public funding is therefore justified by the public nature of knowledge and the high rates of return to public investments in agricultural research.

Traditionally, most agricultural research is publicly funded. However, in recent years, the costs of agricultural technology generation and transfer are shared increasingly with the private sector, particularly in more advanced countries (FAO, 1996b). The proportion of privately funded research is on the order of 30 to 40 per cent of all research expenditures in developed countries (nearly two-thirds in the United States) and about five per cent in the less-developed countries (FAO, 1996b). This increase in private research has to do with protection of markets for research results via patents and intellectual property rights (IPR) as well as recent changes in funding policies (Alston, Norton and Pardey, 1995; Lin, 1998).

Private research is attracted to sectors of the market where research results exist and benefits can be privately appropriated (Alston, Norton and Pardey, 1995). This is typically the case in more developed countries where intellectual property rights are well established and protected for inputs such as agrichemicals, agricultural machinery and seeds (FAO, 1996b). Private investments also include on-farm irrigation systems, land improvements, new tractors and combines, livestock breeds and plant varieties, as well as processing, transport and storage facilities for post-production marketing.

Government, therefore, can provide an environment conducive to investment, through guarantee of rights and law as well as policies encouraging investment, as recognized in the World Food Summit Plan of Action items 2 and 3 (FAO, 1996a). In addition, investments in basic infrastructure, human capital, basic research and resource management will still fall more upon the public sector because of the public goods nature of these investments.

Conclusions and Implications

Concerns over food security are driven by the need to feed an increasing population and to protect the environment. One means of addressing these concerns is to increase the food supply locally by improving agricultural productivity. Although productivity varies across commodities and countries according to stage of economic development, government policy and agronomic-ecological conditions, long-term growth in agricultural productivity depends primarily on technological change, improved input use efficiency and conserving the resource base. All of which, in turn, depend crucially upon investments in agricultural research, extension, and human capital.

From the literature survey, some conclusions can be drawn about the driving forces behind agricultural productivity growth in the Asia-Pacific region. Potential growth due to expansion of land under cultivation or increased input use, with the exception of machinery, is limited. This points to technological progress as the key to growth, driven by agricultural research and extension and improvements in human capital. Policy reforms, on the other hand, while extremely important, may provide only a one-shot boost to agricultural productivity, unlike agricultural research and extension from which the contribution to productivity is long lasting.

Agricultural research intensity ratios are found to be relatively low for developing countries in the Asian-Pacific (Table 10.18), as compared to the two per cent target suggested by Pardey and Alston (1995) and Pinstrup-Anderson, Lundberg and Garrett (1995). Further, public funding of agricultural research and extension has been reduced both nationally and internationally (Anderson and Purcell, 1996).

Table 10.18: Agricultural Research Intensity Ratios (Agricultural Research Expenditures/Value of Agricultural Production)

Region/Country	*Number of Countries*	*1961-65*	*1971-75*	*1981-85*	*Latest Year*
Developing Regions	NA	NA	NA	NA	NA
Sub-Saharan Africa, excluding South Africa	17	0.42	0.67	0.76	0.58
South Africa	1	1.39	1.53	2.02	2.59
Asia and the Pacific, excluding China	15	0.14	0.22	0.32	NA
China	1	0.57	0.44	0.42	0.42
Latin America and the Caribbean	26	0.30	0.46	0.58	NA
West Asia and North Africa	13	0.28	0.50	0.52	NA
Developed countries	18	0.96	1.41	2.03	NA
United States	1	1.32	1.36	1.93	2.22
Australia	1	1.54	3.56	4.52	4.42

Source: Pardey and Alston (1995). 1991 estimate; 1993; 1992; and 1988.

With declining public funding and institutional changes for research, one way to keep up with the growing needs for information and technology is to raise the productivity of public research. Research productivity can be increased with closer collaboration between agricultural research systems by exploiting research synergies and avoiding duplications (Jahnke, Kirschke and

Lagemann, 1987). Further, the feedback between scientists and users is essential for generating the right technology and fully capturing the benefits of its utilization (FAO, 1996b). Finally, existing wide disparities in yields among countries in the same region and between continents suggest that considerable improvements in agricultural productivity could be achieved by transferring technology more effectively and efficiently from research centres to potential users and from existing users to new users.

The funding problems facing public research in developing countries also mean that the private sector will play an increasingly important role in applied and adaptive research. This implies that the role of government is to focus investment on basic research, human capital and infrastructure and to provide an environment and incentives, such as property rights, market reforms, more open policies and a stable economy, conducive to private investment.

CASE STUDY: DEVELOPING COUNTRIES

The combination of rising energy prices, use of feed crops for biofuel, greater world food demand, and stagnant food aid may undermine the food security of low-income countries.

> The use of food crops for biofuels, coupled with greater food demand, has reversed the path of declining price trends for several commodities.
>
> For highly import-dependent or highly food-insecure countries, any decline in import capacity stemming from rising food prices can have challenging food security implications.
>
> Food aid, a key safety net source, has stagnated during the last two decades, and its share has declined relative to total food imports of low-income countries.

Recent hikes in oil prices have raised serious concerns in low-income countries, both because of the financial burden of the higher energy import bill and potential constraints on imports of necessities like food and raw materials. Higher oil prices also have sparked energy security concerns worldwide, increasing the demand for biofuel production. The use of feed crops for biofuels, coupled with greater food demand spurred by high income growth in populous countries, such as China and India, has reversed the long-term path of declining price trends for several commodities.

Worldwide agricultural commodity price increases were significant during 2004-06: corn prices rose 54 per cent; wheat, 34 per cent; soybean oil, 71 per cent; and sugar, 75 per cent. But this trend accelerated in 2007, due to continued demand for biofuels and drought in major producing countries. Wheat prices have risen more than 35 per cent since the 2006 harvest, while corn prices have increased nearly 28 per cent. The price of soybean oil has been particularly volatile, due to high demand growth in China, the U.S., and the European Union (EU), as well as lower global stocks.

The Food and Agriculture Organization of the United Nations (FAO) estimated that the high food prices of 2006 increased the food import bill of developing countries by 10 per cent over 2005 levels. For 2007, the food import bill for these countries increased at a much higher rate, an estimated 25 per cent.

Price Rises will have Greatest Impact on Import-Dependent Countries

The 2006 ERS Food Security Assessment report for developing countries projected a slight increase in food availability during the next decade, mainly because of improvements in Asia. This increased availability is projected to lead to a 5-per cent drop in the number of food insecure people in the 70 low-income countries included in the ERS analysis. But, with the recent surge in food prices, prospects are not so bright for many of the lowest income countries. Projections of food availability consider both domestic production and food imports. Changes in import capacity have direct implications on the food security of low-income countries where food import dependency has increased because of greater demand stemming from income and population growth, as well as slow gains in domestic production. For highly import-dependent or highly food-insecure countries, any decline in import capacity stemming from rising food prices can have challenging food security implications.

Food Price Hikes in 2006 Offset by Record Crops and Higher Export Revenues

In 2006, higher food and oil prices resulted in an estimated decline in total commercial imports by the 70 developing countries. However, most of the expected impact of higher oil and food prices on food security was offset by favourable weather leading to record or above-average crop production, as well as higher export earnings of some of the low-income countries. Higher prices for copper and aluminum brought significant financial gains to some of the poorest countries, such as Zambia, Tajikistan, Guinea, and Mozambique. Increased construction in China, which accounted for 50 per cent of the growth in consumption for copper and aluminum metals, prompted the rise in metal prices, according to an International Monetary Fund (IMF) report.

Strong demand growth for labour in industrial countries and emerging markets also helped offset the impact of food and fuel import price increases in several countries. In Central America, remittances (transfers of money from foreign workers to their home countries) grew to account for 10-20 per cent of Gross Domestic Product (GDP) in 2005, supporting growth in consumption. Asia is the largest recipient of remittances, accounting for 45 per cent of the world total; IMF estimates that remittances contributed to about 10 per cent of GDP in the Philippines and Nepal. Sri Lanka benefited from the economic boom in oil-exporting countries because more than 80 per cent of its migrant workers were working in the oil-exporting Gulf States.

But will export prices for less developed countries continue to grow in the medium term, preventing an erosion in terms of trade for low-income countries? The 2006 IMF Outlook report argues that prices of metals will decline because the reserves of metals are more plentiful than oil reserves. The price trend for agricultural raw materials is less predictable because weather-related shocks will continue to create annual price volatility.

Grains and Oilseeds Crucial in Developing Country Diets

Price increases for grains and oilseeds are of particular concern to low-income countries as these commodities constitute a large share of their citizens' diets. Low-cost grains historically have been a dietary staple in the poorest countries. In low-income Asian countries, grains account for an average of 63 per cent of the diet; in North Africa and Commonwealth of Independent States (CIS—11 former Soviet republics), about 60 per cent. In Sub-Saharan Africa, the region most vulnerable to food insecurity, grains account for nearly half of the calories consumed. The share of grains in the diet is lowest—about 43 per cent—in lower income Latin America. In all regions, the situation varies by country. For example, in Bangladesh, the share is 80 per cent, while in Eritrea and Ethiopia, both among the most food-insecure countries in the world, the share is around 70 per cent.

The vegetable oil share of diets in low-income countries has risen as higher incomes made processed foods more accessible. For example, in Sub-Saharan Africa, the share of vegetable oil increased from less than 8 per cent of the diet in 1980 to 12 per cent in more recent years. In lower income Asian and Latin American countries, the share is now roughly 10 per cent, up from 5-7 per cent in 1980.

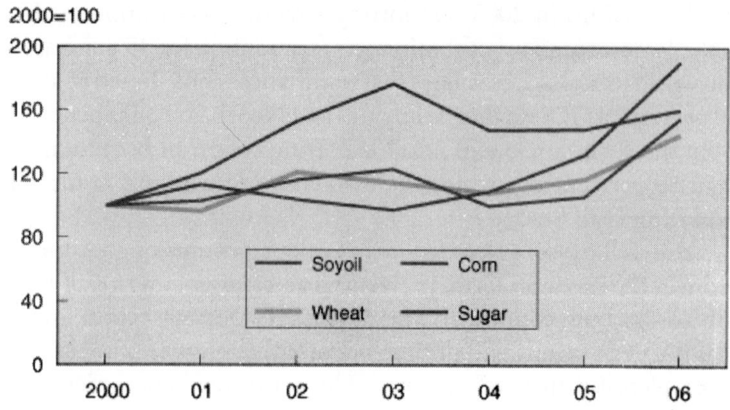

Fig. 10.1: Prices have Increased Significantly since 2000

Source: International Monetary Fund.

Dependence on Imports Rises in Many Developing Countries

Food import dependence in many developing countries has grown during the last three decades, leading to improved and more diversified diets. This trend can be attributed to higher incomes, slow growth in domestic food production, and trade liberalization. For lower income, highly import-dependent countries, however, higher food prices and a larger import bill can be a challenge, particularly for countries with limited foreign exchange availability and high vulnerability to food insecurity.

To identify countries that are highly sensitive to increases in grain prices, ERS ranked the 70 low-income countries by grain import dependence and daily calorie consumption. Six of the low-income countries (Eritrea, Liberia, Haiti, Georgia, Burundi, and Zimbabwe) depend on grain imports for more than 40 per cent of their diets and consume an average of less than 2,200 calories per day. Eritrea, for example, is highly dependent on food imports: 87 per cent of grains, 51 per cent of vegetable oils, and 100 per cent of sugar. Export earnings cover only 25 per cent of Eritrea's import bill; the remainder is filled by external assistance. Eritrea's daily calorie availability of 1,465 in 2005 was among the lowest in the world. Therefore, higher prices and the possibility of a cut in imports could result in a food crisis in Eritrea.

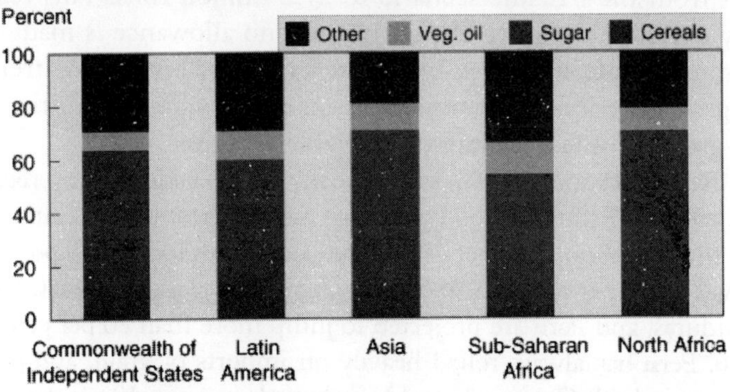

Fig. 10.2: Diet Share among regions, 2006

Source: United Nations, Food and Agriculture Organization.

In the world's least developed countries (50 countries, as defined by the United Nations' FAO, 32 of which are in Sub-Saharan Africa), the import share of production for wheat jumped from 93 per cent in 1980 to more than 130 per cent in 2005. For sugar, the share soared from only 4 per cent in 1980 to more than 65 per cent in 2005. A similar pattern is seen for vegetable oils, with the share rising from about 6 per cent to 80 per cent.

High Prices and Rising Import Dependence Lead to Widening Food Gaps •

Using the ERS Food Security Assessment model, ERS researchers estimated the impact of higher 2007 prices on food security in the 70 low-income countries. The food gap (the amount of food needed to raise consumption of all income groups to the nutritional requirement of roughly 2,100 calories per person) by 2016 was first estimated under the assumption that food prices would rise 1 per cent annually from 2007 to 2016. This baseline scenario results in a projected food gap of 25.2 million tons by 2016.

ERS then estimated the food gap under a price shock scenario, which assumed a nearly 28-per cent increase in grain prices for 2007, (based on actual price movements through July 2007), followed by increases of 1 per cent per year through 2016, as projected in the 2007 USDA baseline. In this scenario, the food gap increases 8 per cent from the baseline scenario to 27.2 million tons. This result may overstate the price impact because no allowance is made for commensurate increases in export earnings, but recent trends suggest that prices for commodities exported by these countries are not growing as fast as grain or vegetable oil prices.

Responses to the 2007 price shock vary considerably by region and country. Estimated food gaps increase the most in Latin America and the Caribbean—24 per cent—compared with less than 9 per cent in Asia and 6 per cent in Sub-Saharan Africa. Food gaps in Guatemala, Honduras, and Peru are projected to jump more than 20 per cent by 2016. Peru has always relied heavily on imports of grain, and grain imports in both Guatemala and Honduras have risen 10 per cent per year since 1990. In fact, in 2006, grain imports exceeded domestic production in Honduras by 30 per cent, and Guatemala by 55 per cent.

In Sub-Saharan Africa, countries most susceptible to economic shocks are often those suffering from political instability, which stifles domestic production. The price shock is projected to have the greatest impact in Cote d'Ivoire, where the food gap jumps an estimated 58 per cent by 2016. This country has been experiencing political problems during the last decade, with grain production virtually stagnant between 1990 and the early 2000s. To maintain grain supplies for a growing population, grain imports rose, and have been virtually equal to production for the past 5 years or so. The 28-per cent price shock is projected to significantly weaken the country's commercial import capacity, worsening food security.

Zimbabwe's grain output has fallen by nearly half since 2000 due to a government-imposed land redistribution programme. To compensate for the shortfall, imports have grown and, just as in Cote d'Ivoire, import dependence has risen. The price shock is projected to result in a 38-per cent increase in Zimbabwe's food gap.

Rising Prices Raise the Cost of Food Aid

Low-income countries, in general, do not have domestic safety net programmes to deal with economic shocks and therefore often rely on external assistance for support. However, in many cases, this assistance is not sufficient to compensate for production shortfalls brought about by higher import costs. For oil-importing developing countries, the $137-billion increase in the energy import bill in 2005 far exceeded the $84 billion of official development assistance they received. Food aid is often critical in mitigating the impact of strict financial constraints and reducing food availability in low-income countries. However, the volume of food aid worldwide has stagnated during the last two decades, and its share has declined relative to both total agricultural exports from food aid suppliers and total food imports of low-income countries. During 1990-2005, food aid received by the 70 low-income countries declined by 2 per cent (in volume) annually.

In 2002-05, food aid accounted for about 9 per cent of grain imports for the 70 low-income countries. The highest share—17 per cent—was in Sub-Saharan Africa, and the share was 10 per cent in lower income Asian countries, 6 per cent in the CIS, and 3 per cent in the low-income Latin American countries. Some low-income countries—like Ethiopia, Sierra Leone, Malawi, and Niger—are so poor that they were financially unable to import grain even under historically lower prices and relied heavily on food aid to augment their food supplies. But food aid quantities fall as prices rise, since the U.S., the major donor of food aid, sets an annual budget for food aid allocations. For many recipient countries, reductions in food aid are more of a problem than higher prices for food imports.

Food Gap, 2016: Baseline vs. Price Shock Scenario

	Base	*Price Shock*	*Percentage Change*
	Million Tons		
Asia	3.62	3.94	8.67
Latin America and Caribbean	1.42	1.76	23.67
Sub-Saharan Africa	20.15	21.36	6.01
Total 70 countries	**25.24**	**27.22**	**7.84**

Source: USDA, ERS.

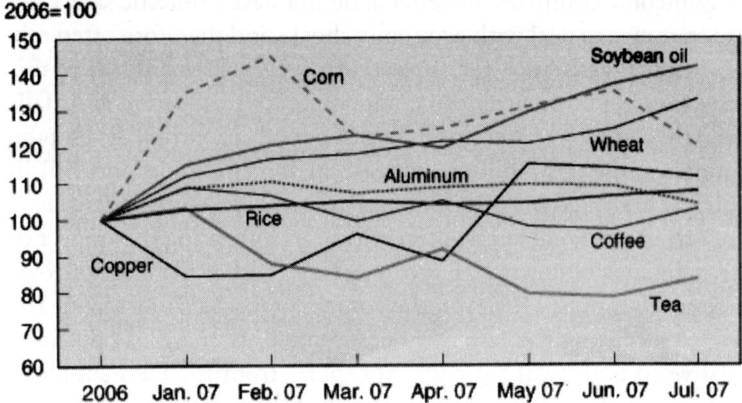

Fig. 10.3: Food Prices in 2007 have risen faster than export prices

Source: International Monetary Fund.

Between 2004 and 2006, global food aid donations averaged around 7.5 million tons per year. This amount was equal to nearly a third of the food gap estimated by ERS. Assuming that average grain prices increased nearly 28 per cent in 2007, followed by increases of approximately 1 per cent per year, as projected in the 2007 USDA baseline, the quantity of global food aid—given a constant 2006 budget—would fall to under 5 million tons by 2016. This amount of food aid would cover only 17 per cent of the projected distribution gap in that year. Global food aid donations covered 25 per cent of the gap in 2006. To maintain the 2006 level of food aid (8 million tons), the global food aid budget would need to rise about 35 per cent over the next decade.

This scenario might actually be understating the severity of the potential price hikes. The ERS model assumed annual increases in grain prices of around 1 per cent from 2008-16. However, as more countries invest in biofuels and if food demand continues to rise in India and China, prices might rise even more steeply. If food aid budgets do not rise in accordance with these price increases, even larger declines in food aid supplies may occur—with severe implications for the most vulnerable countries.

Is There a Silver Lining?

The ERS food security projections are based on several strict assumptions of commodity price trends. But the long-term food security impact of commodity price trends is uncertain because of differences in commodity composition among donor and recipient countries and varying price prospects for exports versus imports. In the long term, high food prices could boost domestic production in developing countries and improve food security. However, net results depend on the magnitude of supply response to the price increases and supporting economic policies, including technology adoption.

While rising energy prices have tightened the budgets of importing countries, they have also encouraged advances in biofuel technology, which could help fill the growing energy needs of developing countries. Investment in biofuel production by low-income countries could promote rural development, since large shares of their populations depend on agriculture for employment and livelihood. Countries such as Colombia and India have adopted production targets for increasing the share of biofuels in their transportation fuel supplies. Other countries are examining alternative biofuel sources appropriate for their particular environment and resource availability. Researchers in Asia, Latin America, and Africa have pointed toward the potential of several indigenous plants, such as jatropha, which grows wild and requires little water or nutrients, and has a relatively high oil yield. Agricultural research in low-income countries has been marginalized by national governments, as well as international development institutions such as the World Bank. However, the interest in biofuels could reverse this trend.

Currently, traditional biofuels such as wood account for about a third of all energy consumed in developing countries. These fuel sources are inefficiently used, however. For example, a kilogram of wood generates only about one-tenth of the heat of a kilogram of liquid petroleum gas. The new sources of biofuels could improve energy efficiency, increase the supply of energy, and boost farm incomes and rural employment where poverty is pervasive.

Success, however, depends on increased investment in new technology consistent with the agricultural sectors of low-income countries. Most low-income countries have poor market infrastructure and weak financial systems. This raises costs of production, particularly for newly introduced biofuel commodities that require dedicated production and distribution facilities. Finally, the financial capacity for investment in low-income countries is limited, so increased investment in biofuel production could distract from food production, thereby intensifying food insecurity.

HOUSEHOLD LIVELIHOOD SECURITY

In the past several years, much progress has been made in understanding the processes that lead to food-insecure situations for households (Frankenberger, 1992). In the 1970s food security was mostly considered in terms of national and global food supplies. The food crisis in Africa in the early 1970s stimulated major concern on the part of the international donor community regarding supply shortfalls created by production failures caused by drought and desert encroachment (Davies, Buchanan-Smith and Lambert, 1991).

This primary focus on lack of food supplies as the major cause of food insecurity was given credence at the 1974 World Food Conference.

The limitations of the food supply focus came to light during the food crisis that again plagued Africa in the mid-1980s. It became clear that adequate food availability at the national level did not automatically translate into food security at the individual and household levels. Researchers and development practitioners realized that food insecurity occurred in situations where food was available but not accessible because of erosion to people's entitlement to food (Borton and Shoham, 1991). "Entitlement" refers to the set of income and resource bundles (e.g. assets, commodities) over which households can establish control and secure their livelihoods. Sen's (1981) theory on food entitlement had a considerable influence on this change in thinking, representing a paradigm shift in the way that famines were conceptualized. Households derive food entitlements from their own production, income, gathering of wild foods, community support (claims), assets, migration, etc. Thus a number of socio-economic variables have an influence on a household's access to food.

Worsening food insecurity came to be viewed as an evolving process in which the victims were not passive to its effects. Social anthropologists observed that vulnerable populations exhibited a sequence of responses to economic stress, giving recognition to the importance of behavioural responses and coping mechanisms in food crises (Frankenberger, 1992). By the late 1980s, donor organizations, local governments and non-governmental organizations (NGOs) had begun to incorporate more extensive socio-economic information in their diagnoses of food insecurity.

The household food security approach that evolved in the late 1980s emphasized both the availability of food and stable access to it; food availability at the national and regional levels and stable and sustainable access at the local level were both considered essential to household food security. Interest was centred on understanding food systems, production systems and other factors that influence the composition of the food supply and a household's access to that supply over time. What was not clear was how nutritional outcomes were factored into food security deliberations.

Work on the causes of malnutrition demonstrated that food is only one factor in the malnutrition equation, and that in addition to dietary intake and diversity, health and disease and maternal and child care are also important determinants (UNICEF, 1990). Household food security is a necessary but not sufficient condition for nutritional security. Researchers identified two main processes that have a bearing on nutritional security. The first involves the household's access to resources for food. This is the path from production or income to food. The second process involves translating the food obtained into satisfactory nutritional levels (World Bank, 1989). A host of health, environmental, cultural and behavioural factors determine the nutritional benefits of the food consumed. This is the path from food to nutrition (IFAD, 1993).

This work on nutritional security demonstrated that growth faltering is not necessarily directly related to failure in household food security. It shifted the emphasis away from simple assumptions concerned with households' access to food, the resource base and food systems by demonstrating the influence of health and disease, caring capacity, environmental sanitation and the quality and composition of dietary intake on nutritional outcomes.

Research carried out in the late 1980s and early 1990s indicated that the focus on food and nutritional security as they were currently conceived needed to be broadened. It was found that food security is but one subset of objectives of poor households; food is only one of a whole range of factors that determine why the poor take decisions and spread risk, and how they finely balance competing interests in order to subsist in the short and longer term (Maxwell and Smith, 1992). People may choose to go hungry to preserve their assets and future livelihoods. It is misleading to treat food security as a fundamental need, independent of wider livelihood considerations.

Thus, the evolution of the concepts and issues related to household food and nutritional security led to the development of the concept of household livelihood security. The household livelihood security model allows for a broader and more comprehensive understanding of the relationships among the political economy of poverty, malnutrition and the dynamic and complex strategies that the poor use to negotiate survival. The model places particular emphasis on household actions, perceptions and choices. Food is understood to be only one of the priorities that people pursue. People are constantly required to balance food procurement against the satisfaction of other basic material and non-material needs (Maxwell and Frankenberger, 1992).

Household Livelihood Security

The NGO CARE USA, realizing the importance of viewing food security in a broader perspective, adopted household livelihood security as its organizing conceptual framework in 1996, understanding the contribution that this framework could make towards improved programming.

Household livelihood security is defined as adequate and sustainable access to income and resources to meet basic needs (including adequate access to food, potable water, health facilities, educational opportunities, housing, time for community participation and social integration). Livelihoods can be made up of a range of on-farm and off-farm activities which together provide a variety of procurement strategies for food and cash. Thus, each household can have several possible sources of entitlement which constitute its livelihood. These entitlements are based on the household's endowments and its position in the legal, political and social fabric of society (Drinkwater and McEwan, 1992). The risk of livelihood failure determines the level of vulnerability of a household to income, food, health and nutritional insecurity. Therefore, livelihoods are secure when households have secure ownership of, or access to, resources and income earning activities, including reserves and assets, to offset risks, ease shocks and meet contingencies (Chambers, 1989).

A livelihood is sustainable, according to Chambers and Conway (1992), when it "can cope with and recover from the stress and shocks, maintain its capability and assets, and provide sustainable livelihood opportunities for the next generation…". Unfortunately, not all households are equal in their ability to cope with stress and repeated shocks. Poor people balance competing needs for asset preservation, income generation and present and future food supplies in complex ways (Maxwell and Smith, 1992). People may go hungry up to a point to meet another objective. For example, de Waal (1989) found that during the 1984/85 famine in Darfur, the Sudan, people chose to go hungry to preserve their assets and future livelihoods. People will tolerate a considerable degree of hunger to preserve seeds for planting, to cultivate their own fields or to avoid selling animals. Corbett (1988), in exploring the sequential ordering of behavioural responses employed in periods of stress, found that in a number of African and Asian countries preservation of assets takes priority over meeting immediate food needs until the point of destitution.

Thus, food and nutritional security are subsets of livelihood security; food needs are not necessarily more important than other basic needs or aspects of subsistence and survival within households. Food-insecure households juggle among a range of requirements, including immediate consumption and future capacity to produce.

Components of Household Livelihood Security

The Relief-Development Continuum

CARE recognizes that the ability of poor households to make a living is not static. A range of intervention options needs to be made available to poor populations facing various circumstances. To enhance the livelihood security of vulnerable populations at different levels, a three-pronged livelihood systems approach has been conceived based on the relief-development continuum: the notion that relief, rehabilitation/mitigation and development interventions are a continuum of related activities, not separate and discrete initiatives. Household food, nutrition and income security can be enhanced by one or a combination of the three intervention strategies described below:

Livelihood Promotion (Development-oriented Programming)

Livelihood promotion involves improving the resilience of household livelihoods so that food and other basic needs can be met on a sustainable basis (i.e. development). Interventions of this type often aim to reduce the structural vulnerability of livelihood systems by focusing on:

- improving production to stabilize yields through diversification into agro-ecologically appropriate crops and natural resource management measures (e.g. soil and water conservation);
- creating alternative income-generating activities (e.g. activities to develop small enterprise);
- reinforcing coping strategies that are economically and environmentally sustainable (e.g. seasonally appropriate off-farm employment);
- improving on-farm storage capacity to increase the availability of buffer stocks;
- improving common property management through community participation.

Promotion-type interventions could also deal with meso-level development, where the linkages between food surplus areas and food deficit areas could be strengthened through investment in regional infrastructure and market organization. Such interventions could help improve the terms of trade for the poor by improving local access to income, enhancing food availability and lowering food prices. In addition, livelihood promotion activities could focus on preventive measures that improve health and sanitation conditions and the population/resource balance to insure that any income and production gains are not lost to disease and unchecked population growth.

Livelihood Protection (Rehabilitation/Mitigation-oriented Programming)

Livelihood protection involves protecting household livelihood systems to prevent an erosion of productive assets or to assist in their recovery (rehabilitation/mitigation). These types of interventions entail timely food and income transfers which can reduce long-term vulnerability resulting from the forced selling of productive assets to meet immediate food and other needs. The negative impacts of livelihood insecurity can be reduced by timely detection of where livelihood and food insecurity are likely to occur and by establishing contingency plans that can be implemented rapidly before a significant erosion of household assets occurs and other erosive coping strategies are activated. The capacity to detect changes in livelihood and food insecurity at an early stage and to respond promptly could considerably reduce the costs of dealing with a full-blown emergency.

Protection-type interventions would include infrastructure improvements or soil and water conservation measures, carried out through food-or cash-for-work or some other means, to enhance the long-term viability and resilience of the communities. Child population from becoming more vulnerable to disease and malnutrition would also fall in this category of intervention approach. Recovery measures such as infrastructure repair and rehabilitation, distribution of seeds and tools, reforestation and repair of water sites would also be included in this set of interventions. The types of intervention pursued would be selected and implemented by the communities themselves.

Livelihood Provisioning (Relief-oriented Programming)

Livelihood provisioning involves providing food and meeting other essential needs for households to maintain nutritional levels and save lives. Interventions of this type usually entail food and health relief for people in an emergency or people who are chronically vulnerable. Targeted food and health relief is critical and should be combined with promotion interventions where possible, to phase out the food transfers. In relief situations where people have left their homes (i.e. situations involving refugees and internally displaced populations), promotion interventions such as health and nutrition education and family planning initiatives will be limited to those activities that can be brought to the camps. Community-focused interventions may be necessary for chronically vulnerable populations (e.g. mother and child health programmes) to allow for the provisioning activities to be taken over by the community on a sustainable basis.

Conclusion

A broadened perspective emphasizing livelihood systems as key determinants of food and nutritional security reveals households as dynamic institutions, where power, control over resources, gender and culture all influence the households' ability to meet basic needs and negotiate survival. Establishing household livelihood security as CARE's organizing framework has allowed CARE to improve programming through holistic diagnosis and design using multisectoral teams, as well as to improve measurement of impact at the household level. While this comprehensive view has made the analysis of food insecurity more complicated, it has enhanced the likelihood of identifying the multiple constraints facing households.

Although it is recognized that the livelihood security framework can still be improved, it nonetheless represents a significant advance from previous conceptual models of food and nutritional security. As experience in its application accumulates, further refinements will be forthcoming.

TOWARDS MOBILIZING SCIENCE FOR GLOBAL FOOD SECURITY

Uncertainties in Climate and Agricultural Production

This paper examines the links between climate and agriculture energy (radiation) and water are essential to agricultural production; they constitute major environmental resources and the development of technologies for their improved management is one of the roles of agricultural research.

Then we examine the losses brought about in current production systems by the natural and human-induced variability of climate (see Box 1 for definitions), and the now well accepted evidence that climate change is one of the factors which has to be reckoned with, in spite of the uncertainties affecting all change scenarios, or perhaps precisely because of the uncertainties.

A major change in perception that occurred over the recent years is the fact that interactions between atmosphere and agriculture are no longer seen as unidirectional (climate impact), but rather that agriculture also affects global climate as one of the sources of greenhouse gases and a sink for CO_2. The feed-backs highlight that agriculture is part of the global environment, and that the issue of sustainable agriculture, due to its links with population and socio-economic considerations is thus a relevant topic also beyond the agricultural community, as was highlighted in the recent Kyoto protocol. Climate change impacts can be understood only in the light of current atmosphere-plant-soil interactions, unless unusual or unexpected combinations of factors should develop, where "unusual" refers to changing averages, the frequency of occurrence of factors, their combination and, possibly their nature as in the case of $CO2$ and UV-B, two factors which had until recently been regarded as "constants". A better understanding of current climate-agriculture interactions remains thus the key to a better understanding of future conditions and impacts.

Large uncertainties are associated with the dynamics of agriculture, as driven by such inter-related factors as population growth (Gommes, 1992), land degradation, international markets, changing diets linked with improving standards of living or other mechanisms, technology and management, etc. Implications for future food security (Bohle et al., 1994; Chen, 1994; EC, 1997) and biodiversity (Emanuel et al., 1985) are thus complex. Our ignorance about future climate, associated with our poor ability to foresee the evolution of world agriculture beyond ten or twenty years are thus a central issue to be considered: we still do not have the adequate tools to bridge the gaps between spatial and temporal scales, and there is an urgent need to reassess some research priorities in the CGIAR (Fresco and Kroonenberg, 1992). We insist on areas of uncertainty where additional research is required, as well as some considerations deriving from the ongoing international climate discussions.

Box 1: Weather and Climate Definitions

Weather describes the condition of the atmosphere at a well defined location and at a given time. Climate, on the other hand, refers to average conditions at the same location. Obviously, adjacent areas tend to undergo similar climate conditions and, therefore, climate can be seen as the average atmospheric conditions over sometimes large areas. It is stressed that variability is as much a characteristic of climate as the averages. Amazingly, there does not appear to be a generally agreed definition of the terms of "variability" and "change", for which Maunder (1994) lists different acceptations. He mentions that the term climate change is also often used in the more restricted sense to denote a "significant" change (that is, a change which has important economic, environmental and/or social effects) in the mean values of a

(*Contd.*)

meteorological element (...) during the course of a certain period of time, where the means are generally taken over periods of a decade or more (Maunder, 1994, p. 39). Maunder defines "fluctuations" as changes in the statistical distributions used to describe climate states (p. 45). As to "variability", one of the definitions proposed is deviations of climate statistics over a given period of time (such as month, season, year) from the long-term statistic, i.e. the departure from the long-term average (p. 56). As with micro-climate, there appears to be a difference in the use of the terms by statistical climatologists and ecologists! The present paper uses "variability" to describe the statistical noise about the average at time scales from days to years, and "change" in the same sense as Maunder, i.e. long-term changes in the average.

Climate as "Resource"

This section presents the view that there is a lot to be gained from looking at climate not only as a hazard, but also as a "resource". Resources must be known, assessed in quantitative terms and properly managed if they are to be used sustainably, and climate is no exception.

To stress the direct link between agricultural production potential and climate, Bernard (1992) uses the concept of climate fertility, coined after soil fertility. The fundamental similarities between climate and soil resources include the following: both contribute to the general production potential of a region, both undergo spatial variations and they can be mapped at different scales. In both cases their deficiencies can sometimes be corrected by adequate management practices. In addition, climate and soil contribute to agricultural production potential in an integrated way, not as separate factors, particularly since soil genesis is also very climate dependent.

Climate Complex

Climate constitutes a "complex", i.e. set variables which behave coherently, essentially as a result of atmospheric physics and dynamics (Sombroek and Gommes, 1996). For instance, rainfall tends to cool the atmosphere because water evaporation absorbs heat; cloudy days are characterised by a low daily thermal amplitude (difference between day and night temperature), relatively high air moisture and low evaporation, etc. In addition, the statistical properties of climate derived from long-term observations ensure that the usual range of variation of the "complex" is known.

Notwithstanding the difficulties of short-term weather forecasts proper, weather thus behaves rather coherently, and this constitutes an essential piece of knowledge which can be applied to improve the output of agricultural systems in terms of amounts and regularity.

The "complex" is also at the basis of agroecological zones (AEZ) interpreted as areas of relative climate stability, associated with typical soils and spectrum of characteristic plants and animals constituting the production system. FAO has bęen constantly developing the AEZ concept as a basic planning tool in agriculture starting in the late seventies (FAO 1978a, 1978b, 1980, 1981). The section below lists the climate variables which are most relevant for plant growth (development) and production. They can all be subdivided into a "normal" or physiological range with a largely predictable effect on plants and animals. The "extreme" range, by definition, covers unusually low or high values. The extreme effects on living organisms are far less predictable, for several reasons:

- their occurrence is they may mechanically damage plants and harm animals;
- their occurrence is rare and therefore less data are available for fine-tuning impact models;
- experimental stations tend to discontinue observations after the occurrence. of extreme
- conditions, thereby further reducing the observation base that would be required for impact assessments.

Climate Resources

Solar Energy and Light

The sun is the primary source of almost all energy stored in organisms in the form of biomass chemical bonds, starting with plant photosynthesis. The maximum amount of solar energy available as light depends essentially on astronomic factors (Hupfer, 1991), where variations of the solar constant (sunspot cycle of about 11 years), the annual and diurnal cycles play the most relevant role. Longer cycles (11,000 to 110,000 years) are associated with the orbit of the earth).

In general, clouds and various aerosol (sulphates, dust, etc.)

can reduce the amount of energy that reaches the ground. Aerosol, including anthropogenic sulphates, have recently been shown to play a significant part in the energy balance of the earth. Dust is often of volcanic origin (e.g. eruption of Mount Pinatubo in 1991) and therefore a-periodic, but the increasing frequency of dry haze in West Africa seem to indicate a link with land degradation.

Finally, clouds constitute one of the major uncertainties in the current climate change scenarios, as a small increase of the planetary albedo could result in global cooling instead of global warming. Light also plays an important qualitative role by triggering the photoperiodic response of Crops and by influencing the reproductive cycle of animals.

Water

While solar energy sets the maximum value of the energy available for plant growth, water determines to what extent the energy can be used. In fact, plants "pay" for the energy they absorb by transpiring water, and similarly water plays an important part in the thermoregulation of animals. The rather direct and almost linear link between actual water consumption and plant production has been very well documented (Chang, 1974; Begun et al, 1991, etc.) and the interactions between transpiration and assimilation have been at the core of plant models from the early stages (de Wit et al.1978; van Keulen and Wolf, 1986). This simple fact is often overlooked in semi-arid areas: all factors which increase biomass (like the introduction of HYV or the use of fertiliser) also increase water consumption, sometimes resulting in agricultural drought under climatically rather average conditions. Rainfall still constitutes the main source of water, and many techniques exist to improve water availability through water harvesting, irrigation, flood recession, cropping and grazing, or breeding, for instance for stronger root development. Less conventional sources like dew and fog may be resorted to locally (Acosta-Baladon, 1996).

Finally, air and soil moisture and water bodies play a very direct role in creating conditions favourable for the development of many pests, diseases, pathogens and their vectors (e.g. egg pod deposition and hatching conditions in desert locusts, liver fluke distribution, etc.)

Wind

At the micro-scale, wind has a less direct effect on plants than solar energy and water. It plays a part in mixing air and homogenising temperatures in canopies, thereby ensuring the continued exchange of CO_2 and water between plants and the atmosphere. It also contributes to the dissemination of pollen in wind-pollinated plants and the movement of migratory pests, but wind is more often associated with negative effects, including excessive desiccation, physical damage to crops, either directly or through abrasion by transported particles.

Heat and Temperature

Temperature is the yardstick used to measure heat, i.e. the energy stored in the thermal motion of particles. Most chemical processes, and therefore biological processes as well, are temperature dependent. Within the limits of the normal physiological range, the speed of biochemical reaction approximately doubles for a temperature increase of 10°C. It is worth noting that the reactions of assimilation (photosynthesis) are globally less dependent on temperature than, for instance, respiration.

In general, higher temperatures are thus associated with higher productivity and shorter biological cycles. This is amply illustrated by the high biomass turnover of the tropical rainforests (where biomass production is paralleled by high rates of decomposition of plant residues), or the short cycles of pests and diseases in warmer climates (for instance, the length of the development of eggs of Diabrotica virgifera, a common maize pest in temperate areas varies from 160 to just 14 as a function of temperature; Schaafsma et al., 1991).

Many qualitative thresholds are temperature dependent (for instance vernalization of winter crops, tuberisation, break of the diapause in insects).

Finally, air and soil temperatures play a major role in the development of growth of cold-blooded animals (earthworms, fish, etc.).

Production Potential and Biodiversity

The energy balance and the water balance of crops are interrelated through crop evapotranspiration. Evapotranspiration is a central concept in the determination of the potential biomass, i.e. the maximum quantity of plant biomass which can be accumulated under a given climate, assuming no interference of limiting factors such as poor soils, water stress or pest attacks. Next to quantity, the timing (calendar) of the production is mostly conditioned by limiting water availability in the warm climates, and by temperatures in the temperate ones.

At the global scale, very direct links can be established between the main characteristics of climate and biological productivity (Lieth, 1972, 1973 and 1975; Uchijima and Seino, 1985; White et al., 1992). Interestingly, curves very similar to the theoretical biomass curves can be obtained with actual crops, as exemplified below with African crop yields (Figure 1) as a function of National Rainfall Indices

Moore (1987) indicates that the biodiversity relates directly to the number of organisms which can make a living out of available resources, which in turn may be dependent on the extent of these resources, the limitations of the physical environment, the way in which resources present themselves for exploitation (habitat heterogeneity), the number of species geographically available, site accessibility, etc. He further states that forest richness is mainly the product of the resource base—water, warmth and solar energy: the total available energy is partitioned among species and limits species richness, as shown, for instance, for temperate forests by Currie and Paquin (1987) in their study on Tree Species Richness (TSR) in the USA, Canada, UK and Ireland (figure 2).

There are many examples of species and ecosystems with narrow ecological amplitudes, the occurrence of which is directly associated with climatic conditions. For instance, on the east coast of the US, the spawning of shad (Alosa sapidissima) peaks at 15°C. Temperature changes could reduce number of repeat spawners and reduce success (Ray, McCormick-Ray and Potter, 1993); mean annual temperature of 11°C appears to be the upper temperature for the formation of ombrotrophic bogs in NW Europe (Schouten, Streefkerk and van der Molen, 1992); prolonged summer chilling (less than 4°C) is lethal to the small white butterfly (Pieris brassicae) and eggs deposited at temperatures above 33°C are infertile 7 (Dennis, 1993).

Most effects described above apply to crops, forest plants,

rangeland, farm animals, fish, etc. As well as and to their competitors, i.e. weeds, pests, fungal and microbial pathogens.

Some are remarkably efficient at utilising the available climatic resources. Their short cycles and easy dissemination by wind and rain splash are an added advantage. Next to the direct effects described above, the following can also be included under indirect effects of climate:

- the development of bush and forest fires;
- the development of pests, including migratory pests, that attack field crops, forests,
- livestock and other farm animals;
- the action of climate on infrastructure;
- the general well-being and health of people (McMichael et al., 1996) and animals,
- including draught animals;
- the trafficability and effect on farm operations and their timing.

Climate Variability and Change: Climate as Hazard

We have so far covered essentially the positive aspects of weather on production. The main hazard associated with weather and climate is random variations 8, which border on unpredictability at all time scales exceeding a couple of days. The reduction of the uncertainty at the scale of weeks to seasons (seasonal forecasts) would constitute a major improvement of food security.

While it is recognised that some extreme climatic factors can provoke massive destruction of infrastructure, crops, livestock, fishing gear, etc. and the loss of human life, far more losses are associated with the chronic and inconspicuous effects of climate variability, like droughts, pest attacks, biodegradation of agricultural materials, products, including agricultural structures. The chronic impact of short-term climate variations (up to several years) is difficult to assess in quantitative terms. After describing some features of climate variability, the sections below conclude that about 10 to 20 per cent of national production can be lost annually due to climate variability, and that the figure can reach 100 per cent in extreme cases in small semi-arid developing countries.

According to Oerke et al. (1994), production losses due to pests, diseases and weeds amount to 15 per cent, 14 per cent and 13 per cent, respectively, on average for the main cereals and potatoes, in the absence of control measures. This refers to actual conditions. When compared with potential yields, the loss reduction is roughly 70 per cent equally distributed between pests, diseases and weeds. Needless to say, pests attacks and diseases are often indirectly conditioned by climatic conditions.

Characteristics of Variability

Variability has a structure, i.e. it exhibits transient behaviours which can be analysed statistically and sometimes used for planning. Without entering into detail, the following examples can be mentioned:

- trends, like the downward trend that affected Sahelian rainfall between the early 1960s and 1984;
- persistence, i.e. the tendency for weather types to occur in clusters: runs of dry and wet days, or runs of dry and wet years etc.;
- pseudo-cycles, often a direct result of persistence. A main characteristic of "cycles" seems to be that they collapse before they reach statistical significance;
- extremes follow well known patterns for each of the climate variables.

Several of the listed characteristics have marked effects on agricultural production and food security. For instance, one of the consequences of persistence is that a "bad" year is more likely to be followed by another "bad" year than by a "good" or "average" year. To some extent, when clusters have a relatively predictable behaviour, this information can be used in agricultural planning.

Atmospheric Pollution

Air pollutants affect life in the immediate surrounding of point sources. Some forms of pollution, like acid rain and ozone, are however known to have significant effects on forest and crop yields over wide areas, particularly in humid climates which improve contact between pollutants and plant surfaces. Tropospheric ozone is singled out because it derives for about half from photochemical reactions involving nitrogen oxides and methane, and because of its effect on crops, particularly legumes.

Direct and Indirect Factors and Complex Interactions

The potential direct negative effects of most climate elements on crops, natural vegetation and forest, and farm animals are well known. They affect all spatial scales from plant organ to the region, through various mechanisms.

For instance, high temperatures increase water stress in all organisms; they induce sterility in certain crops, lead to poor vernalization and increase winter survival of pests in temperate countries. High night-time temperatures are associated with a production loss due to increased respiration loss. In extreme cases, low temperatures can mechanically destroy cell structure (frost); they also contribute to plant desiccation and cause slow growth, particularly during cold waves, etc.

The direct impact of negative climate factors on agriculture, even the spectacular ones (hail, cyclones) is mostly very limited spatially: the main risks lie more with indirect impacts such as conditions favourable for pest and disease outbreaks, fires, etc.

The relative importance of fires and some other factors is illustrated below based on South African plantations data during 1984-85 (Environmental Affairs, 1986), where fires, wind, snow and hail account for half of the area affected by adverse conditions. Drought turned out to be a negligible factor while pests and diseases value, a completely different picture emerges: about 83 per cent of

Table 10.19: Relative Share of Losses (%) in South African Plantations during 1984/85 as a Function of Their Cause (Based on Data in Environmental Affairs, 1986)

	Financial Loss	*Drought*
Area affected	0.2	Negligible
Fungi and rodents	8.2	12.7
Wind, snow and hail	11.7	1.9
Insects	40.9	1.6
Fire	39.0	82.8
Others	Negligible	1.0

make up the other half. If the same results are presented by the damage is to be ascribed to fire only, followed by rodents (12.7%) and by winds (1.9%). In this particular instance, insects and other weather factors played a negligible part.

There are many complex interactions where trends affecting non-climate variables eventually lead to a greater vulnerability of production systems to climate variability. Several examples could be given where population growth has lead to the horizontal expansion of agriculture into marginal areas with low water storage capacity: such areas are more prone to agricultural drought as they cannot "buffer out" short dry spells (Gommes, 1992). The problem will now be perceived as "drought" even if climate remained stable. This is one of the components of the recent 1994 Rwandan genocide (Gommes, 1997).

Another related factor is the switch from traditional crops grown with low water requirements (millet/sorghum) towards crops with high moisture requirements (maize) as a result of changing dietary patterns Long-term effects on production and quality of the diet must also be taken into account when trees or plantation crops suffer damage due, for instance, to violent winds or salinization (due to ocean spray during cyclones, or to other causes).

From Climate Variability to Agricultural Statistics

Climate variability directly and indirectly affects agricultural output (production) through its effects on yields and areas planted. Yields are affected, as indicated, by weather as the main "random" factor, but also by mostly continuous technological trends (including new varieties and management), innovations (including management innovations), agricultural policies (mostly national policies) and extreme factors of various origins. Variation of areas depend more on economic factors. Areas planted vary according to labour availability, level of mechanisation and expected return (prices). Areas harvested are often strongly linked to environmental conditions, including poor weather during the cycle, damage to infrastructure due to extreme conditions, etc. Because of the complexity of the dependence of area-wide yields on different factors, and because of the high level of aggregation of agricultural statistics, it is not always easy to show the effect of climate variability.

In order to isolate the effect of environmental conditions from other factors, the first step is to eliminate the trends in the series. This makes sense only when there is no marked trend in the weather, which happens to be the majority of cases. In addition, trends are not always constant and the detection of trend changes constitutes, per se, a rather difficult technical problem. As an example, some recent time series of yields are shown in figure 3. The countries were chosen only to provide examples of the variety of temporal behaviour of yield time series. The only "clean and easy" series is that of the USA, where a meaningful linear trend can be computed. In Egypt, the variability is relatively low (due to irrigation), but the growth is faster than linear, possibly due to population growth being closer to exponential. Kyrgyzstan and Romania both display a stabilisation or a decrease at the end of Area-wide refers to yields and production by administrative units, from the village level to the national level, as opposed to a field, where conditions can be assumed to be reasonably homogeneous.

Another difficulty stems from the tradition of most national statistical services to report harvested areas instead of planted areas. This results in artificially reducing the effect of weather. the series, clearly associated with the collapse of their economies and the associated lack of inputs. Finally, Saudi Arabia is a clear example of very capital intensive innovation from the eighties onward.

Two factors are actually at work: relatively better soil storage in humid climates, long seasons in humid areas and, of course, the fact that, almost by definition, rainfall variability is higher in low rainfall area.

The "detrended coefficients of variation" were obtained as follows: take the 1961-94 yield time, compute linear trend (regress yield series against time), subtract regression line to obtain residues (departures from trend), compute Standard Deviation of Residues (SDR), express SDR in per cent of the average of the original time series.

Due to the skewed distribution of rainfall, expected amounts are less than the average. According to a global study by Oldeman (1987), dependable rainfall (defined as the amount falling during at least 3 years out of 4) is usually of the order of 80 per cent of the average. For areas where annual rainfall exceeds 100 mm, Le

Houérou et al. (1993) found that the coefficients of variation of annual rainfall increases from 10 per cent (rain forest climate) to more than 50 per cent under arid conditions.

Altogether, due to soil storage and management, agriculture does thus somewhat compensate the natural variability of climate. It remains that, on average, variability is one the main factors why actual yields remain well below the local agro-pedoclimatic potential.

Climate Change

Some Facts

One of the main conclusions of the latest IPCC assessment is that the atmospheric concentrations of greenhouse gases, inter alia carbon dioxide (CO_2), methane (CH_4), and nitrous oxide (N2O) have grown significantly: by about 30 per cent, 145 per cent, and 15 per cent, respectively. These trends can be attributed largely to human activities, mostly fossil-fuel use, land-use change and agriculture *(IPCC, 1996a, summary for policymakers)*

It is also relevant, in this context, to stress that agricultural sources of several GHG are very significant:

- CO_2, an estimated 25 per cent stems from agricultural sources (deforestation: 20%, biomass burning: 5%). The agricultural sources appear to be declining relative to fossil fuel use;
- CH4: there is a lot of uncertainty about the figures. About 70 per cent could be derived from anthropogenic sources, of which 20 per cent each each domestic ruminants, biomass burning and rice production. The remaining 10 per cent is usually assigned to "other waste products".
- Natural wetland could be responsible for about the same emissions as rice fields;
- N_2O, tillage 44 per cent, fertiliser 22 per cent and biomass burning 9 per cent. Agricultural sources seem to be stabilising, while the relative importance of energy is on the increase.

The scenarios developed by IPCC present the following data for 2100: + 1°C with 500 ppmv CO_2 (lowest), + 2.0 to 2.5°C with

725 ppmv CO_2 (most likely) and + 3.5 to 5 °C with CO_2 above 1000 ppmv (worst case). According to Ehsan Masood (1997), if all developed countries kept to their Kyoto target, world temperature would still rise by 2.1°C by 2100. This is only 0.27°C lower than the "Business as Usual scenario" (BAU) resulting from no intervention at all to reduce emissions. This is to say that about 2°C increase by 2100 can be taken for granted.

Under the "virtually certain 'facts' to very probable 'projections'", Mahlman (1997) lists the following:

- cooling effect of climate has considerable inertia, and cannot be reverted over a short period of time;
- cooling effect of sulphate particles is insufficiently quantified;
- significant reduction of the uncertainties will require a decade or more;
- water vapour concentrations will increase in the lower atmosphere, and global mean precipitation could increase by 1.5 to 2.5 per cent per 1°C of global warming;
- sea level rise may reach about 50 cm by 2100.

There is no scientific evidence that the frequency of tropical cyclones, storms or hurricanes would increase, nor should winds in mid latitudes (as opposed to tropical areas).

A Discussion of Potential Impacts

Potential impacts on agricultural production have received a lot of attention (Kaiser and Drennen, 1993; Bazzaz and Sombroek 1996a; Helms et al., 1996; IPCC, 1996b and 1996c;

Smit et al., 1996; EC 1997). Their extent will largely depend on the future concentrations ofCO2, as well as on temperatures, on the internal dynamics of agricultural systems, including their ability to adapt to the changes. Both are unknown, as indicated, because they will eventually depend on the interference of other substances (notably aerosol), on policy measures taken in the ambit of Framework Convention on Climate Change, and on the compliance of countries with the agreed protocols. Note that the scenarios insist on temperature and CO_2, mostly ignoring or mentioning cautious hypotheses for other parameters. This refers, in particular, to the components of potential evapotranspiration (radiation and cloudiness, moisture, wind, extreme temperatures) and the water balance (rainfall, in addition to the previously listed variables) as well as, most importantly, the variability of future climate (Katz et al., 1992). In the words of Reilly (1996), the most "robust conclusion" that does emerge from the studies is that climate change has the potential to change the productivity significantly...

It is also stressed that many changed-climate scenarios are derived from equilibrium models, i.e. they assume that climate has reached an equilibrium under, say, doubled CO_2, when it is obvious that climate will change gradually, and that agriculture will adapt and develop response mechanisms gradually as well. Changed-climate impacts assessments on current agriculture are, therefore, not very useful. Transient model outputs, i.e. model outputs which change gradually over time from the current to some future situation are being developed. In theory, they should be able to forecast weather years ahead, thus actually providing tools for seasonal forecasting. Of course, they still suffer from the difficulty to properly define boundary conditions, including CO_2 concentrations.

There is little doubt that the approach adopted by the IMAGE team (Alcamo, 1994; Alcamo et al., 1994) lends a lot of credibility to their projections: they "train" some components of the global models on past data (1970-90, sometimes longer) and verify that the current situation can be realistically simulated.

In comparison with global impacts on food production and food security (refer to Parry and Carter, 1998, for an overview and the relevant literature), impacts at plant level are relatively easy to assess, although still very uncertain, for direct and indirect effects on plant physiology). They include the following:

- a positive effect of higher temperatures on crops, including longer growing and grazing seasons in some areas, but largely dependent on the relative difference between night-timeand daytime temperatures; shorter crop cycles;
  - CO_2 fertilisation, with a more marked effect on C_3 species than on C_4 plants;
  - improved water-use efficiency;

- modifications of coastal/deltaic agriculture;
- modified crop/animal and pest/disease relations, including new pests and diseases, and
- changes in economic return (including new opportunities);
- modified variability and risk patterns.

Major methodological difficulties are associated with up-scaling (extrapolating local models to the global scale: Körner, 1995; Fischer et al, 1996) and down-regulation (the fact that physiological effects measured under laboratory conditions may overestimate the impact in the field because the response fades away after long exposure times). This being well noted, the following could happen at the global/ecological scale, at least in a first step:

- new agricultural areas become available in currently cold climates, loss of land at high elevations and high southern latitudes, modification of the current crop geopolitical balance;
- loss of carbon stored in peat and soil organic matter, modifying erosion patterns;
- human population movements, increased global insecurity;
- loss of existent biodiversity, and creation of "new" biodiversity;

zonal migration of species, ecosystems, crops and animals. Complex modification of the interactions between species.

Very little is known about the spatial distribution of the more complex impacts. If expressed in terms of Gross Domestic Product from Agriculture (GDPA), and after making due provision for adaptation, impact could generally be positive in developed countries, and negative elsewhere (Fischer et al., 1994 and 1996). The authors also cautiously suggest that by 2060 there may be a relative decrease of hungry people, but an increase in Africa when expressed in absolute terms. In Asia, on the other hand, there would be both a relative and absolute decrease.

Agronomic Research

Improving Climate

Climates can be improved using a variety of traditional and modern methods and techniques, from microclimate manipulation (such as mulching), the orientation of the rows in row-crops and windbreaks through varying levels of water control to artificial climates, for instance in greenhouses where temperature, light and CO_2 can be controlled.

While the techniques like those of frost protection using smoke (fires) and sprinkler, or hail protection and cloud seeding are very "hardware oriented", there is currently a tendency towards more sophisticated use of weather knowledge in models that assist farmers and herders in decision making. Strictly speaking, this is not (micro) climate manipulation, but a way to make optimal use of climate resources.

The dependence of many common pests and diseases on weather can be modelled and their probability of reaching critical levels can be forecasted with good accuracy. However, many farmers and livestock breeders carry out preventive control of pests and diseases, thereby avoiding almost all losses but also, and maybe more importantly, actually insulating their production from weather, and ensuring a better control over their time and capacity to plan. It remains that, at least statistically, agrometeorological pest and disease models have the potential to reduce protection costs while reducing pesticide release into the environment.

Taking Advantage of Climate Knowledge to Manage Variability

The first step in all climate-agriculture work is to know the climate, i.e. to collect long-term data and assemble them into climatic databases. But very often there is a mis-match between biological observations and weather observations: efforts should be made to collect at least basic information from the location of all agronomic experiments, and to ensure that extreme conditions are adequately measured. As indicated above, climate plays a part at the many different levels leading from production or the harvest of wild products (including fish) to consumption, and the effect of weather and climate on all those levels is worth investigating.

It should also be kept in mind that the definition of extreme agrometeorological events is broader (than just weather), as they include as well weather conditions conducive to the development of agents (like pests and diseases) that negatively affect agriculture (definition adopted by WMO). Extreme agrometeorological events thus include, for instance, desert locust outbreaks: rainfall in semi-arid areas can create conditions favourable to locusts, eventually leading to gregarization and swarms spreading over large areas. Fire as well can be included, as risks are very dependent on rainfall, moisture and winds.

The two previous examples stress the need to carry out both a monitoring of conditions favourable to pest, disease, fire, etc. development and, subsequently, to monitor the conditions which control the spread of the extreme agrometeorological event from its source to larger and sometimes distant areas.

Schematically, the use of climate knowledge is relevant for the following "categories":

- pests, diseases types of "organisms": crops, pollen and seeds; livestock, poultry and freshwater fish;
- pests, diseases and parasites; national parks and wildlife;
- monitoring growing and post harvest conditions. This can be done by using models, identifying critical thresholds, forecasting the impact of drought, fires, hail, frost,
- vernalization, extreme agrometeorological factors;
- advice, as basis for decision making: meteorological forecasts, trafficability, farm
- operations, dissemination of pathogens and pollutants, response farming and precision farming, advice to farmers and herders, irrigation and drainage;
- technology (climate as resource): water conservation and harvesting, occult precipitation, artificial climates (greenhouses, stables, tractors and farmhouses), agroclimatic zoning, agroclimatic risk (insurance), microclimate modification, windbreaks;

forecasting: yield forecasting, forecasting quality of production, forecasting phenology (harvest time and labour requirements), rangeland production, international markets as a result of production and resulting prices; methodologies: data technology in the broadest sense (collection, standardisation, software, estimation of missing data, random weather generators, gridding), modeling production, development, impacts...

Forecasting in general deserves a special mention in the light of the interest triggered by the latest 1997/98 El Niño/Southern Oscillation (ENSO), in particular because of the lessons than can be learned..

To start with, El Niño provides a good example of a relatively reliable seasonal forecast, which can be taken advantage of by governments and the agricultural community alike.

Unfortunately, like all forecasts, the actual magnitude, location and other features are affected by error. The methodology of whether to take management decisions, taking into account ENSO information, must be based as much on economic data as on simulated potential agronomic impact scenarios.

Such impact scenarios are not ENSO specific but constitute only a special application of a weather or climate forecast. Current discussions about how to react to El Niño are useful only if they lead to long-term solutions, in particular if efforts are made to improve all seasonal forecasts, if decision/simulation tools to be used by governments and farmers and ranchers are available, and if climate/weather impact on agriculture is seen as much in terms of opportunities (taking advantage of unusually "good conditions", commodity market opportunities and planning, etc.) and more efficient use of climate resources by farmers rather than only in terms of loss mitigation.

The above mentioned decision tools must be developed in collaboration by national climatological services, research and agricultural and livestock extension and tested locally, including a critical evaluation of the impact of the advice on agricultural output in terms of quantities and regularity.

In practice, the decision tools are tables/flow-charts or software that assist farm-level management decision-making based on three types of inputs:

- the measurement of the knowledge of local environmental/ agricultural conditions (reference data
- the measurement of local "decision parameters" by local extension officers, farmers and cattle breeders;
- economic considerations, e.g. cost of inputs vs expected output.

Adapt Species and Production Systems

There are many examples of adaptation of agriculture to extremely difficult climates, for instance, flood recession crops on river banks and irrigation in semi-arid areas and outright deserts (Nile, Niger, Senegal rivers). Another technique uses low mud dams (usually not exceeding a height of 1.5 meters) in terrain depressions to collect run-on water during the very short seasons of the desert margins. As water infiltrates and evaporates, crops are planted at the receding edge of the water and grow on soil moisture during the dry season, thereby enjoying low pest incidence due to low atmospheric moisture and a high production potential due to the virtual absence of clouds. In addition, the harvest is spread over several months, and is predictable.

Livestock is another convenient mechanism to collect the sparse biomass spread over large areas. In semi-arid areas it constitutes virtually the only mechanism for people to make a living in spite of very limited water resources.

More modern techniques are those of precision farming, though still beyond the reach of most developing countries, which adapt management to the micro-variations of the environment, in particular soil features.

The potential of biotechnology is huge; it includes: the breeding of plants and animals better suited to resist abiotic stresses (like high temperatures) through inter-specific crosses the development of morphological adaptations—such as stronger root development and more favourable Leaf Area Index—and physiological improvements to photosynthetic efficiency—like possibly CAM features in C_3 and C_4 plants more specific pest and disease resistance.

Mitigating Climate Change and No-regrets

Conjectured effects of climate change on agriculture are large, but uncertainties are such that specific protection measures (e.g. location-or species-specific) are unlikely to achieve their goal. It is rather through emission reductions, gradual adaptation (including evasion) and preparedness that agriculture will be able to cope with the new environmental setting. Protection is likely to involve structural measures with a sizeable cost.

The uncertainty associated with projections of climate change and assessments of impacts on agricultural potential calls for attentive preparedness, to readily take advantage of beneficial impacts of climate change and increased atmospheric CO_2, to mitigate negative impacts of climate change where they cause loss of productivity, and to cope with the technological and social challenges of changing patterns of land productivity. In essence, this will require addressing many problems which concern farmers, foresters and livestock breeders and decision makers already today.

The prevailing philosophy, particularly in developing countries, has been "no-regrets", i.e. only measures that make economic sense now should be adopted, because they reduce emissions from the agricultural sector or improve resilience of all sectors of agriculture against weather variability. All have a marked management component and could thus often be implemented at minimal cost.

Such measures include:

- improved fertiliser use, as N_2O released into the atmosphere is a loss and constitutes a symptom of inefficient farming. Needless to say, the same applies to nitrates lost to the water table and surface waters;
- improved ruminant digestion through more efficient feeds or, when feasible, a shift to enzymic digesters;
- development of water harvesting and conservation techniques, as well as other improvements to crop-water management as an adaptation to rainfall variability;
- improved rice farming, as higher yields are accompanied by a relatively smaller loss of methane;
- improved soil carbon storage (carbon sink) while at the same time improving soil structure increasing water holding capacity;

- improved low-impact harvesting in forests, reduction of slash-and-burn agriculture, better soil protection;
- a growing of alternative energy crops.

The example of rice provides an interesting illustration of the fact that agricultural emissions of greenhouse gases should be linked to production rather than expressed in absolute amounts, in order to favour the most efficient production systems. Obviously, this criteria should also be kept in mind by plant breeders!

Finally, we mention energy crops as a way to close the carbon cycle, as well as carbon sequestration in soils and biomass. While modern fuels from biomass seem to have real potential in reducing fossil fuel consumption while generating income in rural areas, carbon storage in biomass often needs justifications which are not all relevant for agriculture, such as recreation and tourism, watershed protection, improvement of urban climates.

Some Gaps

Several areas have received insufficient attention in the general field of climate-agriculture research, including both climate variability and change. They include the following:

- the collection of combined data-sets of climate and agronomic information needed for the development of realistic impact assessment tools for current and future climate. The agronomic information should include at least information on varieties, phenology, pests and diseases, management and yields. This is also a point noted by Fischer et al. (1996) when they suggest that agricultural research would benefit from greater attention to macro- and micro-climate in all trials;
- efforts should be made to improve climate (i.e. seasonal) forecasts. While this is a task for climatological research, there are already some cases (El Niño) where the forecasts have achieved a reasonable degree of reliability (Cane et al., 1994). It is up to agronomic research to determine the conditions under which the use of the forecast will improve sustainability of all types of agriculture (from crop

agriculture to inland fisheries) in terms of economic return and food security;

- many global impact assessments are based on models designed for the level of the individual field. They are appropriate for farm and forest management, but inadequate for regional studies, if only because most of the required inputs are meaningless or impossible to obtain at regional scales (Fresco and Kroonenberg, 1992). Methods are needed that will allow to bridge the gap between the field and regional scales, as well as between "sectors" (e.g. combined rangeland species composition and livestock models). This point is highlighted by Leemans and van den Born (1994) who stress that detailed process-oriented models are unsuitable for input data on a coarse spatial grids; the potential interactions between changed climate and other plant responses, for instance to mineral nutrition (Rastetter et al., 1997) need to be further investigated;
- equilibrium global circulation models provide little insight into the dynamics that will lead from the current situation to future situations 30 or even 100 years from now. Transient models should be used instead and tested against recent historical data. A model that cannot represent the current situation is unlikely to be useful in forecasting future situations;
- the question of rates of change: a thorough discussion of impacts on natural vegetation and landscape processes as function of rates of changes is still missing (Walker and Steffen, 1997), as well the links between ecological complexity and resilience.

Partnerships

Overview of Climate-driven Activities in the CGIAR System

- Much research work carried out in the CGIAR system bears a direct relation to climate and climate change:
- Breeding for yield stability in stressful (drought, cold, heat) and variable environments:

- maize and wheat (CIMMYT), barley and durum wheat (ICARDA), legumes (ICARDA:
- adaptation to high altitude), maize (IITA); breeding for earliness: spring wheat (ICARDA), maize (IITA); breeding for increased productivity in flood-prone lowlands (IRRI). WARDA has a holistic approach to "drought resistance", a mix of physiological, phenological and morphological mechanisms for escape, avoidance, resistance and recovery. Breeding should, therefore, be environment specific;
- Models to simulate management: improvement of water use efficiency (ICARDA), model research efficiency and outcomes in desert margins systems (ICRISAT);
- Improved decision making in several areas: (1) use of water resources: water conservation and management (ICARDA), comparison of agroforestry and crop agriculture in respect to sustainable water use (ICRAF), practices and breeds which improve water-use efficiency of rice (IRRI); (2) coastal zone management, fisheries and aquaculture (ICLARM) Climatic and land-resources databases, and conservation of resources: agroecological characterisation (ICARDA); aquatic biodiversity and coral reef conservation (ICLARM);
- baseline data on above-ground biodiversity (CIFOR) Climate and seasonal forecast: IFPRIs medium-term plan proposes "exploratory research" on economic and agricultural implications from medium to long-term climate forecasts;
- Management techniques to reduce CH4 emissions from rice fields (IRRI), development of drought resistant upland rice;
- Management strategies: research into the effect of changing weather patterns on flood-prone riceland (IRRI); improved-impact harvesting of natural forests (CIFOR); alternative land-use strategies (CIFOR) and evaluation of international climate change mitigation policy options (CIFOR).
- Furthermore, several centres have established scientific links with relevant organisations such as IGBP, in

particular with the Global Change and Terrestrial Ecosystems (GCTE) project Focus 3 dealing with agriculture, forestry and soils (Tinker et al, 1996). The main items covered include the effect of global change on key agricultural systems, including food crops and pastures, changes in pests and diseases (with emphasis on weeds), effects on soils, on multi-species agro-ecosystems and on managed forests.

Links between UN and CGIAR on Climate and Climate Change

There has been long-standing collaboration between FAO and WMO on climate and agriculture, often jointly with UNEP, UNESCO in the Interagency Secretariat of Agricultural Biometeorology, etc. (Gommes, 1995), directly or through the WMO Commission on Agricultural Meteorology.

Bilateral contacts of FAO with several CGIAR institutes have mostly centred on agroclimatic data (ICARDA, ICRISAT, CIAT) and the co-sponsorship of several meetings on the agrometeorology of specific crops, starting with rice (IRRI, 1980), sorghum and millet (1982; Virmani and Sivakumar, 1984), groundnut (1985; ICRISAT, 1986), or the characterisation of agricultural environments (Bunting, 1987)...

Several studies carried out under the auspices of the Interagency Secretariat of Agricultural Biometeorology have benefited from the logistic support, including data of the CGIAR centres, for instance the agroclimatology of the humid tropics of Southeast Asia (Oldeman and Frère, 1982).

In 1993, FAO and several CGIAR centres (ICRAF, ICARDA, ILRAD, ICRISAT) have collaborated in an effort to co-ordinate and harmonise databases and software for agroclimatic applications (FAO, 1995).

In an effort to ensure that proper consideration to impacts of climate and climate change will be given in the framework of the Interagency Committee on the Climate Agenda (IACCA), the FAO Council made the recommendation that the CGIAR system should be formally represented in the Committee.

Potential Activities Deriving from the Kyoto Conference

The recent Kyoto Conference (Dec. 1997) and the Kyoto Protocol explicitly recognised the links between climate change issues and sustainable development. In view of the new commitments and options, an increased role of the international agricultural community can be envisaged:

- participation in the development of improved assessment techniques for emissions and sinks of greenhouse gases in the agricultural sector, including terminology issues (e.g., managed and natural "forests");
- participation in the discussion of details of trading emissions, its links with the clean development mechanism, and tools for developing countries to benefit from the trading with emissions;
- assistance to countries in their compliance with new obligations deriving from the UNFCCC and the Kyoto protocol.

Conclusions and Recommendations

This paper has stressed the close links that exist between climate resources and agricultural production potential, including biodiversity. A rapid evaluation of the chronic losses to agricultural production due to climate variability, and the potential losses brought about by climate change was also presented.

It is clear that we do not fully tap the potential of climate resources, and this can be improved with technological, management, institutional and legislative tools. But more than anything else, research has to provide better data, tools and methods to evaluate climate impact at scales ranging from the field to the region and the global scale (Fresco at al., 1997). A good illustration is provided by the IMAGE models which, as stressed by Alcamo (1994), was made possible only by the availability of improved data. At the farm level, crop, livestock, pest and disease models constitute essential management tools; at the regional level, they are indispensable for planning and for long-term impact assessments.

There is ample room for improved collaboration in the field of agronomic and climate research between governments, national and international research centres, as well as the UN system. This collaboration should focus first on the identification of the areas most vulnerable to climate impacts on agriculture, their typification and classification, and mapping. Fertile climates should also be assessed properly, both in terms of production potential and in terms of their resilience and preparedness to cope with increased demand, particularly in areas near to those where the largest impacts are foreseen. Bazzaz and Sombroek (1996b) insist as well on the need to identify large local differences.

Agronomic research must also improve the resilience of production systems and agricultural environments to variability and change, not only in a no-regrets perspective, but also with a view to building agronomically and economically more sustainable systems in the most vulnerable areas. Reilly (1996) suggests that there is a need to map the robustness of current farming systems to variability. He also stresses the importance of genetic variability as a source for adaptation. Similarly, Bazzaz and Sombroek (1996b) stress that modelling has to be more comprehensive to include the feed-backs among biophysical, economic and technological mechanisms. This is also one of the main emerging questions listed by a recent synthesis of GCTE and related research. The authors (Walker and Steffen, 1997) go further as they include environmental, political and institutional feed-backs as well.

New constraints to agricultural productions will no doubt derive from the implementation of the international climate agreements, such as the Montreal protocol (phasing out methyl bromide) and the Kyoto protocol. Countries are committed to report accurately on their emissions from all sectors, and their plans to reduce them. This entails several difficulties, from methodological to institutional. Agronomic research has a role to play in most of them; the CGIAR System and FAO should advocate the fact that, just like energy efficiency is a recognised target, the improved efficiency of agriculture derives directly from the international commitments.

Not only will absolute amounts of greenhouse gases be reduced, but the clean development mechanism should be used to ensure that emissions per unit of production should decrease, this is to say that efficient agriculture should be rewarded. For instance, the intensification of rice cultivation may produce large quantities of methane, but when expressed in terms of unit of methane per unit of rice, properly managed fields are more efficient than low yielding ones. Next to constraints, there will also be new opportunities which agriculture has to prepare itself for in areas such as energy crops, carbon sinks in the form of standing biomass and soil organic matter. And, of course, biotechnological research will contribute to the development of more efficient plants. The CGIAR and international organisations must ensure that improved profit will not be the only criterion adopted by the developers: resilience to stressful environments (where the term is specifically meant to encompass not only the physical environment), more sustainable management techniques and the stability of yields are equally important.

Finally, international and, perhaps more so, national agronomic research have to ensure that national decision makers recognise that climate variability is a fundamental and more immediate concern than climate change, but that it constitutes the conceptual and methodological key to climate change preparedness.

RELEVANCE OF INTERNATIONAL TRADE OF GENETICALLY MODIFIED FOODS

The European Union and the United States have strong disagreements over the EU's regulation of genetically modified food. The US claims these regulations violate free trade agreements, the EU counter-position is that free trade is not truly free without informed consent.

In Europe, a series of unrelated food crises during the 1990s created consumer apprehension about food safety in general, eroded public trust in government oversight of the food industry, and left some consumers unwilling to consider science to be a guarantee of quality.

This has further fueled widespread public concern about genetically modified organisms (GMO), in terms of potential environmental protection (in particular biodiversity), health, and safety of consumers. Critics of GM foods contend that there is evidence that the cultivation of genetically modified plants may lead to environmental changes. Directives such as directive 2001/18/EC were designed to require authorisation for the placing GMO on the market, in accordance with the precautionary principle.

Many European consumers are demanding the right to be informed food they consumed has been genetically modified. Some polls indicate that some Americans would also like labeling, but it has not become a major issue. New EU regulations are expected to require strict labeling and traceability of all food and animal feed containing more than 0.5 per cent GM ingredients. Also Codex Alimentarius published a document to safe guard the GM food in 2003 and further compliances need to be made if the GM food is for the purpose of exporting and importing .

A 2003 survey by the Pew Research Center found that a majority of people in all countries surveyed felt that GM foods were "bad". The lowest scores were in the US and Canada, where 55 per cent and 63 per cent (respectively) were against it, while the highest were in Germany and France with 81 per cent and 89 per cent disapproving. The survey also showed a strong tendency for women to be more opposed to GM foods than men.

In 2002, Oregon Ballot measures gave voters in that state one of the first opportunities in the United States to directly address that issue. The measure, which would have required the labeling of genetically engineered foods, failed to pass by a ratio of 7 to 3.

Friedrich-Wilhelm Graefe zu Baringdorf, member of the German Green Party and vice president of the Landwirtschaftsausschuss (committee of agriculture) of the European Commission said on the 1 July 2003: "In America 55 per cent of the consumers are against GM food and 90 per cent in favour of a clear labeling."

Agricultural Trade Market between USA and Europe

The European Union and United States are in strong disagreement over the EU's ban on most genetically modified foods.

The value of agricultural trade between the US and the European is estimated at $57 billion at the beginning of the 21st Century, and some in the U.S., especially farmers and food manufacturers, are concerned that the new proposal by the European Union could be a barrier to much of that trade.

In 1998, the United States exported $63 million worth of maize to the·EU, but the exports decreased to $12.5 million in 2002.

The drop-off might also be due to falling commodities prices, less demand due to the recession, U.S. maize being priced out of foreign markets by a strong dollar, and importing countries' reaction to the planned invasion of Iraq. Similar European public opposition to Israeli treatment of Palestinians has also affected Israeli food exports. However, American farm industry advocates blame the EU's ban.

European Proposal over Genetically Modified Food

The European Parliament's Committee on the Environment, Public Health and Food Safety proposal, adopted in the summer of 2002 and expected to be implemented in 2003, has deep cultural roots that are difficult to understand for the US agricultural community. It requires that all food/feed containing or derived from genetically modified organisms be labeled and any GM ingredients in food be traced. It would also require documentation tracing biotechnological products through each step of the grain handling and food production processes.

The new European tax, tariff and trade proposal would particularly affect US maize gluten and soybean exports, as a high percentage of these crops are genetically modified in the USA (about 25 per cent of US maize and 65 per cent of soybeans are genetically modified in 2002).

The ultimate resolution of this case is widely thought to rest on labeling rather than food aid. Many European consumers are asking for food regulation (demanding labels that identify which food has been genetically modified), while the American agricultural industry is arguing for free trade and is strongly opposed to labeling, saying it gives the food a negative connotation.

Lori Wallach, director of Public Citizen's Global Watch indicates that American agricultural industry is "using trade agreements to determine domestic health, safety and environmental rules" because they fear that "by starting to distinguish which food is genetically modified, then they will have to distinguish energy standards, toxic standards that are different to those that European promotes."

The American Agricultural Department officials answer that since the United States does not require labeling, Europe should not require labeling either. They claim mandatory labelling could imply there is something wrong with genetically modified food, which would be also a trade barrier. Current U.S. laws do not require GM crops to be labeled or traced because U.S. regulators do not believe that GM crops pose any unique risks over conventional food. Europe answers that the labeling and traceability requirements are not only limited to GM food, but will apply to all agricultural goods. Such labelling has been mandatory for many years in Australia where the U.S. is also arguing against identification of GM products.

The American agricultural industry also complains about the costs implied by labeling.

Official US Complaint with the WTO

The ban over agricultural biotechnology is said by some Americans to breach World Trade Organisation rules. Robert B. Zoellick, the United States trade representative, indicated the European position toward GMO was thought of as "immoral" since it could lead to starvation in the developing world or wars, as seen in some famine-threatened African countries (eg, Zambia, Zimbabwe, and Mozambique) that refuse to accept US aid because it contains GM food.

Zoellick's critics argue that US concern over Third World starvation is merely a cover for other issues. Some money for development aid is used by the American government via the World Food Programme (WFP) to help their farmers by buying up overproduction and giving it to the UN organisation. GM-scepticism interferes with this programme. American farmers lost marketshare in certain countries after changing to genetically modified food because of sceptical consumers.

Another European response to the claims of immorality is that the EU gives 7 times more in development aid than the US, yet its economy is less than 10 per cent bigger than America's, and its GDP/head much lower than that of the US.

In May 2003 the Bush administration officially accused the European Union of violating international trade agreements, in blocking imports of U.S. farm products through its long-standing ban on genetically modified food. Robert Zoellick announced the filing of a formal complaint with the WTO challenging the moratorium after months of negotiations trying to get it lifted voluntarily. The complaint was also filed by Argentina, Canada, Egypt, Australia, New Zealand, Mexico, Chile, Colombia, El Salvador, Honduras, Peru, and Uruguay. The formal WTO case challenging the EU's regulatory system was in particular lobbied by U.S. biotechnology giant Monsanto Company and France's Aventis, as well as by big agricultural groups such as the National Corn Growers Association.

The US move was also interpreted as a sanction against the EU for requesting the end of illegal tax breaks for exporters or face up to $4 billion in trade sanctions in retaliation for Washington's failure to change the tax law, which the WTO ruled illegal four years ago.

Ratification of the Biosafety Protocol by the EU Parliament

In June 2003, the European Parliament ratified a three-year-old U.N. biosafety protocol regulating international trade in genetically modified food, expected to come into force in fall 2003 since the necessary number of ratification was reached in May 2003. The protocol lets countries ban imports of a genetically modified product if they feel there is not enough scientific evidence the product is safe and requires exporters to label shipments containing genetically altered commodities such as corn or cotton. It makes clear that products from new technologies must be based on the precautionary principle and allow developing nations to balance public health against economic benefits.

Jonas Sjoestedt, a Swedish Left member of the EU assembly, said that "this legislation should help the EU to counter recent accusations by the U.S administration that the EU is to blame for the African rejection of GM food aid last year."

The United States did not sign the protocol, saying it was opposed to labeling and fought import bans.

European de facto *Moratorium*

In 1998, a de facto moratorium led to the suspension of approvals of new genetically modified organisms (GMO) in the European Union pending the adoption of revised rules to govern the approval, marketing and labelling of biotech products. Imports and cultivation of already approved GM varieties and food products continued. In July 2003, European environment ministers and the European Parliament agreed to new controls on GMOs that could eventually lead the then 15 members bloc to re-open the Union's markets to new genetically modified products in 2004.

The new labeling and traceability rules, which cover both food and feed, require any products with a GMO content of more than 0.9 per cent to be labelled. Labelling is also required for products that have been derived from GMOs, but where the GM content might no longer be detectable (such as soy oil produced from genetically modified soy).

The threshold for the presence of unapproved GMOs is 0.5 per cent provided that the GMOs have been judged as safe for human health and the environment by the relevant Scientific Committees or the European Food Authority. This amount will be set for 3 years. After 3 years, all food containing non-authorized GMO will be banned.

Animals fed with transgenic cereals are not covered by the labeling requirements.

Traceability of GMO products is mandatory, from sowing to final product. Genetically modified goods will have to carry a special harmless DNA sequence (a DNA code bar) identifying the origin of the crops, making it easier for regulators to spot contaminated crops, feed, or food, and enabling products to be withdrawn from the food chain should problems arise. A series of additional sequences of DNA with encrypted information about the company or what was done to the product could also be added to provide more data.

Following the entry into force of the new regulations, the first genetically modified food product (canned maize) since 1998 was approved for marketing in the European Union in May 2004. While a number of other biotech products have been approved since then, approvals remain controversial. European ministers have continuously failed to reach a decision in support of or against the applications, highlighting the big divide among member states. As a result, the approvals were granted by the European Commission, which is entitled to take a decision in case ministers fail to do so.

Effect of Cultural Differences between US and Europe

The U.S. population has historically placed a considerable degree of trust in the regulatory oversight provided by the U.S. Department of Agriculture and its agencies. There is little tradition of people having a close relationship with their food, with the overwhelming majority of people having bought their food in supermarkets for years. But the 2003 survey by the Pew Research Center showed that even in the U.S., 55 per cent.

In Europe, and particularly in the UK, there is less trust of regulatory oversight of the food chain. In many parts of Europe, a larger measure of food is produced by small, local growers using traditional (non-intensive and organic) methods.

Árpád Pusztai, considered by many to be the leading expert on GM foods, was silenced with threats of a lawsuit after he unexpectedly discovered that rats fed an experimental GM food developed immune system damage and other serious health problems in just ten days. Pusztai later reviewed an industry-sponsored study and found that seven of forty rats fed a GM crop died within two weeks; others developed stomach lesions. The crop was approved without further tests.

In May, when the U.S. filed a challenge with the World Trade Organization (WTO) disputing Europe's GM food policy, Trade Representative Robert Zoellick stated, "Overwhelming scientific research shows that biotech foods are safe and healthy." According to Andrew Kimbrell, director of the Center for Food Safety, "The evidence in the book Seeds of Deception refutes U.S. science and safety claims, and undermines the basis of their WTO challenge."

Kimbrell says, "Author Jeffrey M. Smith's book also presents a compelling argument that nations may use to ban GM foods altogether." Countries gained the right to impose such a ban on September 11, three months after the UN biosafety protocol was signed by 50 nations. "The revelations in the book", says Kimbrell, "are being made public at a pivotal time in the global GM debate, and could tip the scales against the biotech industry."

WTO Decision

The World Trade Organization has made a preliminary ruling that European Union restrictions on genetically engineered crops violate international trade rules. The United States, Canada, and Argentina together grow 80 per cent of all biotech crops sold commercially, by which the EU regulates such crops. The countries argued that the EU's regulatory process was far too slow and its standards were unreasonable given that the overwhelming body of scientific evidence finds the crops safe.

11

Towards Healthy Diet, Nutrition and Physical Fitness

REVISITING NUTRITION

Nutrition (also called nourishment or aliment) is the provision, to cells and organisms, of the materials necessary (in the form of food) to support life. Many common health problems can be prevented or alleviated with a healthy diet.

The diet of an organism is what it eats, and is largely determined by the perceived palatability of foods. Dietitians are health professionals who specialize in human nutrition, meal planning, economics, and preparation. They are trained to provide safe, evidence-based dietary advice and management to individuals (in health and disease), as well as to institutions.

A poor diet can have an injurious impact on health, causing deficiency diseases such as scurvy, beriberi, and kwashiorkor; health-threatening conditions like obesity and metabolic syndrome, and such common chronic systemic diseases as cardiovascular disease, diabetes, and osteoporosis.

HEALTHY EATING GUIDELINES

Healthy Eating Guidelines and Recommendations from around the world:

- USA
- Canada
- UK
- Australia

Healthy Eating

Healthy Eating Guidelines are intended to promote overall health while reducing the risk of developing nutrition-related diseases like cancer and heart disease. They are directed at all healthy individuals over the age of 14. There is nothing difficult about healthy eating. It is simply a common-sense approach to food that is easy to live with, once you get used to it.

REVALUATING NUTRIENT CLAIMS

Many of us are confused by the numerous claims found on packaged food products. How low is the sodium content in a "Low Sodium" chicken stock? What does "Light" Soya Sauce, "Light" cream cheese or "Light" peanut butter really mean?

Nutrient Claims—Basics

Free: This term means that a product contains no amount of, or only trivial or "physiologically inconsequential" amounts of, one or more of these components: fat, saturated fat, cholesterol, sodium, sugars, and calories. Synonyms for "free" include "without," "no" and "zero."

Low: This term can be used to describe foods that can be eaten frequently without exceeding dietary guidelines for one or more of these components: fat, saturated fat, cholesterol, sodium, and calories. Synonyms for low include "little," "few," and "low source of."

Light: This descriptor can mean two things:

1. a nutritionally altered product contains one-third fewer calories or half the fat of the reference food.
2. the sodium content of a low-calorie, low-fat food has been reduced by 50 percent.

The term "light" still can be used to describe such properties as texture and colour, as long as the label•explains the intent. For example, "light brown sugar".

Claims	Requirements
Calories	
Free	Fewer than 5 kcal per serving
Low	40 kcal or less per serving, or per 50 g of the food
Reduced/Less	At least 25% fewer kcal per serving than reference food
Light/Lite	If 50% or more of the kcal are from fat; fat must be reduced by at least 50% per reference amount. If less than 50% of kcal are from fat, fat must be reduced at least 50% or kcal reduced at least 1/3 per reference amount.
Fat	
Free	Less than 0.5g of fat per serving
Low	3g or less per serving, or per 50g of the food
Reduced/Less	At least 25% less per serving than reference food
Light/Lite	If 50% or more of the calories are from fat, fat must be reduced by at least 50% per reference amount. If less than 50% of calories are from fat, fat must be reduced at least 50% or calories reduced at least 1/3 per reference amount.
Sugar	
Free	Less than 0.5g per serving.
Reduced	At least 25% less sugar per serving than reference food
No added sugar, without added sugar, or no sugar added	No sugars are added during processing or packing
Sodium	
Free	Less than 5mg per serving
Low	140mg or less per serving, or per 50g of the food
Very Low	35mg or less per serving, or per 50g of the food
Reduced/Less	At least 25% less per serving than reference food
Light	If food is "Low Calorie" and "Low Fat" and sodium is reduced by at least 50%
Fiber	
High	5g or more per serving. (Foods with high fiber claims must meet the definition for low fat, or the level of total fat must appear next to the high fiber claim.)
Good source of	2.5g to 4.9g per serving
More/added	At least 2.5g more per serving than the reference food
	Other Nutrient Claims
"Healthy"	Products using the term "healthy" in the product name or as a claim on the label must contain, per serving, no more than 3g of fat, 1g of saturated fat, 480mg of sodium, or 60mg of cholesterol. They must also supply

(*Contd.*)

"High", "Rich in" or "Excellent Source"	20% or more of the Daily Value for a given nutrient per serving
"Good Source Of", "More", or "Added"	The food provides 10% more of the Daily Value for a given nutrient than the comparison food. The 10 percent of Daily Value also applies to "fortified," "enriched" and "added" claims, but in those cases, the food must be altered.

Nutrient Claims—the Bottom Line: Remember, these claims are meant to serve as guidelines only. It may seem confusing at times but with some practice, you will be able to quickly scan a food label and learn how a particular food product meets your nutritional needs.

When comparing products, focus on those nutrients that are important to you.

- If you are concerned about your weight, you should compare products based on BOTH calories and fat.
- If you have heart disease or high blood pressure, you should focus on the amount of total fat, saturated fat, trans fat, cholesterol and sodium. Choose products containing less than 20 per cent Daily Values for fat, cholesterol and sodium.
- If you have diabetes, you should pay attention to the amount of carbohyrdate, sugar added as well as fiber.

REVISITING MULTIVITAMINS

For most healthy adults under the age of 50, it is possible to acquire all required nutrients through eating food alone if you follow the 2005 Dietary Guidelines and avoid foods with empty calories.

Table 11.1: 2005 Dietary Guidelines (2000-kcal Diet)

Fruits	at least 2 cups
Vegetables	at least 2 1/2 cups
Calcium-rich foods	3 servings
Grains	at least 3 servings of Whole Grains

Different people face different challenges in reaching optimum nutrition by food alone. We offer some quick and easy solutions to help tackle these challenges.

Challenge 1: Inadequate Fruits and Vegetables

Solutions:

- Eat a serving of fresh fruit at lunch and dinner as dessert
- Include a variety of vegetables for lunch and dinner. Choose dark green, leafy vegetables (such as broccoli, spinach, Chinese bok choy and kale) as well as bright-coloured vegetables (such as bell peppers, tomato, avocado, sweet potato and carrot)
- Use fruits as snacks. Bring to work fruits that are easy to prepare (such as grapes, apple, banana, berries or cut-up melons).

Challenge 2: Inadequate Calcium

Solutions:

- Instead of snacking on cookies, choose low-fat yogurt or low-fat cheese with fruits as snacks throughout the day.
- If you are not a cow's milk fan, try other calcium-rich beverages such as calcium-fortified orange juice, calcium-fortified soy or rice milk, or goat's milk.
- Try other calcium-rich foods such as tofu and canned fish with bones.

Challenge 3: Inadequate Whole Grains

Solutions:

- Choose whole grain bread when making sandwiches
- Have a serving of whole grain breakfast cereal or a bowl of oatmeal for breakfast
- Snack on popcorn instead of chips on movie nights
- Toss in brown rice, wild rice or barley in your soup

Bottom Line
Taking a multivitamin daily is important to ensure optimum nutritional status for a certain population—particularly among pregnant and lactating women, as well as those with specific chronic diseases. For people older than 50 (men and women), a multivitamin or calcium/D supplement may be warranted as foods alone may be not able to deliver adequate calcium and Vitamin D to meet the increased needs. Always speak to your doctor or dietitian before starting a new supplement. As fortified-foods are widely available, the expert panel recommended choosing a multivitamin with ingredients less than 100 percent of the daily value (% DV) to avoid toxicity.

LOW FAT FOODS vs. LOW CALORIE

If you think that low fat means low calories, read on. Often, reduced fat items have more sugar added to enhance the flavor, which contributes calories to the final product. Also, many of us think that by eating the low fat version of a food, we can eat more of it. If you are watching your weight, this will only sabotage your efforts.

Check out the list of foods below to see the difference in calories (if there is any) between common low fat and regular fat foods.

- Reduced Fat Peanut Butter: 2 Tbsp: 190 calories, 12g fat
- Regular Peanut Butter: 2 Tbsp: 190 calories, 16g fat
- Low Fat Wheat Thins: 16 crackers: 130 calories, 4g fat
- Regular Wheat Thins: 16 crackers: 150 calories, 6g fat
- Low Fat Oreos: 3 cookies: 150 calories, 4.5g fat
- Original Oreos: 3 cookies: 160 calories, 7g fat
- Fat Free Fig Newtons: 2 cookies: 100 calories, 0g fat
- Regular Fig Newtons: 2 cookies: 110 calories, 2g fat
- Low fat Fruit-flavored Yogurt: 6 oz: 173 calories, 1.8 g fat
- Regular Fruit-flavored Yogurt: 6 oz: 170 calories, 6 g fat
- Low fat Granola Cereal: ½ cup: 160 calories, 2.2g fat
- Regular Granola Cereal: ½ cup: 210 calories, 6g fat
- Light Tortilla Chips: 1 oz: 132 calories, 4.3g fat
- Regular Tortilla Chips: 1 oz: 141 calories, 7.3g fat
- Fat Free Apple Cinnamon Muffin: Small: 130 calories, 0g fat

- Regular Apple Cinnamon Muffin: Small: 147 calories, 6.9g fat

PHYSICAL FITNESS HEALTH

Nutrition: Diet, Weight Loss, and Health

Nutrition is a science that studies the relationship between diet and health. Wikipedia notes that "There are six main classes of nutrients that the body needs: carbohydrates, proteins, fats, vitamins, minerals, and water. It is important to consume these six nutrients on a daily basis to build and maintain healthy bodily function."

For years, the U.S. Government has employed the "Food Pyramid" as a model of how to consume appropriate amounts of these nutrients. With increasing childhood obesity, it is more important than ever to attempt to eat a balanced diet.

- Hydrate well! Drink several glasses of water each day.
- Weight loss can be achieved by eating the correct quantities of different food groups. Simply eating less is not necessarily the answer.

Balanced Diet, Nutrition, and Obesity

Unhealthy Eating and Nutrition

In general terms it's going to probably depend on the individual. One level nutrition doesn't work for everyone. We come from different backgrounds and different genealogical makeup or whatever you want to call it. You might find that works well for one individual may not work for another.

There is a set of guidelines that the government publishes for 20 or so different vitamins and minerals and nutrient and the carbohydrates and those values or based on population studies where they go out and look at the health and consider what people consume on a regular basis.

To generalize, I would say that good nutrition would be getting the right balance of nutrients necessary for good health.

Nutrients vs. Food Stuffs?

You can look at anything that provides nutrients to the body like carbohydrates, protein, minerals and vitamins. They are the vitamins and minerals that everyone knows about and then there are the ones like micronutrients like selenium, chromium and zinc and some of those that aren't so talked about. But food in general is just a carrier for nutrients. You can take a loaf of bread it…has starch in it and protein and non-fat dry milk, the non-fat dry milk will contain lactose. It will contain a high amount of minerals usually. The non-fat dry milk will contain casing, which is a non-fat dry milk protein. You break down the constituents in the food and each one of those provides nutrients for the body.

Breaking of Bad Eating Habits

If there were an easy answer to the question we wouldn't have the problems we have today like obesity. Right now in the US 60 per cent of the population has a weight problem. "Morbidly Obese" is clinically defined as being 100 pounds or more overweight. In our population, the number of people being morbidly obese is increasing year after year.

The number of people with this weight problem continues to increase every year. In our culture today there is an over abundance of food available. On every corner there is fast food and billboards and everywhere you turn there is an advertisement for fast food. You know starting almost from infancy where you have two working parents they get home from their job and they are more likely to park there kids in front of the TV.

One of the things that I have noticed is the amount and length of the ads seem to be increasing: More and more year after year the cable companies seem to be just filled with everything you can imagine and not very nutritious food. You get exposed to that and it gets ingrained in your thinking about food and, if you will do the research on it, many of those ads are geared toward influencing children. When they go back and do the research on the influence what mom and pop pick off the grocery shelf, they find that the children have a tremendous influence. So they target those ads at the children knowing that they are going to put the pressure on the parents to buy them.

What you can do to change a person's perception of food starts at an early age. You can show a person in black and white what foods are good for them and what isn't and it pretty much comes down to a conscious decision if they want to consume healthy foods or not.

And it certainly would be a value to have a mentor or life coach or fitness trainer or just a friend where there is some kind of relationship when it comes to dealing with eating healthy. The fact is that you need support and one of the reasons there are so many weight loss programmes is that they do something a little different they have meetings and people get together and support each other.

Diet and Weight Loss Support Groups

You know I mentioned Optifast and there is Atkins and when you gauge how much weight people have lost and whether they keep it off, all of those people probably within a 5 year period have gained all that weight back because they have lost their support group. It speaks volumes to me that if people are going to lose weight and keep it off they need a support group. It has to be approached that you are not on a diet to lose weight you are trying to make a lifestyle change. It is going to be a new way of eating and new habits even your daily activities it is something that you are going to do for the rest of your life.

Generational Obesity?

In a way it is endorsement to the children that their eating habits and lifestyle habits are acceptable. Just like any of us what better role models than your parents. If they snack and eat unhealthy then the children will as well.

It is that everyone is trying to answer the question, "why are people getting fatter and fatter," and even Jay Leno makes jokes about people getting fat. You know the notion out there is that it isn't something that people can change it's just that people are genetically predisposed to getting fat. And there is a genetic factor to it but you know that Dr. Phil responds to it like you may be predisposed to it but you don't have to succumb to it.

Fat, Calories, and Weight Loss

Calorie

A calorie is the amount of heat that is required to raise one cubic centimeter of water one degree. It is actually an amount of energy.

Carbohydrate

Carbohydrates are molecular linkages of sugar molecules. If you take a starch, which is a carbohydrate and you link those sugar molecules together. If you look at the ingredients they are always listed in the order of predominance. In that listing you will see an ingredient called maltodextrine. A maltodextrine is a hybrid ingredient that is neither a sugar nor a starch. You know a simple sugar can be like glucose and a starch is a long chain of glucose molecules. You link all those together and you finally get something called a starch. In between where you have the simple sugars and you have the complex substance starch you have these things called maltodextrine.

Fat

It comes back to the whole idea of how many units are in this molecular chain. If you break down a fat you break it down into something called a fatty acid. They can all be broken down into smaller units. In the case of starch it can be broken down into simple sugars or these maltodextrines, which can be broken down into simple sugars.

The point I am trying to make is any of these macronutrients can be broken down into smaller units. Just like starch is broken down into simple sugars, the fat is broken down into fatty acids and the proteins are broken down into peptides or amino acids.

Proteins and Amino Acids

Each one of those macronutrients can be subdivided. In the case of proteins, proteins are made up of amino acids. Not all proteins have all amino acids that are important because there are essential amino acids. If you are consuming proteins and the essential ones are missing you will suffer. You could end up with some disease because those are missing, in some cultures around the world where food isn't so plentiful and they aren't ingesting the right nutrients. You know one that I can think of is called Kwashiorkor. You will see often times where little kids will have the distended tummies. The rest of their bodies are fine and it just comes down to the fact that they have a nutritional deficiency.

Some proteins are absorbed extremely well and an example would be egg albumin, which is the white of an egg rather than the yolk. The egg white protein has an extremely high biological availability and all of the essential amino acids in the right balance. You can take a protein like gelatin and gelatin has the amino acids that it is made of you will find that it is deficient in an amino acid called triptophane and because it is lacking in that it isn't balanced. If it is combined with other sources of protein it is okay.

Balance of Nutrients Thwarts Obesity

The bottom line is if you are looking at fat or protein it is important to look at the composition of them. You can read the declarations of the food labels and especially in snack items the protein will be there but often times the manufacturer is looking for inexpensive ingredients they can find. Often times the protein is inefficient and they don't have the quality and are deficient in amino acids. It is important to know that all fat and proteins are made up of these building blocks and it is important to know to have a balance of all of these building blocks for the fat to be good for you and the protein to be good for you.

Eat More and Lose Weight by Combining Different Foods—A Myth

People say that there are certain foods that take more calories to burn than they provide or that certain food items are going to cause more calories to be burned. It is a misconception. People don't want to put the time and the energy or the money into losing weight. It is a lot of work. People want to lose weight and they know that some of the food they eat is unhealthy and they don't want to put the time and energy into changing things.

It takes planning and time. Instead of visiting the fast food restaurant on the corner on the way home you go to the produce aisle in the grocery store. It might take you a little more time and cost you a little more money but it's worth it. You know the fast food restaurants super size everything. The artists and executives that design the ads know that our mentality is that the more food we can get for our buck then the better we are going to like it. It wasn't so long ago that you would go in and order a soft drink and you would get 8 oz or 12 oz and now it's not uncommon to get 24 or 36oz because they super size everything.

Count of Calories, Carbohydrates or Fat

Let me just go on a little further and we will come back to that. If you look at carbohydrates it is the same scenario. Each gram of carbohydrates contains 4 grams of fat. This is why fat is so important. It is almost twice that of protein and carbohydrates.

One gram of fat contains roughly 9 calories. So if you start talking about the Atkins diet, it depends on how you set up the study. You can get any variety of results you want. You know the Atkins diet is one of my favourites to pick on because the early studies showed that people lost more weight initially and overall the diet was more effective than other diets.

Well I believe that since then they have gone bankrupt. Somewhere along the line people were starting to figure out that it's not all it's cracked up to be. What seems to be the case now when you start looking at the numbers is when you have enough people on the diets it becomes statistically significant. What it seems to boil down to is Atkins restricts your intake to mainly fat and protein and by eliminating carbohydrates from the diet it takes away so many of the food choices that are available.

You know, even lovers of protein and fat what they find that restrictions your variety and choices are taken away and what you do is actually limiting your caloric intake. Just because you don't have the wide variety of choices you can make any more. So it works initially and that is one of the reasons why people are so attracted to it.

Alcohol—Are One or Two Drinks Okay?

Some studies show that a small amount of alcohol ingested on a daily basis may have some positives in reducing your risk for heart disease or may help to lower blood cholesterol levels.

Alcohol Contains Many Calories

Red wine may be preferred because of the antioxidants that you get and the other chemicals that come along with the wine. Obviously there is something in the red wine as opposed to the white that makes it more beneficial. Alcohol is number one a source of calories and you know that it is quite high. The higher the level of alcohol in the beverage the higher the caloric intake is. I believe that one gram of alcohol would be five and a half calories. It isn't as high as fat but not as low as protein and carbohydrates.

There are other aspects of that to think about, if you are trying to lose weight you need to question whether you need the extra calories. There are many other beverages that would provide many more nutrients. If you are trying to lose weight you need to question whether or not you need those extra calories from something that basically has no nutritional value. I would tend to be more negative about consuming alcohol because people tend to get out of hand when consuming it and the damage it can do to families as well as the individual.

So I would never be one to advocate the drinking of alcohol because it has no nutritional value or health value. You know any benefit that alcohol might provide you can get from something else.

Most Diets Fail. Lifestyle Change is Needed.

95 per cent of diets fail and what it really comes down to if you want to lose weight it has to be something that you decide to make as a lifestyle change. You know, a diet is only temporary. You go on it and what are you going to do eventually? You are going to go off it. In my definition that is not a lifestyle change that is a temporary fix. You know that is human nature. You go on the diet and eventually you are going to go off it and revert back to you old eating habits and gain the weight back.

It all comes down to understanding a little bit more to understanding the foods that you are eating and a choice to make a lifestyle change. Also almost all of these diet plans introduce a new way of eating, a way that is abnormal to the way that you are used to eating and we are creatures of habit and we like the foods that we are used to.

And because we are creatures of habit we don't adapt very well to changes like that. We can go on it for a while and because it is so abnormal it just doesn't fit. If you are a busy mom and you are rushing your kids back and forth to school you then all of the sudden you have to prepare these kinds of foods and eat these certain foods it basically forces you off the diet. It all comes down to the fact that you have to make a decision that you are going to change the way you eat and it doesn't' have to be an abrupt change you just need to understand more about what you are eating and what the energy value is and the nutrient value is of the foods you are consuming.

Keeping Track of What You Eat

I know the nutritional value of the foods I am eating. I keep a running tabulation in my mind of the foods I have eaten and what I am going to eat today and how I am going to balance it out. I know that if I have been naughty in eating too many chocolate chip cookies then the next day I am going to watch what I eat.

Our eating habits are so ingrained. How can we change them? If you are doing something healthy for yourself, it can be easier to put aside the unhealthy habits.

When you do something like walk 15 minutes and then you are standing in front of the chocolate chip cookies you are more likely to start thinking, "Should I eat those cookies or shouldn't I?" It becomes a little more easier to make healthy choices. The more healthy choices you make the easier it is to incorporate more.

Exercise Burns Calories

Make Healthy Choices

It's almost like the unhealthy choices don't fit anymore. They are incompatible with the healthy choices. As I kick around health and nutrition with people that are into it like I am, I find that if you do exercise and have more muscle mass you burn more calories when you are at rest. Lean muscle mass has a higher metabolic requirement. When you are just sitting around and your body has more lean muscle mass you are going to burn more calories than if your body contains fatty tissue.

It's kind of a cruel injustice but the fitter you get even at rest you are burning more calories. The basil metabolic requirement on a daily basis may be a very small percent of your total energy needs as compared to other ways you burn energy. The basil metabolic requirement is just how much energy you need to sustain your basic metabolic processes, like breathing, heartbeat and digestion and those things.

Well Balanced Diet

Following the food pyramid is a good place to start and maybe it's a good place to end for some people. If you take all the food somebody eats at the end of the week and then add them all up and how much variety there was, you will find that there really wasn't that much variety.

People generally have a dozen foods they like to eat and they will end up eating the same foods day after day for most of their life and that are where you run into problems. You get stuck in a rut and fail to incorporate a vast variety into your diet and fail to get the nutritional balance that you should be getting. If you know nothing about food but incorporate a lot of variety into your diet the chances of your being malnourished because you don't get the right nutrients goes down hill.

Fruits and Vegetables

My wife does the grocery shopping and she and I like fresh fruit and vegetables. We will just take a big salad bowl and fill it like the diet out there called the Rainbow diet. It's based on all the different colours of fruits and vegetables. So I will take purple grapes and onions and garlic and sprinkle some lettuce and if we have fresh strawberries I will add those cantaloupe and really your imagination is your only limitation. You know, just basically add all your favourite fruits and vegetables and throw in a couple of tablespoons of your favourite dressing and season it to taste. Mix it all up and you have an incorporation of all of that variety. You get all of the vitamins and the nutrients and the minerals that you need in just one meal instead of just ingesting one kind of food.

More Variety = Better Diet

My point is the more variety you can get in your diet the greater the possibility that if you are lacking in something that you are going to get it. I am an advocate of getting variety in your diet. It all comes down to looking at your budget and having some knowledge of getting what you need and looking at the food labels.

Even the restaurants and the fast food chains are starting to offer more nutritious choices, like salads. Subway is one that has really jumped on the bandwagon. You know the one with Jared standing there saying this deep fat fried sandwich contains 45 plus grams of fat I wonder how they got all that fat in there to begin with and compare it to the subway sandwich.

I saw an interview where they were talking with the producer of Sesame Street and they were talking about the cookie monster and how it was presented in a way to get kids to eat more junk food and more cookies. Now they have repositioned that whole programme to where they are starting to teach kids more about nutrition. I am hoping that one of the things that are happening is that there is awareness about nutrition and this obesity epidemic. Some people are just succumbing to obesity and the things that come with it like cancer and heart disease and diabetes. It's good to see some positive changes taking place.

You know that in some developing cultures there is a craving that some people have and I believe it is called Pica. It is where a person will have a craving to eat a particular food item and it doesn't always have to be a food item, it can be dirt or something that isn't a food at all. The theory is that people will have a craving for certain things that will provide a nutrient that is lacking.

In our culture I don't think it is metabolic for food cravings. You know if you are used to consuming sugary sweets and that is all you eat, your metabolism adapts and guides you to the foods you are used to consuming.

An example of that would be someone who has gone on a vegetarian diet and eliminate meat from their diet temporarily. Then they start to reintroduce meat and their stomach is upset. Their stomach is not used to digesting that kind of food. They have adapted to digesting just non-meat items. There are food digestive adaptations to the kinds of food that you eat. One would have to believe that those are the kinds of foods that you get used to.

Do We Become Hungry Because Our Stomach is Empty or is It Because of Something Else?

That is a tricky question. There are people who have studied this and can boil it right down to all kinds of enzymes and mechanisms that kick into play that stimulate appetite or depress appetite. Individual metabolism is so significant individually that I am sure that you can feel that on a general basis.

One thing that I can say is when I go exercise and I get back and sit down I need to replenish my water intake. The next thing that I find is that if I find a combination of fruits to eat it will suppress my hunger because fruits are primarily water and sugar and carbohydrates. But the digestive process is pretty rapid when it comes to breaking down sugars into glucose and the glucose is stored in your body. So digestion of fruits in particular is pretty rapid. I can consume a lot of fresh fruits and it doesn't satisfy my hunger.

Exercise and Appetite

I will still have hunger pains because the digestion is completed so rapidly as opposed to protein, which takes longer. It almost seems like exercise can suppress appetite but I think you have to balance that whole idea with how much exercise you are doing and how many calories your body needs to replace and what kinds of food you are going to consume when you are done.

It is complex to think about why people are gaining weight. Many groups are studying this and trying to help people lose weight. Each of these communities have their own theories and their own recommendations. They all study it in a different way—some try to understand the psychology and some try to understand the nutritional aspects of it. If it was better understood, we probably wouldn't be having the problems we are having today.

Nutrients Decrease the Risk of Some Diseases. Are there Certain Foods Containing these Nutrients that Lend Themselves to Good Health?

The bottom line is there is no magic pill. It wasn't until the 1940's that we as a country started to put together nutritional requirements in relation to disease and when we started to establish the different recommendations.

If you take that historical perspective and go back you find that in the early years there were just a few nutrients for which the recommended daily allowances were established and through the years, through the studies and the whole process of understanding we have continued to add to the list of things that are required. It hasn't been until quite recently that we have learned about trace nutrients like selenium and things like that, that have recently been added to the list. Those levels continue to change as we learn more. One of the things that interest me is the addition to the list; it is almost a never-ending process. I always come back to the concept of nutrition and variety and not getting locked into a few fixed food items.

Basic Nutrients

The level of protein in your diet and a certain amount of carbohydrates to provide energy and a certain amount of fat. Those are the main building blocks and the body requires certain enzymes and vitamins and minerals. A good quality protein contains certain amino acids and then you break it down into smaller blocks called peptides. Basically it just comes down to protein, fat and vitamins and minerals to keep metabolic process continued.

Non-Nutrient

Basically it would be something that didn't contain any calories or a source of protein, carbohydrates or vitamins and minerals. Water would be non-caloric. It is a non-nutrient, but very important.

SCIENCE REFERENCE

Dietitians are health professionals who specialize in this area of study, and are trained to provide safe, evidence-based dietary advice and interventions. Deficiencies, excesses and imbalances in diet can produce negative impacts on health, which may lead to diseases such as cardiovascular disease, diabetes, scurvy, obesity or osteoporosis, as well as psychological and behavioural problems.

Moreover, excessive ingestion of elements that have no apparent role in health, (e.g. lead, mercury, PCBs, dioxins), may incur toxic and potentially lethal effects, depending on the dose. Many common diseases and their symptoms can often be prevented or alleviated with better nutrition.

In general, eating a variety of fresh, whole (unprocessed) plant foods has proven hormonally and metabolically favourable compared to eating a monotonous diet based on processed foods. In particular, consumption of whole plant foods slows digestion and provides higher amounts and a more favourable balance of essential and vital nutrients per unit of energy; resulting in better management of cell growth, maintenance, and mitosis (cell division) as well as regulation of blood glucose and appetite. A generally more regular eating pattern (e.g. eating medium-sized meals every 2 to 3 hours) has also proven more hormonally and metabolically favourable than infrequent, haphazard food intake. There are six main classes of nutrients that the body needs: carbohydrates, proteins, fats, vitamins, minerals, and water.

It is important to consume these six nutrients on a daily basis to build and maintain health. Poor health can be caused by an imbalance of nutrients, either an excess or deficiency, which, in turn, affects bodily functions cumulatively. Moreover, because most nutrients are involved in cell-to-cell signalling (e.g. as building blocks or as part of a hormone or signalling cascades), deficiency or excess of various nutrients affects hormonal function indirectly. Thus, because they largely regulate the expression of genes, hormones represent a link between nutrition and how our genes are expressed, i.e. our phenotype. The strength and nature of this link are continually under investigation, but recent observations have demonstrated a pivotal role for nutrition in hormonal activity and function and therefore in health.

Glossary

Acceptable daily intake (ADI): The amount of chemical that, if ingested daily over a lifetime, appears to be without appreciable effect.

Additives (food additives): Any natural or synthetic material, other than the basic raw ingredients, used in the production of a food item to enhance the final product. Any substance that may affect the characteristics of any food, including those used in the production, processing, treatment, packaging, transportation or storage of food.

Aerobic exercise: Aerobic exercise refers to the kind of fast-paced activity that makes you "huff and puff." It places demands on your cardiovascular apparatus and, over time, produces beneficial changes in your respiratory and circulatory systems.

Algin: A compound which is extracted from algae and used in puddings, milk shakes and ice cream to make these foods creamier and thicker and to extend shelf life.

Allergen (food allergen): A food allergen is the part of a food (a protein) that stimulates the immune system of food allergic individuals. A single food can contain multiple food allergens. Carbohydrates or fats are not allergens.

Ally methyl trisulfide, dithiolthiones: A type of sulfide/thiol found in cruciferous vegetables which may provide the health benefits of lowering LDL cholesterol and of maintaining a healthy immune system.

Alternative agriculture: A range of technological and management option farms striving to reduce costs, protect health and environmental quality, and enhance beneficial biological interactions and natural processes. Alternative agriculture techniques cannot be uniformly applied across all commodities or all regions of the country. Such practices typically require more information, trained labor, time and management skills per unit of production than conventional farming.

Amino acids: Amino acids function as the building blocks of proteins. Chemically, amino acids are organic compounds containing an amino (NH2) group and a carboxyl (COOH) group. Amino acids are classified as essential, nonessential and conditionally essential. If body synthesis is inadequate to meet metabolic need, an amino acid is classified as essential and must be supplied as part of the diet. Essential amino acids include leucine, isoleucine, valine, tryptophan, phenylalanine, methionine, threonine, lysine, histidine and possibly arginine. Nonessential amino acids can be synthesized by the body in adequate amounts, and include alanine, aspartic acid, asparagine, glutamic acid, glutamine, glycine, proline and serine. Conditionally essential amino acids become essential under certain clinical conditions

Anaphylaxis: A rare but potentially fatal condition in which several different parts of the body experience food-allergic reactions simultaneously, causing hives, swelling of the throat and difficulty breathing. It is the most severe allergic reaction to an allergen and requires immediate medical attention when it occurs.

Animal and Plant Health Inspection Service (APHIS): A government agency which resides in the United States Department of Agriculture and governs the field-testing of agricultural biotechnology crops.

Anthocyanidins: A type of flavonoid found in various fruits which provides the health benefits of neutralizing free radicals and possibly reducing the risk of cancer.

Antibiotics: Antibiotics are used in animal agriculture for two reasons. First, to improve the rate of growth and the feed efficiency of animals so they produce more meat or milk on less feed. The second reason is to prevent and treat diseases, just as in humans.

Anticarcinogens: Substances which inhibit the formation of cancers or the growth of tumors. More than 600 chemicals are claimed to be anti-cancer agents. These range from natural chemical constituent present in garlic, broccoli, cabbage and green tea to manmade antioxidants, such as butylated hydroxyanisole (BHA) and derivatives of retinoic acid.

Antioxidant: Antioxidants protect key cell components by neutralizing the damaging effects of "free radicals," natural byproducts of cell metabolism. Free radicals form when oxygen is metabolized, or burned by the body. They travel through cells, disrupting the structure of other molecules, causing cellular damage. Such cell damage is believed to contribute to aging and various health problems.

Ascorbic acid: Also known as vitamin C, it is essential for the development and maintenance of connective tissue. Vitamin C speeds the production of new cells in wound healing and it is an antioxidant that keeps free radicals from hooking up with other molecules to form damaging compounds that might attack tissue. Vitamin C protects the immune system, helps fight off infections, reduces the severity of allergic reactions and plays a role in the synthesis of hormones and other body chemicals. Green peppers, broccoli, citrus fruits, tomatoes, strawberries, and other fresh fruits and vegetables are good sources of vitamin C.

Asthma: Asthma is a chronic medical condition, affecting approximately 10 million Americans (3 to 4 percent of the population). Asthma results when irritants (or trigger substances) cause swelling of the tissues in the air passage of the lungs, making it difficult to breathe. Typical symptoms of asthma include wheezing, shortness of breath and coughing.

Attention Deficit Hyperactivity Disorder (ADHD): Commonly called "hyperactivity," Attention Deficit Hyperactivity Disorder is a clinical diagnosis based on specific criteria. These include excessive motor activity, impulsiveness, short attention span, low tolerance to frustration and onset before 7 years of age.

Basal metabolism: Basal metabolism is the energy (calories) a body burns when completely at rest. Basal metabolism rate (BMR) is the level of energy needed to keep involuntary body processes going. These processes include heartbeat, breathing, generating body heat, perspiring to keep cool, and transmitting messages to the brain. For a sedentary person, BMR accounts for about

60-70 percent of daily energy expenditure; the remaining 30-40 percent is from physical activity and from body heat produced after a meal. Physical activity is responsible for as much as 50-60 percent of the total energy expenditure in people who include frequent aerobic activity into their lifestyles

Beta-carotene: A type of carotenoid found in various fruits and vegetables which provide the health benefit of neutralizing free radicals that may cause damage to cells.

Bias: Bias occurs when problems in study design lead to effects that are not related to the variables being studied. An example is selection bias, which occurs when study subjects are chosen in a way that can misleadingly increase or decrease the strength of an association. Choosing experimental and control group subjects from different populations would result in a selection bias.

Biological activity: The effect (change in metabolic activity upon living cells) caused by specific compounds or agents. For example, the drug aspirin causes the blood to thin, that is to clot less easily.

Biopesticide: A biopesticide is any material of natural origin used in pest control derived from living organisms, such as bacteria, plant cells or animal cells.

Blind (single or double) experiment: In a single blind experiment, the subjects do not know whether they are receiving an experimental treatment or a placebo. In a double blind experiment, neither the researchers nor the participants are aware of which subjects receive the treatment - until after the study is completed.

Bovine spongiform encephalopathy (BSE): Bovine spongiform encephalopathy, or BSE, is also known as "mad cow disease." It is a rare, chronic degenerative disease affecting the brain and central nervous system of cattle. Cattle with BSE lose their coordination, develop abnormal posture and experience changes in behavior. Clinical symptoms take 4-5 years to develop, followed by death in a period of several weeks to months unless the affected animal is destroyed sooner.

Bt (Bacillus thuringiensis): One of the most common microorganisms used in biologically-based pesticides is the

Bacillus thuringiensis or Bt bacterium. Several of the proteins produced by the Bt, principally in the coating the bacteria forms around itself, are lethal to individual species of insects. By using Bt in pesticide formulations, target insects can be controlled using an environmentally benign, biologically-based agent. Bt-based insecticides have been widely used by home gardeners for many years as well as on farms.

Butylated hydroxyanisole (BHA): A phenolic chemical compound used to preserve foods by preventing rancidity. It may also be used as a defoaming agent for yeast. BHA is found in foods high in fats and oils; also in meats, cereals, baked goods, beer, and snack foods.

Caffeic acid: A type of phenol found in various fruits, vegetables and citrus fruits which has antioxidant like activities that may reduce the risk of degenerative diseases, heart disease and eye disease.

Calcium: A mineral that builds bones and strengthens bones, helps in muscle contraction and heartbeat, assists with nerve functions and blood clotting. Teens 18 years and younger should strive to consume about 1,300 milligrams per day. Individuals 50 years and older need about 1,200 milligrams per day. Everyone else should strive for about 1,000 milligrams per day. Milk and other diary foods such as yogurt and most cheeses are the best sources of calcium. In addition, dark green leafy vegetables, fish with edible bones, and calcium fortified foods supply significant amounts.

Carbohydrate: Carbohydrates are organic compounds that consist of carbon, hydrogen and oxygen. They vary from simple sugars containing from three to seven carbon atoms to very complex polymers. Only the hexoses (sugars with six carbon atoms) and pentoses (sugars with five carbon atoms) and their polymers play important roles in nutrition. Carbohydrates in food provide 4 calories per gram. Plants manufacture and store carbohydrates as their chief source of energy. The glucose synthesized in the leaves of plants is used as the basis for more complex forms of carbohydrates. Classification of carbohydrates relates to their structural core of simple sugars, saccharides. Principal monosaccharides that occur in food are glucose and fructose.

Three common disaccharides are sucrose, maltose and lactose. Polysaccharides of interest in nutrition include starch, dextrin, glycogen and cellulose.

Center for Disease Control and Prevention (CDC): The CDC, composed of 11 Centers, Institutes and Offices, aims to promote health and quality of life by preventing and controlling disease, injury and disability. The Center is a component of the U.S. Department of Health and Human Services (HHS).

Catechins: A type of flavonoid found in tea which provides the health benefits of neutralizing free radicals and possibly reducing the risk of cancer.

Cholesterol (dietary): Cholesterol is not a fat, but rather a fat-like substance classified as a lipid. Cholesterol is vital to life and is found in all cell membranes. It is necessary for the production of bile acids and steroid hormones. Dietary cholesterol is found only in animal foods. Abundant in organ meats and egg yolks, cholesterol is also contained in meats and poultry. Vegetable oils and shortenings are cholesterol-free.

Cholesterol (different types): Blood cholesterol is divided into three separate classes of lipoproteins: very-low density lipoprotein (VLDL); low-density lipoprotein (LDL), which contains most of the cholesterol found in the blood; and high-density lipoprotein (HDL). LDL seems to be the culprit in coronary heart disease and is popularly known as the "bad cholesterol." By contrast, HDL is increasingly considered desirable and known as the "good cholesterol."

Clinical trials: Clinical trials undertake experimental study of human subjects. Trials may attempt to determine whether the finds of basic research are applicable to humans, or to confirm the results of epidemiological research. Studies may be small, with a limited number of participants, or they may be large intervention trials that seek to discover the outcome of treatments on entire populations. The "gold standard" clinical trials are double-blind, placebo-controlled studies which employ random assignment of subjects to experimental and control groups unknown to the subject or the researcher.

Collagen hydrolysate: A functional component of gelatin which may help improve some symptoms associated with osteoarthritis.

Control group: The group of subjects in a study to whom a comparison is made in order to determine whether an observation or treatment has an effect. In an experimental study it is the group that does not receive a treatment. Subjects are as similar as possible to those in the test or treatment group.

Correlation: An association, or when one phenomenon is found to be accompanied by another. A correlation does not prove cause and effect. Correlation may also be defined statistically.

Crustacean: Any of the various aquatic arthropods, including lobsters, crabs, shrimps and barnacles. Characteristically have segmented bodies, chitinous exoskeletons and paired, jointed limbs.

Cyclamate: A sweetener which is 30 times sweeter than sucrose, calorie free and heat stable and works synergistically with other sweeteners. It is approved for tabletop use in Canada and more than 50 countries in Europe, Asia, South America and Africa. Since 1970, however, the use of cyclamate has been banned in the United States on the basis of a study that suggested that cyclamates may be related to the development of bladder tumors in rats. Although 75 subsequent studies have failed to show that cyclamate is carcinogenic, the sweetener has yet to be reapproved for use in the United States.

Dextrin: Dextrins are a group of carbohydrates produced by the hydrolysis of starch. They have the same general formula as carbohydrates but are of shorter chain length.

Diallyl sulfide: A type of sulfide/thoil found in onions, garlic, olives, leeks and scallions which may provide the health benefits of lowering LDL cholesterol and of maintaining a healthy immune system.

DNA: Also known as Deoxyribonucleic acid. This is the molecule that carries the genetic information for most living systems. The DNA molecule consists of four bases (adenine, cytosine, guanine and thymine) and a sugar-phosphate backbone, arranged in two connected strands to form its characteristic double-helix.

E. coli: O157:H7: The bacteria Escherichia coli: O157:H7 is a type of E. coli associated with foodborne illness. Healthy cattle and humans can carry the bacteria. It can be transferred from animal to animal and animal to human, and from animal to human on food. Transmission from person to person through close contact is a potential problem, especially among young children in daycare.

Ecologist: An individual who studies the interrelationships between organisms and their environment.

Endocrine disruption: Not considered as an adverse endpoint per se but as a step or mechanism that could lead to toxic outcomes, such as cancer or adverse reproductive effects.

Environmental Protection Agency (EPA): The EPA's mission is to protect human health and safeguard the natural environment—air, water and land—upon which life depends. Through regulation, EPA tries to ensure the human population and the environment are protected from environmental risks and exposures.

Epinephrine: An adrenal hormone that stimulates autonomic nerve reaction. It is used in the treatment of anaphylaxis to open airways and blood vessels.

Experimental group: The group of subjects in an experimental study which receives a treatment.

Fat replacers: Fat replacers are developed to duplicate the taste and texture of fat, but contain fewer calories per gram than fat. Fat replacers generally fall into three categories: carbohydrate-, protein- or fat-based. The ingredients that are used to replace fat depend on how the food product will be eaten or prepared. For example, not all fat replacer ingredients are heat stable. Thus, the fat replacer that worked well in a salad dressing may not work well in a muffin mix.

Fats (dietary fats): Fats are referred to in the plural because there is no one type of fat. Fats are composed of the same three elements as carbohydrates—carbon, hydrogen and oxygen, However, fats have relatively more carbon and hydrogen and less oxygen, thus supplying a higher fuel value of nine calories per gram (versus four calories per gram from carbohydrates and protein). One molecule of fat can be broken down into three molecules of fatty acids and one molecule of glycerol.

Thus, fats are known chemically as triglycerides. Fats are a vital nutrient in a healthy diet. Fats supply essential fatty acids, such as linoleic acid, which is especially important to childhood growth. Fat helps maintain healthy skin, regulate cholesterol metabolism and is a precursor of prostaglandins, hormone-like substances that regulate some body processes. Dietary fat is needed to carry fat-soluble vitamins A, D, E and K and to aid in their absorption from the intestine.

Fertilizer: Any organic or inorganic material, either natural or synthetic, used to supply elements (such as nitrogen, phosphate and potash) essential for plant growth. If used in excess or attached to eroding soil, fertilizers can become a source of water pollution.

Fiber: Dietary fiber generally refers to parts of fruits, vegetables, grains, nuts and legumes that can't be digested by humans. Meats and dairy products do not contain fiber. Studies indicate that high-fiber diets can reduce the risks of heart disease and certain types of cancer. There are two basic types of fiber - insoluble and soluble. Soluble fiber in cereals, oatmeal, beans and other foods has been found to lower blood cholesterol. Insoluble fiber in cauliflower, cabbage and other vegetables and fruits helps move foods through the stomach and intestine, thereby decreasing the risk of cancers of the colon and rectum.

Flavones: A type of flavonoid found in various fruits and vegetables which provides the health benefits of neutralizing free radicals and possibly reducing the risk of cancer.

Folic acid: Folic acid, folate, folacin, all form a group of compounds functionally involved in amino acid metabolism and nucleic acid synthesis. Good dietary sources of folate include leafy, dark green vegetables, legumes, citrus fruits and juices, peanuts, whole grains and fortified breakfast cereals. Recent studies show, if all women of childbearing age consumed sufficient folic acid (either through diet or supplements), 50 to 70 percent of birth defects of the brain and spinal cord could be prevented, according to the U.S. Centers for Disease Control and Prevention (CDC.) Folic acid is critical from conception through the first four to six weeks of pregnancy when the neural tube is formed. This means adequate diet or supplement use should begin before pregnancy occurs. Recent research findings also show low blood folate levels can be associated with elevated plasma homocysteine and increased risk of coronary heart disease.

Food Guide Pyramid: The Food Guide Pyramid is a graphic design used to communicate the recommended daily food choices contained in the Dietary Guidelines for Americans. The information provided was developed and promoted by the U.S. Department of Agriculture and the U.S. Department of Health and Human Services.

Food intolerance: A general term for any adverse reaction to a food or food component that does not involve the body's immune system.

Food preservatives: All preservatives prevent spoilage either by slowing the growth of organisms that live on food or by protecting the food from oxygen. Antimicrobials are preservatives that protect food by slowing the growth of bacteria, molds and yeasts. Antioxidants are preservatives that protect by preventing food molecules from combining with oxygen (air).

Food safety: Food safety is a relative and not absolute matter. Relative food safety can be defined as the practical, certainty that injury or damage will not result from food or ingredient used in reasonable and customary manner and quantity.

Fortified foods: Fortified foods have nutrients added to them that were not present originally. For example, milk is fortified with vitamin D, which helps your body absorb calcium and phosphorus found naturally in milk.

Fructo-oligosaccharides (FSO): A type of prebiotic/probiotic found in Jerusalem artichokes, shallots and onion powder which may improve gastrointestinal health.

Fruit: Fruit is the usually edible reproductive body of a seed plant, especially one having a sweet pulp associated with the seed.

Functional foods: Foods that may provide health benefits beyond basic nutrition. Examples include tomatoes with lycopene, thought to help prevent the incidence of prostate and cervical cancers; fiber in wheat bran and sulfur compounds in garlic also believed to prevent cancer.

Galactose: A monosaccharide occurring in both levo (L) and dextro

(D) forms as a constituent of plant and animal oligosaccharides (lactose and raffinose) and polysaccharides (agar and pectin). Galactose is the sugar derived from digesting lactose ('milk sugar").

Gastronomy: The study and appreciation of good food and good eating, and a culture's culinary customs, style and lore. Any interest or study of culinary pursuits as relates essentially to the kitchen and cookery, and to the higher levels of education, training and achievement of the chef apprentice or professional chef.

Generalizability: The extent to which the results of a study are able to be applied to the general population of people that is comparable to the population studied.

Genome: The total hereditary material of a cell, containing the entire chromosomal set found in each nucleus of a given species.

Glutamate: Glutamate is an amino acid that is necessary for metabolism and brain function, and is manufactured by the body. It is found in virtually every protein food we eat. In food, there is "bound" glutamate and "free" glutamate. Glutamate serves to enhance flavors in foods when it is in its free form and not bound to other amino acids in protein. Some foods have greater quantities of glutamate than others. Foods that are rich in glutamate include tomatoes, mushrooms, parmesan cheese, milk and mackerel.

Glycemic load: The concept of glycemic load was developed to give researchers a more accurate picture of the impact of carbohydrate consumption on the body. The glycemic load calculation takes into account the glycemic index of a specific food as well as the amount of carbohydrate in a serving of that food. To calculate glycemic load, you multiply the grams of carbohydrate in a serving of food by that food's glycemic index. As with glycemic index, glycemic load is a research tool but there are questions about its use as a measure on which to base dietary recommendations for the general population.

Glycerol: A colorless, odorless, syrupy liquid—chemically, an alcohol—that is obtained from fats and oils and used to retain moisture and add sweetness to foods.

Good Manufacturing Practices (GMP): The Food and Drug

Administration's (FDA's) approval mechanism for a process to manufacture a given food or food additive. It is implemented instead of specific regulations (such as, those used to dictate processes in simple food manufacturing, as in beef packing), due to the newness of the technology and may later be superceded (due to further advances in the technology).

GRAS (Generally Recognized as Safe): GRAS is the regulatory status of food ingredients not evaluated by the FDA prescribed testing procedure. It also includes common food ingredients that were already in use when the 1959 Food Additives Amendment to the Food, Drug and Cosmetic Act was enacted.

Health claims: Claims that link food—or food components—in the overall diet with a lowered risk of some chronic diseases. Strictly regulated by the Food and Drug Administration, only health claims supported by scientific evidence are allowed on food labels. Since this information is optional, many foods that meet the criteria don't carry any health claim on their label.

Herbicides: Herbicides are a class of crop protection and specialty chemicals used to control weeds on farms and in forests, as well as in non-agricultural applications such as golf courses, public tracts of land and residential lawns.

Homeostasis: The ability or tendency of an organism or cell to maintain internal equilibrium by adjusting its physiological processes.

Hybridization of crops: The mating of two plants from different species or genetically very different members of the same species to yield hybrids possessing some of the characteristics of each parent. Those (hybrid) offspring tend to be more healthy, productive and uniform than their parents—a phenomenon known as "hybrid vigor."

Hypertension: Hypertension is the persistently elevated arterial blood pressure. It is the most common public health problem in developed countries. Emphasis on lifestyle modifications has given diet a prominent role for both the primary prevention and management of hypertension.

Immune system: The cells and tissues which are responsible for recognizing and attacking foreign microbes and substances in the body.

Immunoglobulin E: The antibody in the immune system that reacts with allergens.

Insecticide: Insecticides are a class of crop protection and specialty chemicals used to control insects on farms and forests, as well as non-agricultural applications such as residential lawncare, golf courses and public tracts of land.

Integrated pest management (IPM): Integrated pest management is the coordinated use of pest and environmental information along with available pest control methods, including cultural, biological, genetic and chemical methods, to prevent unacceptable levels of pest damage using the most economical means, and with the least possible hazard to people, property and the environment.

Lactobacillus: A type of prebiotic/probiotic found in yogurt and some other dairy products which may improve gastrointestinal health.

Lactose: A sugar naturally occurring in milk, also known as "milk sugar," that is the least sweet of all natural sugars and used in baby formulas and candies.

Lecithin: A by-product of the refining for soybean oil and is also found in eggs, red meats, spinach and nuts. Historically, lecithin has been used commercially in food processing as a

National Health and Nutrition Examination Survey (NHANES): A series of surveys that include information from medical history, physical measurements, biochemical evaluation, physical examination and dietary intake of population groups within the United States. The NHANES is conducted by the U.S. Department of Health and Human Services approximately every five years.

Nematodes: Microscopic, wormlike organisms that feed on plant roots.

Neural tube defect: In simple terms, a neural tube defect (NTD) is a malformation of the brain or spinal cord (neurological system) during embryonic development. Infants born with spina bifida, where the spinal cord is exposed, can grow to adulthood but usually suffer from paralysis or other disabilities. Babies born with anencephaly, where most or all of the brain is missing, usually die shortly after birth. These NTDs make up about 5 percent of all U.S. birth defects each year. According to the Centers for Disease Control, the use of sufficient folic acid is enough to eliminate the risk of NTDs.

Nitrogen: A nonmetallic element that constitutes nearly four-fifths of the air by volume, occurring as a colorless, odorless, almost inert diatomic gas in various minerals and in all proteins. It is used in a wide variety of important manufacturing processes, including ammonia, nitric acid, TNT and fertilizers.

No-till farming: A methodology of crop production in which the farmer avoids mechanical cultivation (i.e., only one pass over the field). The plant residue remaining on the field's surface helps to control weeds and reduce soil erosion, but it also provides sites for insects to shelter and reproduce, leading to a need for increased insect control.

Nutrient density: Nutrient dense foods are those that provide substantial amounts of vitamins and minerals and relatively fewer calories. The opposite of nutrient dense is calorie dense which are foods that mainly supply calories and relatively few nutrients.

Obesity, or overweight: Although precise definitions vary among experts, overweight has been traditionally defined as 10 percent to 20 percent above an optimal weight for height derived from statistics. Obesity is defined as body weight being 20% above normal. Some scientists argue that the amount and distribution of an individual's body fat is a significant indicator of health risk and therefore should be considered in defining overweight. Abdominal fat has been linked to more adverse health consequences than fat in the hips or thighs. Thus, calculations of waist-to-hip ratio are preferred by some health experts to help determine if an individual is overweight.

Oligofructose: A soluble dietary fiber that has a sweet flavor and can be used to improve the flavor of low calorie foods and to improve the texture of fat-reduced foods. Oligofructose is also known as fructooligosaccharide, or FOS. A prebiotic, inulin stimulates the growth of intestinal bifidobacteria.

Organic: Organic defines agricultural products that are grown using cultural, biological and mechanical methods prior to the use of synthetic, non-agricultural substances to control pests, improve soil quality an/or enhance processing. The USDA is currently addressing the issue of organic products, and aims to have official rules for what may be considered organic ready for the 1999 spring planting season. Currently organic defines an agricultural process in which farmers use techniques such as crop rotation, cultivation, mulching, soil enrichment and the "encouragement" of predators and microorganisms which naturally keep pests away. The now widely accepted definition allows farmers to use natural pesticides, but nothing synthetic.

Outcomes research: A type of research increasingly used by the health industry which provides information about how a specific procedure or treatment regimen affects the subject (clinical safety and efficacy), the subject's physical functioning and lifestyle, and economic considerations such as saving or prolonging life and avoiding costly complications.

Palatable: Acceptable or agreeable to taste.

Pectin: A natural gelling agent found in ripe fruit. Pectin is an important ingredient in making jams and jellies. Some fruits have high pectin levels (e.g., citrus fruit, blackberries, apples and red currants) but others are low in pectin (e.g., strawberries) so lemon juice is added to strawberry jam to help the set.

Phenylalanine: An amino acid that is one of the components of the low-calorie sweetener aspartame. Phenylalanine also occurs naturally in such protein-containing foods such as chicken, beef, milk and vegetables.

Phytate: A chemical complex (large molecule) substance that is the dominant (i.e., 60 to 80%) chemical form of phosphorous within cereal grains, oilseeds, and their by-products. Monogastric animals (e.g., swine) cannot digest and utilize phosphorus within phytate, because they lack the enzyme known as phytase in their digestive system, so that phosphorus (phytate) is excreted into the environment. When phytase enzyme is present in the ration of a monogastric animal, at a high enough level, the monogastric animal is then able to digest the phytate (thereby releasing that phosphorus for absorption by the animal).

Placebo: Sometimes casually referred to as a "sugar pill," a placebo is a "fake" treatment which seems identical to the real treatment. Placebo treatments are used to eliminate bias that may arise from the expectation that a treatment should produce an effect.

Polyols: A type of sweetener used in reduced-calorie foods. They differ from intense sweeteners in that they are considered nutritive; that is, they do contribute calories to the diet. Polyols are incompletely absorbed and metabolized, however, and consequently contribute fewer calories than sucrose. The polyols commonly used in the United States include sorbitol, mannitol, xylitol, maltitol, maltitol syrup, lactitol, erythritol, isomalt and hydrogenated starch hydrolysates. Most are approximately half as sweet as sucrose; maltitol and xylitol are about as sweet as sucrose. Polyols are found naturally in berries, apples, plums and other foods. They also are produced commercially from carbohydrates such as sucrose, glucose, and starch for use in sugar-free candies, cookies and chewing gum. Along with adding a sweet taste, polyols perform a variety of functions such as adding bulk and texture, providing a cooling effect or taste, preventing the browning that occurs during heating and retaining the moisture in foods.

Prevalence: The number of existing cases of a disease in a defined population at a specified time.

Proanthocyanidins: A type of tannin found in cranberries, cranberry products, cocoa and chocolate which may provide the health benefits of improving urinary tract health and of reducing the risk of cardiovascular disease.

Protein: Chemically, a protein is a complex nitrogenous compound made up of amino acids in peptide linkages. Dietary proteins are involved in the synthesis of tissue protein and other special metabolic functions. In anabolic processes they furnish the amino acids required to build and maintain body tissues. As an energy source, proteins are equivalent to carbohydrates in providing 4 calories per gram. Proteins perform a major structural role in all body tissues and in the formation of enzymes, hormones and various body fluids and secretions. Proteins participate in the transport of some lipids, vitamins and minerals and help maintain the body's homeostasis.

Randomization, or random assignment: A process of assigning subjects to experimental or control groups in which the subjects have an equal chance of being assigned to each group. Randomization is used to control for known, unknown and difficult-to-control-for variables.

Random sample: A random sample is a procedure to select subjects for a study in which all individuals in a population being studied have an equal chance of being selected. using a random sample allows the results of the study to be generalized to the entire population. The term random also applies to assignments within controlled studies, or the division of subjects into groups. Random assignment ensures that all subjects have an equal chance of being in the experimental and control groups, and increases the probability that any unidentified variable will systematically occur in both groups with the same frequency. Randomization is crucial to control for variables that researchers may not be aware of or cannot adequately control, but which could affect the outcome of an experimental study.

Rapid assays: These diagnostic tests use emerging technology to identify and remove impurities from foods before they reach the consumer. There are two major types of rapid assays. Antibody-based assays link a "familiar" characteristic on a pathogen's surface (the antigen) to a substance known as an antibody. When this connection is made, the test registers "success." Similarly, nucleic acid-based assays use the unique genetic materials of the cells to detect a pathogen.

Reliability: Whether a test or instrument used to collect data, such as a questionnaire, gives the same results if repeated on the same person several times. A reliable test gives reproducible results.

Research design: How a study is set up to collect information, or data. For valid results, the design must be appropriate to answer the question or hypothesis being studied.

Retrospective study: Research that relies on recall of past data, or on previously recorded information. Often this type of research is considered to have limitations, because the number of variables that cannot be controlled, and because memory is not infallible.

Risk factor: A risk factor is anything statistically shown to have a relationship with the incidence of a disease, however it does not necessarily infer cause and effect.

Saccharin: Saccharin, the oldest of the non-nutritive sweeteners, is currently produced from purified, manufactured methyl anthranilate, a substance occurring naturally in grapes. It is 300 times sweeter than sucrose, heat stable and does not promote dental caries. Saccharin has a long shelf life, but a slightly bitter aftertaste. It is not metabolized in the human digestive system, is excreted rapidly in the urine and does not accumulate in the body.

Saponins: The functional component of soybeans, soy foods and soy protein-containing food which may lower LDL cholesterol and may contain anti-cancer enzymes.

Selective breeding: This process allows for the transfer of only one or a few desirable genes, thereby permitting scientists to develop crops with specific beneficial traits and those without undesirable traits. Current technology allows scientists to alter one plant characteristic at a time, thereby not spending years trying to develop the tastiest and hardiest plants.

Sodium nitrite: A salt used in smoked or cured fish and in meat-curing preparation. It acts as a preservative and color fixative. Can combine with chemicals in the stomach to form nitrosamine, a carcinogenic substance.

Soy protein: The protein found in soybeans and soy-based foods which when consumed at the level of 25 grams per day may reduce the risk of heart disease.

Stanol/sterol esters: A functional component found in wood oils, corn, soy and wheat which may reduce the risk of coronary heart disease by lowering blood cholesterol levels.

Starch: Starches are complex carbohydrates (polysaccharides), composed of chains of glucose molecules, which plants use to store food energy. It is a nutrient that is naturally abundant in foods such as rice, wheat and potatoes.

Statistical significance: The probability of obtaining an effect or association in a study sample as or more extreme that the one observed if there was actually no effect in the population. Based on the hypothesis that if there truly is no effect, the results of a study are unlikely to have occurred. A P value of less than five percent (P<0.05) means the result would occur less than five percent of the time if there were no effect, and is generally considered evidence of a true treatment effect or a true relationship.

Sucralose: Sucralose is the only low-calorie sweetener that is made from sugar. It is approximately 600-times sweeter and does not contain calories. Sucralose is highly stable under a wide variety of processing conditions. Thus, it can be used virtually anywhere sugar can, including cooking and baking, without losing any of its sugar-like sweetness. Currently, sucralose is approved in over 25 countries around the world for use in food and beverages. In the US, sucralose is FDA-approved for use as a tabletop sweetener and in 15 different food and beverage categories, including carbonated soft drinks, low-calorie fruit drinks, apple sauce and other products.

Sugar: Although the consumer is confronted by a wide variety of sugars—sucrose, raw sugar, turbinado sugar, brown sugar, honey, corn syrup—there is no significant difference in the nutritional content or energy each provides, and therefore no advantage of one nutritionally over another. There also is no evidence that the body can distinguish between naturally occurring or added sugars in food products.

Sulfites: Sulfiting agents are sometimes used to preserve the color of foods such as dried fruits and vegetables, and to inhibit the growth of microorganisms in fermented foods such as wine. Sulfites are safe for most people. A small segment of the population, however, has been found to develop shortness of breath or fatal shock shortly after exposure to these preservatives. Sulfites can provoke severe asthma attacks in sulfite-sensitive asthmatics. For that reason, in 1986 the FDA banned the use of sulfites on fresh fruits and vegetables (except potatoes) intended to be sold or served raw to consumers. Sulfites added to all packaged and processed foods must be listed on the product label.

Synergistic effect: The effect achieved by the combination of two or more substances or organisms which neither alone could accomplish.

Thermal effect of food: The increase in energy expenditure associated with the processes of digestion, absorption and metabolism of food; represents approximately 10% of a person's total energy expenditure and includes facultative thermogenesis and obligatory thermogenesis; often called diet-induced thermogenesis (DIT).

Toxicologist: A scientist who studies the nature, effects and detection of poisons and the treatment of poisoning.

Traditional crop breeding: For traditional crop breeding, breeders mix thousands of genes in order to transfer the protein products to enhance one or a few genetic traits. Therefore, the odds of something undesirable being transferred unintentionally are far greater in traditional breeding than in biotechnology.

Partially hydrogenated vegetable oils were developed in part to help displace highly saturated animal and vegetable fats used in frying, baking and spreads. However, trans *fats, like saturated fats, raise blood LDL cholesterol levels (the so-called "bad" cholesterol). High consumption of* trans *fats may also reduce the HDL or "good" cholesterol levels. In January 2006, FDA revised food labeling regulations to require that the amount of* trans *fat in a product be declared on the Nutrition Facts panel.*

Type 1 diabetes: Results from the body's failure to produce insulin, the hormone that "unlocks" the cells of the body, allowing glucose to enter and fuel them. It is estimated that 5-10% of Americans who are diagnosed with diabetes have type 1 diabetes.

Umami: In addition to the four main taste components (sweet, sour, salty and bitter), there is the additional taste characteristic called "umami" or savory. One of the food components responsible for the umami flavor in foods is glutamate, an amino acid.

Validity: The extent to which a study or study instrument measures what it is intended to measure. Refers to accuracy or truthfulness in regard to a study's conclusion.

Vegetarian: According to the Vegetarian Resource Group, less than 1 percent of Americans are true vegetarians. Such people never eat meat, fish or poultry, although they may eat foods derived from animals such as dairy products and eggs (lacto-ovo vegetarians). There are even fewer vegans, strict vegetarians who avoid all animal-derived foods — even honey.

Vitamins: Vitamins are organic compounds that are nutritionally essential in small amounts to control metabolic processes and cannot be synthesized by the body. Vitamins are usually classified by their solubility, which to some degree determines their stability; occurrence in foodstuffs; distribution in body fluids, and tissue storage capacity. Each of the fat-soluble vitamins A, D, E and K has a distinct and separate physiologic role. Several have antioxidant properties to depress the effects of metabolic byproducts called free radicals, which are thought to cause degenerative changes related to aging. Most of the water-soluble vitamins are components of essential enzyme systems. Many are involved in the reactions supporting energy metabolism. These vitamins are not normally stored in the body in appreciable amounts and are normally excreted in the urine. Thus, a daily supply is desirable to avoid depletion and interruption of normal physiologic functions.

Water: Although deficiencies of energy or nutrients can be sustained for months or even years, a person can survive only a few days without water. Experts rank water second only to oxygen as essential for life. In addition to offering true refreshment for the thirsty, water plays a vital role in all bodily processes. It supplies the medium in which various chemical changes of the body occur, aiding in digestion, absorption, circulation and lubrication of body joints. For example, as a major component of blood, water helps deliver nutrients to body cells and removes waste to the kidneys for excretion.

Whole grains: The whole kernel of grain which includes the bran (outer shell), germ (nutrient rich core) and endosperm (starchy portion). The health benefit provided by whole grains is the reduced risk of cardiovascular disease which results from the combination of fiber, vitamins, minerals and phytochemicals found in whole grains.

Xenobiotics: Synthetic chemicals believed to be resistant to environmental degradation. A branch of biotechnology called bioremediation is seeking to develop biological methods to degrade such compounds.

Bibliography

Adams, M.R., 1982, *Kick start for Village Vinegar in Papua New Guinea*, AT Journal, 9, (2), IT Publications, London, UK.

Agricultural Research, Livelihoods, and Poverty: Studies of Economic and Social Impacts in Six Countries Edited by Michelle Adato and Ruth Meinzen-Dick (2007),Johns Hopkins University Press Food Policy Report (Brief)

Aguilera, Jose Miguel and David W. Stanley. *Microstructural Principles of Food Processing and Engineering*. Springer, 1999.

Andrews et al (2005). "Salmonella spp.", *Foodborne Pathogens: Microbiology and Molecular Biology*. Caister Academic Press.

Asiedu, J.J., 1989, *Processing Tropical Crops*, MacMillan Press Ltd, London.

ASTM MNL14 The Role of Sensory Analysis in Quality Control, 1992

Axtell, B., 1983, *The Orange Hill Estate: a Successful Small Industry in St. Vincent*, AT Journal, 10, (2).

Bacteriological analytical manual online. 2001. 8th ed. + updates. FDA

Bales, C.W. and Ritchie, C.S. (eds.) 2009. *Handbook of clinical nutrition and aging*. 2nd ed. Totowa, NJ: Humana.

Barbara Santich (1996). *Looking for Flavour*. Wakefield Press. pp. 118–119.

Barron, F.H. and J.D. Burcham. (2003). "Metal Containers." In *Encyclopedia of Agricultural, Food, and Biological Engineering*. D.R. Heldman, Ed. New York: Marcel Dekker. pp. 636-642.

Battaglia, R., Pfannhauser, W., and Murkovic, M. (eds.) 2001. *Who's who in food chemistry. Europe*. 2nd ed. rev. expanded.

Berlin; NY: Springer, 241 p.

Bazzaz, F.A., and W.G. Sombroek, 1996b. Global climatic change and agricultural production: an assessment of current knowledge and critical gaps. In: F. Bazzaz and W. Sombroek (Eds.), 1996a, 199-235.

Beeton, Isabella (1998) [1861]. *The Book of Household Management* (Facsim. reprint of: London, 1861 ed.). Lewis: Southover.

Bengston. 1924. Studies on organisms concerned as causative factors in botulism. Hyg. Lab. Bull. 136: 101

Bentley, R, Meganathan, R., Biosynthesis of Vitamin K (menaquinone) in Bacteria, *Bacteriological Reviews*, 1982, 46(3):241-280. Review.

Berdanier, C.D.*CRC desk reference for nutrition*. 2006. 2nd ed. Boca Raton, FL: CRC Press. 518 p.

Bertolli, Paul. *Cooking by Hand*. New York, NY: Clarkson Potter/ Publishers, 2003.

Bidault, B. and Gattegno, I., 1984,*Le Point sur la Transformation des Fruits Tropicaux*, GRET (Groupe de Recherche et D'échanges Technologiques), Paris, France.

Bohle, H.G., T.E. Downing and M.J. Watts, 1994. Climate change and social vulnerability. Towards a sociology and geography of food insecurity. Global Envir. Change, 4(1):37-48.

Bourque, R.A. (2003). "Secondary Packaging." In *Encyclopedia of Agricultural, Food, and Biological Engineering.* D.R. Heldman, Ed. New York: Marcel Dekker. pp. 873-879.

Burdock, G.A. 2002. *Fenaroli's handbook of flavor ingredients*. 4th ed. Boca Raton, FL: CRC Press. 1834p.

C. Corbridge "Phosphorus: An Outline of its Chemistry, Biochemistry, and Technology" 5th Edition Elsevier: Amsterdam 1995.

Cane, M.A., G. Eshel and R.W. Buckland, 1994. Forecasting Zimbabwean Maize yield using eastern equatorial Pacific sea surface temperature. Nature 370:204-205.

Carpenter, Ruth Ann; Finley, Carrie E. *Healthy Eating Every Day*. Human Kinetics, 2005.

chemistry.about.com

Chinnan, M.S. and D.S. Cha. (2003). "Primary Packaging." In

Encyclopedia of Agricultural, Food, and Biological Engineering. D.R. Heldman, Ed. New York: Marcel Dekker. pp. 781-784.

Claude Bourguignon, *Regenerating the Soil: From Agronomy to Agrology*, Other India Press, 2005

Collinson, M. (editor): *A History of Farming Systems Research*. CABI Publishing, 2000.

Cousin et al (2005). "Foodborne Mycotoxins: Chemistry, Biology, Ecology, and Toxicology", *Foodborne Pathogens: Microbiology and Molecular Biology*. Caister Academic Press.

Crosby, Alfred W.: *The Columbian Exchange : Biological and Cultural Consequences of 1492*. Praeger Publishers, 2003 (30th Anniversary Edition).

da Motta, Silvana; Lucia M. Valente Soares. "Survey of Brazilian tomato products for alternariol, alternariol monomethyl ether, tenuazonic acid and cyclopiazonic acid <internet>". Retrieved on 13 August 2007.

Davidson, Alan. *The Oxford Companion to Food*. 2nd ed. UK: Oxford University Press, 2006.

Davis, Mike, *Late Victorian Holocausts: El Niño Famines and the Making of the Third World*, London, Verso, 2002

De Vries, John (1997), *Food Safety and Toxicity*, CRC Press, pp. 70,

Definition: Confit. *American Heritage Dictionary*. Dictionary.com. http://dictionary.reference.com/browse/confit. Retrieved 2008-09-20. "A condiment made by cooking seasoned fruit or vegetables, usually to a jamlike consistency"

Dickson, A. G. (1984) pH scales and proton-transfer reactions in saline media such as sea water. *Geochim. Cosmochim. Acta*, *48*: 2299–2308.

Dietary supplement fact sheets. Office of Dietary Supplements, National Institute of Health.

Domestic Preservation of Fruit and Vegetables, 1954, Ministry of Agriculture and Fisheries, Her Majesty's Stationery Office, 49 High Holborn, London, UK.

Doyle, Michael P. (2007). *Food Microbiology: Fundamentals and Frontiers*. ASM Press.

Dutt, Romesh C. *The Economic History of India under early British Rule*, first published 1902, 2001 Routledge.

Egan, H., Kirk, R.S., and Sawyer, R., 1981, *Pearson's Chemical Analysis of Foods,* Churchill Livingstone, London.

Environmental Affairs, 1986. Report of the Director-General: Environmental Affairs for the period 1 April 1984 to 31 March 1985. Environmental Affairs Authority, Republic of South Africa, Pretoria, 100 pp.

FAO agrometeorology Series Working Paper N. 13. FAO, Rome. 313 pp.

FAO, 1978a. Report on the agro-ecological zones project. Vol.1: Results for Africa. World Soil Resources Report 48/1. FAO, Rome, 158 pp. and 8 tables.

FAO, 1980. Report on the agro-ecological zones project. Vol.4: Results for south-east Asia. World Soil Resources Report 48/4. FAO, Rome, 39 pp. and 13 maps.

FAO, 1994. AGROSTAT-PC. Digital version of the FAO annual Production Yearbooks.

Fellows and A Hampton, 1992, *Small Scale Food Processing: a guide to appropriate equipment*, IT Publications, 103-105 Southampton Row, London WC1B 4HH, UK

Fellows, P.J., 1993, *Food Processing Technology*, Woodhead Publishing, Cambridge, UK

Ferrando, R., 1981, *Traditional and Non-Traditional Foods*, FAO Publications, Via delle Terme di Caracalla, Rome, Italy.

Fischer, G., and H. van Velthuizen, 1996. Climate change and global agricultural potential project: A case study of Kenya. IIASA Working Paper WP-96-71, Laxenburg, Austria. 96 pp.

Fischer, G., K. Frohberg, M.L. Parry and C. Rozenzweig, 1996. The potential effects of Climate Change on World Food Production and Security. In: F. Bazzaz and W. Sombroek (Eds.), 1996a, 199-235.

Food and Agriculture Organization of the United Nations. *The State of Food Insecurity in the World 2005*.

Food code. 2001. U.S. Department of Health and Human Services, Public Health Service, Food and Drug Administration.

Ford Runge and Benjamin Senauer, "How Biofuels Could Starve the Poor," *Foreign Affairs*, May/June 2007.

Francis, F.J. (2000). "Harvey W. Wiley: Pioneer in Food Science and Quality." In *A Century of Food Science.* Chicago: Institute of Food Technologists. pp. 13-14.

French–English food glossary". *At Home With Patricia Wells.* Patricia Wells, Ltd.. http://www.patriciawells.com/glossary/atoz/c.htm.

Fresco, L.O. and S.B. Kroonenberg, 1992. Time and spatial scales in ecological sustainability. Land Use policy, 155-168.

Galdston, I., *Human Nutrition Historic and Scientific* (New York: International Universities Press, 1960)

Garrison, R.H. *The nutrition desk reference.* 1995. 3rd ed. New Canaan, CT: Keats Pub. 663 p

Genady Golubev and Nikolai Dronin, *Geography of Droughts and Food Problems in Russia (1900-2000)*, Report of the International Project on Global Environmental Change and Its Threat to Food and Water Security in Russia (February, 2004).

Glewwe, P., Jacoby, H., & King, E. (2001). Early childhood nutrition and academic achievement: A longitudinal analysis. Journal of Public Economics, 81(3), 345-368.

Gommes, R. 1997. Some aspects of climate variability and food security in sub-Saharan Africa. Bull. Soc. Royale Sciences D'Outremer, Brussels. In press.

Gommes, R., and F. Petrassi. 1994. Rainfall variability and drought in sub-Saharan Africa since 1960. FAO Agrometeorology Series Working Papers N. 9, 100 pp.

Granum PE (2005). "Bacillus cereus", *Foodborne Pathogens: Microbiology and Molecular Biology*. Caister Academic Press.

Greenough, Paul R., *Prosperity and Misery in Modern Bengal. The Famine of 1943-1944*, Oxford University Press 1982

Guernsey, L. (1993). Many colleges clear their tables of steak, substitute fruit and pasta. Chronicle of Higher Education, 39(26), A30.

Hall, L. M. McCroskey, B. J. Pincomb, C. L. Hatheway. 1985. Isolation of an organism resembling Clostridium baratii which produces a type F botulinal toxin from an infant with botulism. J. Clin. Microbiol. 21: 654–655.

Hansson, I. (1973) A new set of pH-scales and standard buffers for seawater. *Deep Sea Research*, *20*: 479-491.

Hazard Analysis Critical Control Point. U.S. Food and Drug Administration, Center for Food Safety and Applied Nutrition. Variety of information on HACCP including HACCP for land and seafoods, education and training, and information from both other governmental and non-governmental sources.

Helms, S., R. Mendelsohn and J. Neuman, 1996. The impact of climate change on agriculture, Editorial essay. Climatic Change, 33:1-6.

Hohn, Thomas M.. "Trichothecene-resistant transgenic plants <internet>". Retrieved on 13 August 2007.

Home Scale Processing and Preservation of Fruits and Vegetables, 1977, Central Food Technology Research Institute, Mysore, India.

How long can someone survive without water?. Retrieved on 2007-05-14.

Hudault, S.; J. Guignot and A.L. Servin (July 2001). "*Escherichia coli* strains colonizing the gastrointestinal tract protect germfree mice against *Salmonella typhimurium* infection." *Gut 49*:47-55.

Hui, Y.H. (ed.) 2006. *Handbook of food science, technology, and engineering*. 4 volumes. Boca Raton, FL: Taylor & Francis.

Humphery, Kim. *Shelf Life: Supermarkets and the Changing Cultures of Consumption*. Cambridge University Press, 1998.

Hutchinson, B.S. and Greider, A.P. (eds.) 2002. *Using the agricultural, environmental, and food literature*. New York: Dekker. p. 533

Ihekoronye, A.I., and Ngoddy, P.O., *Integrated Food Science and Technology for the Tropics*, 1985, Macmillan Press Ltd., London, UK.

International Food Information Service. 2005. *Dictionary of food science and technology*. Oxford, UK: Blackwell. 413p.

J. Carlson (1931) Hunger *The Scientific Monthly* 33:77-79.

Jay, J.M., 1978, D van Nostrand, *Modern Food Microbiology,* New York.

Johnson, R. K. (2000). *The 2000 Dietary Guidelines for Americans: foundation of US nutrition policy*. - British Nutrition Foundation

Nutrition Bulletin 25. p241-248

Jurgens, Marshall H. *Animal Feeding and Nutrition*. Kendall Hunt, 2001.

Kanarek, R. B., & Swinney, D. (1990/2). Effects of food snacks on cognitive performance in male college students. Appetite, 14(1), 15-27.

Kennedy, John F. and Joaquim M. S. Cabral (1993). *Recovery Processes for Biological Materials*. John Wiley & Sons Ltd.

Kim, J. and Wilemon, D. (2002), Sources and assessment of complexity in NPD projects. R&D Management, 33 (1), pp. 16-30.

Koen et al. (2001), Providing clarity and a common language to the 'fuzzy front end'. Research Technology Management, 44 (2), pp.46-55

Kripke, Gawain. *Food aid or hidden dumping?*. Oxfam International, March 2005.

L. Hatheway, L. M. McCroskey. 1987. Examination of faeces for diagnosis of infant botulism in 336 patients. J. Clin. Microbiol. 25: 2334–2338.

Land use and cover change. Open Science meeting proceedings, 29-31 January 1996, Royal Academy of Arts and Sciences, Amsterdam. LUCC Report series N.1, Institut Cartogràfic de Catlunya, Barcelona, Spain. 143 pp.

LeBlanc, Steven, *Constant battles: the myth of the peaceful, noble savage*, St. Martin's Press (2003) argues that recurring famines have been the major cause of warfare since paleolithic times.

Lester R. Brown, "Beyond the Oil Peak" and "Stabilizing Climate" in Plan B 2.0: Rescuing a Planet Under Stress and a Civilization in Trouble (New York: W.W. Norton & Company, 2006).

Lester R. Brown, "Distillery Demand for Grain to Fuel Cars Vastly Understated: World May Be Facing Highest Grain Prices in History," *Eco-Economy Update*, 4 January 2007.

Lester R. Brown, "*Massive Diversion of U.S. Grain to Fuel Cars is Raising World Food Prices,*" *Eco-Economy Update*, 21 March 2007.

Lester R. Brown, "*The Short Path to Oil Independence: Gas-Electric*

Hybrids and Wind Power Offer Winning Combination," Eco-Economy Update, 13 October 2004.

Lester R. Brown, *Outgrowing the Earth* (New York: W.W. Norton & Company, 2005).

Li, F. Q. *et al.*. "Production of Alternaria Mycotoxins by Alternaria alternata Isolated from Weather-Damaged Wheat <internet>". Retrieved on 13 August 2007.

Lippard, S. J. and Berg, J. M., Principles of Bioinorganic Chemistry, University Science Books: Mill Valley, CA, 1994.

List of Canadian acceptable common names for fish and seafood. Canadian Food Inspection Agency.

Ljungh A, Wadstrom T (editors) (2009). *Lactobacillus Molecular Biology: From Genomics to Probiotics*. Caister Academic Press.

MacDonald, I. and Low, J., 1984, *Fruit and Vegetables*, IT Publications, London, UK.

Madigan MT, Martinko JM (2006). *Brock Biology of microorganisms*, 11th ed., Pearson.

Magdoff, Fred; Foster, John Bellamy; and Buttel, Frederick H. *Hungry for Profit: The Agribusiness Threat to Farmers, Food, and the Environment*. September 2000.

Mahan, L.K. and Escott-Stump, S. eds. (2000) *Krause's Food, Nutrition, and Diet Therapy*. 10th ed. (Philadelphia: W.B. Saunders Harcourt Brace)

Malik, S., McGlone, F., Bedrossian, D., & Dagher, A. (2007) *Cell Metabolism* 7:400-409.

Malnutrition Is Cheating Its Survivors, and Africa's Future article in the *New York Times* by Michael Wines, December 28, 2006

Managed food service contractors react quickly to the demands of their clients achievement: A longitudinal analysis. Journal of Public Economics, 81(3), 345-368.

Manual of clinical dietetics. 2000. Chicago: American Dietetic Association, 874p.

Marasas, Walter F. O.. "Fumonisins: Their implications for human and animal health <internet>". Retrieved on 12 August 2007.

Mason, John. *Sustainable Agriculture*. Landlinks Press: 2003.

McCabe, B.J., Frankel, E.H., and Wolfe, J.J. (eds.) 2003. *Handbook of food-drug interactions*. Boca Raton, FL: CRC Press. 567p.

McGee, Harold. *On Food and Cooking: The Science and Lore of the Kitchen*. New York: Simon and Schuster, 2004.

Mead, Margaret. *The Changing Significance of Food*. In Carole Counihan and Penny Van Esterik (Ed.), Food and Culture: A Reader. UK: Routledge, 1997.

Merson, Michael H.; Black, Robert E.; Mills, Anne J. *International Public Health: Disease, Programs, Systems, and Policies*. Jones and Bartlett Publishers, 2005.

Messer, Ellen; Derose, Laurie Fields and Sara Millman. *Who's Hungry? and How Do We Know?: Food Shortage, Poverty, and Deprivation*. United Nations University Press, 1998.

Michael Givel (December 2005) *Philip Morris' FDA Gambit: Good for Public Health?* Journal of Public Health Policy (26): pp. 450-468.

Nachamkin I and Guerry P (2005). "Campylobacter Infections", *Foodborne Pathogens: Microbiology and Molecular Biology*. Caister Academic Press.

National Academy of Sciences - National Research Council Academy of Life Sciences. "The Health Effects of Nitrate, Nitrite and N-Nitroso Compounds". Washington DC: National Academy Press, 1981.

National Health Service (2005) *Five a day - a guide to healthy eating* NHS Press (http://www.5aday.nhs.uk/)

Nelson, D. L.; Cox, M. M. "Lehninger, Principles of Biochemistry" 3rd Ed. Worth Publishing: New York, 2000.

Nelson, P.E. and Tressler, D.T., 1982, *Fruit and Vegetable Juice Processing*, AVI Publications, Conn., USA.

Nesbakken T (2005). "Yersinia enterocolitica", *Foodborne Pathogens: Microbiology and Molecular Biology*. Caister Academic Press.

Nestle, M. (1998) *Animal v plant foods in human diets and health - Proceedings of the Nutrition Society*

Nicklas, Barbara J. *Endurance Exercise and Adipose Tissue*. CRC Press, 2002.

Nishibuchi M (2005). "Vibrio spp.", *Foodborne Pathogens: Microbiology and Molecular Biology*. Caister Academic Press.

Nollet, L.M.L. 2004. *Handbook of food analysis.* 2nd ed. rev/exp. New York: Marcel Dekker. 3 vols.

Nordstrom, DK *et al* (2000) Negative pH and extremely acidic mine waters from Iron Mountain California. *Environ Sci Technol*, *34*, 254-258.

Notermans, A. H. Havellar. 1980. Removal and inactivation of botulinum toxin during production of drinking water from surface water. Antonie van Leeuwenhoek 46: 511–514.

Novaķ et al (2005). "Clostridium botulinum and Clostridium perfringens", *Foodborne Pathogens: Microbiology and Molecular Biology*. Caister Academic Press.

Nutrient lists - USDA national nutrient database for standard reference, Release 18

Nutrition Analysis Tool v2.0 (NATS 2.0). Developed and maintained by the Department of Food Science and Nutrition, University of Illinois at Urbana-Champaign.

NutritionData (ND). A searchable database that generates nutritional labels. A majority of data from USDA. Sources are referenced.

Official methods for the microbiological analysis of foods. The compendium of analytical methods. 5 vols. Methods used by Health Canada, Agriculture and Agri-Food Canada, and the Canadian Food Inspection Agency.

Ohye, W. J. Scott. 1957. Studies in the physiology of Clostridium botulinum type E. Aust. L. Biol. Sci. 10: 85–94.

Oliver, J., Channel Four (2005) *Jamie's School Dinners - Documentary produced for channel four* Television Programme.

Olver, L. 1999, 2008. *The food timeline*. The history of food + recipes.

ORO Stacks QR65 .C64 1995

Ortega Y (2005). "Food and Waterborne Protozoan Parasites", *Foodborne Pathogens: Microbiology and Molecular Biology*. Caister Academic Press.

Otten, J.J., Hellwig, J.P., and Meyers, L.D. (eds.) 2006. *Dietary DRI reference intakes [:] The essential guide to nutrient requirements*. Washington, D.C.: The National Academies Press. 543p.

Paoli et al (2005). "Listeria monocytogenes", *Foodborne Pathogens:*

Microbiology and Molecular Biology. Caister Academic Press.

Parekh, Sarad R. *The Gmo Handbook: Genetically Modified Animals, Microbes, and Plants in Biotechnology*. Humana Press, 2004.

Paston-Williams, Sara (2005). "Morecambe Bay shrimps". *Fish: Recipes from a Busy Island*. London: National Trust. p. 140.

Patten, Marguerite (February 2001) (in En). *Basic Basics: Jams, Preserves and Chutneys Handbook* (2004 reprint ed.). Grub Street Books.

Paul, A.A. and Southgate, D.A.T., 1985, *The Composition of Foods*, Her Majesty's Stationery Office, 49 High Holborn, London, UK.

Philip J. Hilts. *Protecting America's Health: The FDA, Business, and One Hundred Years of Regulation*. New York: Alfred E. Knopf, 2003.

Pimentel David, Pimentel Marcia, *Computer les kilocalories*, Cérès, n. 59, sept-oct. 1977

Potter, N.N. and J.H. Hotchkiss. (1995). *Food Science, Fifth Edition*. New York: Champman & Hall. pp. 24-68.

Potter, N.N. and J.H. Hotchkiss. (1995). *Food Science, Fifth Edition*. New York: Chapman & Hall. pp. 478-513.

Provencher, L. & Riechert, S. E. (1991) Short-Term Effects of Hunger Conditioning on Spider Behavior, Predation, and Gain of Weight *Oikos* 62:160-166

Quiros, R.D., Madrigal, A., Samuals, L., Aguilar, A., Orfiz, F., Fernandez, R. and Cooke, R., 1980, *Fruit and Vegetable Processing*, Appropriate Technology in Costa Rica; A Case Study, Tropical Science, 22 (2).

Regulatory Fish Encyclopedia. U.S. Food and Drug Administration, Center for Food Safety & Applied Nutrition.

Rehm BHA (editor). (2009). *Microbial Production of Biopolymers and Polymer Precursors: Applications and Perspectives*. Caister Academic Press.

Reid, G.; J. Howard and B.S. Gan (September 2001). "Can bacterial interference prevent infection?" *Trends in Microbiology* 9(9):424-428.

Remminghorst and Rehm (2009). "Microbial Production of Alginate: Biosynthesis and Applications", *Microbial Production of Biopolymers and Polymer Precursors*. Caister Academic Press.

Remminghorst and Rehm (2009). "Microbial Production of Alginate: Biosynthesis and Applications", *Microbial Production of Biopolymers and Polymer Precursors*. Caister Academic Press.

Renewable Fuel Association, "*Ethanol Biorefinery Locations*"

Richard H. Grove, "Global Impact of the 1789–93 El Niño," *Nature* 393 (1998), 318-319.

Richards GP (2005). "Food- and Waterborne Enteric Viruses", *Foodborne Pathogens: Microbiology and Molecular Biology*. Caister Academic Press.

Ron Nielsen, *The little green handbook*, Picador, New York (2006)

Ron Nielsen, *The Little Green Handbook: Seven Trends Shaping the Future of Our Planet*, Picador, New York (2006)

Rucker, R.B., Suttie, J.W., McCormick, D.B., and Machlin, L.J. 2001. *Handbook of vitamins*. 3rd ed. rev. exp. NY: M. Dekker. 600p.

Rural Home Economic Food Preparation, Series 1, Food Preservation, Series 2, Labour Saving Ideas, Series 3, FAO, Via delle Terme di Caracalla, 00100 Rome, Italy.

Russell E. Walter, *Soil conditions and plant growth*, Longman group, London, New York 1973

Ruth Berolzheimer (ed) et al. (1969). *Culinary arts institute encyclopedic cookbook (revised),*. Chicago USA.: Culinary arts institute. p. 830.

S. Smith, G. Hobbs. 1974. Genus III Clostridium Prazmowski 1880, 23. In R. E. Buchanan, N. E. gibbons (eds.), Bergey's Manual of Determinative Bacteriology, 8th edition. William & Wilkins, Baltimore. pp. 551–572.

Salamini Francesco, Oezkan Hakan, Brandolini Andrea, Schaefer-Pregl Ralf, Martin William, *Genetics and geography of wild cereal domestication in the Near East*, in Nature, vol. 3, ju. 2002

Saltini A.*Storia delle scienze agrarie*, 4 vols, Bologna 1984-89

Salunkhe, D.K. and Kadam, S.S. 1995. *Handbook of fruit science and technology : production, composition, storage, and processing.* NY: M. Dekker. 611 p.

Schaible UE, Kaufmann SH (2007). "Malnutrition and infection:

complex mechanisms and global impacts". *PLoS Med* **4** (5): e115. Provencher, L.; Riechert, S.E. (1991) Short-Term Effects of Hunger Conditioning on Spider Behavior, Predation, and Gain of Weight *Oikos* 62:160-166

Scherz, H. and Senser, F. (compilers) *Food composition and nutrition tables*. 2000. 6th ed. Stuttgart: Medpharm Scientific Publ. 1182p.

Schor, Juliet; Taylor, Betsy (editors). *Sustainable Planet: Roadmaps for the Twenty-First Century*. Beacon Press, 2003.

Sen, Amartya, *Poverty and Famines : An Essay on Entitlements and Deprivation*, Oxford, Clarendon Press, 1982

Shephard, Sue. *Pickled, Potted, and Canned: How the Art and Science of Food Preserving Changed the World*.

Shih and Wu (2009). "Biosynthesis and Application of Poly(gamma-glutamic acid)", *Microbial Production of Biopolymers and Polymer Precursors*. Caister Academic Press.

Shih and Wu (2009). "Biosynthesis and Application of Poly(gamma-glutamic acid)", *Microbial Production of Biopolymers and Polymer Precursors*. Caister Academic Press.

Shils *et al.* (2005) *Modern Nutrition in Health and Disease*, Lippincott Williams and Wilkins.

Smith and Fratamico (2005). "Diarrhea-inducing Escherichia coli", *Foodborne Pathogens: Microbiology and Molecular Biology*. Caister Academic Press.

Smith, J. and Hong-Smith, L. (eds.) 2003. *Food additives data book*. Oxford: Blackwell Science. 1016p.

Smith, Preston G. and Reinertsen, Donald G. (1998) *Developing Products in Half the Time*, 2nd Edition, John Wiley and Sons, New York, 1998.

Sommerville, Keith. Why famine stalks Africa, BBC, 2001

Soriano, J.M.; S. Dragacci. "Occurrence of fumonisins in foods <internet>". Retrieved on 12 August 2007.

Spiller, G.A. *Handbook of lipids in human nutrition*. 1996. Boca Raton, FL: CRC Press. 233 p.

Spurlock, M. *Supersize Me - A film of epic Proportions* Columbia Tristar

Srivastava, H.C., The History of Indian Famines from 1858-1918,

Sri Ram Mehra and Co., Agra, 1968.

Steven, M.D. and J.H. Hotchkiss. (2003). "Package Functions." In *Encyclopedia of Agricultural, Food, and Biological Engineering.* D.R. Heldman, Ed. New York: Marcel Dekker. pp. 716-719.

Stewart GC (2005). "Staphylococcus aureus", *Foodborne Pathogens: Microbiology and Molecular Biology.* Caister Academic Press.

Suen, C. L. Hatheway, A. G. Steigerwalt, D. J. Brenner. 1988, Clostridium argentinense sp.nov.: a genetically homogeneous group composed of all strains of Clostridium botulinum type G and some nontoxigenic strains previously identified as Clostridium subterminale or Clostridium hastiforme. Int. J. Sys. Bacteriol. 38: 375–381.

Suresh and Mody (2009). "Microbial Exopolysaccharides: Variety and Potential Applications", *Microbial Production of Biopolymers and Polymer Precursors.* Caister Academic Press.

Suresh and Mody (2009). "Microbial Exopolysaccharides: Variety and Potential Applications", *Microbial Production of Biopolymers and Polymer Precursors.* Caister Academic Press.

Tannock GW (editor). (2005). *Probiotics and Prebiotics: Scientific Aspects.* Caister Academic Press

The Fund for Peace and Foreign Policy, "The Failed States Index 2007," *Foreign Policy*, July/August 2007.

The nutriBase nutrition facts desk reference. 2nd ed. 2001. New York: Avery Books. 947p.

The Nutrition Source. Detailed information on nutrition related subjects including: carbohydrates, protein, fiber, calcium and milk, and type 2 diabetes. Developed and maintained by the Department of Nutrition, Harvard School of Public Health.

Thiollet, J-P, *Vitamines & minéraux* (Paris, Anagramme, 2001)

Thomas J. Moore. *Prescription for Disaster: The Hidden Dangers in Your Medicine Cabinet.* New York: Simon & Schuster, 1998.

Thomas, Midge (2002-09-02). *Best kept secrets of the Women's Institute: Jams, pickles & chutneys* (1st ed.). Simon & Schuster.

Tindall, H.D., 1983, *Vegetables in the Tropics*, MacMillan Press Ltd., London

Turner, B.C., 1970, *Home Wine Making and Brewing*, Boots

Company Ltd., London, UK.

U.N. Food and Agriculture Organization, *The State of Food Insecurity in the World 2006* (Rome: 2006).

U.N. Food and Agriculture Organization, *The State of Food Insecurity in the World 2006* (Rome: 2006).

U.S. Department of Agriculture, *2007 Agricultural Outlook Forum*, March 2007.

U.S. Department of Agriculture, *USDA Agricultural Projections to 2016* (Washington, DC: February 2007).

U.S. Food and Drug Administration. (1993). *Everything Added to Food in the United States.* Boca Raton, FL: C.K. Smoley (c/o CRC press, Inc.).

U.S. Food and Drug Administration. (1993). *Everything Added to Food in the United States.* Boca Raton, FL: C.K. Smoley (c/o CRC press, Inc.).

U.S. House of Representatives – Committee on Agriculture, Subcommittee on Livestock, Dairy, and Poultry, *Review of the Impact of Feed Costs on the Livestock Industry*, 8 March 2007.

Ulrich, Karl T. and Eppinger, Steven D (2004) *Product Design and Development*, 3rd Edition, McGraw-Hill, New York, 2004

Umezawa, M., Kogishi, K., Tojo, H., Yoshimura, S., Seriu, N., Ohta, A., et al. (1999). High-linoleate and high-alpha-linolenate diets affect learning ability and natural behavior in SAMR1 mice. The Journal of Nutrition, 129(2), 431-437.

V. Holdeman, J. B. Brooks. 1970. Variation among strains of Clostridium botulinum and related clostridia. Protocols of the first U.S-Japan conference on Toxic Microorganisms. pp. 278–286

Valentas, K.J.; Rotstein, E. and Singh, R.P. *Handbook of food engineering practice*. 1997. Boca Raton, FL: CRC Press. 718 p.

Valla et al (2009). "Bacterial Cellulose Production: Biosynthesis and Applications", *Microbial Production of Biopolymers and Polymer Precursors*. Caister Academic Press.

van Ergmengem. 1897. Uber einen neuen anaeroben Bacillus und seine Beziehungen Zum Botulismus. Zentralbl. Hyg. Infektionskr. 26. 1–8.

van Wyk, B-E. 2005. *Food plants of the world[:] An illustrated guide.*

Portland, OR: Timber Press. 480p.

Varma, J.K. & K.D. Greene, M.E. Reller, S.M. DeLong, J. Trottier, S.F. Nowicki, M. DiOrio, E.M. Koch, T.L. Bannerman, S.T. York, M.A. Lambert-Fair, J.G. Wells, P.S. Mead (2003), "An outbreak of *Escherichia coli* O157 infection following exposure to a contaminated building", *JAMA 290*(20): 2709-2712.

Vaughan, J.G. and Judd, P.A. 2003. *The Oxford book of health foods*. Oxford: Oxford University Press. 188p.

Vavilov Nicolai I. (Starr Chester K. editor), *The Origin, Variation, Immunity and Breeding of Cultivated Plants. Selected Writings*, in Chronica botanica, 13: 1-6, Waltham, Mass., 1949-50

Vavilov Nicolai I., *World Resources of Cereals, Leguminous Seed Crops and Flax,* Academy of Sciences of Urss, National Science Foundation, Washington, Israel Program for Scientific Translations, Jerusalem 1960

Vidal O, Longin R, Prigent-Combaret C, Dorel C, Hooreman M, Lejeune P (1998), "Isolation of an Escherichia coli K-12 mutant strain able to form biofilms on inert surfaces: involvement of a new ompR allele that increases curli expression", *J. Bacteriol. 180*(9): 2442–9.

Vogt, R.L. & L. Dippold (2005), "*Escherichia coli* O157:H7 outbreak associated with consumption of ground beef, June-July 2002", *Public Health Reports 2*: 174–178

W. Eklund, F. T. Poysky M. E. Peterson, L. W. Peck, Brunson. 1984. Type E botulism in salmonids and conditions contributing to outbreaks. Aquaculture 41: 293–309.

W. Eklund, M. E. Peterson, F. T. Poysky, L. W. Peck, J. F. Conrad. 1982. Botulism in juvenile Coho salmon (Onocorhynchus kisutch) in the United States. Aquaculture 27: 1–11

W. Hauschild. 1989. Clostridium botulinum. In M. P. Doyle (ed.), Food-borne Bacterial Pathogens. Marcel Dekker, New York. Pp. 111–189

Wald, G.; Jackson, B. (1944) Activity and Nutritional Deprivation *Proceedings of the National Academy of Sciences of the United States of America* 30:255-263

Walter C. Willett and Meir J. Stampfer. 2003. Rebuilding the Food Pyramid. *Scientific American* January 2003.

Watson, A.M (1974), 'The Arab agricultural revolution and its diffusion', in The Journal of Economic History, 34,

Watson, A.M (1983), ' Agricultural Innovation in the Early Islamic World', Cambridge University Press

Webley, D. J. *et al.*. "Alternaria toxins in weather-damaged wheat and sorghum in the 1995-1996 Australian harvest <internet>". Retrieved on 13 August 2007.

Wells, Spencer: *The Journey of Man : A Genetic Odyssey*. Princeton University Press, 2003.

Whitley, J., O'Dell, B., & Hogan, A. (1951). Effect of diet on maze learning in second-generation rats. folic acid deficiency. Journal of Nutrition, 45(1), 153.

Wickens, G.M.(1976), 'What the West borrowed from the Middle East', in Introduction to Islamic Civilization, edited by R.M. Savory, Cambridge University Press, Cambridge

Williams, C.N., Uzo, J.O. and Peregrine, W.T.H., 1991, *Vegetable Production in the Tropics*, Longman Press, London, UK.

Winogradsky Serge, *Microbiologie du sol. Problèmes et methodes. Cinquante ans de recherches,* Masson & c.ie, Paris 1949

Wiseman G (2009). "Real-Time PCR: Application to Food Authenticity and Legislation", *Real-Time PCR: Current Technology and Applications*. Caister Academic Press.

Woo-Cumings, Meredith, *The Political Ecology of Famine: The North Korean Catastrophe and Its Lessons*PDF (807 KiB), ADB Institute Research Paper 31, January 2002.

Wood, B.J.B., (ed), 1985, *Microbiology of Fermented Foods*, Elsevier, London.

Wood, C.A., 1992. "The climatic effects of the 1783 Laki eruption" in C. R. Harrington (Ed.), The Year Without a Summer? Canadian Museum of Nature, Ottawa, pp. 58– 77

Zeebe, R. E. and Wolf-Gladrow, D. (2001) *CO2 in seawater: equilibrium, kinetics, isotopes*, Elsevier Science B.V., Amsterdam, Netherlands

Zempleni, J., Rucker, R.B., McCormick, D.B., and Suttie, J.W. (eds.) 2007. *Handbook of vitamins*. 4th ed. Boca Raton, FL: CRC Press. 593p.

Index